RESPIRATORY CARE PRACTICE

Respiratory Care Practice

Edited by

THOMAS A. BARNES, ED.D., R.R.T.

Director, Respiratory Therapy Program
Associate Professor of Respiratory Therapy
College of Pharmacy and Allied Health Professions
Northeastern University
Boston, Massachusetts

In Consultation With

ALAN LISBON, M.D.

Co-Chairman, Respiratory-Surgical Intensive Care Unit
Beth Israel Hospital
Assistant Professor of Anaesthesia
Harvard Medical School
Boston, Massachusetts

Illustrations by

JODY L. FULKS, M.S., A.M.I.

Columbus, Ohio

YEAR BOOK MEDICAL PUBLISHERS, INC.

Chicago • London • Boca Raton • Littleton, Mass.

2   3   4   5   6   7   8   9   0   KC   92   91   90

Library of Congress Cataloging-in-Publication Data

Respiratory care practice.

Includes bibliographies and index.
1. Respiratory therapy.   I. Barnes, Thomas A.
[DNLM: 1. Respiratory Therapy.   WB 342 R4346]
RC735.I5R483   1988   615.8'36   87-23208
ISBN 0-8151-0490-1

Sponsoring Editor: Richard H. Lampert
Associate Managing Editor, Manuscript Services: Deborah Thorp
Production Project Manager: Gayle Paprocki
Proofroom Supervisor: Shirley E. Taylor

This book is dedicated to my wife and children, who bring unbounded joy and tranquility to my life. Diane, Tom, and Tracy

CONTRIBUTORS

THOMAS A. BARNES, ED.D., R.R.T.
Director, Respiratory Therapy Program
Associate Professor of Respiratory Therapy
College of Pharmacy and Allied Health Professions
Northeastern University
Boston, Massachusetts

RICHARD K. BEAUCHAMP, R.C.P.T., R.P.F.T.
Applications Engineering Manager
Medical Graphics Corporation
St. Paul, Minnesota

GEORGE G. BURTON, M.D.
Director, Kettering Institute of Respiratory Diseases
Kettering Medical Center
Kettering, Ohio

EDWARD P. DIDIER, M.D.
Consultant in Anesthesiology
Mayo Clinic
Associate Professor of Anesthesiology
Mayo Medical School
Rochester, Minnesota

F. HERBERT DOUCE, M.S., R.R.T.
Director and Assistant Professor, Respiratory Therapy Division
School of Allied Medical Professions
The Ohio State University
Columbus, Ohio

RAYMOND S. EDGE, ED.D., R.R.T.
Professor and Head
Department of Cardiopulmonary Sciences
School of Allied Health Professions
Louisiana State University Medical Center
New Orleans and Shreveport, Louisiana

ROBERT R. FLUCK, JR., M.S., R.R.T.
Clinical Coordinator, Respiratory Care and Advanced
  Cardiorespiratory Science Programs
Associate Professor
State University of New York
Health Science Center at Syracuse
Syracuse, New York

DONNA L. FROWNFELTER, P.T., R.R.T.
Assistant Director, Respiratory Care Services
Rush-Presbyterian-St. Luke's Medical Center
Instructor, Internal Medicine
Rush Medical College
Instructor, Programs in Physical Therapy
Northwestern University Medical School
Chicago, Illinois

ROBERT M. KACMAREK, PH.D., R.R.T.
Director, Respiratory Care Department
Massachusetts General Hospital
Boston, Massachusetts

GLEN G. J. LOW, M.ED., R.R.T.
Assistant Professor of Respiratory Therapy
College of Pharmacy and Allied Health Professions
Northeastern University
Boston, Massachusetts

JON O. NILSESTUEN, PH.D., R.R.T.
Director, Respiratory Therapy Program
Associate Professor
School of Allied Health Sciences
University of Texas
Health Science Center at Houston
Houston, Texas

TIMOTHY OP'T HOLT, M.H.P.E., R.R.T.
Assistant Professor and Director of Clinical Education
Department of Respiratory Care and Cardiopulmonary Sciences
College of Allied Health Professions
University of South Alabama
Mobile, Alabama

PATRICK F. PLUNKETT, ED.D., R.R.T.
Director, Perfusion Technology Program
Associate Professor of Respiratory Therapy
College of Pharmacy and Allied Health Professions
Northeastern University
Boston, Massachusetts

JOSEPH L. RAU, JR., PH.D., R.R.T.
Associate Professor
Department of Cardiopulmonary Care Sciences
Georgia State University
Atlanta, Georgia

J. DOUGLAS VANDINE, R.R.T.
Technical Specialist
Nellcor Corporation
Hayward, California
Senior Respiratory Therapist
Stanford University Hospital
Stanford, California

JEFFREY J. WARD, M.ED., R.R.T.
Director, Respiratory Therapy Program
Rochester Community College/Mayo
Rochester, Minnesota

Mary E. Watson, Ed.D., R.R.T.
Director of Clinical Education
Respiratory Therapy and Perfusion Technology Programs
Associate Professor of Respiratory Therapy
College of Pharmacy and Allied Health Professions
Northeastern University
Boston, Massachusetts

Carl P. Wiezalis, M.S., R.R.T.
Director, Respiratory Care and Advanced Cardiorespiratory
Science Programs
Associate Professor
State University of New York
Health Science Center at Syracuse
Syracuse, New York

William V. Wojciechowski, M.S., R.R.T.
Associate Professor and Chairman
Department of Respiratory Care and Cardiopulmonary Sciences
College of Allied Health Professions
University of South Alabama
Mobile, Alabama

John W. Youtsey, Ph.D., R.R.T.
Professor and Chairman
Department of Cardiopulmonary Care Sciences
Georgia State University
Atlanta, Georgia

PREFACE

This book was written to provide a text that could be read and studied progressively, following a path not unlike that taken when administering respiratory care, and similar to the sequence of topics found in professional courses taught by respiratory care schools. The text includes comprehensive discussions of the knowledge, principles, concepts, and skills necessary to administer respiratory care. This book was designed to be used by students preparing for both the entry level and advanced practitioner examinations administered by the National Board for Respiratory Care.

Twenty experienced respiratory care practitioners were assembled by the editor and asked to accomplish collectively what would be impossible to accomplish individually. The mission for the group of primarily full-time respiratory care educators was to present, in an organized manner, the concepts that must be mastered before entering the profession. The focus was placed on those principles and skills necessary to be a safe respiratory care practitioner. Authors were asked to include material that they expected their own students to know about an assigned topic. An early commitment was made by the editor and publisher to produce a text with high-quality medical illustrations and photographs, using a uniform style and format throughout the book.

This book was written for anyone who will be actively involved in administering respiratory care. It should be read by students in respiratory therapy schools and also by students in nursing, physical therapy, emergency paramedical, and physician assistant schools if their career plans involve treating patients with respiratory disorders. The text should serve as a resource for experienced respiratory care practitioners who need to review techniques for pulmonary function testing and various therapeutic modalities of respiratory care. Physicians and house staff who are involved with patients requiring respiratory care would benefit from reading the text in order to better understand the therapeutic modalities, procedures, and equipment that they have ordered for their patients.

Topics that have been identified by the profession as necessary for entry into the field as an advanced respiratory care practitioner have been included in this book. This profile of practice was determined by reviewing several studies conducted by the National Board for Respiratory Care, the American Association for Respiratory Care, and the University of Texas Health Science Center at Dallas Curriculum Project. A set of detailed chapter specifications was prepared by the editor and subsequently embellished by the chapter authors based on their knowledge and interpretation of the profile of practice of advanced practitioners at entry into the field. Also, over 600 self-assessment examination questions published by the National Board of Respiratory Care and the American Association for Respiratory Care were reviewed by the editor and compared against the specifications for each chapter and appendix. The four sections of the text were organized in a fashion similar to the way a clinician approaches the delivery of respiratory care. The first section, "Patient Assessment, Diagnosis, and Care Plan," covers concepts that lead to the development of a respiratory care plan. Section II, "Therapeutic and Emergency Modalities," covers the theoretical and scientific basis for respiratory care. Section III, "Respiratory Care Equipment," presents representative examples of equipment and procedures for safe operation. Section IV, "Strategies for Modifying Respiratory Care," deals with concepts involved in ongoing assessment and the necessary changes required in the initial respiratory care plan.

Five appendixes provide support for the text and include a useful learning technique for understanding the purpose of specific drugs (Appendix A, "Major Drug Families"). Appendix B, "Applied Mathematics for Respiratory Care," presents many examples of calculations required by practitioners, and derives and reinforces many of the concepts presented by chapter authors. Appendixes C and E, "Infection Control" and "Pulmonary Function Normal Values," add to the knowledge base needed to be a safe practitioner.

A referenced self-assessment examination with 362 questions covers all 20 chapters of the text. The examination was designed to provide a means for the reader to quickly assess his or her understanding of the material presented in each chapter. While it is not possible with 10 to 20 questions to test all the principles included in a chapter, the reader's understanding of some of the more important concepts can be self-analyzed by using Appendix D.

A large page format has been used with this text to allow a larger space for diagrams of pneumatic circuits and control panels of equipment. Also, wherever possible, photographs have been enlarged to show details of the equipment.

Case studies, clinical narratives, and descriptions of early historical developments have been used in the text to help the reader apply the examples provided to similar but slightly different clinical problems. Photographs of both historically significant and modern equipment prepare the reader to work with respiratory care devices in laboratory and hospital settings. Over 150 tables compile and summarize physical data, clinical signs and symptoms, therapeutic indications, contraindications, and complications of respiratory care.

Labeled photographs and diagrams in the equipment section combine with detailed step-by-step procedural outlines to take the "guesswork" out of assembling equipment for patient use. In many instances photographs and illustrations indicate application or attachment of the equipment to the patient.

This book presents what 20 experienced respiratory care educators believe students should know prior to entering the field as advanced respiratory care practitioners. Several of the chapter contributors have authored books on the topics they cover in a single chapter in this text. Fortunately, they have the experience to organize very complex areas of practice into a presentation of the most important concepts and principles needed to administer respiratory care. Both beginning and experienced practitioners should benefit from the years of experience of the contributing authors.

Several well-referenced chapters in this text will lead the reader to journal articles and reports that help to clarify some of the more controversial technical questions. The equipment section provides the reader with a way to learn more about representa-

tive types of equipment. The reader's interest should be held, since the text was designed to combine "need-to-know" information with over 400 medical illustrations and photographs that address the concepts and principles related to safe administration of respiratory care.

My appreciation is extended to my wife and children for their support over the several years during which this text was planned and brought to fruition. Special thanks go to Rosemary Demirjian, who typed the entire manuscript and organized the references for many of the chapters. Personal thanks go to the contributing authors who have truly made this a national project and for the many hours they dedicated to writing excellent manuscripts. Jody L. Fulks and Thomas B. Steinhoff did an outstanding job preparing the illustrations for this text and deserve recognition for the way they worked so closely with the authors and editor to create hundreds of excellent drawings. Many thanks to Gerald Schrader for photographing several pieces of equipment shown in the text and for sharing his extensive technical knowledge of photography. Several persons too numerous to list individually, who are employed by companies that manufacture the equipment shown in this text, worked hard to locate or produce photographs for many of the chapters, and this book would not have been possible without them.

My appreciation is extended to Richard H. Lampert, Vice President, Editorial, Year Book Medical Publishers, for his great enthusiasm for this book and his expert advice. The copyediting of the manuscript was supervised by Deborah Thorp, who did an excellent job and tirelessly gave her attention to large and small details with equal skill. Gayle Paprocki is thanked for keeping the project on schedule and for the excellent page design. Special thanks go to former Year Book editors Diana L. McAninch and Stephany S. Scott for their help during the critical early stages of this project.

The contribution of Dr. Alan Lisbon is acknowledged for his critical and timely review of the manuscript as a medical consultant to the editor. I wish to thank a good friend, Dr. George G. Burton, for reviewing the chapter specifications, overall design, and preliminary manuscripts for this book. His extensive knowledge as a physician, author, and editor combined with his experience in respiratory care have contributed significantly to this text.

Thomas A. Barnes, Ed.D., R.R.T.

CONTENTS

SECTION I

Patient Assessment, Diagnosis, and Care Plan

Patient Assessment Procedures

George G. Burton, M.D.

It is appropriate that an introductory textbook covering the specifics of respiratory care practice begin with material dealing with the "front end" of the therapist-patient interface: assessment of the patient and his complaint. In an era of diagnosis related groups (DRGs) and cost effectiveness, efficiency of care is a byword. In that setting, assessment of the patient must be performed accurately, quickly, and thoroughly.

The beginning student will benefit from selecting role models early in his training, and none is better than the physician or lead therapist who consistently seems most attuned to the dynamic, ever-changing patient scenario. The student will sense that his role model enters the information-gathering setting with well-defined goals in mind, and that nothing escapes his attention. All of the examiner's senses are brought into play—sight, sound, smell, and touch. Even extrasensory perception sometimes appears to be operative! He works quickly, but leaves the patient with the impression that he has been visited and examined by one who truly cares about him. The respiratory therapist has temporarily set aside all other considerations in the interest of learning as much as possible, in the short time allowed, about the patient and his respiratory disorder.

It would be naive to suggest that all patient complaints are straightforward, or that the pathophysiology responsible for the complaints is simple and easy to understand. Indeed, we will shortly see that this is not the case. Early in their careers, medical students and house officers are taught to overlook nothing in their history-taking and physical examinations. A typical format for the history-taking portion of such an approach is found below. Clearly, while such an approach may be informative, it is also impractical in a 26-minute therapy session. The usual therapist bedside assessment must be performed in less than 5 minutes. Although it centers on the respiratory system, it must cover other systems as well, as we shall see. With experience, the student will develop a facility for simultaneously assessing the patient and at least beginning therapy, a capability that may seem farfetched to him at present.

THERAPY-TARGETED PATIENT ASSESSMENT

A key to all this is "therapy-targeted patient assessment." A brief case presentation will be illustrative.

A 15-year-old boy was seen following admission to the hospital for cough and fever. The patient denied any previous respiratory history. He was not a smoker. Two days prior to admission, he developed a sore throat and chills. The day before admission, he complained of mild chest pain, developed fever of 102°F, and had a cough productive of thick, reddish-brown ("rusty") sputum. A chest x-ray in the emergency department revealed a left lower lobe pneumonia. Chest examination revealed crackles at the left lung base posteriorly. The remainder of the physical examination was normal except for fever (103°F) and dehydration of the mucous membranes. Ultrasonic aerosol therapy and percussion and postural drainage procedures were instituted, and were well tolerated by the patient.

This kind of assessment, with its historical and physical findings, mandates therapy, which in turn (1) requires patient cooperation and (2) effects change in patient complaints and (perhaps) physical findings. Knowing exactly what to expect out of a therapy session allows one to be more efficient with the assessment procedure itself. In this case, the therapist expects the findings of pneumonia in the left lower lobe, and targets his examination to that area accordingly.

Initial Assessment

The initial, or baseline, assessment, of course, will take longer than the periodic one. A fairly complete respiratory history can usually be obtained from the appropriate section of a patient's chart, and the student must learn how to extract this information. Many times, however, the physician has not had time to write out this information, dictate it, or have it typed. Examples of this include interfaces with patients in the emergency room or involvement in the admission of new acutely ill patients. In these situations, the therapist must be prepared and able to perform a quick, therapy-targeted history and physical examination. The baseline physical examination will serve as a reference point for future evaluations; it must be fairly rigorous and complete. Detailed outlines of the complete respiratory history and physical examination appear below.

COMPREHENSIVE HISTORY: ADULT PATIENT[1]

1. Date of history.
2. Identifying data, including at least age, sex, race, place of birth, marital status, occupation, and perhaps religion.
3. Source of referral, if any.
4. Source of history, which may be the patient or relative or friend, for example, together with the practitioner's judgment of the validity of his reporting. Other possible sources include the patient's medical record or a referral letter.
5. Chief complaints, when possible in the patient's own words.
6. Present illness: This is a clear, chronological narrative account of the problems for which the patient is seeking care. It should include the onset of the problem, the setting in which it developed, its manifestations, its treatments, its impact on the patient's life, and its meaning to the patient. The prin-

cipal symptoms should be described in terms of their (1) location, (2) quality, (3) quantity or severity, (4) timing (i.e., onset, duration, and frequency), (5) setting, (6) factors that have aggravated or relieved these symptoms, and (7) associated manifestations. Relevant data from the patient's chart, such as laboratory reports, also belong in the present illness, as do significant negatives (i.e., the absence of certain symptoms that will aid in differential diagnosis).

7. Medical history.

- General state of health.
- Childhood illnesses, such as measles, rubella, mumps, whooping cough, chicken pox, rheumatic fever, scarlet fever, polio.
- Immunizations, such as tetanus, pertussis, diphtheria, polio, measles, rubella, mumps.
- Adult illnesses.
- Psychiatric illnesses.
- Operations.
- Injuries.
- Hospitalizations not already described.
- Allergies.
- Current medications, including home remedies, nonprescription drugs, and medicines borrowed from family or friends. When a patient seems likely to be taking one or more medications, survey one 24-hour period in detail: "Take yesterday, for example. Starting from when you woke up, what was the first medicine you took? How much? How often in the day did you take it? What are you taking it for? What other medicines . . .?"
- Diet. Use a similar line of questioning: "Let's look at yesterday. Starting from when you woke up, what did you eat or drink first? . . . Then what? . . . And then?"
- Sleep patterns, including times that the person goes to bed and awakens, difficulties in falling asleep or staying asleep, snoring, observed apneic spells and daytime naps.
- Habits, including exercise and the use of coffee, alcohol, other drugs, and tobacco.

8. Family history.

- The age and health, or age and cause of death, of each immediate family member (i.e., parents, siblings, spouse, and children). Data on grandparents or grandchildren may also be useful.
- The occurrence within the family of any of the following conditions: diabetes, tuberculosis, heart disease, high blood pressure, cerebrovas-

cular accident, kidney disease, cancer, arthritis, anemia, headaches, mental illness, or symptoms like those of the patient.

9. Psychosocial history: This is an outline or narrative description that captures the important and relevant information about the patient as a person:

- His lifestyle, home situation, significant others.
- A typical day—how he spends his time from when he gets up to when he goes to bed.
- Important experiences, including upbringing, schooling, military service, job history, financial situation, marriage, recreation, retirement.
- Religious beliefs relevant to perceptions of health, illness, and treatment.
- His view of the present and outlook for the future.

10. Review of systems.

- General—Usual weight, recent weight change, weakness, fatigue, fever.
- Skin.—Rashes, lumps, itching, dryness, color change, changes in hair or nails.
- Head.—Headache, head injury.
- Eyes.—Vision, glasses or contact lenses, last eye examination, pain, redness, excessive tearing, double vision, glaucoma, cataracts.
- Ears.—Hearing, tinnitus, vertigo, earaches, infection, discharge.
- Nose and sinuses.—Frequent colds, nasal stuffiness, hay fever, nosebleeds, sinus trouble.
- Mouth and throat.—Condition of teeth and gums, bleeding gums, last dental examination, sore tongue, frequent sore throats, hoarseness.
- Neck.—Lumps in neck, "swollen glands," goiter, pain in the neck.
- Breasts.—Lumps, pain, nipple discharge, self-examination.
- Respiratory.—Cough, sputum (color, quantity), hemoptysis, wheezing, asthma, bronchitis, emphysema, pneumonia, tuberculosis, pleurisy, tuberculin test; last chest x-ray film.
- Cardiac.—"Heart trouble," high blood pressure, rheumatic fever, heart murmurs; dyspnea, orthopnea, paroxysmal nocturnal dyspnea, edema; chest pain, palpitations; past electrocardiogram or other heart tests.
- Gastrointestinal.—Trouble swallowing, heartburn, appetite, nausea, vomiting, vomiting of blood, indigestion, frequency of bowel movements, change in bowel habits, rectal bleeding

or black tarry stools, constipation, diarrhea, abdominal pain, food intolerance, excessive belching or passing of gas, hemorrhoids, jaundice, liver or gallbladder trouble, hepatitis.
- Urinary.—Frequency of urination, polyuria, nocturia, dysuria, hematuria, urgency, hesitancy, incontinence; urinary infections, stones.
- Genitoreproductive.
  Male.—Discharge from or sores on penis, history of venereal disease and its treatment, hernias, testicular pain or masses; frequency of intercourse, libido, sexual difficulties.
  Female.—Age at menarche; regularity, frequency, and duration of periods; amount of bleeding, bleeding between periods or after intercourse, last menstrual period; dysmenorrhea; age of menopause, menopausal symptoms, postmenopausal bleeding; discharge, itching, venereal disease and its treatment; last Papanicolaou smear, number of pregnancies, number of deliveries, number of abortions (spontaneous and induced); complications of pregnancy; birth control methods; frequency of intercourse, libido, sexual difficulties.
- Musculoskeletal.—Joint pains or stiffness, arthritis, gout, backache. If present, describe location and symptoms (for example, swelling, redness, pain, stiffness, weakness, limitation of motion or activity). Muscle pains or cramps.
- Peripheral vascular.—Intermittent claudication, cramps, varicose veins, thrombophlebitis.
- Neurologic.—Fainting, blackouts, seizures, paralysis, local weakness, numbness, tingling, tremors, memory.
- Psychiatric.—Nervousness, tension, mood, depression.
- Endocrine.—Thyroid trouble, heat or cold intolerance, excessive sweating, diabetes, excessive thirst, hunger, or urination.
- Hematologic.—Anemia, easy bruising or bleeding, past transfusions and possible reactions.

Periodic Assessment

Periodic assessment of the patient will occur at intervals of time ranging from minutes in the critically ill patient to weeks or months in the outpatient setting. Clearly, an *interval* history will be necessary: "Are you feeling better? Less short of breath? Is it easier to cough?" Change of symptoms and signs is as important in the periodic assessment as the symptoms and signs themselves. Finally, the laboratory data in the subsequent assessment will also, hopefully, reflect patient improvement. Comparative data will document improvement in such measurements as blood gas analysis, pulmonary function tests, chest x-rays, and sputum Gram's stain. The physical findings also will reflect change: fewer wheezes, less rales, reduced fever, etc.

Students should understand that completeness and accuracy is the desired goal of periodic assessment. To achieve these goals, the basic assessment skills must first be learned and practiced in an unhurried, nonpressured setting. Only after a great deal of familiarity with the basic assessment tools has been gained should the student begin work on the speed required in the periodic or interval assessment.

Appropriate Responses

It is reasonable for the student to inquire about appropriate responses to patient assessment data, but probably premature at this stage. Some responses must (1) be immediate, without physician direction, (2) be immediate but only with a physician order, and (3) be slowly thought out and gradually applied. An example in the first category would be the prompt initiation of cardiopulmonary resuscitation. The second would be administration of bronchodilator aerosol in an asthmatic patient in the emergency room; and the third might be illustrated by the therapist who, by protocol, can initiate a program of breathing exercises and exercise conditioning for a patient in a pulmonary rehabilitation program. In each of these settings, the acuity of the situation will mandate the speed of response. In each situation, the degree of physician "supervision" will vary. The good therapist will be quick to analyze and respond to each situation on an individual basis. The success of all these therapeutic ventures depends heavily on good therapist assessment techniques.

STANDARDIZED ASSESSMENT FORMATS

Weed (S-O-A-P) System

The tendency to believe that all good assessment comes out of the earpieces of a stethoscope must be avoided. As we will see, the stethoscope is but one tool in the total armamentarium. The author believes that this tool is overutilized at the expense of some others. The notion that the patient has something

worthwhile to say about his problem has led to the development of a more humanistic, problem oriented system of patient assessment. This is the so-called Weed system of patient evaluation.[7]

The Weed system has four portions (1) *Subjective*, (2) *Objective*, (3) *Assessment*, and (4) *Plan*. The acronym S-O-A-P has been given to this format.

1. The *Subjective* evaluation of his status by the patient ("I am very short of breath today; I am more short of breath than yesterday; I am coughing less than yesterday.")

2. The *Objective* findings consist of data such as temperature, intake and output, auscultatory findings, and laboratory data.

3. The *Assessment* is the therapist's or physician's evaluation of what the subjective or objective data really mean. For instance, an assessment could be that the pneumonia is improving, that the asthma is worsening, or that there is no change in the patient's conditions.

4. The *Plan* reflects what the physician/therapist team intends to do about the data thus far accumulated, e.g., "We will increase the inhaled bronchodilator aerosol treatments to every 4 hours."

The author highly recommends the use of the Weed (S-O-A-P) system to beginners and experts alike. It has the distinct advantage of being patient and problem oriented; it takes the patient concerns into account and gives, at least, a notion that ongoing evaluation and planning are taking place. In addition, it is a structured way to evaluate the patient and his disease process, and anyone interested in looking at the chart can quickly be brought up to date on the thinking of the respiratory care team. This is not often possible by reading standard "progress notes" and trying to infer from them what was actually intended by (or accomplished by) the physician orders.

Modified Weed System

Limitations of the Weed system revolve around the fact that patients often have more than one complaint. For instance, it is perfectly possible to have exertional dyspnea and productive cough in a patient with chronic bronchitis and emphysema. If one is too vigorous in the application of the Weed system, then one needs to keep records of two S-O-A-Ps: S-1, O-1, A-1, P-1 (dyspnea) and S-2, O-2, A-2, P-2 (productive cough). Clearly this is burdensome when one realizes that the United States Public

Health Service has stated that, "beyond age 55, each average American has 2.3 chronic illnesses." With more than one complaint, then, the system begins to break down. Because of this, many workers have developed a modified Weed system that collapses various objective complaints under one heading (i.e., cough and exertional dyspnea) and then goes ahead to list the other components as if the objective data, assessment, and planning were focused on that joint complaint. An example of such charting is seen in Table 1–1.

Treatment-to-Treatment Charting

Even the modified Weed system is too cumbersome for treatment-to-treatment charting. In response to the need to communicate to therapists what has transpired to date, many different approaches have been developed. Figure 1–1 shows a form that is currently used in our department for charting the effects of bronchodilator or aerosol therapy, ultrasonic therapy, and chest physical therapy. The "Comment" section is reserved for both patient and therapist comments and for suggested changes in therapy. While this type of charting is very helpful, the complete S-O-A-P format is urged for the initial examination and assessment of the patient.

Other charting tools have been developed and utilized with varying degrees of success. Most of them stress the physical examination findings and exclude the patient's subjective complaints and pertinent laboratory data. Each department will have its own assessment tools, but the student is encouraged to consider the S-O-A-P protocol as a paradigm of completeness against which all other assessment tools must be judged.

THE CHIEF RESPIRATORY COMPLAINT

Most patients arrive at the hospital with a major concern or symptom as the initiating force precipitating their hospitalization. Historically, this has been recorded as the "chief complaint." The major respiratory complaints are *dyspnea* and *cough*. In one form or the other, these concerns are present in 80% to 90% of the patients on a respiratory care service. Symptoms of chest pain or discomfort, sputum production, weight loss, hemoptysis, and peripheral edema constitute the chief complaints of the remainder of the population. In our high technology era, with its focus on speed of diagnosis and efficiency of treatment, it is well to not only record but to react to the patient's major complaint with care and compassion.

Cough

The easily recognized sound of coughing may represent a protective mechanism to guard the airway (as in aspiration), or it may represent an effective mechanism to clear material from the airway (as with sputum production in chronic bronchitis). Indeed, cough, and not ciliary clearance, appears to be the most important mechanism of airway clearance in patients with chronic bronchitis. Many respiratory illnesses first evidence themselves as cough. Among these clinical conditions are postnasal drip, asthma, bronchitis, pneumonia, tuberculosis, and lung cancer. The cough symptoms may last for hours or years and may range in severity from a nusiance "tickle in the throat" to disabling racking paroxysms that continue day and night. Students should seek to qualify and quantify the cough symptoms as carefully as possible for meaningful comparisons to be made in the course of therapy.

In the past, coughing was thought to be rude and unsanitary, and anecdotes abound of patients quietly coughing bloody sputum into handkerchiefs behind their fluttering fans. In Kansas City, brick

TABLE 1–1.

Use of the Modified Weed System in a Complex Case

DATE PROBLEM ENTERED	PROBLEM NO.	ACTIVE PROBLEMS	INACTIVE PROBLEMS
1–7–86	1	Exertional dyspnea	
1–8–86	2		Migraine headaches
1–7–86	3	Hemoptysis	
1–7–86	4		Recurrent pyelonephritis

On 1/10/86, the above patient was seen, and since time was of the essence, priority was given to the problems bothering the patient that day, namely persistent hemoptysis and migraine headaches. The charting on that day was as follows:

Migraine headaches
    S—Headaches "worse than ever" (patient's own words)
    O—BP 140/80 left arm, sitting. Neurological exam normal
    A—Patient worried about persistent hemoptysis
    P—Reassurance; CT scan of head

Hemoptysis
    Subjective (S): Continues to cough up approximately 2 oz of bright red blood, mostly in the morning
    Objective (O): Crackles persist at right apex posteriorly
    Assessment (A): Persistent hemoptysis, not improved
    Plan (P): Bronchoscopy is scheduled for this afternoon

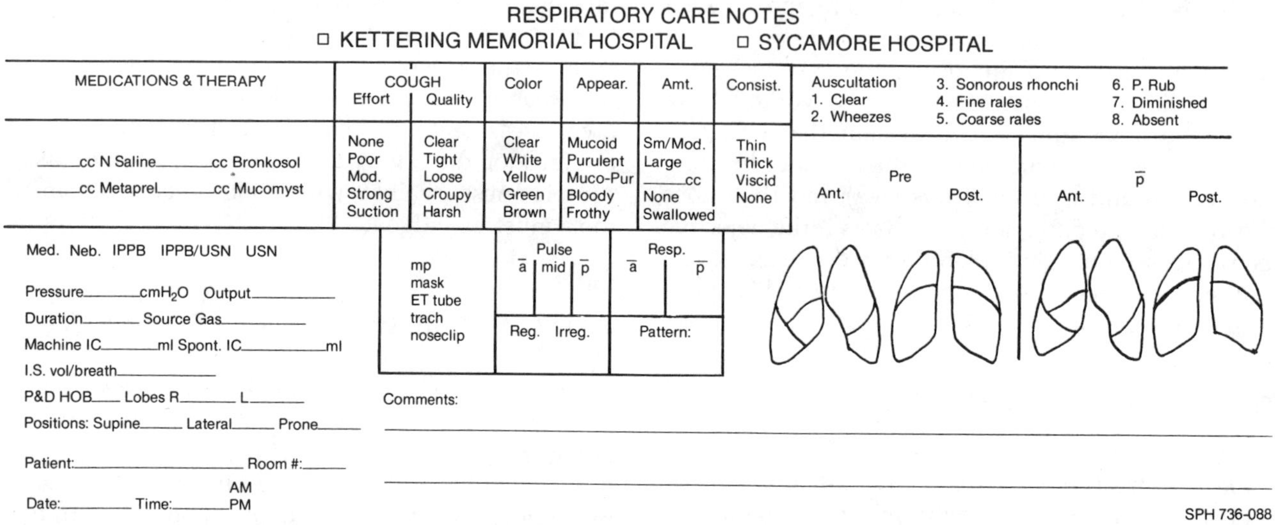

RESPIRATORY CARE NOTES

☐ KETTERING MEMORIAL HOSPITAL　☐ SYCAMORE HOSPITAL

MEDICATIONS & THERAPY	COUGH		Color	Appear.	Amt.	Consist.	Auscultation 1. Clear 2. Wheezes	3. Sonorous rhonchi 4. Fine rales 5. Coarse rales	6. P. Rub 7. Diminished 8. Absent
	Effort	Quality							

____cc N Saline____cc Bronkosol

____cc Metaprel____cc Mucomyst

| | None Poor Mod. Strong Suction | Clear Tight Loose Croupy Harsh | Clear White Yellow Green Brown | Mucoid Purulent Muco-Pur Bloody Frothy | Sm/Mod. Large ____cc None Swallowed | Thin Thick Viscid None | Pre Ant. Post. | | p̄ Ant. Post. |

Med. Neb. IPPB IPPB/USN USN

Pressure____cmH2O Output____

Duration____ Source Gas____

Machine IC____ml Spont. IC____ml

I.S. vol/breath____

P&D HOB____ Lobes R____ L____

Positions: Supine____ Lateral____ Prone____

Patient:____ Room #:____

Date:____ Time:____ AM/PM

mp mask ET tube trach noseclip

Pulse: ā | mid | p̄　Resp.: ā | p̄

Reg. Irreg.　Pattern:

Comments:

SPH 736-088

FIG 1–1.
Respiratory care charting form. (Courtesy of Kettering Medical Center, Kettering, Ohio.)

paving stones are imprinted with the words, "Don't spit on the sidewalk," another allusion to the public's hygienic concern over the coughing-expectoration symptom.

Many patients accept mild to moderate cough (and for that matter, shortness of breath) symptoms as a fact of life. They ascribe the symptom(s) to cigarette smoking, industrial exposure, air pollution, the residuals of viral infection of the upper airways, postnasal drip, and a host of other causes, and not to the more significant conditions listed above. Thus, it is not unusual to obtain a history of cough of *years'* duration before more dramatic symptoms, such as hemoptysis, chest pain, or severe dyspnea, bring the patient to medical attention.

The cough symptom should at least initially be described as to severity, length, frequency, inciting factors (if known), relationships to body position, smoking, known allergens or other inciting factors, past attempts (successful or unsuccessful) at therapy, and type and volume of sputum production. The latter description, type of sputum production, may point to a specific diagnostic entity (Fig 1–2). In hospitalized patients, the volume, color, and consistency of expectorated sputum should be charted frequently, and the relationship of sputum production to respiratory therapy treatments should be noted. A few short examples of typical charting notations will illustrate this point.

Case 1.—A 28-year-old housewife, a 2-pack/day cigarette smoker for the past 12 years, was admitted to the hospital because of cough productive of large amounts of thick, yellow, tenacious sputum of 2 weeks' duration. Her cough was so severe that she could not sleep, talk, or eat without racking cough paroxysms. She had been on tetracycline therapy for one week as an outpatient without improvement. The chest x-ray showed no acute infiltrates although the basilar bronchovascular markings were accentuated. Arterial blood gas analyses (ABGs) with the patient breathing room air showed a Pa_{O_2} of 55 mm Hg and Pa_{CO_2} of 46 mm Hg.

A bronchial hygiene program directed to modifying her sputum production was instituted. Systemic hydration, bronchodilator therapy, sodium iodide, antibiotics, and ultrasonic aerosol therapy were used. Within 48 hours, her sputum was no longer yellow. It was less viscid, and the 24-hour sputum volume had increased from less than 0.5 oz to more than 2 oz.

Comment.—In this case, typical of patients with chronic bronchitis, we see the effects of good bronchial hygiene on thick, tenacious secretions. Note that with such a program, the patient's secretions actually increased in volume, at least temporarily, and became less purulent, probably as a result of less mucostasis and control of her bronchitis with antibiotics.

Case 2.—A 4-year-old boy with cystic fibrosis, has been hospitalized three times in the past year for respiratory problems, twice with pneumonia on chest x-ray. He had been compliant with a home therapy regimen of bronchodilators, systemic (oral) hydration, and periodic antibiotics. He came to the hospital on this occasion with a dry, nonproductive cough, an

Type of Sputum	Lung Abscess	Acute Bronchitis	Chronic Bronchitis	Pneumonia	Pulmonary Edema	Bronchiectasis	Tuberculosis	Lung Cancer	Pulmonary Infarction	Bronchial Asthma	Cystic Fibrosis	Aspiration Pneumonia
Mucoid (white or clear)			X							X		
Mucopurulent		X	X								X	
Purulent (yellow or green)	X	X		X		X						X
Fetid	X					X					X	X
Bloody		X		X	X	X	X	X	X			
Frothy, sometimes pink					X							

FIG 1–2.

Sputum characteristics in clinical conditions. (From Burton GG, Hodgkin JE: *Respiratory Care: a Guide to Clinical Practice*, ed 2. Philadelphia, JB Lippincott, Co. 1984. Used with permission.)

oral temperature of 101°F, and left anterior chest pain. A chest x-ray showed a consolidated left lower lobe.

The patient did not improve with inhaled bronchodilator and ultrasonic aerosol therapy. The cough worsened and interfered with his sleep. On the third hospital day, chest physical therapy (postural drainage and percussion) was started. By the fifth hospital day, he still was not improved, and therapeutic bronchoscopy was performed. A large mucus plug was removed from the left lower lobe bronchus. Cultures from a bronchial aspirate grew out large numbers of *Pseudomonas aeruginosa* and staphylococcal organisms. The infiltrate and fever were not present by the seventh day, and he was discharged on the ninth day.

Comment.—Here we see a patient in whom cough signaled localized airway obstruction (in this case, a large mucus plug in the left lower lobe bronchus). As one writer has expressed it, cough is "the janitor and housekeeper of the airways and lungs . . . ." In this case, cough acted as a doorkeeper announcing the presence of a mucus plug that may have otherwise gone unnoticed. This case illustrates the scope of several therapeutic interventions that were needed before improvement occurred.

Case 3.—A 36-year-old man with cough-variant asthma came to the outpatient chest clinic complaining of a 2-year history of chronic cough, worse with exercise and on exposure to cold air. There was no family or personal history of allergies. He was not a smoker. Chest x-rays and pulmonary function tests done 3 months previously were unremarkable. He categorically stated that he never wheezed and with the exception of cough, he was in good health. He reported a chronic postnasal drip.

Physical examination was entirely normal. On the second hospital day, he was brought to the pulmonary function laboratory, where flow volume loop analysis was performed before and after treadmill exercise (Fig 1–3). After exercise, he coughed and wheezed until he was treated with inhaled bronchodilator medication. A bronchial provocation test with methacholine was also positive. He was treated with a theophylline-containing bronchodilator and aerosolized cromolyn sodium and improved greatly.

Comment.—This patient's cough was finally diagnosed as being due to an atypical kind of asthma, in which cough (and not wheezing) is the predominant symptom. Asthma in one form or another is ultimately found to be present in more than one-fourth of patients with persistent cough. Chronic postnasal drip is another frequent cause of cough. When the cause of the cough is accurately identified and treated, virtually all of the patients improve.[4]

Dyspnea

The sensation of difficult or uncomfortable breathing is called dyspnea. It is a poorly understood sensation; it is *not* a sensation of pain, choking, or coughing. The shortness of breath that normal individuals feel with severe exercise comes closest to what patients describe with mild exertion or with no exertion at all. One must be sure that the patient really *means* dyspnea, and not fatigue, weakness, chest discomfort, chest pain, or faintness when being questioned about his "shortness of breath."

A useful concept of dyspnea is that of inequality between requirement to breathe ("must breathe")

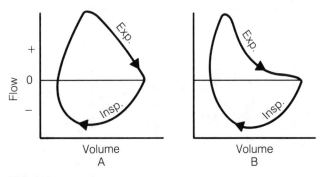

FIG 1–3.
Flow/volume loop in a 36-year-old male with exercise-induced asthma. **A,** before exercise. **B,** after exercise.

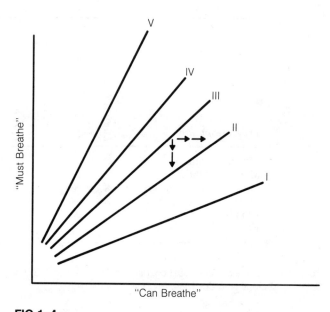

FIG 1–4.
Must Breathe/Can Breathe Concept of Dyspnea. Roman numerals stand for dyspnea grades (I = none, V = severe). Arrows represent direction of clinical improvement. Note that reduction in the "must breathe" requirement causes relief of dyspnea (lower dyspnea grade) as surely as increase in the "can breathe" capacity.

and ability to breathe ("can breathe"). First, it is important to rate dyspnea as to severity (mild, moderate, severe, or on a 1 to 5 scale, with 1 being "appropriate dyspnea" and 5 being "dyspnea with any activity or at rest"). No dyspnea exists when the ventilatory requirements are modest and the ventilatory capacity, e.g., the maximum voluntary ventilation (MVV), is normal. However, now consider a 300-lb man with severe bronchitis, who is short of breath with the mildest exertion. His "must breathe" requirement is high; because of his obesity he is moving about twice the mass of most people. His "can breathe" capacity is reduced; because of his bronchitis, his MVV is reduced to 30% of predicted. This patient's "must breathe" requirement outstrips his "can breathe" capability, and dyspnea on exertion exists.

This concept of dyspnea is useful when thinking about treatment (Fig 1–4). Here we see that reducing the "must breathe" requirement is every bit as helpful as increasing the "can breathe" capability of relieving dyspnea. Both types of maneuvers move the patient across dyspnea grades.

The historical "fingerprints" of the various causes of dyspnea and their severity and onset/offset histories are found on pages 11–14.

Chest Pain

Respiratory care practitioners will, from time to time, work with patients who experience chest pain, and several types should be recognized.

Angina Pectoris

This type of chest pain is most typically precordial (over the heart). It may be precipitated by exercise, and may radiate to the neck, shoulders, and arms (usually the left). However, these classic symptoms of coronary artery insufficiency and relief of the pain by nitroglycerin are not always present. There is no tenderness to palpation over the area of pain. The student should always check blood pressure, cardiac rate, and rhythm before any therapy (except oxygen therapy) is given to such patients.

Pleuritic Chest Pain (Pleurisy)

The pain associated with inflammation of the pleura is often sharp, gnawing, nonradiating, localized, and worsened by deep breathing or coughing. There is usually no tenderness over the affected area. A characteristic friction rub may be heard over the pleuritic area, said to sound like "creaking shoe leather."

Chest Wall Pain

Severe pain and tenderness will develop over areas of trauma, e.g., over fractured ribs. The key to this type of pain is that it always is accompanied by *tenderness* over the affected area. Tietze's syndrome consists of painful swelling and tenderness over one or more costochondral cartilage. Another example of chest wall pain is that associated with "shingles" (herpes zoster) and its associated neuritis.

Less Common Respiratory Complaints

Weight Loss

Weight loss may accompany clinical depression, tuberculosis, chronic infection, malignancy, or end-stage chronic obstructive pulmonary disease. Signs of clinical malnutrition are now routinely sought for and treated as part of pulmonary rehabilitation programs, as well as in the weaning process of ventilator patients (see Chapter 19). Pulmonary patients who complain of weight loss should be questioned about after-eating fullness or epigastric discomfort, since hiatal hernia and peptic ulcer disease are not uncommon in patients with chronic lung disease.

Hemoptysis

Coughing of blood is a symptom of respiratory disease in 2% to 3% of patients entering a busy hospital internal medicine service. Hemoptysis may reflect thoracic carcinoma, certain bacterial pneumonias, tuberculosis, and pulmonary vascular diseases, such as Wegener's granulomatosis. Blood-streaked sputum should be promptly examined for the acid-fast organisms of tuberculosis and the atypical cells of malignancy. Despite the startling appearance of bloody sputum, less than 1% of patients with hemoptysis experience life-threatening exsanguination.

Peripheral Edema

Swelling of the lower extremities in chronic pulmonary patients may reflect the presence of cor pulmonale, or right ventricular hypertension. Although cosmetically unattractive, therapy rarely needs to be on an emergency basis. Treatment of the underlying lung disease may resolve the cor pulmonale, even without diuretic therapy. More generalized edema may reflect hypoalbuminemia, as in severe liver disease. Left ventricular failure typically produces pulmonary, and not peripheral, edema.

Subcutaneous Emphysema

This finding occurs when air leaks from the thoracic cavity into the subcutaneous tissues, where it is seen as tissue swelling and crepitation. It may accompany a pneumothorax, but not always. This finding, though alarming, is rarely life-threatening in and of itself.

THE BASELINE (INITIAL) HISTORY

How did the patient's course progress from a state of well-being (health) to one of discomfort (dis-ease)? This question must be answered clearly, to understand both the patient and the tempo of the pathologic process affecting him. The baseline history-taking session will gather and process this important information. Obviously, the complete historical inventory is more important in chronic, less acute situations than in respiratory emergencies, where the therapist would do well to "treat first, and ask questions later!"

Historical Fingerprints of Respiratory Disease

Beginners frequently have difficulty in organizing historical data in a cogent, nonmeandering way, and this is reflected in rambling, often incoherent case presentations, morning reports, and progress notes on the hospital chart. The author has found that most clinical histories divide themselves into one of several time/severity patterns, or "historical fingerprints." The beginning student should not be satisfied until he can reduce the patient's history to one of these time/severity patterns.

In the illustrations that follow (see Figs 1–5 to 1–9), note that severity of symptoms is on the vertical axis and that the time, expressed without dimension, e.g., hours, days, or years, is on the horizontal axis. The Gaensler scale (Table 1–2) for severity of dyspnea allows at least some quantitation of this common problem. I know of no similar scale for severity of cough or chest pain. Let us now look at several short case histories to observe how the various "fingerprints" are developed.

Onset by Crisis

Case 1 (tension pneumothorax).—A 35-year-old white man had been in good health until the night of Sept. 12, 1985, when he developed severe left-sided chest pain and incapacitating dyspnea (Fig 1–5). Any activity made him very short of breath, and the paramedics were summoned. The patient was a non-smoker with no history of heart or lung disease. He denied angina, cough, orthopnea, paroxysmal nocturnal dyspnea, or hemoptysis. Immediately before the onset of the severe shortness of breath, he had been lifting a 100-lb sack of flour from the floor to a storage compartment in his barn. On admission to the hospital, he was severely short of breath, pale, and cyanotic, and complained of left-sided chest pain. Auscultation over the left side of the chest relieved markedly diminished breath sounds. There was hyperresonance to percussion on the left side of the chest as well.

Case 2 (pulmonary embolism).—A 70-year-old woman came to the hospital on Dec. 12, 1986, after

TABLE 1–2.*

Classification of Dyspnea by Degree of Severity in the Evaluation of Permanent Impairment

CLASS I	CLASS II	CLASS III	CLASS IV	CLASS V
Dyspnea only on severe exertion ("appropriate" dyspnea)	Can keep pace with person of same age and body build on the level without breathlessness, but not on hills or stairs	Can walk a mile at own pace without dyspnea, but cannot keep pace on the level with a normal person	Dyspnea present after walking about 100 yards on the level, or upon climbing one flight of stairs	Dyspnea on even less activity, or even at rest

*From Burton GG, Hodgkin JE: *Respiratory Care: A Guide to Clinical Practice*, ed 2. Philadelphia, JB Lippincott Co, 1984. Used with permission.

falling at home and injuring her right hip. An x-ray in the emergency room showed a comminuted fracture, which was treated conservatively by immobilization, traction, and casting. On the third postoperative day, she developed sudden severe shortness of breath with precordial chest pain. It was noted that her right leg was swollen and warm. Her respiratory rate was elevated at 30/min and she was mildly cyanotic. Auscultation of her lungs was unremarkable. A ventilation perfusion lung scan was nonspecific, but later a pulmonary arteriogram showed a large pulmonary embolus in the left main pulmonary artery.

Comment.—These cases, one of a tension pneumothorax (case 1) and the other acute pulmonary embolism (case 2), share the same historical configuration, i.e., sudden, or crisis, onset, with no historical antecedent or early sign of the developing condition. The "fingerprint" of this historical pattern appears in Figure 1–5. Crisis onset illnesses are usually dramatic, as in these patients. In some of them, e.g., those with pneumothorax, relief with treatment may be as dramatic as the crisis onset, but this is not invariably the case. Crisis onset illnesses include acute myocardial infarction (chest pain), allergic reactions (bronchospasm), some pneumonias (fever,

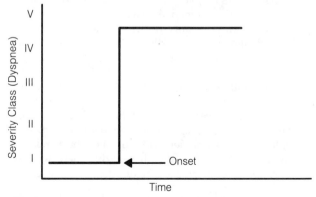

FIG 1–5.
Historical fingerprint: crisis onset dyspnea.

dyspnea), pleurisy (chest pain), aspirated foreign bodies (dyspnea), and pneumothorax and pulmonary embolism, as illustrated above.

Intermittent Symptomatology

Case 3 (bronchial asthma).—A 16-year-old-boy presented to the emergency room with severe wheezing and shortness of breath of 1 day's duration (Fig 1–6). He had had similar episodes of wheezing and shortness of breath in the past after eating seafood. The night of admission, he had eaten some clams and thereafter developed a rash that involved his face, trunk, and extremities. About 3 hours after eating the clams, he began to note severe shortness of breath and mild nonproductive cough. One brother and his maternal aunt had hay fever and bronchial asthma.

Comment.—This case resembles the crisis-onset pattern in the relative rapidity with which symptoms developed, but differs in that the patient has had these symptoms before. Note the symptom-free intervals between episodes and the related rapid offset of symptoms as well (see Fig 1–6). The intermittent pattern occurs most classically in asthma, but can occur with chronic bronchitis (cough and sputum production), congestive heart failure (dyspnea, orthopnea, or paroxysmal nocturnal dyspnea), angina pectoris (chest pain with exercise), tuberculosis (intermittent hemoptysis), myasthenia gravis (dyspnea), or recurrent aspiration (cough, dyspnea).

Progressive Symptomatolgy

Many lung conditions have a more subtle onset, during which progressive damage to pulmonary tissues causes little symptomatology early in the course, and later, more progressive (and perhaps) rapid worsening with more disease. This relationship is depicted in Figure 1–7. In this hypothetical, conceptual illustration, increasing impairment from disease is plotted against increasing disability. Early

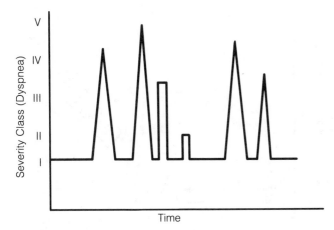

FIG 1–6.
Historical fingerprint: intermittent symptomatology.

in the course of progressive pulmonary disease, symptoms are often not noted because of the enormous physiological functional reserve of the lung and the patient's inclination to disregard symptoms such as mild cough and shortness of breath. These symptoms are often shrugged off by victims of pulmonary disease as being due to cigarette smoke, obesity, age, upper respiratory tract infection, or air pollution, when in fact these symptoms point to early (and possibly treatable) pulmonary dysfunction.

Case 4 (panacinar emphysema).—A 40-year-old white woman came to the hospital complaining of severe shortness of breath at rest (class IV dyspnea). She had been a 2-pack/day cigarette smoker for 20 years, but had not complained of cough or dyspnea until about 3 years earlier when she began to notice

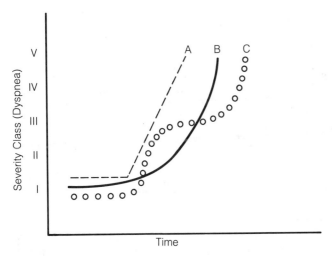

FIG 1–7.
Historical fingerprint: progressive pattern (note variations *A, B,* and *C*).

that she could not keep up with people of her same age when walking up hills or stairs. About 2 years ago, it became impossible for her to walk much at all even at her own pace without shortness of breath, even when walking on the level. She had lost 20 lb over the past 6 months. Cough had not been much of a problem compared to progressive exertional dyspnea. Examination showed evidence of clinical malnutrition. She appeared cachectic.

She was breathing only in the braced position, with her arms bent on a table in front of her. There was severe tachypnea (respiratory rate, 30/min) and use of accessory muscles. The lungs were hyperresonant to percussion. Breath sounds were decreased and there was expiratory prolongation throughout all lung fields. A chest x-ray showed pulmonary hyperexpansion with attenuation of the vascular markings bilaterally and some bullous change at both bases. Pulmonary function tests showed severe airways obstruction with a reduced diffusion capacity.

Case 5 (pulmonary fibrosis).—A 60-year-old female came to the physician's office complaining of slowly progressive shortness of breath of about 3 years' duration associated with cough. She was not a cigarette smoker and denied any industrial exposure. Chest x-rays over the last few years showed an increasing reticulonodular pattern in both lungs. Two months prior to admission, she began to have joint pain and swelling suggestive of rheumatoid arthritis. A chest x-ray demonstrated a diffuse pattern in both lung fields. A rheumatoid factor test and antinuclear antibody test (ANA) were positive. Pulmonary function tests revealed a reduced vital capacity, total lung capacity, and diffusion capacity suggestive of restrictive pulmonary disease with diffusion blockade. It was suspected that the patient's pulmonary fibrosis represented involvement of her lungs with rheumatoid arthritis (fibrosing alveolitis).

Case 6 (high permeability pulmonary edema—adult respiratory distress syndrome).—A 40-year-old alcoholic man presented to the emergency room with abdominal pain of 3 weeks duration associated with nausea, vomiting, and diarrhea. He was admitted for a possible bleeding duodenal ulcer, but it soon became clear that he was suffering from acute pancreatitis. On the third hospital day, be began to complain of mild shortness of breath. Physical examination revealed that he was dyspneic. At that time, his pulmonary examination and chest x-ray were unremarkable. Over the next 2 days, he became acutely and progressively more short of breath with severe hypoxia refractory to oxygen therapy, and a progressive "whitening out" of his chest x-ray. When he was no longer able to be oxygenated on 50% oxygen, he was intubated and positive end-expiratory pressure (PEEP) therapy was begun.

Comment.—Cases 4 to 6 all have one thing in common—progressive worsening of symptomatology. This may occur in various ways (see Fig 1–7), but respiratory function and symptomatology *never* return to normal baseline. Conditions that fall into this category include uncomplicated emphysema (dyspnea), pulmonary fibrosis (dyspnea), metastatic neoplastic interstitial disease (dyspnea), carcinoma of the lung (dyspnea, chest pain, cough, hemoptysis), treated tuberculosis (cough, hemoptysis, especially pattern "7C"), and pulmonary vascular hypertension (dyspnea).

Mixed Patterns

The righthand portion of Figure 1–7,C suggests that effective therapy, though not "curing" the basic process, e.g., emphysema or pulmonary fibrosis, may result in considerable symptomatic improvement. Thus, the use of mucolytics may facilitate sputum clearance in such patients, as diuresis may improve lung compliance in patients with chronic congestive heart failure though the low cardiac state itself remains. Symptomatic exacerbations and remissions are thus not rare, even in "chronic" conditions such as cystic fibrosis and emphysema.

Case 7.—A 70-year-old man with known pulmonary emphysema came into the hospital with acute worsening of his (usually moderate) chronic shortness of breath. In the 3 days prior to admission, he had cough productive of yellow purulent sputum and moderate swelling of his ankles. He was now short of breath even at rest. Prior to the current episode, he had been able to move about his house at his own speed, albeit slowly.

A Gram's stain of his sputum showed many white blood cells and gram-positive diplococci. A chest x-ray showed pulmonary overexpansion with increased bronchovascular markings at the bases, but no acute infiltrate suggesting pneumonia. The patient was treated as having a bronchitic exacerbation of his chronic obstructive pulmonary disease, with vigorous bronchial hygiene, intravenous hydration, and antibiotics. Seven days later he was discharged without oxygen and much improved.

Comment.—Almost any combination of historical patterns is possible, but the infectious (bronchitic) exacerbations of chronic obstructive pulmonary disease and cystic fibrosis are the most well-known of the mixed pattern historical fingerprints (Fig 1–8). Figure 1–9 shows a mixed historical pattern wherein sudden worsening is superimposed on a progressive disease such as the adult respiratory distress syn-

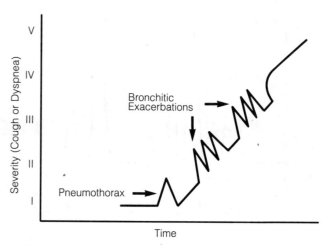

FIG 1–8.
Historical fingerprint: mixed patterns of disease.

drome. Such a mixed pattern may be called "worse on bad," a dyspnea pattern that occurs in severely ill patients who deteriorate rapidly despite intensive respiratory care. It may be illustrated by the worsening of dyspnea or alveolar-arterial oxygen gradient in an already dyspneic patient, e.g., from a pneumothorax occurring with the use of "super-PEEP" in a patient with adult respiratory distress syndrome (ARDS).

Additional Baseline Data

In addition to determining the historical fingerprint of the patient's illness, some additional background data should be assessed. A brief family and

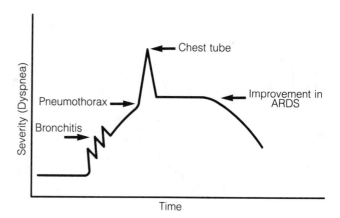

FIG 1–9.
Historical fingerprint: exacerbations in ARDS. The arrows represent and define bouts of acute bronchitis and pneumonia. A spontaneous pneumothorax occurred at a time when only *class II* dyspnea was present. The improvement in severe dyspnea with the placement of a chest tube thoracostomy is noted.

smoking history, allergy history, environmental exposure history, and treatment response history should be taken. The last item is often overlooked by beginners who should understand that many respiratory conditions tend to be chronic. Thus, it is appropriate to ask what medications the patient has used previously and to inquire if they were beneficial or not.

Compliance History

Another baseline piece of data may be called the compliance history. Has the patient been following his previously outlined treatment program? If, for example, the patient has been counseled not to smoke, his carboxyhemoglobin level should be normal. If he has been given a theophylline-containing bronchodilator but has a low or nonexistent serum theophylline level, he is either not taking his medication correctly or too small a dose was prescribed. Other markers of patient compliance include eosinophil suppression in asthmatics, equipment cleanliness and good return demonstrations of its use, and weight reduction in patients who have been placed on reducing diets.

THE INTERVAL HISTORY

From the standpoint of the treating therapist, the events of the intervening minutes or hours since the last respiratory care procedure may be even more important than the precision of the baseline history, the foregoing section notwithstanding. Indeed the "R.T. progress notes" (see Figure 1–1) constitute nothing more than a short, concise record of what was done to (and for!) the patient during a therapy session and an impression as to the results of that therapy. Another type of interval history is that of the record of an intervening potentially stressful (albeit short-term) event: exercise, sleep, surgery, an extensive laboratory study, or a trip to the radiology department come to mind as examples.

Although the student must become proficient in organizing data if he is to be able to "present cases" to his superiors or colleagues, his skill in recording and assessing the interval history are even more important in ensuring his long-term success as a participant in the health care process. Careful records must be kept for scientific and operational (as well as for medicolegal) purposes.

There are three ways that the interval history needs to be documented: before, during, and after therapy. Here is an example:

Before.—A 30-year-old man with asthma in room 565 has severe wheezing and dyspnea. His respiratory rate is 30/min, and his pulse is 120/min and regular. Wheezes were heard in all lung fields.

During.—A medicated nebulizer treatment was given using 0.3 ml of metaproterenol in 2.0 ml of normal saline by therapist John Jones between 3:15 and 3:25 P.M. Halfway through the treatment, his dyspnea improved, his respiratory rate dropped to 22/min, and his pulse fell to 90/min. He coughed up about 5 ml of thick, tenacious mucus.

After.—At the end of the treatment, the patient felt much improved and his chest was clear to auscultation. His pulse was 82/min. His oxygen therapy at 3 L/min was resumed.

What we see here are the five classic elements of a good reporter's story: who, what, why, when, and where. The story can be embellished but not shortened, without suffering from incompleteness. Note that there are really two "who's"—the patient and John Jones, the therapist. Note also that the patient was given the treatment by the therapist; the patient did not give the treatment to himself. The example above also illustrates something else in the good interval note—an attempt at quantifiable documentation: the exact medication dosage, pulse, respiratory rate, sputum volume and characteristics, and auscultatory findings. The old quick notation "Patient took treatment well" will just not suffice in our current reimbursement and medicolegal environment.

New or Previously Unrecognized Pathology

Contrary to popular opinion, people can become sicker in the hospital! Pulmonary emboli, septicemia, hypotension, and pneumonia are just a few of the conditions that can develop in hospitalized patients, and *not* as results of therapy. A caution is therefore necessary: no matter how complete the *baseline history*, it is entirely possible that something new may develop, and therapists should be willing to add new diagnoses to their problem lists as necessary. The S-O-A-P 1, S-O-A-P 2 approach has been mentioned in this regard, and the historical fingerprint of this type of situation has been described (see Figs 1–8 and 1–9).

Adverse Reactions to Therapy

The list of things that can go *wrong* with therapy seems at times to be longer than things that can go *right!* These complications of therapy are discussed elsewhere, but remember how carefully the *interval history* must document exactly what happened and what was done about it. An example may be helpful.

Before.—A 70-year-old woman with emphysema, in room 1002, is hospitalized for acute bronchitis. She is confused and combative, and a bronchodilator medication, isoetharine, is given by an IPPB device. At 10 A.M., before therapy, her heart rate is 100/min and her respiratory rate is 12/min. Her breath sounds are decreased bilaterally and there are coarse crackles at the left base.

During.—Initially treatment is uneventful. At 10:15 A.M., she becomes pale, sweaty, and her heart rate increases to 130/min. Breath sounds are no longer heard in the right chest. At 10:17 A.M., she loses consciousness. A "code 99" is called.

After.—The therapist inserts an oropharyngeal airway and administers 100% oxygen by mask. The CPR team arrives at 10:19:30 A.M. and manual cardiac massage is begun. An ECG monitor is applied and a sample for ABG is drawn. Chest auscultation again reveals absent breath sounds in the right chest, and a Clagett needle thoracostomy tube is inserted in the right clavicular line, in the sixth interspace.

Here we have documented a dreaded complication of pressure ventilation, a pneumothorax. Note that the record quickly and appropriately switches from a report of the treatment to a chronology of the complication. This record will serve the hospital well in any alleged malpractice proceeding that may develop. Again, the "who, what, when, why, and where" has stood us in good stead, but now a "how" has been added.

Good charting, like good therapy, takes practice and time. It is a learned skill that every entering student must master. If he has had any training as a news reporter, it will stand him in good stead.

ANATOMY OF A HOSPITAL CHART

As in all interpersonal relationships, communication in the delivery of health care is essential to success. Considering that the patient is "in the system" from the time he enters the hospital lobby or emergency room until the time he leaves, a careful record of all that transpires must be available to the (literally) dozens of health care workers who care for him from dawn to dusk, every minute of the day, every day of the week. Despite all the current interest in automated data entry and retrieval, and the considerable impact that computer technology is making in other aspects of the health care field, the hard facts are that the majority of patient data must still be manually entered in the hospital chart.

Thus, the hospital record serves as the primary source of information about the patient at any given time during his hospital stay. In general, respiratory care workers are granted ready access to any and all portions of the chart, both for the gathering of background information as described above and for the ongoing recording of their diagnostic and treatment interventions. The beginning therapist must remember that many health care workers besides himself need to "get at the chart." He should always be kind and courteous in waiting his turn in line when others are standing by. Because of the pressures for chart access, many departments have gone to in-the-room or in-department charting notes that can be kept with the therapist during the duty rotation. These then may be entered into the chart with adhesive backing at the end of shift (see Fig 1–1).

This section of the chapter introduces the beginning student to the format of a typical hospital chart, developing in the process a "road map" to the various sections, with brief descriptions as to what one might expect to find therein. There will be variability between hospitals as to the precise format of the patient record, but the following comments will suffice by way of introduction.

The order of content listing in the patient chart, as it exists on the care unit, may be somewhat different than when the chart is finally assembled for permanent record in the medical records department. The ordering of information is for convenience of the health care team, and it should not come as a surprise that the physician orders and clinical records often appear in the front of the chart, while the history and physical examination, as well as consultation reports, may come somewhere later. In this section, utilization of the format employed at our hospital, the Kettering Medical Center, is presented.

Patient Data

At the beginning of every chart, as well as on the outside of the chart binder, is data that identifies the patient as to name, physician of record, and room number. Inside the chart is a data sheet that customarily contains the patient's name, hospital record number, address, home phone, social security number, date of birth, age, marital status, religious preference, race, and occupation. The name and address of his next of kin, as well as his employer and insurance coverage, is listed, as is space for the room number, admission date, discharge date, and primary and secondary diagnoses. Also, on the face sheet of most charts is space for listing of surgical procedures, complications of care, preexisting or nosocomial infection problems, and space for the various necessary signatures documenting the patient's care.

Physician Orders

In our hospital, physician orders comprise the next section of the chart. These are blank-ruled pages where physician orders are recorded. This form is in triplicate so that copies can easily be sent to the pharmacy, laboratory, and other centers within the hospital without having to copy the main order sheet. Orders are listed chronologically, with the most recent orders usually at the front of the section. In some care areas, printed *standing orders* are used, and these are noted with the date and time of the physician "writing" the order. When working in critical care areas, it is particularly important to note the time as well as the date of the orders, to make sure that the most current orders are being followed.

Clinical Records

The next section of our typical chart records shift-to-shift descriptions of vital signs, such as weight, temperature, pulse, blood pressure, respiratory rate, and nursing observations of patient care. In this section, one may find records of nursing attendance, patient ambulation, and more or less a diary of the patient's many activities during the day. The clinical records may serve as a relatively untapped source of information regarding much of what goes on in a patient's busy schedule.

Intake/Output Records

These important records of fluid intake and output are usually located in or near the clinical records. In critically ill patients, intake and output may be charted on an hourly basis, but usually this is done on an 8-hour shift basis. Since adequate hydration is so important in respiratory care, the intake/output record is often a veritable "gold mine" of information for the therapist who would like to know why a patient's sputum is so thick, or conversely, why the patient seems to forever be slipping into and out of a state of pulmonary edema.

Medications

Every hospital record has a section for "listed medications" in which the patient's oral and parenteral medications are listed. Interestingly, in most hospitals, the respiratory therapy medications are not listed here, as we will see. Since the possibility of cross-reaction between medications exists, the entering student should be familiar with this portion of the chart, if only to explain some of the potentially adverse medication reactions that he may encounter.

Laboratory Reports

This section of the chart usually documents the results of tests performed in the clinical laboratory. Increasingly, these are being reported in tabular, chronologic form by periodic computer update. This makes it possible to serially assess progress of various laboratory parameters with ease. Arterial blood gas reports often appear in this section of the chart, as do reports from the bacteriology laboratory and, sometimes, from the pulmonary function laboratory as well.

X-Rays and Scans

A separate section of the chart is often devoted to the report of radiologic and nuclear medicine studies, such as chest x-rays, computerized tomography scans, and angiograms. The respiratory therapy student will often want to look at the report of an x-ray, at least, if not the x-ray itself. This is the section where these reports would be found.

ECG/EEG

In this section of the chart, the reports and tracings of electrocardiograms and other electrophysiological studies are reported. This section is particularly important in dealing with patients suffering from cardiac disease. Cardiac rhythm strips are often recorded in this section as well.

History, Physical Examination, and Consultation Reports

This section of the chart contains the history, physical examination, and consultation reports dictated by physicians involved in the patient's care. While these reports are being typed, handwritten short summaries are often left here as well. Also in this section of the chart, on a daily or even hourly basis, progress reports may be written by the physicians involved in the patient's care. This section of the chart is not to be written on by anyone other than physician personnel, except under conditions approved by the medical staff. It is, however, not inviolate, and is often referred to by nurses and therapists in the course of their care of the patient.

Respiratory Therapy and Physical Therapy Progress Notes

This is a section of the chart in which the various therapists record documentation of their care of the patient. We have discussed formatting of these reports, and have stressed the importance of brevity and accuracy in these notes, if they are to be of help to the members of the health care team.

Circumstance will often dictate which part of the chart the therapist should study. The therapist's perusal of the record must be efficient, and handling of the information must be done in the strictest confidence to protect the patient and patient-physician relationship. The contents of hospital charts should never be treated as idle hospital gossip. The access granted by most modern hospitals to physicians and other members of the health care team should be treated with the utmost respect and gravity.

In short, we have described a record that may be from 1 to 2 in. thick. For patients who have stayed in the hospital for long periods, the chart may be divided into volumes. The therapist must have some idea as to what is important and what is not. We have stressed the importance of the therapist's own particular contribution to the medical record, specifically that of the therapist progress notes. If the therapist wants to get an idea of what the physician is thinking, a look at the history and physical and daily progress notes may be helpful.

THE PHYSICAL EXAMINATION

First Impressions—The Intuitive Edge

Efficiency is as important in diagnosis and assessment as it is in therapy. Clearly the therapist cannot afford the luxury of sitting down and taking a complete history and performing an exhaustive inspection—palpation, percussion, and auscultation of the chest at the beginning and end of every therapeutic session. What can be done in the interest of time without sacrificing accuracy? The answer lies in the ability to utilize one's sensory facilities *continuously* from the initial chart pick-up at the nurses' station to the "sign-off" at the end of charting. I have described this information-gathering routine in another publication, under the rubric "The View From the Door."[2] Recently, a growing literature has described development of the "sixth sense" and described its obvious advantages, most particularly in a work entitled "The Intuitive Edge."[2, 3]

It is a great temptation to let the stethoscope and the blood gas report be the major diagnostic evaluative tools, probably because so much effort is spent on ensuring that the student become familiar with them. Not to diminish their importance, the student should, however, use *all* of his senses to precondition himself to what the stethoscopic findings and the blood gas results might be. Table 1–3 summarizes some of these observations, which can be made more rapidly than a reading of this material will indicate, and suggests possible clinical correlations of importance.

The physical examination of the respiratory patient should be performed in the therapeutic as well as diagnostic content. The therapist comes as a participant in the overall care saga, and accordingly, confirmation of what he or she has garnered from chart review, oral reports, and the "view from the door" should be made. This confirmation will include an assessment of cardiac rate and rhythm, blood pressure, respiratory rate and pattern, and temperature. These physical findings are commonly referred to as "vital signs."

Blood Pressure

The patient's blood pressure is recorded with a sphygmomanometer (Fig 1–10) and the systolic (higher) and diastolic (lower) numbers recorded. These values reflect the cardiovascular pressure head that perfuses body tissues. Normal values range between 110–130/70–80 mm Hg. The tech-

TABLE 1–3.

Clinical Implications of Signs and Observations

OBSERVATION	CLINICAL IMPLICATIONS
Patient chart	
1. Chart is in great demand at nurses' station	1. Patient may be critically ill, or at least a lot is going on with him (laboratory tests or procedures)
2. Pulse rate, temperature	2. Cardiovascular status, evidence of infection, inflammation, or atelectasis
3. "Flags" on chart cover	3. Notification of drug allergies, isolation, other warnings, and notifications
4. Medication sheet	4. See page 17
Attendant garb	
1. Isolation gowns, caps, masks, gloves	1. Patient may have a contagious disease, e.g., tuberculosis, hepatitis, or be immunosuppressed, e.g., patients with AIDS, or be colonized or infected with organisms with high potential for causing nosocomial infection, e.g., *Pseudomonas, Staphylococcus*
2. Lead-shielded aprons	2. Portable x-ray equipment in use
Patient position	
1. Supine	1. Normal eupneic breathing, or orthodeoxia as in pulmonary fibrosis
2. Erect or head-up	2. Possible orthopnea
3. Braced shoulders	3. The so-called emphysematous habitus
4. On one side	4. Possible pleurisy, fractured ribs, or pleural effusion
5. Trendelenburg	5. Shock
6. Postural drainage positions (see Chapter 7).	6. Airway secretions are probably present, e.g., bronchietasis, cystic fibrosis
Family in room	
1. Facial expression, tears, laughter, degree of animation of family members	1. A good indication of the gravity of the immediate situation; family is usually willing to leave the room while therapy is carried out
Equipment in room	
1. Oxygen	The patient receiving oxygen therapy presumably would be hypoxemic without it; the patient on a ventilator presumably would hypoventilate or become hypoxemic without it, etc. The various pieces of respiratory care equipment are discussed in the appropriate sections of this textbook. The presence of such equipment should bias the observer as to what he might (or might not) find in his examination, e.g., if suction apparatus is present, and the suction trap is full of thick tenacious mucus, he should expect to find the adventitious breath sounds associated with airway secretions, crackles, and rhonchi (or if suctioning has been successful absence of crackles and rhonchi).
2. Aerosol generators	
3. Sputum cups	
4. Face masks and tents	
5. Ventilators	
6. Facial CPAP masks	
7. Suction apparatus	
8. Hemodialysis units	
Markings on the chest	
1. Markings made with indelible ink	1. Usually the areas of shielding for external radiation therapy; implies that the patient has cancer
2. Surgical tape, incisions, sutures	2. A surgeon has been there, in the remote or recent past!
3. Puncture marks	3. In the emergency room, the patient may be a stabbing victim. In the hospital ward, think of the possibility that the patient may have had a thoracentesis or pleural biopsy

(Continued)

TABLE 1–3. *Continued*

OBSERVATION	CLINICAL IMPLICATIONS
Chest tubes	
1. Connected to drainage, not bubbling	1. Probable drainage of fluid in the chest (pleural effusion, emphysema, or hemothorax), or of air in the pleural space (pneumothorax)
2. Connected to drainage, bubbling	2. Reflects a bronchopleural fistula or tear or leak in the visceral pleura
Breathing sounds	
1. Stridor	1. Upper airway obstruction, croup, or laryngitis.
2. Gurgling sounds	2. Fluid, food (aspiration?), or mucus in the upper airway
3. Cough	3. See pages 7–9
4. Wheezing	4. In severe bronchospasm, may be loud enough to hear without a stethoscope
5. Crescendo snoring with apneic spells	5. May reflect obstructive sleep apnea
Sputum	
1. Volume	The diagnostic implications of sputum appearance are discussed in Figure 1–2. Figure 1–2 relates the gross appearance of sputum to various disease states
2. Consistency and viscosity	
3. Purulence	
4. Presence or absence of blood	
Bedside Chart	
1. Heart rate and rhythm	It is ridiculous *not* to be aware of these life-critical parameters during the care of the sick. Utilization of these data is also time saving, since independent measurement of the parameters before, during, and after therapy is needless duplication.
2. Vascular pressures	
3. Ventilatory parameters	

nique of blood pressure measurement is more easily learned at the bedside than described in a textbook; it basically involves listening for emerging (systolic) and disappearing (diastolic) sounds with a stethoscope placed over the brachial artery, as the sphygmomanometer cuff is decompressed.

Hypertension commonly results from arteriosclerotic heart disease. One blood pressure reading, however, "does not make a day," and occasionally elevated blood pressures may reflect anxiety, pain, or other discomfort on the part of the patient. Persistent diastolic blood pressure readings of more than 90 mm Hg in adults are worrisome.

Hypotension may reflect cardiogenic or septic shock, or hypovolemia. Blood pressures lower than 100/60 in adults may represent one of these conditions.

From a therapeutic standpoint, elevated blood pressure should (at least temporarily) restrain the treating therapist from administering β-agonist bronchodilator drugs or from performing any pain-

ful procedure. Hypotension, on the other hand, should caution him against the use of high ventilator pressures or positive end-expiratory pressures (PEEP). These cautions are repeated in Chapters 6 and 10.

Heart Rate and Rhythm

Space does not permit an extensive discussion of pulse rate or cardiac rhythm. The pulse may be ascertained by counting the number of pulsations felt over a carotid, brachial, radial, or femoral artery over an interval of time, and multiplying to determine the rate/minute, i.e., (rate at 15 seconds × 4) or (rate at 30 seconds × 2). Hypotensive patients, of course, may have such faint, thready peripheral pulses as to preclude pulse measurement, and heart rate in such patients must be determined by auscultation over the heart or by analysis of an electrocardiographic rhythm strip.

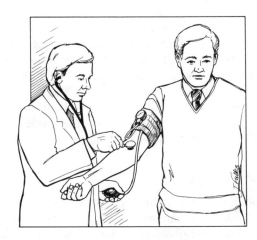

TABLE 1–4.

Life-Threatening Cardiac Arrhythmias

Paroxysmal atrial tachycardia
Rapid atrial fibrillation
Supraventricular atrial tachycardia
Frequent ventricular extrasystoles (>10/min)
Ventricular tachycardia
Ventricular fibrillation
Chaotic supraventricular tachycardia
Sinus bradycardia
Nodal rhythm
Cardiac standstill

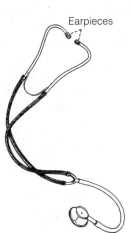

Earpieces

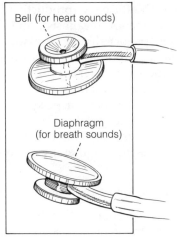

Bell (for heart sounds)

Diaphragm
(for breath sounds)

FIG 1–10.
Sphygmomanometer for measuring blood pressure. A stethoscope is used to listen for emerging (systolic) and disappearing (diastolic) sounds.

Tachycardia (ventricular rate greater than 100/min) and *bradycardia* (ventricular rate less than 60/min) are common enough to warrant brief discussion. Pulse rates in excess of 120/min are *relative* contraindications for administration of sympathomimetic drugs such as the β-agonist bronchodilator agents. Tissue hypoxia is another common cause of tachycardia, and, for that matter, of bradycardia. Obviously, discretion is called for. The best advice for the beginner is: "When in doubt, ask."

The beginning respiratory therapy student is not expected to recognize more than the simplest and most significant of cardiac arrhythmias. These cardiac rhythms described in Table 1–4 can be life-threatening, and should be reviewed in a standard cardiology textbook. As the therapist improves his skills and begins to work more in critical care areas, his familiarity with other cardiac rhythms will improve.

Respiratory Rate and Pattern

The casually obtained respiratory rate, i.e., counting breaths for 15 seconds and multiplying times 4 is essentially worthless in evaluating patient condition; more accurate and sophisticated (and unfortunately, more expensive) assessment tools have been developed.[5, 6] The normal frequency range of respiration rates for adults is so large (9 to 30 breaths/min, depending on age, weight, and metabolic rate) as to preclude much use in the clinical setting. As has been described elsewhere, a change in respiratory rate or rhythm is of much more importance.[1, 2]

Increases in respiratory rate may reflect hypoxia, fever, pain, or psychological disturbances. Decreases in rate may reflect improvement in oxygenation status on the one hand, or hypoventilation (as in narcotic overdosage) on the other. The general dictum that reduction in breathing rate reflects improvement in dyspnea is fairly accurate, as is the converse, i.e., that tachypnea reflects worsening respiratory status, with the above provisions. For example, recent works suggest that patients whose spontaneous ventilatory rate exceeds 30/min will not tolerate respirator weaning.

The normal individual, whatever his age or metabolic status, demonstrates no positional preference for breathing. He is comfortable breathing while prone, supine, sitting, or standing, or in either lateral decubitus position. He may change position occasionally, and take a sigh or two each minute. These movements, however, are casual and not associated with any untoward effort. Clinical conditions associated with dyspnea in various body positions are described in Table 1–5.

The length of expiration is slightly longer than inspiration (I:E ratio of 3–5:6) in adults. In neonates and small infants, the I:E ratio is nearer to 1:1. Tidal volumes, of course, are small in neonates (in pre-

TABLE 1–5.

Causes of Dyspnea Related to Preferred Body Position

KIND OF DYSPNEA	CLINICAL CORRELATIONS
Orthopnea (must sit up to breathe; often occurs at night as paroxysmal nocturnal dyspnea)	Congestive heart failure
Obstructive sleep apnea (periodically stops breathing, particularly when lying on back)	Obesity—obstructive sleep apnea syndromes
Emphysematous habitus	COPD
Platypnea	Pleural effusion, dyspnea associated with various body positions
Orthodeoxia	Pulmonary fibrosis, dyspnea is improved when patient is lying flat

mature infants as little as 5 ml) compared to more than 500 ml in adults. Assessment of the I:E ratio at the bedside is helpful in dyspnea assessment, in that patients with obstructive pulmonary disease have prolonged expiration while patients with restrictive pulmonary diseases (such as pulmonary fibrosis), breathe rapidly and shallowly and have I:E ratios closer to 1:1. Less commonly seen patterns of breathing include the crescendo respiratory efforts of obstructive sleep apnea, the totally irregular pattern of breathing seen in central nervous system disturbances (*Biot* breathing), and the waxing and waning breathing patterns of congestive heart failure (*Cheyne-Stokes* breathing).

Temperature

Though most of us have been brought up to believe that the normal oral temperature is 98.6°F (37°C), the fact of the matter is that a range of 96.5° to 99.4°F (35.8° to 37.4°C) is more realistic. These variations are caused by circadian cycles (daytime-nighttime variation, menstrual/ovulation cycles) and alterations in activity. In respiratory patients, unless proved otherwise, oral temperatures above 99.4°F (37.4°C) are thought to represent infection or atelectasis. Because so many patients cannot or will not permit the taking of oral temperatures, rectal (sometimes called core) temperatures are often recorded. Normal temperatures range between 97.5° and 100.4°F.

The therapist may be tempted to think *all* temperature elevations in his (respiratory) patients will reflect respiratory infections. Although this may be the case, he should recall that other sites of infection potentially exist, such as the urinary tract, central nervous system, and from intravascular devices such as intravenous and arterial catheters. The pulmonary system should be suspected as the cause of fever when there is radiographic evidence of infection or airway obstruction (pneumonia or atelectasis) or change in sputum volume or character.

General Findings

Notation of the patient's state of consciousness (alert, drowsy, comatose), mood (happy, sad, cooperative, uncooperative), nutritional state, hydration, cough efficiency (productive, nonproductive), tissue oxygenation (cyanosis), and systemic perfusion (rubor, pallor) should be made. Therapists should not equate an order for bronchodilator therapy via medication nebulizer with one for intravenous antibiotics. Since patient cooperation is so important to the success of many aspects of bronchial hygiene therapy, some notation of the patient's state of consciousness, and his cooperation (or lack of it) with the respiratory therapy, is certainly worthwhile.

Inspection of the Chest

Inspection of the chest, if possible, is performed with the patient seated comfortably. Inspection is the first step in the formal initial chest examination. Customarily, inspection needs to be done thoroughly once, since the findings do not usually change in the course of therapy. In the traditional sequence, inspection of the chest is followed by palpation, percussion, and auscultation. In practice, unfortunately, only the latter technique—auscultation—receives much attention, and the stethoscope becomes an almost natural extension of the therapist's arm!

In infants, the chest is more or less circular when viewed from above downward. As the child grows, the chest increases in lateral diameter, so that the lateral dimension of the chest is more than its anteroposterior dimension. With advancing age, or in the presence of obstructive pulmonary disease, the chest may increase in anteroposterior diameter. In patients with kyphoscoliosis, or in patients who have had a pneumonectomy, the chest may be asymmetrical. These configurations, as viewed looking down on the chest from above the patient's head, appear in Figure 1–11.

The adult thorax is normally symmetrical when

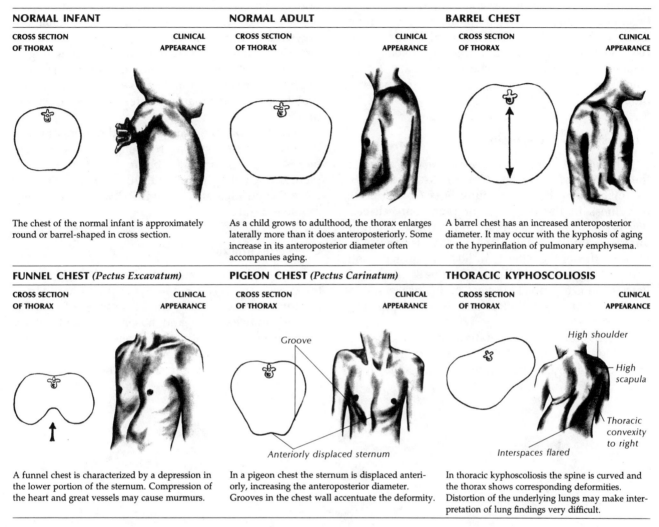

NORMAL INFANT		NORMAL ADULT		BARREL CHEST	
CROSS SECTION OF THORAX	CLINICAL APPEARANCE	CROSS SECTION OF THORAX	CLINICAL APPEARANCE	CROSS SECTION OF THORAX	CLINICAL APPEARANCE
The chest of the normal infant is approximately round or barrel-shaped in cross section.		As a child grows to adulthood, the thorax enlarges laterally more than it does anteroposteriorly. Some increase in its anteroposterior diameter often accompanies aging.		A barrel chest has an increased anteroposterior diameter. It may occur with the kyphosis of aging or the hyperinflation of pulmonary emphysema.	

FUNNEL CHEST *(Pectus Excavatum)*		PIGEON CHEST *(Pectus Carinatum)*		THORACIC KYPHOSCOLIOSIS	
CROSS SECTION OF THORAX	CLINICAL APPEARANCE	CROSS SECTION OF THORAX	CLINICAL APPEARANCE	CROSS SECTION OF THORAX	CLINICAL APPEARANCE
A funnel chest is characterized by a depression in the lower portion of the sternum. Compression of the heart and great vessels may cause murmurs.		In a pigeon chest the sternum is displaced anteriorly, increasing the anteroposterior diameter. Grooves in the chest wall accentuate the deformity.		In thoracic kyphoscoliosis the spine is curved and the thorax shows corresponding deformities. Distortion of the underlying lungs may make interpretation of lung findings very difficult.	

FIG 1–11.
Deformities of the thorax. (From Bates B: *A Guide to Physical Examination and History Taking*, ed 4. Philadelphia, JB Lippincott Co, 1987. Used with permission.)

viewed from any aspect. Asymmetry may be caused by pulmonary parenchymal conditions themselves, such as unilateral atelectasis or pneumothorax, or by deformities such as kyphoscoliosis, pectus deformities of the sternum, or rib injuries. Abdominal protuberance or retraction should also be looked for, as in obesity or with use of the abdominal accessory muscles of respiration. Reduced or absent movements of one hemithorax may reflect pain from fractured ribs or disease of the pleura or underlying lung, diminished diaphragmatic excursion, or unilateral pneumothorax. Scars of trauma or past surgeries should be noted.

Normal tidal breathing, as viewed at the bedside, is easily carried out regardless of body position. It is effortless, rhythmic, and not associated with visible muscular effort. The diaphragm and internal intercostal muscles that affect normal resting ventilation do so without much fuss or ceremony. When the work of breathing increases, the so-called *accessory muscles of respiration* (the platysma, sternocleidomastoids, external intercostals, and even the trapezius muscles) are used and it becomes clear that dyspnea (difficult breathing) is present.

Palpation of the Chest Wall

If the patient complains of chest wall pain or discomfort, palpation of the spine and bony thorax may reveal tenderness over specific areas. This finding may reflect underlying pathology in the sternum, spine, or ribs, and should be noted on the chart. It is sometimes helpful to inquire whether deep breathing aggravates the pain or discomfort as in patients with costochondritis, fractured ribs, or pleurisy. Such tender or painful areas are usually best avoided when performing chest percussion, for example, or when positioning the patient for postural drainage.

Diagnostic Chest Percussion

The use of percussion to localize wall studs in the building of a house is known to anyone who has installed wallboard or hung heavy pictures. Its usefulness in the diagnosis of pulmonary disease (Fig 1–12), whatever its utility in the construction industry, is limited. Only the largest of lesions, e.g., pleural effusions greater than 500 ml, lobar consolidations, and severe air trapping can be so discerned. Percussion is essentially useless in the localization of small infiltrates, small effusions, or small pneumothoraces.

Percussion *is* useful in determining the extent of diaphragmatic motion at the extremes of inspiration and expiration. This observation, with a determina-

tion of thoracic expansion and mobility, should always be recorded as part of the initial evaluation. Low-riding, immobile diaphragms are seen in obstructive pulmonary disease with air trapping (Fig 1–13). Asymmetrical "diaphragmatic" borders are seen in phrenic paralysis, unilateral pleural effusions, and unilateral parenchymal infiltrates (such as pneumonia).

Hyperresonance is noted over the thorax in conditions associated with air trapping. Flatness or dullness to percussion may be noted over areas of pleural thickening or pleural effusion, or over any consolidated area such as with atelectasis or pneumonic infiltrate.

Chest Auscultation

Although auscultation of the chest may not be the most precise way of studying pulmonary structure and function, it has the advantages of low (essentially no) expense and absolute patient safety. When combined with the evaluation techniques listed earlier in this chapter, and when performed in a fairly vigorous manner soon to be described, its

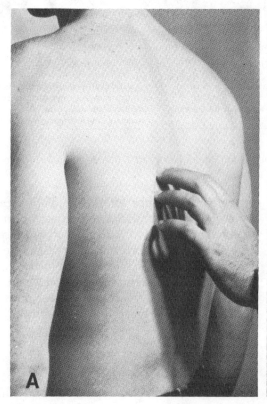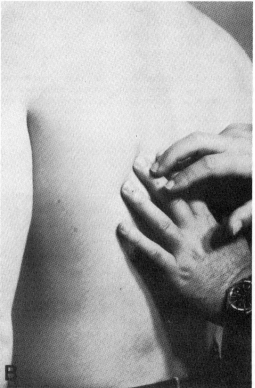

FIG 1–12.
Immediate (A) and mediate (B) chest percussion technique. (From Burton GG, Hodgkin JE: *Respiratory Care: A Guide to Clinical Practice*, ed 2. Philadelphia, JB Lippincott Co, 1984, p 291. Used with permission.)

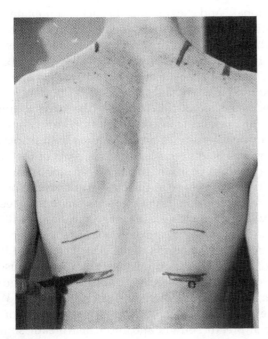

FIG 1–13.
Range of normal thoracic excursion with deep inspiration. The upper line marks the limit of percussion resonance with forced expiration. The lower line marks the limit of percussion resonance with maximum inspiration. (From Burton GG, Hodgkin JE: *Respiratory Care: A Guide to Clinical Practice*, ed 2. Philadelphia, JB Lippincott, 1984, p 292. Used with permission.)

place in the therapist's armamentarium is justly secure. (Respiratory therapists and nurses, in the not-too-distant past, were sometimes snidely referred to as "little doctors" for *daring* to auscultate the chests of their patients; fortunately, those days are over.)

Absolute quiet is necessary for optimal auscultation of the chest. Unfortunately this state of affairs is sometimes not attainable in the noisy intensive care unit, but it should be diligently sought. Noisy conversation should be hushed, radios, television, monitor alarms, infusion pump alarms, and telephones should be silenced; the doorway to the hall should be closed, and the best stethoscope available should be used.

One should avoid breathing heavily on the stethoscope tubing, which can produce a soft, roaring sound not unlike a legitimate breath (lung) sound. The bell should be firmly and flatly pressed on the chest wall to filter out extraneous sounds such as those caused by hair on the chest. If this is not done, sounds that mimic a pleural friction rub may be heard. Movement of tendons and muscles may mimic some friction rubs and crackles, but usually disappear when the subject relaxes completely. Furthermore, bona fide crackles are often modified by coughing, while the sounds from joint, muscle, and tendon motion are not.

Stethoscopes

First introduced by Laennec in 1816, the stethoscope allowed description of the major categories of disease that still form the basis of modern classification. His "auscultation" consisted of listening to such acoustic phenomena as stridor, cough, sighs, and wheezes through a hollow tube at some distance from the patient. Earlier, by the time of Hippocrates, direct application of the listening ear to the chest had formed the basis of clinicopathologic determinations.

The earpieces of the stethoscope should conform to the shape and size of the listener's external auditory canals, and the proximal ends of the stethoscope should be angled in the general direction of these channels, so that extraneous voice sounds are excluded. Most clinicians prefer stethoscopes with two separate sound-conducting tubes from the chest piece to each ear. The diaphragm of the chest piece is almost exclusively used in auscultation of the adult chest, since it more accurately transmits the majority of breath sounds, which fall within the range of 80 to 800 cycles/second. The bell of the chest piece is helpful in examination of children and thin-chested individuals, as it may fit between the ribs, producing an acoustic seal that excludes extraneous sounds.

When judged by the standards of high-fidelity reproduction, the stethoscope is far from perfect. Its response to the whole range of frequencies (pitch) and loudness (intensity) emitted by the heart and lungs is uneven at best, even in the most optimal conditions and in the hands of the most skilled observer. At some frequencies, the loudness of sound transmission may vary as much as 50 dB between brands of stethoscope. These problems notwithstanding, the stethoscope can be used both for quantitative and qualitative assessment of breath sounds.

Fortunately, adventitious breath sounds are loud enough to be heard through any stethoscope, though normal breath sounds are nearer the threshold of hearing, and may not be heard unless the foregoing precautions are taken.

Procedure

A systematic approach to auscultation improves the efficiency and accuracy of the whole operation. One should begin at the apex of one lung, comparing the sounds with those on the opposite side. Normal breath sounds are not generated by breaths of normal tidal volumes, and deeper breaths must be taken if any sound is to be generated. Be careful not to have the patient hyperventilate himself into unconsciousness. One breath over each area should suffice, at least initially. Beginners tend to make the mistake of listening over one lobe or segment for long periods of time, hoping for some hidden truth to be revealed. While this approach may be helpful in cardiac auscultation, it is not in the pulmonary setting. Likewise, auscultation over the scapulae, spine, and sternum is unrewarding. Right to left comparison of breath sounds is as important as the sounds themselves. Remember to keep that stethoscope moving!

One complete respiratory (inspiration/expiration) cycle should be listened to at each auscultatory site:

1. The presence (or absence) of breath sounds in the area should be noted. Decreased breath sounds (see below) are probably the most ominous of all breath sounds. Yet in a recent study, there was a 30% interobserver error in reporting this finding alone.

2. The intensity and duration of each phase of respiration (inspiration:expiration) should be noted, e.g., "3:2, inspiration louder."

3. The presence, timing, nature, and quality of normal and adventitious (added) breath sounds should be recorded.

4. When describing breath sounds, it is wise to take a musician's approach and to discern timing, pitch, and loudness.

Also, for purposes of convenience, we will divide each phase of respiration into three phases: early, middle, and late. Thus we will describe a total of six possible time windows: early, middle, and late inspiration, and early, middle, and late expiration.

The term *pitch* refers to the acoustic frequency of sounds that reach the ears. Like the pitch of a musical note, the lower the pitch the lower the frequency; the higher the frequency the higher the pitch. Normally, breath sounds heard over the chest have a low pitch due to the filtering of higher frequencies by lung and chest wall tissue.

Finally, the term *intensity* refers to the loudness, or amplitude of breath sounds and correlates with the speed of gas flow. The amount of energy (intensity) lost in transit depends on the distance between the source of sound and the chest wall and the path of transmission. For example, sounds produced in

the lobar and segmental bronchi dominate the breath sounds heard over the central regions of the chest. Breath sounds originating over the trachea are best heard over the sternum.

One final concept must be mastered if one is to thoroughly understand the genesis of normal breath sounds, and it is this: because the driving (intrapleural) pressures are not uniform throughout the chest, the intensity of breath sounds with respect to timing will be different in different parts of the lung. In the upright position, the airways at the apices will fill earlier than those at the base. Thus, apical breath sounds decrease in intensity as inspiration proceeds. Conversely, sounds heard over the bases will increase in intensity to a maximum of 50% of the vital capacity. Breath sounds at the periphery of the lung are of shorter duration during expiration because of the reverse in the direction of airflow and the drop in airflow rate and, therefore, sound intensity. With these thoughts in mind, a graphic description of normal breath sounds and bronchial breath sounds can be made (Table 1–6).

Normal Breath Sounds

The sounds heard over normal functioning lungs are called *vesicular breath sounds*. They have a relatively low frequency (less than 500 cycles per second) and generally are quiet. Unlike adventitious sounds, which may (and often do) change from minute to minute, breath to breath, and cough to cough, normal breath sounds are constant between contralateral lobes and from instant to instant. The inspiratory-expiratory ratio as heard through the stethoscope is approximately 5:2, in contrast to the inspiratory:expiratory ratio of chest wall motion, which is closer to unity (5:6). Inspiration is louder, longer, and higher pitched than expiration (see Table 1–6).

Laennec thought that vesicular breath sounds were produced by "friction of air against the lining of the airways." More recent studies of gas flow through the lungs have allowed us to make certain assumptions about how breath sounds are actually produced and where in the tracheobronchial tree they originate. It is believed, for example, that sound waves are produced in the lung either by rapid fluctuations in gas pressure in the airways or by oscillations of lung tissues themselves. Bulk airflow is slow and laminar in the terminal or small airways. In the alveoli, in fact, gas exchange is carried out by molecular diffusion, rather than by gas flow in the traditional sense. Breath sounds depend (like

TABLE 1–6.

Normal and Bronchial Breath Sounds*

TYPE	LOCATION WHERE TYPICALLY HEARD	PITCH	AMPLITUDE (LOUDNESS)	INSPIRATION-EXPIRATION RATIO	DESCRIPTION	GRAPHIC ILLUSTRATION
Vesicular	Over most of chest except major airways	Low	Moderate	3:1	"Breezy" (sound of wind in trees)	
Tracheal	Over trachea	Very high	Very great	5:6	Loud, harsh "tubular"	
Bronchial	Over major central airways	High	Great	2:3	Hollow tubular	
Bronchovesicular	Over major central airways	Medium	Moderately great	1:1	"Breezy," tubular, "tent-shaped"	

*From Burton GG, Hodgkin JE: *Respiratory Care: A Guide to Clinical Practice* ed 2. Philadelphia, JB Lippincott Co. 1984. Used with permission.

those from any wind musical instrument) on the effects of rapid movement of air across and through small orifices. Because there is little or no turbulent airflow in the terminal airways and the alveoli, these regions must be "silent" with respect to the generation of breath sounds. Thus, the old concept of alveolar, or vesicular, breath sounds needs to be revised. They are better called "normal breath sounds."

Vesicular breath sounds, which are normally heard over the greater part of the thorax, are modified where the trachea or bronchi lie close to the chest wall (as in the right upper lobe anteriorly). Vesicular sounds increase in intensity as tidal volume increases, and disappear when lung tissue ceases to be ventilated (as in atelectasis or pneumonia). They are diminished in emphysema and absent over a pneumothorax. They may be diminished or absent when pleural effusion or pleural thickening separates the lung from the chest piece of the stethoscope.

The term *bronchial breathing* correctly describes the source of sounds over the trachea and first few generations of bronchi. Within these large airways, break-up of gas flow occurs at the bifurcations, producing turbulence and breath sounds of equal intensity, during both inspiration and expiration.

Bronchial (or tubular) breath sounds are louder and higher pitched than vesicular breath sounds. Expiration is louder, longer, and of higher pitch than vesicular breath sounds. The inspiratory-expiratory ratio is closer to 1:1, and expiration may even be longer than inspiration, e.g., 5:6. In addition, there is a short but definite pause between the phases, at the instant of zero flow (end inspiration) (see Table 1–6). Bronchial breath sounds are normally heard only over the trachea and large bronchi; everywhere else they suggest the presence of pulmonary consolidation (e.g., lobar pneumonia, tuberculosis, or pulmonary infarction). In patients with a pleural effusion, bronchial breath sounds may be heard just above the effusion because of parenchymal compression. The term *bronchovesicular breathing* is used to describe breath sounds with hybrid characteristics, intermediate between *normal* and *bronchial breath sounds*. Such sounds are heard over areas of consolidation, where the lumen of the airway connecting the lesion with the larger airways is patent, as over a cavity.

In summary, one should expect to hear *bronchial breath sounds* in the parasternal and intrascapular areas. Expiration sounds persist longer than inspiration, and the sounds are more hollow or "tubular" than normal breath sounds. Bronchial and bronchovesicular breath sounds may also be heard over consolidated areas of lung in the periphery, as in pneumonia. Normal breath sounds may be described as ones in which inspiration is longer than expiration and in which the intensity-timing relationship depends on the sequence of gas filling—first at the apex, last at the bases.

Adventitious (or Added) Breath Sounds

These sounds, which always reflect underlying pulmonary abnormalities, are of two basic kinds: (1) *crackles*—discrete, noncontinuous sounds, and (2) *wheezes*—continuous musical sounds of greater duration. The terminology for lung sounds is changing, and the student may at first be confused with hold-overs from older nomenclature:

> Crackles
> > Rales (fine, medium, dry, coarse)
> > Rubs (friction, pleural, pericardial)
>
> Wheezes
> > Rhonchus (sonorous, low pitched)
> > Wheeze (high pitched, diminishing)

Crackles

While the modifying adjectives seen above may have meaning for the observer, it is better to communicate descriptions of these sounds in terms of pitch, loudness, and timing in relation to events in the respiratory cycle, location, and persistence (modification with deep breathing or coughing).

The sound of crackles can be mimicked by rolling a lock of hair between one's fingers, near to the external auditory canal. The timing of crackles can be related to the origin of the sounds: early inspiration (as in bronchitis or bronchiectasis); midinspiration (atelectasis); late inspiration (pneumonia, congestive heart failure, pulmonary fibrosis, and tuberculosis). Crackles which disappear with deep breathing or coughing, are sometimes referred to as atelectatic. Loud gurgling and bubbling sounds heard during both inspiration and expiration have been called the "death rattle." These sounds may be produced by secretions in the large airways, as in pulmonary edema or in terminally ill patients who cannot cough up their secretions.

Wheezes

These high-pitched sibilant, piping, or whistling sounds result from partial obstruction of airways. The walls of such airways are thought to oscillate between closed and open positions, thus generating the sounds. These musical sounds can be heard during either inspiration or expiration, although they are usually louder during expiration. Wheezes vary in pitch, but no clear inferences as to the site of airways obstruction can be made from pitch alone. Some wheezes have a tendency to become higher (and quieter) with the passage of the expiratory phase, which may reflect the effects of progressive dynamic compression of the airways as expiration proceeds.

Wheezes may be called monophonic or polyphonic, depending on the purity of musical tone produced, but these descriptions are not used much. The disappearance of a wheeze may be cause for rejoicing or consternation; the former as bronchial obstruction is relieved, the latter as it progresses to complete airway closure. Thus, it is not uncommon to hear physicians rejoice at the reappearance of wheezes in an asthmatic who previously was not doing well.

Wheezes are the hallmarks of airway obstruction and thus may be heard in any condition wherein airway caliber is compromised: foreign body aspiration, tumor obstruction, asthma, bronchitis, or any of the obstructive pulmonary diseases.

Rhonchi are lower pitched, sonorous sounds that usually suggest the presence of airway secretions in larger airways. As such, these sounds occur early in the respiratory cycle. Coughing may clear the obstructing mucus, blood, or aspirate, so the effect of this maneuver (and of tracheal suctioning) should be noted.

Pleural Friction Rubs

Normal pleural surfaces move noiselessly against each other during respiration. When these surfaces are inflamed, as in pleurisy, a characteristic grating, creaking sound may occur, which has been said to sound like that of old shoe leather. Friction rubs are sometimes heard over pneumonic infiltrates (with pleural extension), over pulmonary infarcts, and in pleurisy per se. They usually disappear when pleural effusion develops. The sounds of a characteristic pleural friction rub may be heard in both expiration and inspiration. They sound close to the ear (as, indeed, they are!); they are low pitched and usually limited to a discrete area of the chest wall.

CLINICAL ASSESSMENT OF THE CHEST PHYSICAL EXAMINATION

Physical signs of some selected respiratory diseases are described in Table 1–7. These findings must be assessed in light of the history obtained and whatever laboratory data are at hand. Such data will include the results of the clinical and bacteriologic evaluation, chest x-rays, and pulmonary function data (see Chapter 3).

Be as quantitative as possible. A good way to assess the patient's complaint of dyspnea is to walk

TABLE 1–7.

Physical Findings in Selected Pulmonary Diseases*

CONDITION	DESCRIPTION	PERCUSSION NOTE	TACTILE FREMITUS VOICE SOUNDS, WHISPERED VOICE SOUNDS	BREATH SOUNDS	ADDED SOUNDS
Normal *Pleura* *Alveoli* *Bronchus*	The tracheobronchial tree and alveoli are clear; the pleurae are thin and close together; the mobility of the chest wall is unimpaired	Resonant	Normal	Vesicular, except perhaps for bronchial breath sounds near the large bronchi	None, except perhaps for a few transient, inspiratory crackles at the bases after recumbency or sleep
Pulmonary consolidation (e.g., lobar pneumonia) *Deflated airway* *Alveoli filled with fluid, red and white cells*	A consolidated lung is dull to percussion but, as long as the large airways are clear, fremitus, breath, and voice sounds are transmitted as if they came directly from the larynx and trachea; abnormally deflated portions of the lungs produce crackles	Dull	Increased, with bronchophony, egophony, whispered pectoriloquy	Bronchial	Crackles
Bronchitis *Bronchial constriction* *Deflated airway*	In bronchitis, there may be partial bronchial obstruction from secretions or constrictions; abnormally deflated portions of lung may produce crackles	Resonant	Normal	Normal or prolonged expiration	Wheezes or crackles
Emphysema *Overinflated alveoli with destruction of walls*	A hyperinflated lung of emphysema is hyperresonant; the overfilled air spaces muffle the voice and breath sounds	Hyperresonant	Decreased	Decreased vesicular, often with prolonged expiration	None, or signs of bronchitis
Left-sided heart failure *Swollen mucosa (sometimes)* *Deflated airway*	In left-sided heart failure, some alveoli in the dependent portions of the lungs are deflated abnormally during expiration; the bronchial mucosa may be edematous	Resonant	Normal	Normal or sometimes prolonged expiration	Crackles at lung bases; sometimes wheezes

(Continued)

TABLE 1–7. *Continued*

CONDITION	DESCRIPTION	PERCUSSION NOTE	TACTILE FREMITUS VOICE SOUNDS, WHISPERED VOICE SOUNDS	BREATH SOUNDS	ADDED SOUNDS
Pleural fluid or thickening *Pleural fluid or thickening* 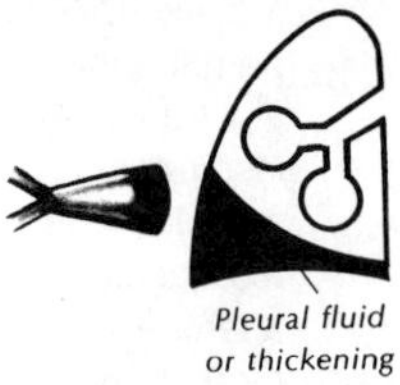	Pleural fluid or fibrotic thickening muffles all sounds	Dull to flat	Decreased to absent; however, when fluid compresses the underlying lung, bronchophony, egophony, and whispered pectoriloquy may appear	Decreased vesicular or absent; however, when fluid compresses the lung, a bronchial quality may appear	None unless there is underlying disease
Pneumothorax 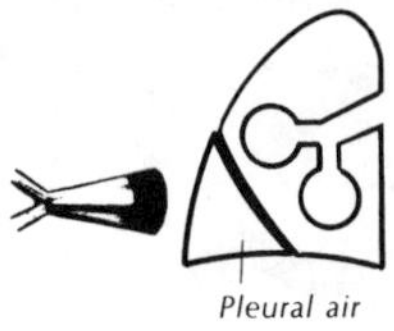 *Pleural air*	Free pleural air of pneumothorax may mimic obstructive lung disease but is usually unilateral and may shift trachea to opposite side; air-filled pleural space gives hyper-resonant percussion note but muffles voice and breath sounds	Hyperresonant	Decreased to absent	Decreased to absent	None
Atelectasis 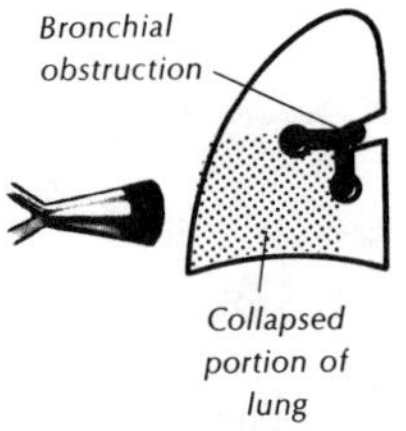 *Bronchial obstruction* *Collapsed portion of lung*	A collapsed or atelectic lung is dull to percussion; bronchial obstruction (shown here but not always present) prevents transmission of breath and voice sounds; the trachea may shift to the same side	Dull	Decreased to absent	Decreased vesicular or absent	None

*From Bates B: *A Guide to Physical Examination*, ed 3. Philadelphia, JB Lippincott Co, 1983. Used with permission.

down the hall or climb a flight of stairs with him. Further, a quick bedside estimate of airflow limitation can be made of assessing either the "match test" or the *forced vital capacity time*. In the former test, the patient is asked to blow out a lighted paper match 15 cm (6 in.) from his open mouth, not with pursed lips. If he cannot do this, significant airflow obstruction is present.

In the forced vital capacity time test, the patient is asked to exhale rapidly from a maximal lung inflation position, while the examiner listens to breath sounds with a stethoscope, over the back in the midscapular line. All sound should cease in less than 4 seconds.

RECORDING THE RESULTS OF THE EXAMINATION

Hospital convention will determine the nature of therapist's communication in the medical record. Both the narrative and graphic types of communication were earlier described.

Reports of *special studies* such as the recording of "ventilator checks," weaning parameters, or optimal PEEP studies are usually recorded on departmental forms designed for those purposes.

Whatever the setting, the record must constitute a clear resumé of the events that preceded the patient's admission to the hospital and of what occurred thereafter. The medical record is a legal document, discoverable as evidence and thus capable of subpoena as well. This in itself should cause the beginning therapist to be cautious and to err on the side of completeness, if at all.

As one begins, the sheer enormity of the data-gathering enterprise should not discourage the earnest student. Practice will make perfect, as suggested by the inspiration given to his students by Sir William Osler:

> Learn to see, learn to hear, learn to feel, learn to smell, and know that by practice alone can you become expert. Medicine is learned by the bedside and not in the classroom. Let not your conceptions of the manifestations of disease come from words heard in the lecture room or read from the book. See, and then reason and compare and control. But see first.
>
> Do not waste the hours of daylight in listening to that which you may read by night. But when you have seen. Read. And when you can, read the original descriptions of the masters who, with crude methods of study, saw so clearly.
>
> To study medicine without books is to sail an uncharted sea, while to study medicine only from books is not to go to sea at all.

REFERENCES

1. Bates B: *A Guide to Physical Examination*, ed 3. Philadelphia, JB Lippincott Co, 1983, pp 2–5.
2. Burton GG: Practical physical diagnosis in respiratory care, in Burton GG, Hodgkin JE: *Respiratory Care: A Guide to Clinical Practice*, ed 2. Philadelphia, JB Lippincott Co, 1984.
3. Goldberg P: *The Intuitive Edge Understanding Intuition and Applying It In Everyday Life*. Los Angeles, JP Tarcher Inc, 1983.
4. Loudon R, Murphy RLH: Cough. *Am Rev Respir Dis* 1984; 130:663.
5. Tobin MJ, Chadha TS, Jenouri G, et al: Breathing Patterns: I. Normal subjects. *Chest* 1983; 84:202.
6. Tobin MJ, Chadha TS, Jenouri G, et al: Breathing Patterns: II. Diseased subjects. *Chest* 1983; 84:286.
7. Weed LL: *Medical Records, Medical Education, and Patient Care*. Cleveland, Cleveland Press of Case Western Reserve University, 1969.

SUGGESTED READING

Burton GG.: Practical physical diagnosis in respiratory care, in Burton GG, Hodgkin JE (eds): *Respiratory Care: A Guide to Clinical Practice*, ed 2. Philadelphia, JB Lippincott Co, 1984.

Cousins N: *Anatomy of an Illness as Perceived by the Patient*. New York, WW Norton & Co, Inc, 1981.

Delp MH, Manning RT: *Major's Physical Diagnosis*, ed 9. Philadelphia, WB Saunders Co, 1981.

Goldberg P: *The Intuitive Edge*. Los Angeles, JP Tarcher, Inc, 1983.

Pulmonary Function Testing Procedures

Richard K. Beauchamp, R.C.P.T., R.P.F.T.

Respiratory therapy is generally directed toward restoring or altering the *function* of the pulmonary system. It is essential that respiratory therapy practitioners have a thorough understanding of the methods used to measure pulmonary function and its response to therapeutic intervention. This chapter describes the pulmonary function measures most commonly employed in respiratory therapy. Those measures are spirometry, peak flow, lung volumes, respiratory muscle force, expired gases, and blood gases. In each case, discussion will focus on the equipment, the procedure, and data reduction.

The discussion of equipment will survey the variety of devices available for each test, and describe the function, capabilities, and limitations of those devices. In addition, the necessary calibration and quality assurance techniques will be outlined.

Each test procedure will be delineated step by step, with special emphasis on those aspects that are critical for optimal results. In a few cases, we will also attempt to dispel some pervasive misconceptions about proper methodology.

The sections on data reduction will relate the processes by which the data derived during each test is translated into the appropriate numeric or graphic results.

SPIROMETRY MEASUREMENTS

The term *spirometry*, as used in the following discussion, denotes a constellation of measurements derived from three maneuvers known as the slow vital capacity (SVC), forced vital capacity (FVC), and maximal voluntary ventilation (MVV). As generally defined, SVC (or simply VC) is the maximum volume of air exhaled from the point of maximum inspiration, FVC is a vital capacity performed with a maximally forced expiratory effort, and MVV is the volume of air expired in a specific period during repetitive maximal respiratory effort.[22] The FVC may also be accompanied by a maximally forced inspiratory effort (FIVC), in which case the entire maneuver (when plotted appropriately) is termed a flow-volume loop. The measurements commonly derived from these maneuvers are shown in Table 2–1.

Equipment

A bewildering variety of devices is available for measurements of spirometry, which, despite a diversity of specific operating principles, can be divided into two broad categories: (1) volume devices and (2) flow devices.

Volume devices measure spirometric events by recording changes in the size of a chamber into which the subject breathes. These devices can be further categorized, on the basis of the type of chamber used, as (1) water seal spirometers, (2) dry, rolling seal spirometers, and (3) bellows spirometers.

The water seal spirometer (Fig 2–1,A) consists of a cylindrical chamber, or "bell," suspended in a water-filled sleeve. As a subject breathes, the cylinder is displaced in the water, which both serves to seal the cylinder against loss of gas, and to provide a medium through which the cylinder can move easily. The dry, rolling seal spirometer (Fig 2–1,B) also consists of a cylindrical chamber but, rather than the entire cylinder moving, the walls of the cylinder are stationary while a plate which forms one end of the

TABLE 2–1.

Measurements Commonly Derived From Spirometric Maneuvers

ACRONYM	DEFINITION*	UNITS	EXAMPLE(S)
	Slow Vital Capacity		
VC	Vital capacity; the maximum volume of air exhaled from the point of maximum inspiration (the sum of ERV and IC)	L or ml	
ERV	Expiratory reserve volume; the maximal volume of air exhaled from the end-expiratory level	L or ml	
IC	Inspiratory capacity; the maximum volume of air inhaled from the end-expiratory level	L or ml	
	Forced Vital Capacity		
FVC	Forced vital capacity; vital capacity performed with a maximally forced expiratory effort	L or ml	
FEV_t	Forced expiratory volume (timed); the volume of air exhaled in the specified time (in seconds) during the performance of the FVC	L or ml	$FEV_{0.5}$ FEV_1 FEV_3
$FEV_t/FVC\%$	Forced expiratory volume (timed) to forced vital capacity ratio, expressed as a percent	%	FEV_1/FVC FEV_3/FVC
FEF_x	Forced expiratory flow at a point in the FVC ("instantaneous flow"); modifiers refer to the percent of the FVC already exhaled when the measurement is made	L/sec	$FEF_{25\%}$ $FEF_{50\%}$ $FEF_{75\%}$
FEF_{x-y}	Forced expiratory flow between two points in the FVC ("averaged flow"); modifiers may refer to either percents of the FVC (as in $FEF_{25\%-75\%}$ or to absolute volume (e.g., ml, as in $FEF_{200-1200}$)	L/sec	$FEF_{25\%-75\%}$ $FEF_{200-1200}$
FEF_{max}	The maximal forced expiratory flow achieved during an FVC (also often termed PEFR, for peak expiratory flow rate).	L/sec or L/min	
MTT	Mean transit time	sec	
	Flow-Volume Loop		
FIVC	Forced inspiratory vital capacity. The maximal volume of air inspired with a maximally forced effort from a position of maximal expiration	L or ml	
FIV_t, FIF	All of the measurements listed for the expiratory FVC can be measured for the inspiratory effort as well; I is substituted for E in the acronyms	Same as expiratory	$FIF_{50\%}$ $FIF_{25\%-75\%}$ FIF_{max}
E/I Ratios	Ratio of expiratory value for a given measure to the corresponding inspiratory measure; most commonly flows		$FEF_{50\%}/FIF_{50\%}$ FEF_{max}/FIF_{max} *(Continued)*

TABLE 2–1.   *Continued*

ACRONYM	DEFINITION*	UNITS	EXAMPLE(S)
	Maximum Voluntary Ventilation		
MVV_x	Maximum voluntary ventilation; the volume of air expired in a specified period during repetitive maximal respiratory effort; the respiratory frequency is indicated by a numerical qualifier; if no qualifier is given, an unrestricted frequency is assumed	L/min	MVV MVV_{100}

*The definitions in this table are taken, in large part, from the following source, although a number of additions and alterations are made herein. Modified from Joint Committee on Pulmonary Nomenclature: Pulmonary Terms and Symbols—Report of the ACCP-ATS. *Chest* 1975; 67:583–592.

cylinder moves. The cylinder is sealed by a collar of Silastic or similar material attached at one edge to the moving plate and at the other to the cylinder wall. As a subject breathes, the movable plate is displaced along the "rolling seal" of the Silastic collar. The bellows spirometer (Fig 2–1,C) consists of two plates, one stationary and one movable, connected by a pliable material. Most commonly, this connection is achieved by an accordion-folded vinyl plastic bellows (hence the name). As the subject breathes, the movable plate is displaced. In one type of bellows spirometer, the "wedge" spirometer, the two plates are hinged on one side, such that the movable plate is displaced vectorially. In all these types of spirometers, volume is measured directly as the displacement of the movable component. In many cases, volume devices also provide a flow output derived by differentiation of the volume signal.

Flow devices, or pneumotachographs (on the other hand), measure volume indirectly as the integral of flow. There are at least four types of pneumotachographs, which differ in the principle utilized for measuring flow. The four types are: (1) differential pressure, (2) "hot wire" (anemometer), (3) ultrasonic, and (4) turbine. In its simplest model (Fig 2–2), a differential pressure pneumotachograph measures flow based on the relationship:

$$\dot{V} = dP/R$$

where $\dot{V}$ is flow, dP is a pressure drop across a resistive element, and R is the resistance of that element. If R is fixed and known, $\dot{V}$ can be derived by measuring dP with a differential pressure transducer. While this simple model is useful for understanding the principle of differential pressure pneumotachography, the model on which an actual device of that type is constructed is considerably more complex. A discussion of the complexities of differential pressure pneumotachograph function is outside both the scope of this chapter and probably the interest of the beginning practitioner. For the reader who is interested, there are a number of published reviews of the subject, such as the recent one by Dawson.[8]

The second type of flow device, the hot wire anemometer, is predicted on the assumption that flow can be measured by the rate at which a heated element, usually a very thin platinum wire, is cooled by the stream of gas. Flow is proportional to the current required to sustain the temperature of the element.

In ultrasonic pneumotachographs (Fig 2–3), gas is passed across struts to create turbulent waves, or vortices, which then pass through the path of high-frequency sound waves sent between two crystals opposite each other in the flow tube, thereby creating pulses. Flow is proportional to the number of pulses.

In turbine devices (Fig 2–4), gas flow causes a vane or louvered wheel to turn, and flow is proportional to the velocity of the vane or wheel. (Strictly speaking, a turbine device measures quanta of volume, but turbines are commonly grouped with flow devices.) Thus, whereas flow devices are similar in that they measure flow as the primary signal (which is then integrated to derive volume), they vary widely in the method of measuring flow.

Capabilities and Limitations

Whatever the type of device, and whatever the functional construct employed, any clinical spirometry instrument should meet certain performance standards for the characteristics of accuracy, precision, range, linearity, frequency response, and resis-

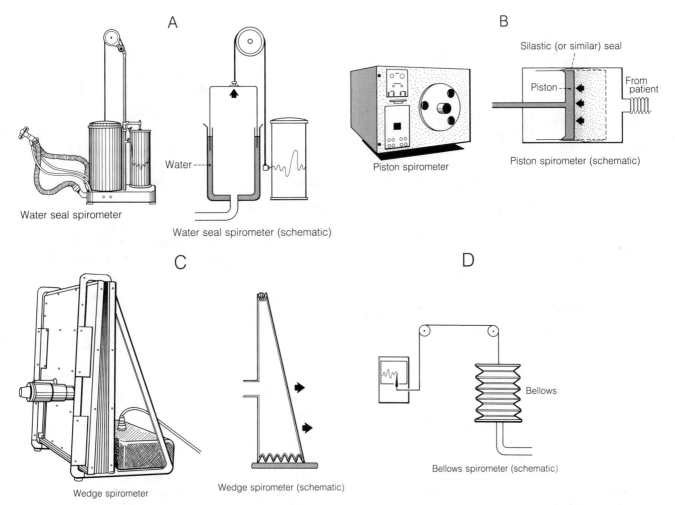

A

Water seal spirometer

Water ---

Water seal spirometer (schematic)

B

Silastic (or similar) seal

Piston

From patient

Piston spirometer

Piston spirometer (schematic)

C

Wedge spirometer

Wedge spirometer (schematic)

D

Bellows

Bellows spirometer (schematic)

FIG 2–1.
Volume displacement spirometers. In each case, the arrow shows the direction of movement. **A,** water seal spirometer. The device diagramed here is the prototypic design of water seal spirometers; more recent designs have eliminated the counterweighted pulley necessitated by the relatively heavy bell, substituting a very lightweight plastic bell which moves on guide rods. **B,** dry, rolling seal. Two types of bellows spirometer: wedge **(C)** and regular **(D).** In most devices of all three types, a recording pen, which then traces on a moving paper record, may be attached directly to the moving component ("direct writing"), as shown here for the water seal spirometer. Alternatively, the devices may use a potentiometer or transducer to translate the movement of the displaceable component into an electrical signal, which can be displayed on a variety of recorders and/or video devices.

tance. Familiarity with these standards is helpful in discussing the capabilities and limitations of particular spirometry devices.

A framework for such standards is provided in the 1979 statement on standardization of spirometry by the American Thoracic Society (ATS).[11] That statement recommends minimal performance standards for the most common spirometric tests; the standards that should be met by any particular device depend on the test(s) for which it is to be used.

For measuring VC, an instrument should:

• Accumulate volume for at least 30 seconds.

• Be capable of measuring volumes of at least 7 L.
• Measure volume independent of flows (be linear) for flows between 0 and 12 L/sec.
• Have an accuracy of at least ±3% of reading or 50 ml, whichever is greater.

Measurement of FVC requires the same features with one exception and one addition:
• The instrument need accumulate volume for only 10 seconds
• "End of test" will occur when the average flow over a 0.5-second interval is less than 50 ml/sec,

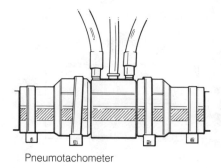

Pneumotachometer

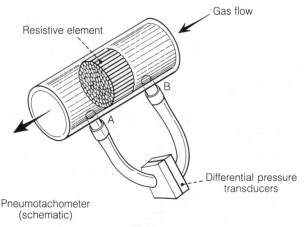

Pneumotachometer
(schematic)

FIG 2–2.
Model of a differential pressure pneumotachograph. Flow is measured as the pressure drop between *A* and *B*, which are ports leading to a differential pressure transducer. The resistive element may consist of a mesh screen or screens, a network of parallel capillary tubes, or other device.

or when the volume change in a 0.5-second interval is less than 25 ml (this requirement, and the one for "start of test" below, presumably apply to devices providing automated data reduction).

Standards for measurement of timed forced expiratory volume(s) (FEV_t) are the same as for FVC, with the additional requirements that:

- Resistance to air flow at 12.0 L/sec should be less than 1.5 cm H_2O/L/sec
- The "start of test" for purposes of timing will be determined by the back extrapolation method (see "Data Reduction" section below) or a method shown to be equivalent.

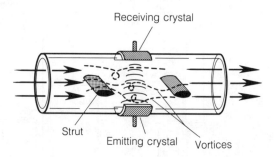

FIG 2–3.
Model of an ultrasonic pneumotachograph. Flow is measured as the number of pulses created by vortical flow between the emitting and receiving crystals.

If flows are to be determined, the device should fulfill the above criteria and provide accuracy of:

- ±5% of reading or 0.1 L/sec, whichever is greater, for $FEF_{25\%-75\%}$.
- ±5% of reading or 0.2 L/sec, whichever is greater, for "instantaneous" flow (e.g., $FEF_{50\%}$).

When a spirometry device is used to determine MVV, it should:

- Have a response that is flat within ±10% up to 4 Hz at flows of up to 12 L/sec over the volume range
- Measure for 12 to 15 seconds
- Have a time-base accuracy of ±3%
- Have an overall accuracy of ±5% of reading at signals of up to 250 L/min produced with stroke volumes of up to 2 L
- Produce less than ±10 cm H_2O pressure at the mouthpiece at stroke volume of 2 L at 2 Hz

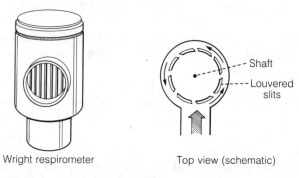

Wright respirometer   Top view (schematic)

FIG 2–4.
Model of a turbine device. The turbine itself may be a louvered wheel, vane(s), or propeller attached to a shaft. The turbine rotates in proportion to the volume of air moving across it. (The louvered wheel in this example is shown in three-quarters view.)

The ATS standards also require that devices measuring FVC and FEV$_t$ provide a tracing, in either a volume-vs.-time or flow-vs.-volume format, for the entire forced expiration. In the volume-vs.-time format, the recorder should:

- Display the entire FVC maneuver at a constant speed.
- Be up to speed before expiration is begun.
- Record for at least 10 seconds after the start of the maneuver.

The standards stipulate the tracing must be stored and available for recall, implying display on a cathode-ray tube (CRT) or other screen is acceptable, provided there is magnetic storage with the capability to retrieve the display. Tracings recorded on paper should provide:

- Time axis speeds of at least 2 cm/sec, with higher speeds preferred
- Volume axis deflections of at least 10 mm/L of volume
- Flow axis deflections of at least 4 mm/L/sec of flow.

According to the standards, a graphic recording is not required but is highly recommended for "screening" spirometry, unless abnormal, or for follow-up studies in subjects who have had baseline study with tracing.

The foregoing standards are provided in detail because they have gained wide acceptance, and should be familiar to anyone evaluating spirometers or performing spirometry. However, as stressed in the ATS statement itself, these instrument specifications are intended as *minimum* recommendations, a fact seemingly forgotten by many practitioners and equipment manufacturers. Therefore, as noted earlier, while the ATS standards provide a framework for the performance specifications required by spirometry devices, a number of exceptions or additions are invited.

There are at least five exceptions to be considered. *First,* as recognized by the task force that formulated the ATS standards, a volume capacity of 7 L may be inadequate if inspiration preceding expiration is measured (see "Procedure" section). *Second,* the 0 to 12 L/sec flow range may be inadequate, particularly for testing populations with a significant number of younger, taller subjects whose maximal flows often exceed 12 L/sec. In fact, even the two studies cited by either the ATS task force or a subsequent Epidemiology Standardization Project to justify the 12 L/sec recommendation demonstrated peak flows over 11.75 L/sec in 8.4% of coal miners tested, and over 12 L/sec in 7.1% in a group of asbestos workers, two groups likely to contain significant numbers of subjects with *reduced* peak flow.[10] The *third* and by far most serious exception is to the minimal volume accumulation time of 10 seconds. The Epidemiology Standardization Project demonstrated in its own study that 18% of subjects with chronic obstructive lung disease did not complete a forced expiratory maneuver within 10 seconds. Our experience suggests the percentage is significantly greater. *Fourth,* the specified criteria for "end of test" may cause marked underestimation of FVC in many subjects with obstruction who may continue to exhale for many seconds, accumulating significant volume, at flows below 50 ml/sec. *Fifth,* the suggestion that a graphic recording, or spirograph, may not be necessary in some contexts seems indefensible. Whatever the application, spirometry can never be properly assessed without a graphic display of the maneuver. On the basis of these factors, we suggest clinical spirometry be performed with a device that has a volume capacity of 9 L or more, a flow ceiling of 16 L/sec or more, no time limit, no automatic flow threshold below which the test is terminated, and that provides a graphic record. Many of the available spirometry devices possess these characteristics.

There are at least two other factors in addition to those in the ATS statement that should be considered. The first has to do with the characteristic of precision, which, as applied to analytic devices, describes the reproducibility of repeated measurements of a given input. For example, if two spirometers both meet accuracy requirements by always measuring a 5-L input to within ±3% but device A does so with values ranging from 4.85 to 5.15 while device B only varies from 4.99 to 5.01, device B has more precision. While not addressed in the ATS standards, precision represents an additional desirable feature in spirometry devices.

The second performance standard to consider is actually a set of recommendations concerning automated devices. In the years since the ATS statement was issued, more and more spirometers have been interfaced to computers and microprocessors to provide automatic data reduction. As we will discuss again in the section on calibration and quality assurance of spirometry devices, the performance characteristics discussed to this point apply to a spirometry system as a whole, including recorders and computers, as well as the measuring device. It is probably worthwhile to discuss those computer characteristics that affect the performance of spirometry systems, specifically the resolution and sampling rate of the analog-to-digital converter (ADC). The resolution of an ADC, which is the range of the input signal divided by the size of the ADC, determines how small a volume or flow the system can detect. The Epidemiology Standardization Project recommends a minimal resolution of 0.02 L.[10] The accuracy of computerized data reduction is also influenced by the frequency at which the ADC "samples" the input signal (sampling rate). If the ADC receives only a few data points during a rapidly changing event, accuracy may be compromised. On the other hand, the higher the sampling rate, the greater the amount of computer memory required. One way to balance the need for accuracy with the constraints of computer memory size is to sample at a high frequency during the initial portion of an FVC maneuver while the flow profile is changing precipitously, and then to decrease the sampling rate. The Epidemiology Standardization Project recommends a minimal sampling rate of 60 Hz for peak flow and 15 Hz for all other measures.[10]

With all of the above standards in mind, we can turn to an examination of the capabilities and limitations of particular types of spirometry devices. The first step in such an examination is determination of the degree to which a particular device meets the aforementioned performance standards. A 1980 study, which evaluated a number of spirometry devices, provides valuable information.[12] While the number of manufacturers of spirometry equipment has increased dramatically since that study, all of the newer devices are similar enough to the devices tested that the categorical findings are still applicable.

In general, volume devices (water seal, dry rolling seal, and bellows spirometers) are more accurate, precise and linear than are flow devices. They are probably preferable when one's primary concern is to measure volume very accurately or to measure small volumes. In terms of the other performance specifications, volume devices vary considerably according to type and even manufacturer. For example, of the equipment tested in the 1980 study, one wedge spirometer had the lowest resistance of all volume devices, while another wedge device had the highest resistance of all volume devices.[12] Therefore, the practitioner should refer to the published manufacturer's specifications for a given device to determine its effective range, resistance, frequency response, etc.

There are several additional considerations be-

yond the scope of the outlined performance specifications that represent limitations or disadvantages, albeit generally minor ones, to volume devices. First, the fact that mechanical movement of all or part of the volume chamber is required means volume devices have some degree of inertia, which may result in a slow response to the initial portion of a forced maneuver. This problem is minor, and probably has no significant effect on clinical measurements in water seal spirometers with plastic bells, dry rolling seal spirometers, and vertically suspended wedge spirometers. However, the effect of inertia is of sufficient magnitude in some water seal spirometers with metal bells and some horizontally mounted wedge or bellows spirometers to cause clinically significant errors in FEV_1, flows, and/or MVV. Second, because they are closed systems with a finite and rather limited capacity, volume devices are generally not suitable for continuous monitoring. Third, as will be discussed again in the "Data Reduction" section below, when gas is expired into a volume device, it is assumed the gas cools from body temperature to room (ambient) temperature, with a consequential loss of humidity. A mathematical or electronic correction is generally applied, it is believed, to restore the volume to the value it occupied in the subject's lungs. This assumption may not be valid since gas may not cool completely to ambient temperature at all points during expiration. At least one group has questioned the practice,[19] although others have shown the effect to be of no practical concern, with the maximal error introduced being approximately 2% in FEV_1.[12] An elaborate formula has been proposed to improve the correction.[13]

Flow devices, as already mentioned, are, as a group, less accurate, precise, and linear than are volume devices. The magnitude of these deficits, however, is markedly different between types of devices, and, again, among similar devices made by different manufacturers. Some of the newest differential pressure pneumotachographs, with linearization attempted mathematically via computer, substantially decrease the inaccuracy and flow dependency that have characterized these devices in the past, while many of the hot wire anemometers and ultrasonic and turbine devices on the market remain grossly inaccurate. The inaccuracy of these devices is due primarily to alinearity in the generated flow signals at very high and very low flows.

In addition to this fundamental limitation of many flow devices (that they are simply inaccurate), there are a number of other limitations as well. Some of these considerations are not particularly germane to spirometric measurements, but are included here because the same devices are often used in other applications. First, both differential pressure pneumotachographs and hot wire devices are affected by the physical properties of the gas measured. In differential pressure pneumotachographs, the pressure drop across the resistive element, and hence, the measured flow, is affected by gas viscosity (a more complete version of the equation given earlier is $\dot{V} = d\mathrm{P}/(81\mathrm{n/r}^4)$, with 1 being the length of the tube through which the gas is flowing, n being viscosity, and r being the radius of the tube). In hot wire devices, the rate at which the element is cooled is affected by the density of the cooling gas. As a result, differential pressure pneumotachographs and hot wire devices are generally unsuitable for applications involving a significant component of a gas with high or low viscosity or density relative to room air (such as helium). A second limitation is that, although flow devices overall have better frequency response than do volume devices, differential pressure pneumotachographs have some peculiar frequency response problems relative to large pressure changes. This characteristic may cause problems if the device is to be used for monitoring in a positive pressure ventilator circuit.[8] Third, while measurements derived from ultrasonic devices are largely unaffected by gas composition, temperature, or humidity, their accuracy can be affected by excess moisture on the struts or ultrasonic crystals,[35] so that these devices should probably not be used for continuous monitoring in high humidity circuits.

Provided the accuracy of a particular device has been demonstrated as outlined in the "Calibration and Quality Assurance" section that follows, flow devices may offer some advantages for particular applications. First, flow devices have several practical advantages in that they tend to be smaller, more portable, and easier to disinfect or sterilize than volume devices. Second, as a rule, flow devices have better frequency response than volume devices, resulting in a better ability to measure rapidly changing flows. Third, as they have no inherent volume limit, they are, with the provisos discussed above, generally well-suited for continuous monitoring or measurement of large volume events (e.g., exercise testing).

As we have already mentioned, spirometry devices often include or are interfaced with recorders and/or computers. The characteristics of these devices also affect the overall performance of the system. A full discussion of the capabilities and limitations of recorders will not be attempted (the interested reader is referred to a recent review by Snow[39]), but two observations will be made. First, while a recorder cannot improve the inherent performance characteristics of a spirometry device, a poor recorder can decrease the overall performance of a system. Thus, it is important that the precision, linearity, frequency response, etc., of the recorder be at least as good as those of the measuring device.

One often cited example in which the performance of a spirometer may be compromised by a recorder's performance characteristics is the use of X-Y recorders to trace FVC maneuvers in the flow-vs-volume format. Such a recorder has physical limits to its ability to track high acceleration, particularly if set for large deflections. This limitation of "slewing speed" can result in blunting and, therefore, underestimation of peak flows.

A second observation concerning recorders is a personal recommendation. In our experience, the single most useful recorder for spirometry is a two-channel strip recorder with volume displayed on one channel and flow on the other, yielding both volume and flow vs time (see "Data Reduction" section for an example of such a tracing). Although rarely found in commercial systems, this recording format provides all the information contained in both the volume-time and flow-volume format.

Computers, like recorders, should enhance rather than degrade the overall performance of a spirometry system. There are, however, a number of software limitations in many commercial spirometry systems that should be considered in addition to the hardware specifications of the ADC discussed earlier. The most significant of these limitations are problems of determination, including determination of end-expiratory level during SVC maneuvers, and "start of test," "end of test," and flow aberrations during FVC maneuvers. It is imperative that anyone performing spirometry with an automated system understand these sources of potential error, and always evaluate physical recordings and computer output for evidence of their having occurred. When one of these misdeterminations does occur, the operator must be prepared to recalculate the results manually.

The most common approach to computer determination of an end-expiratory level, by which to separate an SVC into IC and ERV, is to average the lung volume at end-expiration of some number of breaths preceding the VC maneuver. While this approach is probably acceptable for a constant end-expiratory level, or even one that has slight random variation around a given point, it does not work for a steadily increasing level, as is frequently seen in volume devices, due (presumably) to a low respiratory exchange ratio. Criteria for "start of test" and "end of test" of FVC maneuvers are found in the ATS standards delineated earlier. Automated systems often employ these criteria. The application of "back extrapolation" to determine the point (t_o) from which time measurements are made is easily performed by the human eye and, in most cases, by computer algorithm. Some microprocessors, however, are unable to correctly extrapolate (t_o) in some subjects with unusual expiratory flow patterns. In such cases, FEV_t and associated measurements may be significantly miscalculated. The "end of test" criteria are, as we have seen, probably flawed even when applied correctly because they are inappropriate in subjects with significant obstruction. Additional problems often arise when the criteria are incorporated into computerized systems, due to the difficulty in distinguishing true flow decay from momentary hesitations, flow transients such as coughing, spirometer resonance, or a host of other occurrences that are not actually signals of the end of an FVC maneuver, but that are sensed as such by the computer. A false termination of this sort would obviously result in an underestimation of FVC and, for reasons discussed later, an overestimation of volume-dependent flows. The solution to this last problem is simply to program the computer to continue accumulating volume until the operator signals the test should be terminated. Fortunately, manufacturers are increasingly adapting this approach.

The last problem of determination we will mention has to do with determination of flows during flow aberrations. When measuring an instantaneous flow, a computer simply determines the flow signal at the designated point (e.g., 50% of VC). If that point falls during a cough or other flow transient, the measured flow may be misleading. Although the ideal FVC would not contain such events, many subjects cannot, for pathophysiological reasons, perform a forced expiration without terminal coughing, "saw-toothing," etc. Such events do not necessarily invalidate a maneuver, but do require that the affected flow(s) be recalculated.

Any discussion of the capabilities and limitations of spirometry devices, particularly one aimed at beginning practitioners, should end with a warning. There are many commercially available (and, alas, widely used) instruments that are demonstrably inaccurate. While their use is problem enough, what is more disturbing is the attitude on the part of many that such devices (which are often much less expensive than good devices) are "good enough" for a particular application. A recent review[40] addressed this attitude in a statement worth repeating here:

> Some spirometry devices are patently crude. There is absolutely no justification for using such an instrument on the grounds that it is "good enough for screening" or it is "good enough for an office instrument." No pulmonary function testing equipment is good enough. Testing is fraught with enough uncertainties. Adding to them with the use of poor equipment is unconscionable.

Calibration and Quality Assurance

All devices used for spirometry measurements must be evaluated periodically for adherence to the performance characteristics described below. Before using a particular device for the first time, whether the equipment is newly purchased or already in use in a setting to which the practitioner is new, one should ensure the device has been shown to fulfill all the requirements. Ideally, the user himself should measure the performance characteristics in all the categories, but determination of frequency response and resistance is beyond the resources of many institutions. For these characteristics, one should at least review the manufacturer's *published* performance specifications. There is, however, sometimes a significant disparity between the performance of a device on a workbench in the hands of the engineer who designed it and its performance in a "real life" clinical setting. Accordingly, users without the resources to test such features themselves should also contact other users of the device (names are usually available from the manufacturer) for their experiences with it.

Once the inherent characteristics of a device are determined, the user must be capable of periodically calibrating and/or checking its accuracy, linearity, and precision. Whereas one can allow that determination of frequency response and resistance are legitimately outside the purview of some users, any user without the relatively simple and inexpensive equipment to perform regular minimal quality assurance procedures for accuracy, linearity, and precision simply should not perform spirometric testing.

Before outlining the specific approaches to quality assurance in spirometry devices, a few general principles should be noted. First, the signals for volume and flow should be a physical input, not electronic simulations. Such electronic signals, provided by many systems, are useful in making quick checks for drift between subjects or in providing calibration marks on tracings, but do not suffice as true calibration or quality control signals. Furthermore, one should never rely on an internal or self-calibration routine: *at some point the device output must be compared to an external, physical volume, or flow input.* Second, the system must be calibrated as a whole; the known input must be retrieved as the output of whatever device is used to derive values during testing, whether a digital display on the spirometer itself, a recorder, or a computer. Third, the system should be calibrated with all filters, hoses, adapters, etc., which will be in place during actual testing. With these principles in mind, we can discuss a few specific approaches to quality assurance.

The simplest and perhaps most commonly recommended approach to calibration and quality assurance is use of a large, calibrated syringe to check volume and a stopwatch to check time, the two primary determinants of spirometric indices. The syringe should have a capacity of 3 L or more, since lesser volumes would tend to mask small errors. The procedure is as follows:

1. If the device has an electronic temperature correction (or "BTPS") feature, turn control to 37°C (or 0 correction). (The significance of this correction is discussed in "Data Reduction".) Likewise, if the system is computerized, enter 37°C to prevent mathematical "correction." If the device is a differential pressure pneumotachograph with heated element, turn off the heater.

2. Connect the calibrated syringe to the system *exactly* as a human subject would be connected, with all filters, hoses, adaptors, etc., which will be in place during actual testing.

3. Inject the known volume at slow, moderate, and fast rates, taking approximately 0.5, 3, and 10 seconds to empty a 3-L syringe, and obtain a tracing or reading for each injection.[10] This procedure assesses both accuracy and linearity. The use of a range of flows is believed by many to be necessary only in systems employing flow devices, but we recommend it for all systems. Although volume devices are generally linear, the entire system in which one is used may not be linear due to a recorder, microprocessor, or component of the tubing system that responds differently at low and high flows.

4. If inspiratory values are to be measured, the known volume should also be drawn back through the system in a similar fashion.

5. All injections should, as previously discussed, yield readings that are within 3% or 50 cc (whichever is greater) of the known volume input.

For a 3-L syringe, therefore, all readings should fall between 2.91 and 3.09 L. If all readings are systematically higher, the appropriate attenuation or gain control should be adjusted and the procedure repeated. If systematically lower readings are produced, one should first check the system for leaks. If none are found, adjust the appropriate attenuation or gain control and repeat the procedure. If some readings are too low and others too high, repeat the procedure. If the same pattern of error persists, the device is alinear and should not be used until the error can be rectified.

6. Check the time base (generally the X axis) of the recorder by determining how far the pen or paper moves in a 10-second interval, timed with a high-quality stopwatch. While no specific guidelines for accuracy of recorder speed are generally accepted, it seems reasonable to apply a limit of ±3% of predicted movement. If in error, most recorders would require internal adjustment by the manufacturer or a biomedical engineer.

7. Once the volume and time signals have been carefully checked, the output of computerized systems can be evaluated by comparing the values generated by the computer to ones calculated manually from the tracings. Small discrepancies will almost always be present due to the ability of the computer to discriminate more exactly than the human eye, but significant discrepancies should lead one to suspect an error in the computer software.

The above procedure may be used both for calibration and (excepting the adjustments in step 5) for quality control in many systems. Some systems, however, may have a calibration routine peculiar to that system, and, in such cases, the procedure outlined should be used only for quality assurance after the manufacturer's calibration protocol has been performed. In either case, when used for quality assurance in a computerized system with separate calibration and testing modes, the above procedure should be done in the test mode to simulate how the system handles signals during actual testing.

A number of other approaches to calibration and quality assurance have been suggested by various groups, and are sometimes employed. One variation of the above procedure is to use a device that delivers a known volume of heated (37°C), humidified air, in which case step 1 is omitted. A second alternative is use of devices which, by means of explosive decompression through pinhole resistors, provide not only a known volume but also known signals for FEV_t, $FEF_{25\%-75\%}$, and even some instantaneous flows. A third and rather peculiar suggestion by at least one group is to initially confirm the accuracy of equipment by performing tests in 10 to 20 healthy individuals, checking that the measured values fall within the predicted ranges, and repeating the testing "in the same healthy individuals every morning before diagnostic studies are performed."[3] Considering that the intrasubject coefficient of variation for some spirometric variables is 6% or more, this last suggestion is strongly discouraged.

The discussion to this point has centered on calibration of volume and time. Brief mention should be made of flow signal calibration and quality assurance. Paradoxically, additional assessment of flow accuracy is less important in flow devices than in volume devices because an accurate integrated volume response at different flows, as described above, documents accurate primary flow measurements. Calibration or quality testing of flow as differentiated by volume devices can be performed using a variety of devices, including calibrated mechanical flow generators and rotameters. Such determinations are complicated by the fact that, particularly at high flows, a 7- or even 10-L capacity provides very little accumulation time during which to make adjustments.

The final point concerning calibration and quality assurance is the frequency with which such procedures should be performed. As regards volume calibration, the minimal frequency required is somewhat dictated by the type of device. Volume devices with recording pens attached directly to the moving component are the least likely to change calibration, but even in these devices, the development of leaks, damage through mishandling, or other untoward events may alter their performance. Devices of this type should be calibrated or checked at least weekly[3, 10] but preferably daily. Flow devices and volume devices with electrical connections to recorders or computers should be calibrated at least daily, and in some settings as often as every 2 to 4 hours, or even before each test.[10] In our experience, hot wire devices are the least stable and, if used at all, represent one case in which the device should be calibrated with a volume signal before every test. In addition to volume calibration on the foregoing schedule, time and flow calibration should be performed at least quarterly.[3]

Procedure

Spirometry has long suffered from the misperception it is a simple test; in fact, the term *simple spirom-etry* is often used to distinguish forced expiratory maneuvers from more thorough pulmonary function profiles. There is, however, nothing simple about spirometry. From the physiology of forced expiration to the correct interpretation of spirometric indices, spirometry, in all its aspects, is a complex undertaking. In no aspect is the complexity of spirometry more manifest than in the proper methodology for its performance. The pervasive belief that spirometry is simple to perform is one of several lines of evidence to the fact that it is, as often as not, poorly done. The detail of the following discussion is offered in the hope it will inculcate in the beginning respiratory therapy practitioner an appreciation of the subtleties of spirometry which is necessary if the test is to yield all the information it contains about the status of the respiratory system.

We will first discuss several procedural steps that are common to the SVC, FVC, and MVV, and then outline the procedure for each maneuver. For any or all of the maneuvers, the following preliminary steps should be taken.

1. Have the subject loosen any tight clothing that might constrict the neck, chest, or upper abdomen. Such articles would include neckties, collars, brassieres, and girdles.

2. Explain the procedure thoroughly to the subject. The subject will be less apprehensive if he knows exactly what to expect, and less time and effort will be wasted on unacceptable maneuvers. Following each attempt, tell the subject *specifically* what should be done to correct any deficiencies on subsequent attempts.

3. Position the subject properly. Conventional wisdom, as well as the ATS statement and Epidemiology Standardization Project, holds that adults may be tested either sitting or standing, while children generally generate better values when tested standing. A 1976 study[33] showed adults actually have slightly higher values sitting, while a 1984 study,[42] suggesting a sequencing bias in the earlier study, demonstrated higher standing values. Seated testing offers the minor advantage that the subject will not fall if he experiences dizziness or syncope (fainting) during the test. If testing is performed with the subject seated, he should be instructed to sit as erect as possible, with both feet on the floor (not with legs crossed). If tested standing, the subject should stand as erect as possible, and a chair into which he can be quickly lowered if he does become light-headed should be placed immediately behind him. In performing bedside testing of a subject who can neither sit on the edge of the bed nor

stand, the head of the bed should be raised and the subject positioned so he is sitting up as straight as possible. Occasionally, spirometry may be performed with the subject in some other particular position, such as lying supine, prone, on one side, or even upside down in a circle-electric bed, either because the subject is fixed in that position by traction or the like, or to investigate positional abnormalities such as those occurring with diaphragm dysfunction. In such cases, the position should be clearly noted on any report of, or other reference to, the resulting values. Whatever the subject's body position, his chin should be slightly elevated and his neck extended. Many subjects tend to move their chins down toward the chest during testing, which may affect performance.

4. If the subject wears loose-fitting dentures, they should be removed to prevent leaks or occlusion to flow should they slip. If the dentures fit securely, the subject will probably do better with them in place.

5. Have the subject insert the mouthpiece correctly. The most common type of mouthpiece used for spirometry is a disposable cardboard cylinder. This type of mouthpiece should be placed *between* the teeth (or gums) with the lips closed tightly around it. For subjects who are unable to maintain a good seal around such a cylinder, flanged rubber or plastic mouthpieces are available (and widely used for other tests such as diffusion and plethysmography) which can be used to help eliminate leaks. These mouthpieces are positioned so that the flanges are inside the mouth between the lips and teeth (gums). Proper placement of the mouthpiece is very important.

6. Apply a nose clip. There is considerable controversy as to whether a nose clip is necessary for FVC maneuvers unless the preceding inspiration is to be recorded. While absence of a nose clip probably makes a difference in only a few cases, there seems little reason not to routinely use one to avoid the possibility.

The SVC Maneuver

For this test, the subject should first be instructed to relax during the tidal breathing preceding the VC maneuver. Differentiation of IC and ERV from the VC requires a reliable, stable end-expiratory level, which will be achieved only if the subject is relaxed and breathing at true functional residual capacity (FRC). In our experience, ERV is second only to PEFR as the most variable of routine pulmonary function measures, and this variability is largely due to failure to establish such a reference point through relaxed tidal breathing. The subject should then be instructed that, when asked to do so, he should *completely* fill his lungs and *completely* empty his lungs. Most subjects will feel both full and empty before they actually are, and there are physiologic reasons for these misleading sensations. We have always found it useful to tell the subject something to the effect "you are going to think you're full and empty before you really are, so keep pulling in and blowing out as long as I tell you to, even though it doesn't feel to you as if you are moving any air."

Following these instructions, and the other six preparatory steps outlined above, proceed with the following steps.

1. Activate any recorder(s) and/or computer(s) as necessary. An SVC maneuver is usually recorded at slow paper speed (approximately 1 mm/sec) to facilitate calculation (as discussed later), as well as to enhance visualization of the end-expiratory level.

2. Have the subject breathe normally for several breaths until a stable end-expiratory level is established. In a subject with an erratic end-expiratory level or one who is obviously anxious, having him take a deep breath, *slowly* let it out, and resume normal breathing will often help relax him and stabilize end-expiration.

3. Have the subject inspire to TLC, coaching him with some simple, repeated phrase such as "deeper, deeper, deeper . . ." or "more, more, more. . . ."

4. Have the subject expire to RV at a slow to moderate flow, again coaching him with repeated exhortations to exhale completely.

5. Allow the subject to resume normal breathing for a couple of breaths, then remove mouthpiece and relax.

6. Repeat the procedure two or more times until reproducible results are obtained. There are no established criteria for reproducibility of VC measurements as distinct from FVC measurements; it seems reasonable to apply the ATS criteria for FVC reproducibility, so that the best two of at least three attempts should be within ±5% or 100 ml, whichever is greater.

There is some disagreement as to whether an SVC should be performed as an inspiration followed by expiration or the other way around. While there are a number of theoretical concerns in considering these two alternatives, including the fact that a deep inspiration precipitates bronchospasm in some subjects (which might alter the expiratory limb), in practice there is seldom any difference between the two approaches.

The FVC Maneuver

The instructions to the subject for an FVC maneuver should include an explanation of the need for complete inspiration and expiration such as that given above for an SVC maneuver. In addition, and perhaps most important, the subject should be instructed to exhale as forcefully as possible, using his thoracic and abdominal muscles to "blast" out the air. The maneuver should then be demonstrated. Experience has shown that, even with a comprehensive verbal explanation, many subjects do not understand the degree of force appropriate to the FVC maneuver, and subjects invariably do better when a demonstration is included in the instructions.

1. Have the subject take a maximal inspiration (to TLC). This step may be accomplished either by having the mouthpiece in place and inspiring from the system or by taking the deep breath and then inserting the mouthpiece. There is some contention as to which approach is preferable. The former is discouraged by some as a possible source of cross-contamination, but we have, for reasons discussed below, used that approach for years with many different systems and have never found an unwelcome organism in routine cultures of the equipment. Others echo this record.[10] Such considerations aside, some spirometry devices simply do not permit inspiration through the system. For three reasons, we strongly recommend that inspiration be made with the mouthpiece in place and that equipment that allows such be used. The first reason is that many subjects, particularly older or debilitated ones, cannot maintain maximal inspiration and may lose considerable volume in the process of getting the mouthpiece inserted. Second, proper placement of the mouthpiece, as described earlier, may take some adjustment, and requires close inspection by the tester, all of which is difficult to achieve quickly with the subject holding his breath. Third, correct "back extrapolation" to determine (t_o) (see "Data Reduction" section), as well as determination of certain other aberrations, requires graphing of the inspiratory plateau immediately preceding expiration. This approach requires that volume devices be placed near midposition to allow room for both inspiration and expiration. As discussed in the exceptions to ATS recommendations, a 7-L device is often inadequate.

2. Once the subject has achieved maximal inspiration and, if necessary, inserted the mouthpiece, activate any necessary recorder(s) and/or computer(s). As mentioned in the discussion of ATS guidelines, FVC maneuvers should be recorded at a fairly fast paper speed of at least 2 cm/sec.

3. Have the subject exhale forcefully, using a simple injunction such as "Blow!" to elicit an instant, concerted effort from the subject.

4. Encourage the subject to continue blowing until he is *completely* empty. That a subject is empty can probably best be assessed by monitoring a volume versus time tracing of the maneuver. After the initial steep, curvilinear rise almost perpendicular to the time axis, the volume tracing curves and begins to approach a line parallel to the time axis. The subject is empty when the tracing levels off. The plateauing should, however, occur gradually; an abrupt flattening likely represents premature termination or an occlusion by the subject's tongue or dentures, or glottic closure. One often encounters the recommendation that FVC maneuvers be terminated after some arbitrary time interval, such as 10 seconds. The basis for such recommendations is the belief that prolonging expiration will cause syncope. In our experience, very few subjects actually suffer syncope or even significant dizziness from a prolonged FVC maneuver. On the other hand, routinely terminating FVC maneuvers at 10 seconds will result in gross underestimation of FVC, and, therefore, overestimation of the FEV_1/FVC ratio and volume-dependent flows, in many subjects with obstructive lung disease. It seems unreasonable, therefore, to introduce a categorical error into tests of a large group of subjects to avoid the possibility of syncope in the occasional subject. If a particular subject exhibits an untoward reaction of any kind, testing can be modified for that subject.

5. If the FVC maneuver is being performed as a flow-volume loop, when the subject is empty, have him inhale forcefully back to TLC. Alternatively, a flow-volume loop may be performed by having the subject expire slowly, then perform the maximal inspiration, followed by the maximal expiration. This approach may be preferable in subjects with significant obstructive defects, in whom airway collapse accompanying forced expiration may reduce forced inspiratory volume.

6. Evaluate the maneuver for acceptability. The ATS statement, cited earlier for equipment specifications, also addresses some points of procedure, including enumeration of ten criteria for an acceptable FVC maneuver. These criteria are listed in Table 2–2.

TABLE 2–2.

ATS Criteria for Acceptability of an FVC Maneuver

Acceptability will be determined by the tester's observations that the subject performed the test:
1. With an understanding of the instructions
2. With a smooth, continuous exhalation
3. With apparent maximal effort
4. With a good start
5. Without coughing
6. Without glottis closure
7. Without early termination
8. Without a leak
9. Without an obstructed mouthpiece
10. Without an unsatisfactory start of expiration

7. Repeat the procedure until at least three acceptable maneuvers are obtained. In addition to the criteria listed above for acceptability of an individual maneuver, the ATS statement also stipulates that the "two best of the three acceptable curves should not vary by more than ±5% of reading or ±100 ml, whichever is greater." The statement does not make clear if this criteria applies to only the FVC or to all measurements derived from the maneuver. It seems reasonable to apply it at least to the FVC and FEV_1.

The ATS statement contends that "at least three acceptable tests are required to ensure that maximal effort and cooperation are obtained and that the tests provide an accurate reflection of the subject's pulmonary function." The statement goes on to suggest, however, that "there is no need to obtain more than three acceptable tests." This latter suggestion, which is repeated by the Epidemiology Standardization Project, is based on review of a number of studies that purport to demonstrate that subjects fatigue beyond three attempts, and subsequent values become progressively worse. We believe this conclusion is unfortunate for two reasons. First, it has led to the belief in many quarters that proper technique requires only three attempts, rather than three *acceptable* attempts. Obtaining three acceptable maneuvers often requires several more attempts. The second problem is that even three acceptable maneuvers may not yield a subject's best effort. In our experience, some subjects improve with successive maneuvers, and in those subjects, in particular, performing more than three maneuvers will often produce significantly better final values. For example, if on three successive, acceptable attempts a subject's FEV_1 is 3.00, 3.15, and 3.30 L, there is every reason to believe continued testing will yield higher values, even though the two best of these three values are within ±5% of one another. On the

other hand, if a subject's values on three acceptable attempts are 3.00, 2.99, and 3.01 L, it is unlikely that continued testing would be useful.

While we have long recommended doing more than three acceptable maneuvers, we did so in opposition to an overwhelming consensus of opinion. A recent study,[43] however, has confirmed our position and underscored the need to do more than three maneuvers. Ullah and colleagues had subjects perform either 10 or 20 FVC maneuvers, measuring PEFR, FEV_1, and FVC, and found that the highest value for one or more of the variables frequently occurred after the third acceptable attempt. They concluded:

> The self-evident truth that the subjects cannot exceed their maximum value, but may do less well, clearly is not attacked by these findings; but the assumption derived from it, that repeated attempts must give results which are negatively skewed, is now untenable. We have shown that the highest value in the first few attempts is not necessarily the highest value achieved—in fact, half of the patients achieved the highest values in the fourth and subsequent attempts in the series of 10.
>
> If only the patients' best values are to be used, then more than three measurements are required.

There are two additional phenomena that affect the decision as to how many trials should be performed in certain subjects: (1) negative effort dependence, and (2) precipitated bronchospasm. The practitioner should be familiar with these concepts both because the occurrence of either has in itself certain pathophysiological significance, and because they color how a subject's test results should be handled. Negative effort dependence is a reflection of the increased airways collapsability sometimes associated with obstructive lung diseases. It is manifested by forced expired volumes (particularly FEV_1) and midflows (such as $FEF_{25\%-75\%}$) which are higher when the subject blows with moderate force than when he blows with maximal force. Or perhaps more simply stated, the FEV_1 goes down as the PEFR goes up. This pattern differs from that of normal subjects whose timed volumes and flows increase with increased effort up to a point, and then, excepting PEFR, become independent of greater effort.

Precipitated bronchospasm occurs, generally in asthmatics, when the act of doing an FVC induces bronchospasm. In such cases, all values get progressively worse with each subsequent maneuver in a subject who reports feeling no different or who complains of tightness as opposed to fatigue. There is occasionally an onset of audible wheezing.

Both of these phenomena raise a question as to

how many maneuvers should be done. When negative effort dependence is suspected, enough trials should be performed to establish that the pattern is present. The tester might even have the subject deliberately exert different degrees of submaximal effort to help document it. In the case of precipitated bronchospasm, we recommend continuing testing until the subject's values "bottom out," and are reproduced at that level. Both of these patterns, despite the dramatic impact they may have on a given subject's assessment by spirometry, are not widely recognized or understood. As a result, there is certainly no consensus of opinion as to how their occurrence should be handled; the above recommendations are our personal ones. These phenomena also raise questions about which values should be reported, a problem that will be addressed in the discussion of data reduction.

As a final thought on the FVC procedure, the four most important considerations are that the subject (1) inspire maximally, (2) exhale as forcefully as possible, (3) continue expiration until empty, and (4) perform enough trials to ensure optimal results have been obtained. Failure to achieve one or more of these objectives is the most frequently observed procedural deficiency.

The MVV Maneuver

In explaining the MVV maneuver, the tester should instruct the subject to breathe deeply and rapidly, over and over, imitating the type of breathing encountered during severe exercise.[10] The MVV, like the FVC, must also be demonstrated. Make clear to the subject that he will be required to continue the maneuver for several seconds, and that he might get dizzy toward the end of the test.

1. Connect the subject to the system, and allow him to breathe normally for a few breaths to ensure proper mouthpiece placement and that no leaks are present.

2. Have the subject begin breathing deep and fast, coaching him for maximal effort. Most subjects achieve maximum values for MVV at respiratory frequencies between 70 and 120 breaths per minute,[3] but exact rate and depth are not important as long as any deficiency in one is made up in the other.

3. As soon as the proper breathing pattern is established, activate appropriate recorder(s) and/or computer(s). Tracings of MVV maneuvers are usually made at moderate recorder speeds of about 0.5 cm/sec. Particularly in the case of computers, activation should not occur until the proper pattern is

established to avoid including submaximal excursions in the accumulated volume.

4. Encourage the subject to sustain maximal effort throughout the MVV maneuver. It is generally useful to help the subject maintain a steady rhythm by calling out a cadence with, for example, "in, out, in, out."

5. Continue the maneuver for the desired length of time. The single most common measurement interval for MVV is probably 12 seconds, but one encounters recommendations for intervals of 6 to 15 seconds.

6. Repeat the maneuver at least once, or more times if necessary for reproducible results, allowing the subject to rest a few minutes between runs. Most subjects will be unable to tolerate more than two or three MVV maneuvers, making proper instruction and coaching even more important to minimize the number of trials.

In closing this discussion of spirometry procedures, we would like to address an issue only intimated up to this point. That issue is the importance of the tester's role in spirometric (and, indeed, most pulmonary function) testing. No other single factor is more critical in obtaining good spirometry than is the competence of the person administering the test. Any person performing spirometry should possess at least two characteristics. The first characteristic is one essentially of attitude, which makes the person capable of performing the test correctly, and which was recently described by Sobol:[40]

> It takes a special type of person to administer spirometric tests correctly. Patients are occasionally uncooperative and frequently uncomprehending. The technician should be a mixture of saint and drill sergeant to get proper performance out of the patient. It takes patience, understanding, good humor, and warmth to deal with those undertaking the test, but it also takes firmness, insistence and frequently all the qualities of a martinet to get spirometry performed correctly. Once having explained and demonstrated the procedure to the patient, it is insufficient merely to allow the patient to perform the maneuver the way his inclination directs. Much exhorting is necessary, especially near the end of the effort. The exhortation should be loud and insistent. Occasionally there will be a patient, notably a child, an elderly or debilitated person, or one with a language barrier who cannot perform adequately. The test must then be abandoned. With a technician who has the proper qualities, this is a rare occurrence; but if it happens, the technician must be mature enough to inform the physician of failure. He should never be allowed to base his interpretation on improperly performed studies.

The second characteristic is a combination of proper training and a certain innate analytic sense, both of which make the person capable of evaluating the test correctly to determine what, if anything, a subject did wrong, what should be done differently on subsequent trials, and under what circumstances a particular aberration may be acceptable. These characteristics are recited here to impress upon the beginning practitioner the importance of his role when performing spirometry.

Data Reduction

Before describing the calculation of specific indices from the spirometric maneuvers, two general considerations are worthy of note. First, for most spirometric parameters (other than volume-dependent flows, which, as discussed later, may be spuriously elevated), the largest value obtained is reported. While there are reasons to believe the mean value of several maneuvers may be more reproducible and therefore more useful for serial comparison, the implicit purpose of spirometry is to measure the subject's best performance. Second, by convention, all volumes and flows derived from spirometry are adjusted to compensate for the loss which is assumed to occur as gas moves from the lungs into the measuring device, therein cooling and losing moisture. As mentioned earlier, this practice has been questioned by some, but we feel the practice to be well founded, and it is, at the very least, common practice. The beginning practitioner, therefore, should be familiar with this concept, which applies to all of the primary calculations described below.

While in the lungs, gas is said to be at BTPS, an acronym for *body temperature pressure saturated*. After being exhaled into a spirometry device, gas is described as being at ATPS, for *ambient temperature pressure saturated*. The adjustment then is referred to as ATPS to BTPS correction, and the function by which it is made is the BTPS correction factor. This factor is calculated by the equation

$$[(P_B - P_{H_2O} \text{ at } T)/(P_B - 47)] \times [310/(273 + T)]$$

where P_B is barometric pressure, T is ambient temperature in degrees centigrade, and (P_{H_2O} at T) is partial pressure of the water vapor at that ambient temperature. More conveniently, the factor can be taken from a list (Table 2–3).

Spirometry performed on most older devices, as well as many of the simpler new devices, requires application of the BTPS correction factor. However, as noted in the discussion of the calibration and

TABLE 2–3.

ATPS to BTPS Conversion Factors for the Normal Range of Ambient Temperatures*

TEMPERATURE	BTPS FACTOR
20	1.102
21	1.096
22	1.091
23	1.085
24	1.080
25	1.075
26	1.068
27	1.063

*While these factors are also affected by barometric pressure, that effect is sufficiently small to ignore at or close to standard barometric pressure (760 mm Hg). If the barometric pressure is significantly different, the factor should be calculated using the formula given.

quality assurance procedures, many devices provide automatic electronic correction, in which case mathematical correction is obviously unnecessary. Some simpler devices attempt correction to BTPS by providing recording paper with gradations adjusted for one assumed ambient temperature, a practice that may introduce an error of several percentage points. When using such a device, the practitioner is urged to take the true reading and correct it mathematically for the actual ambient temperature.

We will now turn to consideration of the specific calculations made from the three spirometric maneuvers. Table 2–1 will remind the reader of the indices that are routinely derived from each maneuver.

SVC Calculations

The measurements of VC, IC, and ERV, as illustrated in Figure 2–5, are straightforward once the end-expiratory line is drawn. Determining this line can be somewhat problematic when the end-expiratory level is nonlinear. If end-expiration is wildly erratic on a particular trial, that trial should probably not be used to calculate IC and ERV, although VC would still be valid. However, some variation around a line of best fit does not necessarily invalidate a trial. Figure 2–6 provides examples of end-expiratory line determination.

The largest measured VC is reported. Indeed, in our practice, the largest VC obtained by any means, whether an SVC, FVC, or IVC performed during the

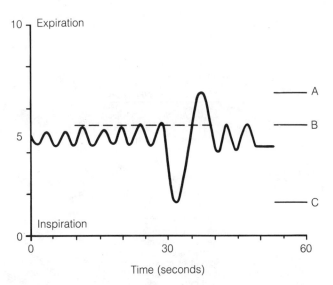

FIG 2–5.
Calculation of components of SVC. The idealized end-expiratory level is shown by the dotted line. The VC is the volume between A and C, the IC is the volume between B and C, and the ERV is the volume between A and B.

course of diffusion, distribution or other tests, is reported for VC, and used in subsequent calculations of other lung volumes, etc. As noted earlier, ERV is often variable while IC is reproducible; occasionally, the opposite is true. We recommend that whenever ERV or IC is reproducible while the other is not, the largest value for the reproducible parameter be reported, and subtracted from the largest VC value to drive the other parameter.

FVC Calculations

The combination of variables that can be derived from an FVC maneuver is largely dependent on the format in which it is recorded, and discussion will be divided on that basis.

Time-vs.-Volume Format.—The traditional time versus-volume format allows measurement of FVC, timed volumes FEV_t such as FEV_1, averaged flows FEF_{x-y} such as $FEF_{25\%-75\%}$, and mean transit time (MTT). Instantaneous flows FEF_x such as PEFR and $FEF_{50\%}$ cannot be reliably measured from a volume-time curve. One occasionally encounters the claim that these flows can be measured by tangents drawn to the volume curve, but such estimations are notably poor.

The measurements of FVC and FEV_t are shown in Figure 2–7. In order to optimize FEV_t measurements, t_o should be determined by the "back extrapolation" method recommended in the ATS guide-

lines (Fig 2–8) and mentioned previously. The ATS statement implies that application of this procedure may be invalid if the extrapolated volume exceeds 10% of the FVC or 100 ml, whichever is greater. Averaged flows can be calculated by either of two equivalent methods, as demonstrated in Figure 2–9. The calculation of MTT is really feasible only with computerized data reduction (Fig 2–10).

These calculations are further complicated by selection of the curve from which the reported values are to be taken. Here again, the ATS statement provides guidelines, which have been widely accepted, resulting in a consistent, if somewhat arbitrary, rule for selection of the values to be reported. The FVC and FEV_1 should be measured on each of at least three acceptable forced expiratory curves. Flows—$FEF_{25\%-75\%}$ and any other averaged flow, or instantaneous flows if available from an additional flow-volume or flow-time tracing or computer—are calculated from the curve with the greatest sum of FVC and FEV_1 (what the ATS statement terms the *best curve*). The rationale for this approach reflects a concept already mentioned: flows measured at increments of relative volume will be spuriously increased if the FVC on which they are based is an underestimate of the subject's "true" FVC. This effect, probably best explained graphically, is illustrated in Figure 2–11. Measurement of flows from the curve with the greatest sum of FVC and FEV_1 is intended to help ensure flows are not calculated from a truncated maneuver.

Despite the usefulness of these guidelines, there are two points with which we take issue, and on which basis we make additional recommendations that are strictly our own and do not reflect the ATS guidelines. First, it seems reasonable to report the highest PEFR recorded rather than the one associated with the "best curve" as implicitly suggested by the ATS guidelines. The reason for this recommendation is that PEFR, like FVC and FEV_1, and unlike other flows, is a variable for which a subject cannot artificially exceed his own best value. Second, the ATS statement does not mention negative effort dependence, but does imply that in the presence of precipitated bronchospasm the highest FVC and FEV_1 be reported. For both these phenomena, simply reporting the largest FVC and FEV_1 and "best curve" flows may present a misleading picture. At the very least, if the best values are reported, a note should be included explaining the circumstances, and specifying, in the case of negative effort dependence, the values associated with the most maximal effort, or, in the case of induced bronchospasm, the values at which the subject "bottomed out." It seems

A

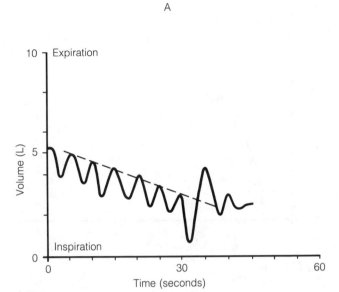

B

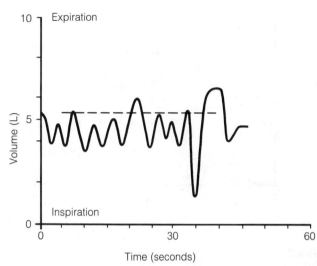

C

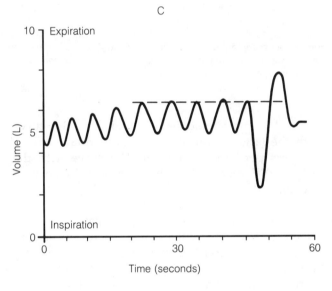

FIG 2–6.
Determinations of end-expiratory level, represented by dotted line in each case: **A,** increasing level (possibly due to low respiratory exchange ratio). **B,** acceptable variation around a line. **C,** decreasing level, as would be seen in a subject "settling down."

more appropriate, however, to report the lower values, with a note specifying the submaximal effort or initial values.

Flow-vs.-Volume Format.—FVC and instantaneous flows can be measured in this format. Timed volumes cannot be measured in the flow-volume format as such, but some devices add time marks which allow measurement of one or more time intervals, e.g., 0.5, 1.0, and 3.0 seconds. Averaged flows and mean transit time cannot be measured from flow-volume tracings in any case because of the ab-

sence of a continuous time base. The calculation of flow-volume parameters is shown in Figure 2–12.

When maneuvers are recorded in the flow-volume format without time marks, the ATS criteria for "best curve" obviously cannot be applied, since no FEV_1 is available to add to FVC. A reasonable solution for this oversight has been proposed by Boushey and Dawson.[3] They recommend:

1. The FVCs of the curves considered for selection must be within 5% of the maximal FVC observed.

2. The maximal inspiratory volumes should be

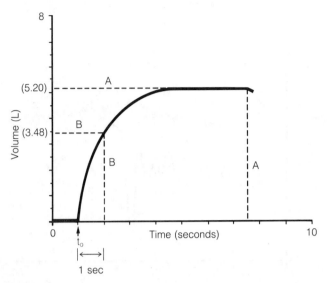

FIG 2–7.
Measurement of FVC and FEV_t in the volume-time format. FVC is the maximum volume, shown here by *dotted line A* (5.20 Liters in this example). FEV_t is determined as the volume expired at the specified time (t) from t_o (see Figure 2–8). Shown here, by *dotted line B*, is measurement of FEV_1, which is the volume expired at one second from t_o (3.48 Liters in this example).

assumed to be identical, and the flow-volume loops should be considered to be superimposed at TLC; the volume intervals for maximal flow points (e.g., $FEF_{50\%}$) should be taken from the largest observed FVC.

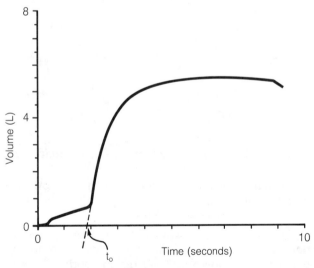

FIG 2–8.
Determination of t_o, by which to begin measurement of time for FEV_t measurements. A line *(dotted line)* is drawn through the steepest portion of the volume-time curve; the point at which this line intercepts the time line (X-axis) is t_o.

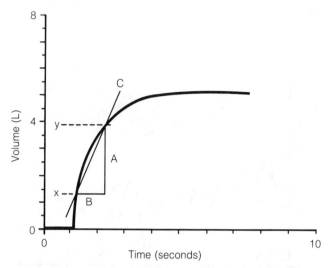

FIG 2–9.
Measurement of FEF_{x-y}. The first step is to locate the points specified by *x* and *y*. The case illustrated here is $FEF_{25\%-75\%}$; *x* is 25% of the FVC (1.3 Liters in this case), *y* is 75% of FVC (3.9 Liters). FEF_{x-y} is then calculated either as (1) the volume represented by *x − y (A)* divided by the time required to expire the volume *(B)*, or (2) the slope of a line *(C)* drawn through points *x* and *y*. Method 2 has the twofold advantage of allowing one to always use 1 second for *B*, so that *A* is the value for FEF_{x-y} without any division being necessary, and allowing one to expand *A* and *B* in cases in which one or both may be too small to resolve accurately (e.g., with very high or very low flows).

3. All data should be reported from the curve with the largest sum of FVC (in liters) and $FEF_{50\%}$ (in liters per second), or from the curve with the largest FVC that appears to have been made with maximal effort.

Volume and Flow-vs.-Time Format.—As mentioned earlier, the single most useful format in which to record spirometry is probably with volume and flow on separate channels of a strip recorder, thereby providing volume-vs-time and flow-vs-time tracings. This format provides the data of both the volume-time and flow-volume formats. The volume-time parameters are calculated exactly as described for that format above. Calculation of instantaneous flows in this format is illustrated in Figure 2–13.

MVV Calculations

Only one parameter, the MVV itself, is normally calculated from the MVV maneuver. An MVV is normally recorded as inspiratory and expiratory excursions against time, from which the MVV can be calculated in one of two ways. The first is to mea-

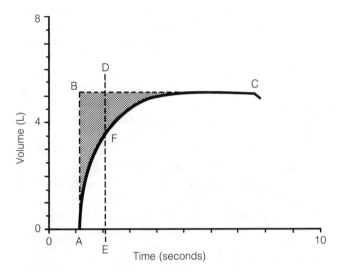

FIG 2–10.
Determination of mean transit time (MTT). The area enclosed by a line drawn up from t_o, and one drawn back from FVC (*ABC*, the shaded area, in this example) is integrated, and a line *(DE)* drawn such that the area *AEF* is equal to the area *FDC*. The point at which *DE* crosses the time axis is the MTT in seconds.

sure the volume of each excursion, add the volumes, and multiply the sum by 60 over the number of seconds for which excursions were counted. The second method is shown in Figure 2–14. A few devices record only the expirations during an MVV maneu-

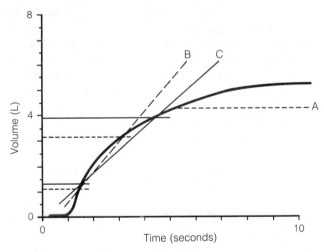

FIG 2–11.
Effect of truncated volume on volume-dependent flows. If a subject terminates an FVC maneuver prematurely, as illustrated by *dotted line A*, flows determined at percentages of the FVC will be artifactually increased. This example illustrates the effect on $FEF_{25\%-75\%}$. The *dotted line B* is the line drawn through the points representing 25% and 75% of the truncated volume, while *line C* is the 25–75 line for the full volume. As can be seen, the $FEF_{25\%-75\%}$ value derived from *B* would be (artifactually) larger than that derived from *C*.

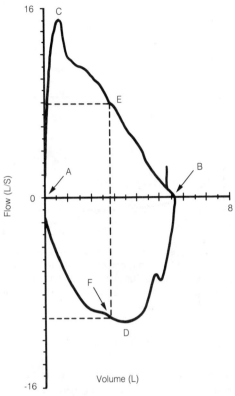

FIG 2–12.
Determination of flow-volume parameters. The FVC is the volume between *A* and *B* (5.60 Liters in this example). The FIVC is the volume between *B* and *A*; the FVC and the FIVC are equal in this example, but will often differ in clinical subjects. The FEF_{max} (PEF[R]) is represented by point *C* (15.2 L/sec in this example), the FIF_{max} (PIF[R]) by point *D* (10.3 L/sec in this example). FEF_x is determined by locating point x (a percent of FVC), and reading the flow at that point. In this example, line *EF* is drawn through 50% of the FVC; point *E* is the $FEF_{50\%}$ (7.8 L/sec in this example), and point *F* is the $FIF_{50\%}$ (10.1 L/sec in this example).

ver, producing a stepped pattern, in which case one simply measures the accumulated volume, and extrapolates it to 60 seconds as outlined above. The MVV value is sometimes expressed with the breathing frequency at which it was generated as a subscript, e.g., 150_{100} where 150 is the MVV and 100 the breathing frequency during the maneuver.

PEAK FLOW MEASUREMENTS

A disturbing recent trend in clinical pulmonary medicine has been the advent of the widespread use of independent measurements of peak expiratory flow (rate) (PEFR). While PEFR measured incident to an FVC maneuver (in which case it is more properly termed FEF_{max}) can provide valuable information,

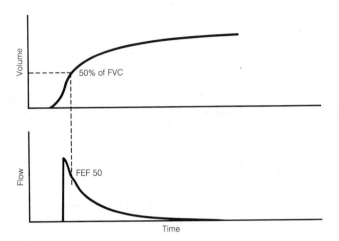

FIG 2–13.
Example of FVC recorded in volume and flow-vs.-time format, illustrating calculation of FEF$_x$. The percent of FVC represented by x is located on the volume-time tracing, and the flow occurring at the corresponding point in time on the flow-time tracing is determined. The measurement of FEF$_{50\%}$ is shown here.

PEFR measured alone can be misleading. We have included a discussion of PEFR measurements because such measurements have become so commonplace, but will preface that discussion with an explanation of the reasons PEFR measured by itself can be misleading.

Some of the parameters derived from the forced vital capacity maneuver, such as the FEF$_{25\%-75\%}$, are often said to be "effort independent." This designation refers to the fact these parameters are largely determined late in the maneuver, after equilibration of the pressures inside and outside the airways, at what is termed the "equal pressure point" (EPP).

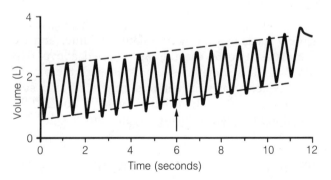

FIG 2–14.
Calculation of MVV by averaging excursions. For MVV maneuvers with fairly linear end-expiratory and end-inspiratory levels, the MVV can be computed by drawing lines (the *dotted lines* shown here) through the end-expiratory and end-inspiratory points, taking the volume at the median time (shown here by the *arrow*), and multiplying that volume times the number of excursions times 60 over the number of seconds for which excursions were counted.

When the EPP is reached, the airways partially collapse due to the loss of a positive transmural pressure difference, and beyond that point air flow is determined by the elastic recoil pressure of the lungs, a factor over which the subject has no control. According to the EPP model, airway collapse occurs at the same point regardless of how hard the subject blows (at least above a certain threshold), so that terminal flows will be the same no matter how much initial effort is increased; hence, the term "effort independent." On the other hand, flows that are primarily determined before the EPP is reached *are* affected by the degree of muscular effort generated by the subject, and, therefore, are termed "effort dependent." Of all the parameters measured from a forced expiration, PEFR is the most effort dependent. This characteristic of PEFR has several implications.

The first implication is that PEFR, when measured independently of other parameters, may not measure what it is intended to measure. The reason all flows, including PEFR, are measured in the first place is that they are believed to reflect the two factors that become abnormal in obstructive lung disease, namely airway caliber and lung elasticity. The more effort-independent parameters, such as FEV$_1$ and FEF$_{25\%-75\%}$, are determined primarily by these two factors, so that abnormalities in these parameters can be interpreted as evidencing airflow limitation, and, thus, an obstructive defect. Peak flow, however, because it is largely determined by the strength of the thoracic muscles, is not necessarily a measure of airway caliber and/or recoil. Decreases in PEFR may reflect thoracic muscle dysfunction rather than a true obstructive defect, and changes in PEFR may simply represent changes in thoracic muscle function. Conversely, in subjects with strong thoracic musculature, PEFR may be well maintained in the presence of significant obstruction. Indeed, it is not uncommon in the course of bronchoprovocation testing with exercise or bronchoconstrictive agents to see significant changes in FEV$_1$, FEF$_{25\%-75\%}$, and values derived from measures of airway resistance, with little or no change in PEFR.

The second implication of the effort dependence of PEFR has far greater practical significance. As the term *effort dependent* implies, PEFR is determined not only by the mechanical factors of airway caliber, elastic recoil, and thoracic muscle strength, but also by the subject's motivation. As a result, changes in PEFR may not represent any physiologic alteration at all, but simply a difference in how the subject feels. For example, if a subject thinks an asthmatic episode is beginning, PEFR may be reduced or reduced further by his anxiety. Similarly, following medication, the subject may feel better, whether due to actual physiologic improvement or a placebo effect, and any recorded improvement in PEFR may be disproportionate to the degree of functional improvement.

The third implication is that PEFR can be highly variable. It is not uncommon in the course of pulmonary function testing of even healthy, cooperative subjects to see significant variability in PEFR, despite good reproducibility of other parameters such as FEV_1. A number of studies have documented this greater variability of PEFR.[7, 20, 34, 37, 41] In our own lab, we have recorded cases in which, during sequential FVC maneuvers, PEFR varied by *as much as 64%* while FEV_1 varied by less than 1%!

In short, PEFR measurements have the potential for frequent false positive and false negative results, as well as overwhelming variability. These problems have led a number of authors to conclude that PEFR should not be used as a substitute for the FVC maneuver.[34, 35] At the very least, if such measurements are to be made, anyone utilizing the results should be fully cognizant of the attendant limitations.

Equipment

Much of the current interest in PEFR stems from the fact it can be measured with simple, portable, and inexpensive devices which, as a group, are generally termed *peak flowmeters*. Many other types of devices, such as those designed for general spirometry, may also measure peak flow, but the discussion here will focus on dedicated peak flowmeters. Several such devices are available. It is probable, however, that any new devices will utilize one of the principles described herein. The Wright peak flowmeter has a rotating vane that measures flow as the distance the vane turns and moves a needle on a face dial. A spring stop keeps the needle at the peak reading until reset. This device has a range of 60 to 1,000 L/min. The Wright peak flowmeter is a durable device, while the three other widely used peak flowmeters are made of plastic and are essentially for single-patient use. Two of the three, the Mini-Wright peak flowmeter (Armstrong Industries) and Pulmonary Monitor (Vitalograph Ltd.), operate through linear displacement of a spring-loaded piston, which moves a marker along a column with graduated markings. The Mini-Wright provides a range of 60 to 800 L/min, with measurement of higher flows possible by re-

moval of two plastic plugs. The third such device, the Assess peak flowmeter (Health Scan), operates as a rotometer, with PEFR measured as the distance a floating ball in a column is displaced by air flow directed through a precisely drilled orifice. Two scales are provided that, together with a removable resistor, allow measurement of flow from 80 to 520 L/min.

The most significant limitation to these devices is the well-documented[5, 9, 31, 32] inaccuracy and imprecision of the Mini-Wright and Pulmonary Monitor, which are probably related to their use of a single expanding spring to measure flow. It is often argued that accuracy is not particularly important in peak flow meters because they are generally used to detect trends, but at least one study has demonstrated significant intrainstrument variability in these two devices, suggesting limited utility even in the detection of trends.[9] A second obvious limitation of all but the standard Wright peak flowmeter is the range of flowrates that can be measured. All three of the "nondurable" meters have ranges that are too low at the upper end for testing relatively normal subjects, and the Pulmonary Monitor is too high at the lower end for discriminating changes in subjects with severe peak flow limitation.

Peak flowmeters do not lend themselves to calibration, since little if any adjustment is possible. Quality assurance is probably best achieved by connecting the peak flowmeter in series behind a pneumotachograph system, which is itself known to be accurate, and comparing the simultaneous maximum values of flow maneuvers directed through the tandem system. The test maneuver could be produced by exhalation of a human subject or by use of a calibrating syringe, and should cover the range of flowrates the device is designed to measure. The readings from the peak flowmeter should agree with those from the pneumotachograph to within ±5% or 12 L/min, whichever is greater (see ATS guidelines discussed in "Spirometry Measurements"). Many commercial devices are available that produce a range of calibrated flow rates, but most produce negative (inspiratory) flow, so they are of no use with expiratory peak flowmeters. One alternative approach, used in some published evaluations of peak flowmeters, is to determine the PEFR of a trained subject, using some other validated device, and then use that subject's PEFR to provide quality control of individual peak flowmeters. Based on the inherent variability of PEFR discussed above, we would strongly discourage this approach.

Procedure

The procedure for PEFR measurement is essentially the same as that for an FVC maneuver described previously, with the obvious difference that it is unnecessary to continue the maneuver beyond the initial expulsion which determines PEFR. The steps of that procedure most applicable to determination of PEFR are briefly recounted here.

1. Have the subject loosen any constrictive clothing.
2. Explain and demonstrate the procedure. Due to its extreme effort dependence, PEFR, more than any other forced expiratory measure, suffers from lack of the type of explanation and demonstration emphasized earlier.
3. Have the subject sit or stand erect with chin elevated and neck extended.
4. If subject has loose fitting dentures, have him remove them.
5. Have subject take a maximal inspiration (to TLC) and insert the mouthpiece of the peak flowmeter.
6. Have subject exhale as forcefully as possible.
7. Record reading and reset meter.
8. Repeat procedure until subject exerts what appears to be maximal effort, and duplicates that value at least once to within ±5%.

The reader should review the discussion of general spirometry and FVC procedures for a more detailed explanation of these instructions and the rationale on which they are based.

Data Reduction

In most cases, peak flow measurements are simply read directly from scales on the meter, and the highest value of the several attempts recorded. For some applications, the results are graphed to assess the presence of patterns such as cyclical variations. Occasionally, subjects are required to measure and record PEFR determinations themselves in order to obtain data at the precise moment certain symptoms appear or during a particular external event, such as exposure to cold air or occupational irritants. It often falls to the respiratory therapy practitioner to instruct these subjects in the use of the peak flowmeter and record keeping. The practitioner should realize the necessity of providing careful instruction and having the subject demonstrate competence at

the procedure, since errors by the subject add one more variable to the already high variability of PEFR measurements. In a study specifically designed to examine this variable, it was found that 69% of the readings made by subjects were within ±10% of the readings made simultaneously by a physician.[17] On the basis of the 69% accuracy rate, the authors conclude that subjects can monitor their own PEFR. However, the converse of a 69% accuracy rate is that 31%, or almost a full third, of the readings made by subjects were misread by more than 10%.

LUNG VOLUME MEASUREMENTS

To quantitate the total volume of a subject's lung (total lung capacity, or TLC), it is necessary to measure the volume left in the lungs after exhalation of the VC. Once this residual volume (RV) is known, the TLC can be partitioned into a number of functional subcompartments, which are summarized in Table 2–4. In practice, the RV is usually not measured directly; rather, by convention, it is determined indirectly by measuring the functional residual capacity (FRC) and subtracting the ERV. This practice is based on the fact FRC is more reproducible than RV, owing to what determines both. The FRC, representing the volume of the lungs at the end of a tidal expiration, is the normal resting level of the respiratory system, representing the point at which the tendencies of the chest wall to pull outward and the lungs to pull inward are balanced. Hence, the respiratory system seeks this level, as long as the subject is relaxed, making FRC a highly reproducible volume. The RV is effort dependent as well as physiologic, being dependent on the ERV, which is highly variable. As we will discuss below, making multiple determinations of a static lung volume (FRC or RV) is often impractical. Therefore, more reliable results are obtained when FRC is measured directly, and RV is computed using a reliable ERV value taken from a series of SVC maneuvers.

There are a number of methods available for measuring FRC. The following discussion will focus on the three most widely employed methods: (1) helium dilution (equilibration), (2) nitrogen washout, and (3) plethysmography. The helium dilution method, also termed the closed circuit method, and the nitrogen washout, or open circuit method are similar in that they are based on the same basic principle of gas dilution, and in that they both measure only those lung units in communication with the trachea. These gas dilution methods do not measure

TABLE 2–4.

Compartments of ("Static") Lung Volume

ACRONYM	DEFINITION	DERIVATION
FRC	Functional residual capacity: The volume of air remaining in the lungs at the end of a normal expiration. When measured via plethysmography, this end-expiratory volume is termed thoracic gas volume, or TGV	
RV	Residual volume: The volume of air remaining in the lungs after a maximal expiration (i.e., vital capacity)	FRC − ERV or TLC − VC
TLC	Total lung capacity: The volume of air in the lungs with maximal inspiration	FRC + IC or RV + VC
RV/TLC%	Residual volume to total lung capacity ratio, expressed as a percent	

piratory lung volumes are termed *thoracic gas volume* (TGV) to distinguish them from the *functional residual capacity* (FRC) measured by the gas dilution techniques. By measuring both an FRC and a TGV and subtracting the former from the latter (TGV − FRC), one can quantitate the volume of nonventilated lung.

Helium Dilution (Equilibration)

There are at least two major variants of the helium dilution or equilibration method for measuring lung volumes: (1) the oxygen bolus, or oxygen consumption method, and (2) the volume-stabilized, or constant volume method. The former allows the volume of the system to decrease as the subject consumes oxygen, while the latter maintains a constant system volume by adding oxygen at a rate equal to the subject's oxygen consumption. The oxygen bolus method has a number of potential problems, and, as far as we know, is not widely employed. We will, therefore, focus our discussion on the more conventional volume-stabilized method.

those lung units subtending occluded airways or otherwise sequestered. The plethysmographic method, which measures all compressible gas in the thorax, does measure noncommunicating lung units as well. Plethysmographic measurements of end-ex-

Equipment

The helium dilution system, as illustrated in Figure 2–15, includes a spirometer, helium analyzer, oxygen supply, two-way valve and breathing circuit

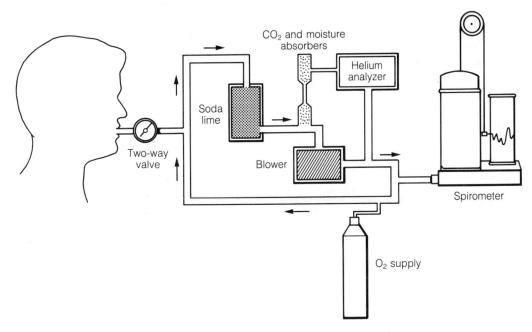

FIG 2–15.

Schematic of helium dilution system, showing spirometer, helium analyzer (katharometer), oxygen supply, two-way valve ("patient valve"), blower (variable speed circulation pump), CO_2 absorber (soda lime), and CO_2 (soda lime) and moisture absorbers (Drierite) for helium analyzer. The arrows show the path of gas through the circuit.

which, in turn, includes a blower, or circulating pump, and CO_2 absorber. The most commonly used type of helium analyzer is a katharometer, which is a type of thermal conductivity detector. Such detectors are based on the principle that conduction of heat through a gas occurs at a rate determined by the nature of the gas. The gas to be analyzed is brought into contact with a heated electrical resistor in which resistance is related to temperature. Heat is conducted away from the element at a rate dependent on the thermal conductivity of the gas, thereby changing the element's resistance. The resistance of this sampling element is compared to the resistance of an identical reference element exposed to gas that does not contain the constituent to be measured (in this case helium). The electrical potential between the two resistor elements is proportional to the concentration of that constituent. The thermal conductivity of helium is about 8 to 10 times greater than O_2 and CO_2, making its detection in respiratory gases fairly simple. However, the thermal conductivity of helium is influenced by background gases and moisture. As a result, high concentrations of O_2 in the sample should be avoided, while both CO_2 and moisture are usually removed chemically from the gas entering the katharometer. The purpose and function of the other system components will become obvious in discussion of the procedure.

Calibration and quality assurance of a helium dilution system involves a number of considerations, including determination of system deadspace, system linearity and overall system accuracy, as well as checking for leaks, and, in some systems, setting the blower speed. Determination of system deadspace can be made from the actual test procedure in many systems (see "Data Reduction" section), while in others a separate procedure is required. To determine dead space:

1. Turn on blower, set spirometer's recorder to slow speed, and eliminate any automatic volume correction for temperature by setting temperature correction feature to 37°C (or BTPS correction to 0).
2. Zero the helium analyzer by pulling through room air.
3. Empty the spirometer completely, and close the valve to which the subject would be connected during testing ("patient valve") to seal the system.
4. Add a small amount of helium (the exact amount will depend on the particular sys-

tem, but should be an amount that will result in a three-fourths to full-scale deflection of the helium meter).
5. Open the patient valve, empty the spirometer again, and close the patient valve.
6. Allow the helium meter to stabilize and record reading (He_1).
7. Add room air in an amount sufficient to reduce the helium meter reading to approximately half of the initial reading (in some systems this step is accomplished by an automated valve, while in others it is necessary to open the patient valve, pull air in by expanding the spirometer, and close the patient valve).
8. Again allow the helium meter to stabilize and record reading (He_2).
9. Determine from the recorder tracing the volume (V) of air added in step 7.
10. Calculate dead space as:
$$(V \times He_2)/(He_1 - He_2).$$

In the above procedure for determining dead space, as well as the actual determination of lung volume, the accuracy of the helium meter is not particularly important, while linearity is critical. It is important, therefore, to periodically demonstrate system linearity. The procedure for assessing system linearity is the same as that for determining dead space, except that in step 7 volume is added in several smaller increments of approximately 1 L each, with a stabilized He_2 reading taken after each volume addition. After five or so such volume additions, the dead-space is calculated from each cumulative V and corresponding He_2. These several dead space values should agree very closely with no upward or downward trend. While there are other approaches to evaluating linearity of the helium analyzer alone, this approach checks linearity of the entire system.

The most important quality check of a helium dilution or any lung volume system is the demonstration of overall system accuracy in measuring volume. Overall system accuracy is determined by performing a helium dilution procedure on a calibrated 3-L or larger syringe in precisely the same manner a subject would be tested. The system is prepared as described in the "Procedure" section, with the one difference that in systems with an electronic correction of volume for temperature the correction feature is set to 37°C (or 0 BTPS correction), or in automated systems with mathematical correction 37°C is entered for the (ambient) temperature. The plunger of the calibrated syringe is set at a point of known volume, preferably 0.5 L less than the maximum volume; the syringe is connected to the system as a subject would be; the patient valve is opened and tidal breathing is simulated by moving the plunger of the syringe in and out between the initial position and the maximum position until the helium meter readings stabilize. This reading is recorded and the measured volume of the syringe is calculated by the appropriate formula (see "Data Reduction" section). In automated systems, the results should be generated by the computer or microprocessor to again check the performance of the entire system as it will be used in testing actual subjects.

One problem with this quality assurance procedure in automated systems is that some such systems automatically apply one or more "corrections" to the measured volume to eliminate the effects of certain physiologic phenomenon which, of course, would not be present in an inanimate calibrating syringe. These correction factors are outlined in the discussion of data reduction. In automated systems, it would be necessary to consult the manufacturer's literature to determine which, if any, of these corrections are being factored into the final computed value, and, if present, to restore the computed value to its uncorrected state. One exception is the correction for "valve dead space" which would be made for syringe determinations as well as for tests on human subjects.

An additional factor concerning this quality assurance procedure is worthy of note. In some calibrating syringes, the total volume is greater than the displaceable volume due to areas between plunger stops and the end of the barrel, and/or the volume of the syringe's connection nozzle. Thus, while a syringe may deliver 3 L when evacuated into a spirometer, it may contain, say, 3.2 L of dilutional volume. Some syringe manufacturers provide an "FRC volume" or "dilution volume" value for each syringe, while others do not. The practitioner should make certain, for this procedure, he uses a syringe with a known *total* volume. This known volume and the value determined by the above procedure should agree to within ±0.05 L.[10]

Helium dilution systems should also be checked regularly for leaks. To do so:

1. Add a small amount of helium and enough air to put the spirometer at midposition.
2. Close the patient valve.

3. Turn on the blower.
4. Allow helium meter to stabilize.
5. Turn on recorder at slow speed.
6. Leave the system running in this mode for several (5 to 10) minutes, during which the recorder tracing reflecting spirometer volume should remain steady, and the helium meter reading should remain constant.

If either the volume tracing or helium concentration is not stable, the source of the leak should be identified and corrected before the system is used for further testing. The presence of a leak will also become obvious during testing by the failure of the helium concentration to stabilize.

A final consideration in the calibration of helium dilution systems is the need, in some systems, to adjust the blower speed. This step is generally required only in systems built around water seal spirometers that employ a weight placed on top of the spirometer bell to offset the force of the blower. With the weight in place, the spirometer bell at midposition, and the patient valve open, the blower speed is adjusted until the bell is exactly balanced.

Procedure

As intimated earlier, there are two slightly different approaches to the constant volume helium dilution procedure, the more conventional "two-reading" method and a "three-reading" method which provide simultaneous determination of system dead space. The two methods differ in only step 8 of the procedure.

1. Check and, if necessary, replace the chemical moisture and CO_2 absorbers. (The most commonly used moisture absorber, indicating Drierite, is blue, and turns pink as it become saturated. The soda lime generally used for CO_2 removal turns from white to blue.)
2. Ensure an adequate O_2 supply.
3. Turn on blower.
4. Flush system with room air until the helium meter stabilizes at lowest value (should be close to zero).
5. Zero helium meter.
6. Empty spirometer and close patient valve.
7. Inscribe a mark with the recorder to denote the initial spirometer volume (V_1).
8. Add enough helium to produce a helium meter reading of 13% to 15%. The amount of helium

required varies, depending on system deadspace, from about 0.5 to 2 L; then,

- For the three-reading method, open patient valve, empty spirometer, close patient valve, allow helium meter to stabilize, and record reading He_1;
- For the two-reading method, go to step 9.

9. Add 4 or 5 L of room air (see step 7 in deadspace procedure), inscribe a mark with recorder to denote volume of gas added (V_2), allow helium meter to stabilize and record reading He_2.

10. Have subject sit erect, insert mouthpiece, and apply nose clip. It is important that the subject be situated comfortably in a position he can maintain for the duration of the test. If the subject is not comfortable, he will be more likely to move around during the test, increasing the chance for a leak around the mouthpiece.

11. Allow the subject to become accustomed to the mouthpiece by breathing normally for 30 seconds or so, encouraging him to relax. As already mentioned, it is critical that the subject be relaxed to help ensure he is breathing at "true" FRC. In a subject who seems not to be, having him take a deep breath and exhale slowly will often facilitate matters. However, a deep inspiration can precipitate bronchospasm in some asthmatic subjects, which in turn may alter FRC.

12. Activate the recorder at slow speed (approximately 1 mm/sec).

13. When the subject is relaxed, open patient valve (switching subject into system) at the end of a normal expiration. End-expiration generally has to be adjudged by watching the subject's chest excursions. While the operator should attempt to catch the subject exactly at end-expiration, if a "switch-in error" does occur, it can be corrected in the calculation of FRC. Correction of "switch-in errors" is described in the *Data Reduction* section below.

14. Turn on the oxygen supply and adjust flow so as to keep the subject's end-expiratory level stable at V_2. (The amount of oxygen required will obviously be equal to the subject's metabolic oxygen uptake, and, therefore, will generally be approximately 3.5 ml/min/kg of body weight.) It may be necessary to readjust the flow several times during the course of the test.

15. Record helium meter readings at regular intervals of 15 to 30 seconds until equilibration occurs. Equilibration is variously defined as helium meter readings which fluctuate by no more than 0.02%

during a 30-second interval[10] or 0.05% in 1 minute.[15] Ideally, the reading should completely stabilize. In some subjects with significant "slow spaces" (lung units with increased compliance and/or which subtend airways with increased resistance), equilibration may take longer than the test can be reasonably continued in a clinical subject. It is customary, although not necessary, to terminate the test at 7 minutes if equilibration has not occurred.

16. During the test, have the subject periodically take a deep breath and slowly exhale. These breaths will both hasten equilibration and help to alleviate the anxiety many subjects experience during this test.

17. When equilibration is achieved, record the final helium meter reading (He_3), close the patient valve, and turn off recorder.

Ideally, the test should be repeated to ensure reproducibility. While one author suggests the best reproducibility one can expect for duplicate tests is ± 0.52 L,[44] our experience and the recommendation of the Intermountain Thoracic Society[23] suggest that when done properly, there should be less than 0.25 L difference between the two values. The average of the two values is reported. A minimum of 5 minutes in normal subjects and 15 to 20 minutes in subjects with significant obstructive disease should be allowed between tests to permit washout of residual helium in the subject's lungs.

Data Reduction

Two equations, one for the two-reading method, the other for the three-reading method, are presented below. The formulae are based on the principle that in a closed system, volume and the concentration of an inert gas, such as helium, are linearly and inversely related. In other words, the product of spirometer volume (V_s) and helium concentration at the beginning of the test is equal to the product of spirometer volume plus lung volume (V_L) and helium concentration at the end of the test, or

$$V_s \times He_2 = (V_s + V_L) \times He_3$$

solving for V_L,

$$V_L = V_s \times (He_2 - He_3)/He_3$$

In the two-reading method, V_s includes not only the volume of gas added to the spirometer (V_2 in the test procedure) but the deadspace V_{DS} of the system as well. Therefore, in the two-reading method,

$$V_L = [(V_2 + V_{DS}) \times (He_2 - He_3)]/He_3$$

In the three-reading method, the formula for calculating deadspace is incorporated into the calculation of V_L, making a separate determination of deadspace unnecessary. Therefore, in the three-reading method

$$V_L = [V_2 \times He_1 \times (He_2 - He_3)]/[He_3 \times (He_1 - He_2)]$$

Once the V_L is calculated by one of the above formulas, a number of adjustments have been suggested as being necessary to make V_L equal to the subject's FRC. We endorse only three of these "corrections," but will describe the others as some of them are widely used. The three adjustments that should be made are (1) correction of switch-in error (SIE), if present, (2) application of the BTPS correction factor, assuming the system does not provide automatic electronic or mathematical correction, and (3) subtraction of the patient valve volume, including the volume of any tubing and/or mouthpiece on the patient side of the valve. As described in the procedure section, a switch-in error occurs when a subject is turned into the system during inspiration or expiration, rather than at end-expiration, resulting in measurement of a volume above, or occasionally below, FRC. Detection of such errors is illustrated in Figure 2–16. The quantity of the valve deadspace (V_{DS}) should be stated in the manufacturer's literature; if not, it can be determined by filling the apparatus with water which is then poured into a graduated beaker and measured. The value to be reported for FRC, then, is calculated as

$$FRC = (V_L \pm SIE - V_{DS}) \times BTPS$$

Of the additional adjustments to FRC that we do not endorse, the most common is subtraction of a constant to correct for what is thought to be helium absorption into the bloodstream. The suggestions for correction range from 0.06 to 0.105 L. Two far less common adjustments are those for the presumed effects of the respiratory exchange ratio in concentrating helium in the lungs relative to the spirometer, and of changes in the concentration of nitrogen in the spirometer at the end versus the beginning of the test. The net suggested adjustment for both effects together is 0.10 L subtracted from V_L.

Nitrogen Washout

The multiple-breath nitrogen washout method for lung volume determinations utilizes the gas dilution principle in a manner different from that of the helium dilution (equilibration) maneuver. Rather than measuring lung volume by determining dilution of an inert gas introduced into the lungs as part of a closed circuit, the open circuit nitrogen washout method has the subject inhale 100% oxygen through one side of a two-way valve and exhale through the other side until all of the resident nitrogen in the

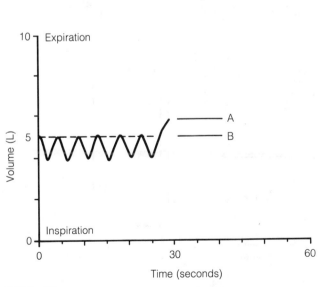

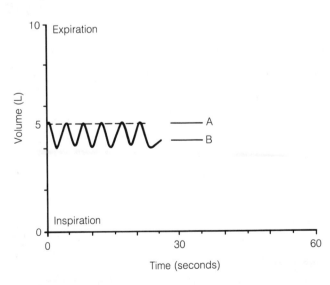

FIG 2–16.
Examples of switch-in errors for gas dilution lung volumes. **A,** subject was turned in to the system below FRC; the volume represented by the difference between *A* and *B* would be *added* to the measured volume. **B,** the subject was turned in above FRC; the volume represented by the difference between *A* and *B* would be *subtracted* from the measured volume.

lungs is "washed out." Measurement of the expired volume and its concentration of nitrogen permits calculation of the volume the nitrogen occupied in the lungs at the point the washout was initiated. Traditionally, the expired gas is actually collected in a large chamber. Newer automated systems use computers to sum the volume and nitrogen concentration of individual expirations, obviating the need to physically collect the expirate. Both the traditional and automated approaches will be discussed.

Equipment

Common to both approaches is the nitrogen analyzer. As with the helium dilution maneuver, a number of devices capable of discriminating nitrogen are available, but one type of dedicated analyzer is very widely used because of its simplicity, stability, and rapidity of response. In the case of nitrogen, this dedicated analyzer is an emission spectrometer, which operates by drawing a sample through a pin valve into a chamber where a high-voltage current

ionizes the sample, causing the nitrogen to emit a blue light which is selectively filtered onto a photocell; the output of the photocell is then proportional to the concentration of nitrogen. The major limitation of this type of device is the sensitivity of the analyzer to fluctuations in the pressure created by the vacuum pump used to pull the sample into the ionization chamber. The device is also affected by excessive water vapor in the sample.

Traditional Method.—The remainder of a typical gas collection nitrogen washout circuit is shown in Figure 2–17, and includes an oxygen source, two-way valve, gas collection chamber, two switching valves, recording spirometer and recorder, in addition to the nitrogen analyzer. The collection chamber is usually a large (Tissot) spirometer or Douglas-type bag with a capacity of 120 L. The recording spirometer is used to monitor end-expiration and determine switching errors. This regular spirometer may have its own recorder, or the signal from it might be dis-

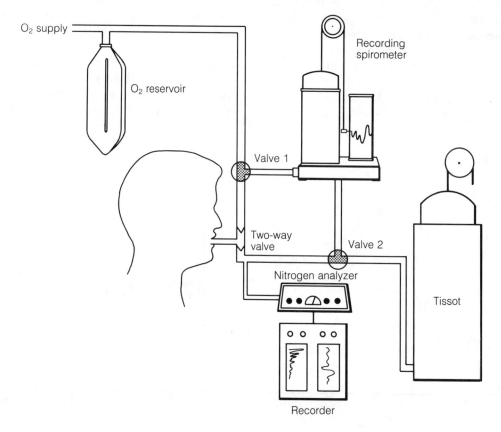

FIG 2–17.
Schematic diagram of a traditional nitrogen washout system showing oxygen reservoir, two-way valve, gas collection chamber (Tissot), two switching valves (valve 1 and valve 2), recording spirometer (in this case with its own recorder, although the type of strip-

chart recorder mentioned in the text for displaying output from this spirometer and the nitrogen analyzer is also shown), recorder and nitrogen analyzer.

played on the second channel of a strip chart recorder also used to display the nitrogen readings. The recorder used to display nitrogen concentrations might be a strip recorder as just mentioned, or a biaxial recorder with time base (X-Y-T).

Conventionally, the entire collection circuit (the Tissot spirometer or Douglas bag, all valves and the tubing connecting them) is flushed with oxygen just prior to use, the result of which does not represent deadspace. An alternative approach eliminates the need to flush the circuit with oxygen, but requires determination of the circuit volume which is treated as deadspace. Considering the comparative effort involved, as well as the fact the deadspace changes with the Tissot bell position and water level, the conventional approach seems preferable. If, however, one wishes to use the alternative approach, collection circuit deadspace can be determined in the following manner, as described by Jalowayski and Dawson:[21]

1. The Tissot spirometer is washed 10 times with air, the gas analyzed for its nitrogen content, and the bell lowered fully.
2. A 15-L anesthesia bag is filled with 100% O_2 and attached to the tubing at valve 2 (see Fig 2–17). The bag is emptied completely into the Tissot spirometer to determine the volume of oxygen added (V_{bag}).
3. The gases in the bag-spirometer system are mixed by alternately filling and emptying the bag from the spirometer at least 15 times. The bag is again emptied into the spirometer and the volume checked for leakage.
4. The nitrogen analyzer is connected to the outlet port of the spirometer, and the final nitrogen concentration is measured.
5. The deadspace V_{DS} is calculated from the formula

$$V_{DS} = V_{bag} \times [(F_2 - F_{bag})/(F_1 - F_2)]$$

where F_1 and F_2 are the initial and final nitrogen concentrations, respectively, in the Tissot spirometer, and F_{bag} is the initial nitrogen concentration in the oxygen-filled bag.
6. The deadspace thus determined will only be valid if the position of the fully lowered Tissot bell and the level of water in the Tissot remain unchanged. Any changes necessitate repeat measurement of the deadspace.

In addition, the deadspace between the two valves (see Fig 2–17) must be quantified, which can be done by filling the apparatus with water and pouring it into a graduated beaker.

Automated Method.—An example of an automated nitrogen washout system is illustrated in Figure 2–18. It consists of an oxygen source with automated switching and demand valve apparatus, pneumotachograph, expiratory valve, recorder, and microprocessor or computer with associated electronics, in addition to the nitrogen analyzer.

One point related to calibration that is peculiar to automated systems concerns the phase delay between the signals from the pneumotachograph and nitrogen analyzer. As each breath is expired, the integrated volume is derived almost immediately from the pneumotachograph, while the nitrogen analysis is delayed by the time it takes for the sample to traverse the sampling circuit and to be analyzed. The pneumotachograph and analyzer signals must be matched by determining and applying a correction for this delay. The manufacturer's instructions for any automated nitrogen washout system should include provision for determining such a correction factor.

Whichever method is used, there are at least three common points of calibration and quality assurance. First, the nitrogen analyzer must be carefully calibrated. Unlike the helium dilution procedure, where the analyzer need not be accurate as long as it is linear, the nitrogen washout method requires a critically accurate analyzer. The analyzer is calibrated by first occluding the needle valve to get a zero reading, then sampling room air and adjusting to the specified value, and then positioning the needle valve according to the manufacturer's instructions. It is also advisable to sample a calibrated gas with a nitrogen concentration in the range of 5% to 10%. This step is particularly important with the traditional method, in which expired nitrogen is quantified by a solitary determination which tends to be in the lower range. Second, the recorder (or other display device) should be calibrated during this process, such that the difference between 0% and room air nitrogen is a fairly large deflection (at least 10, or preferably 20 cm). Third, and most important, the overall accuracy of any nitrogen washout system, just like any helium dilution system, *must* be assured by performing a washout on a calibrating syringe of known volume. As in the case of helium dilution, the practitioner should (1) make certain he knows the total volume of the syringe, as opposed to its displaceable volume, (2) perform the quality assurance washout with the system config-

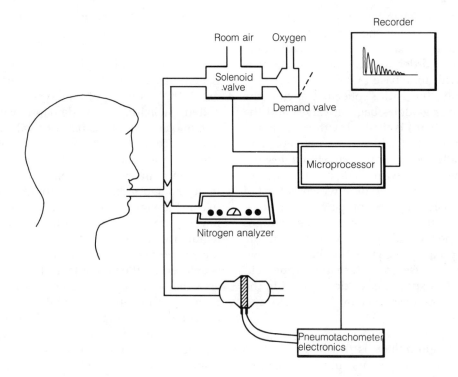

FIG 2–18.
Schematic of an automated nitrogen washout system. The solenoid valve can be controlled by the microprocessor to initiate the washout (switch the subject from breathing room air to breathing oxygen) at an end expiration. The volume signal from the pneumotachometer and the nitrogen signal are summed to determine the volume of nitrogen eliminated with each breath. The output of the nitrogen analyzer can be displayed to provide the conventional nitrogen-vs.-time plot.

ured as it would be for testing a human subject, and (3) override any physiologic corrections. The physiologic corrections usually applied to nitrogen washouts are subtraction of the volume of nitrogen excreted by blood and tissues and the BTPS factor. As prescribed for the helium dilution maneuver, if data reduction is computerized, the practitioner must be aware of which if any corrections are being made and apply them in reverse when performing washout of a syringe volume. In those systems which calculate nitrogen excretion based on weight or body surface area (see "Data Reduction" section), it may be possible to eliminate all physiologic correction by entering "37°C" for temperature, and "0" for weight and height.

Procedure

One composite procedure for the traditional method and automated method will be outlined, with the considerations peculiar to each method noted in the appropriate steps.

1. Ensure an adequate oxygen supply. In traditional systems, the oxygen reservoir bag is filled immediately prior to the test.

2. If a traditional system is being used, flush the system with either air or oxygen depending on which approach is being used (see discussion in previous section).

3. Explain the procedure to the subject, remembering the crucial importance of the subject's being relaxed.

4. Have the subject sit erect, insert the mouthpiece, and apply the nose clip. As with the helium dilution procedure, the subject should be situated comfortably to reduce the likelihood of a leak due to fidgeting.

5. Allow the subject to adjust to mouthpiece until he appears relaxed (see step 11, page 58). In systems such as the traditional one illustrated in Figure 2–17, which include a separate monitoring spirometer or other means of displaying breathing prior to initiating the washout, this judgment can be made by observing the displayed respiratory pattern for stability. This display also provides the means of determining if a switch-in error occurs when the washout is initiated.

6. Activate the recorder. This test is best recorded at a slow speed (1 mm/sec).

7. Initiate the washout at the end of an expira-

tion. In a traditional system, the washout is initiated by simultaneously turning both valves shown in Figure 2–17, so that the subject is inspiring from the oxygen supply and expiring into the collection device. Automated systems generally provide for automatic switching at the onset of an inspiration once the operator has designated a stable respiratory pattern.

8. If a traditional system is being used, watch the oxygen reservoir bag throughout the procedure to ensure there is an adequate flow of oxygen.

9. Continue washout until one of the following occurs:

- Expired nitrogen falls below a target value, variously suggested as 1.2%, 1.5%, or 3%.
- A leak is detected.
- The collection device reaches capacity.
- The washout period reaches 7 minutes.

Leaks in an open circuit nitrogen system are less easily detected prior to testing than are those in a closed circuit helium system. Leaks in the inspiratory side of a nitrogen system are often made manifest during the washout as a failure of the expired nitrogen to fall below an elevated level and/or by failure of inspired gas to read 0% nitrogen. A leak by the patient around the mouthpiece (pulling in room air containing approximately 79% nitrogen) will cause a significant rise in expired nitrogen above that of the immediately preceding breaths. While there is no reason other than convention to terminate a helium dilution at 7 minutes, there are effects of prolonged oxygen breathing in some subjects which should cause at least minor concern about prolonging a nitrogen washout beyond 7 minutes.

10. Determine a final alveolar nitrogen (N_{2A}) reading by having the subject blow to RV following a normal inspiration and recording the peak concentration. In a traditional system, the valve to the collection device is first turned so as to direct this ERV into the smaller spirometer.

11. Remove the subject from mouthpiece and turn off recorder.

12. If a traditional system is being used, measure the volume and nitrogen concentration contained in the collection device (the sampling line of the nitrogen analyzer is moved to the sampling port of the Tissot spirometer or Douglas bag).

The nitrogen washout, like the helium dilution, ideally should be repeated, after an appropriate interval, to ensure reproducibility. The two measurements should agree to within ± 0.4 L.[21]

Data Reduction

For nitrogen washouts performed with a traditional system by the conventional approach (flushing system with oxygen), the lung volume (V_L) washed out is calculated as

$$V_L = [V_E (N_{2end} - N_{2inspired} - V_{N2tissue})]/[0.81 - (N_{2A} - N_{2inspired})]$$

where V_E is the volume expired during the washout, N_{2end} is the nitrogen concentration in the collection device at the end of the washout, $N_{2inspired}$ is the nitrogen concentration in the oxygen supply ("pure" medical oxygen may contain as much as 1% nitrogen), N_{2A} is the final alveolar nitrogen concentration, and $V_{N2tissue}$ is the volume of nitrogen excreted by body tissues during the course of the washout. At least four equations have been proposed for deriving the volume of excreted nitrogen, two based on the assumption the volume is a function of the duration of the washout, one based on the assumption it is a function of the body mass of the subject, and one based on the assumption it is a function of both. The four equations are:

1. $V_{N_2 tissue} = 0.05 \times t$
2. $V_{N_2 tissue} = 0.1209 \times t^{1/2} - 0.0665$

where t is the duration of the washout in minutes,

3. $V_{N_2 tissue} = (BSA \times 96.5) + 35$

where BSA is body surface area in square meters.

4. $V_{N_2 tissue} = (0.1209 \times t^{1/2} - 0.0665) \times (W/70)$

where W is weight in kilograms.

For washouts performed by the alternative approach (treating the circuit as deadspace), Jalowayski and Dawson[21] provide the following formula (symbols have been changed to agree with earlier usage):

$$V_L = [(V_E + V_{DS1}) \times (N_{2end} - N_{2inspired}) - (V_{DS2} \times N_{2 tissot}) - V_{N_2 tissue}]/0.81 - N_{2A}$$

where V_{DS1} is the volume of dead space (V_{DS}) as calculated in the procedure described on page 61, V_{DS2} is the dead space between the two valves, and $N_{2tissot}$ is the nitrogen concentration in the Tissot at the beginning of the washout.

Whichever approach is used to derive V_L, corrections for switch-in error and BTPS are applied to arrive at FRC:

$$FRC = (V_L \pm SIE) \times BTPS$$

In automated systems, volume is derived by summing the product of volume and nitrogen concentration of each breath.

Plethysmography

Measurement of lung volumes by whole body plethysmography represents several advantages over measurements by the gas dilution techniques. First, as already observed, plethysmographic measurements include nonventilated lung, meaning such measurements provide a truer quantification of lung volume in the presence of obstructed airways or noncommunicating cavitation. Actually, a number of studies in the last few years have questioned this longheld belief, suggesting plethysmographic measures of volume may overestimate true lung volume in subjects with severe obstructive defects. Recognizing a number of flaws in those studies, however, we investigated the accuracy of plethysmographic lung volumes in the presence of severe obstruction by comparing plethysmographic volumes in a group of patients to those measured (planimetered) from chest radiographs, which provide a nonfunctional standard. In our patients, whose degree of obstruction was considerably worse than that at which measurement errors are purported to occur, the mean difference between plethysmographic and planimetered TLC was 0.06 (± 0.41) L (with mean values of 7.75 and 7.69 L, respectively), or 0.8 (± 5.1) %. We believe, therefore, the contention that plethysmographically determined volumes are more accurate in the presence of obstruction remains a valid one.

The second advantage of plethysmography is the rapidity with which determinations can be made. Whereas a helium dilution or nitrogen washout may take 15 minutes or longer (including setup), an individual plethysmographic determination of thoracic gas volume (TGV) takes only seconds. This difference is significant not only for the time saved, but also because some subjects, particularly those with resting dyspnea, are unable to tolerate the sensation of breathing on a mouthpiece with nose occluded for as long as 7 minutes. Such subjects can, however, generally tolerate the plethysmographic maneuver.

Third, plethysmographic measures of lung volume offer the advantage of being readily repeatable. Because of the time required and the need to allow the alveolar gas composition to return to normal between tests, helium dilution and nitrogen washout procedures are generally repeated only once or, regretfully, not at all, reliance being placed on a single measurement. With plethysmography, on the other hand, any number of repeat determinations can be performed in rapid succession.

Equipment

An archetypal whole-body plethysmograph is schematized in Figure 2–19. It consists of a cabinet—generally with approximately a 600-L capacity—in which the subject sits, a pneumotachometer fitted with a shutter device that can be activated to occlude the subject's breathing, a pressure transducer connected to a tap between the mouthpiece and shutter, and a volume-measuring device attached to the singular egress from the cabinet. Three types of plethysmographs have evolved, categorized by the type of volume-measuring device used. The three types are commonly termed volume, pressure, and flow. Most plethysmographs also contain a vent, which can be opened and closed as needed.

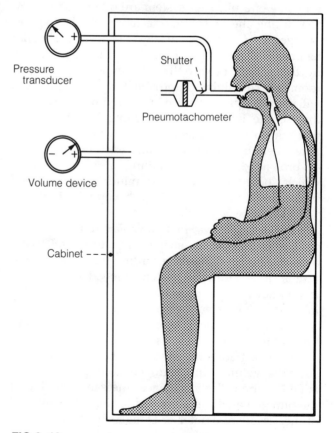

FIG 2–19.
Schematic diagram showing the basic components of all plethysmographs.

A volume plethysmograph measures volume change within the cabinet directly by means of a spirometer. A pressure plethysmograph substitutes a second pressure transducer, which is calibrated such that a known volume injected and withdrawn from the cabinet produces a given pressure change. Despite relying on an indirect measure of volume, the pressure plethysmograph benefits from the better frequency response of pressure transducers relative to spirometers. Indeed, the pressure plethysmograph is far and away the most widely used type, at least in clinical settings, and will be the focus of our discussion here. Flow plethysmographs employ a second pneumotach built into the wall of the cabinet. While flow plethysmographs have a number of theoretical advantages over volume and pressure plethysmographs, certain technical difficulties have precluded their widespread use.

The three types of plethysmographs operate in the same essential manner. In all three, changes in a subject's lung volume are measured as the changes induced in cabinet volume (or pressure) by movement of the subject's chest wall. As the subject inspires, his chest expands, decreasing the cabinet volume (or increasing cabinet pressure) proportionately; as he expires, the opposite occurs. Such changes in "box" volume (pressure) can be measured either while the subject breathes through the pneumotachometer or while he makes respiratory efforts against the closed shutter. The former yields a reading of box volume vs. flow, which is used to determine airway resistance, while the latter yields box volume (pressure) versus mouth pressure, which provides the determination of lung volume with which we are concerned here. These readings are displayed on a biaxial recorder, which must have very good frequency response, such as an oscilloscope. How changes in box volume (pressure) versus mouth pressure translate into a measure of lung volume will be described in the discussion of data reduction.

Plethysmograph calibration consists of calibrating the pneumotachometer, mouth pressure transducer, and box volume (pressure) device individually. Pneumotachometer calibration in this context is different from that described in previous sections. In this case, actual flow, rather than integrated volume, is the measured commodity. Accordingly, the pneumotachometer is calibrated with a rotameter or electronic flow calibrator. Routine plethysmographic maneuvers employ low flows, so that the pneumotachometer should generally be calibrated in the range of ± 3 L/sec. A flow of, say, 1 L/sec is applied, and the oscilloscope or other recorder trace adjusted for the desired deflection (commonly 1 cm/L/sec) for flow during opened shutter maneuvers. Whatever setting is chosen, the value for liters per second of flow per centimeter (or inch) of deflection becomes the flow calibration factor to be used in calculation of results. (This factor is used in calculation of airway resistance measures, but not, as we are discussing here, calculation of lung volumes).

Mouth pressure, which in most plethysmograph systems replaces flow on the Y-axis during closed shutter panting, is calibrated by applying a known pressure, generated through a manometer, to the mouth pressure transducer. The value for pressure per centimeter (or inch) of deflection (commonly 5 to 10 cm H_2O per centimeter) becomes the mouth pressure calibration factor.

Box volume (pressure), at least in most commercially available plethysmographs, is calibrated by means of a piston pump which alternately injects and withdraws a known volume, usually 30 to 50 ml. The box volume (pressure) calibration factor is the ml of volume per centimeter of deflection (commonly 10 to 20 ml/cm).

Quality assurance of the integrated performance of a plethysmograph system used for lung volume determinations is achieved in one or both of two ways. First, one or more normal subjects (nonsmokers with a negative respiratory history) with reproducible FRC by gas dilution are used as the standard. The gas dilution and plethysmographic determinations should be made in close time proximity, and (in a normal subject) should agree to within $\pm 10\%$.[23] Second, accuracy of plethysmograph volume measurements may be assured by use of an "isothermal bottle," which can be constructed as shown in Figure 2–20. To use it, one operator sits with it in the plethysmograph, disconnects from the pneumotachograph/shutter apparatus the line leading to the mouth pressure transducer, connects that line to the open port out of the bottle, and, with a second operator manning the controls, holds his breath and pumps the bulb to generate mouth pressure vs. box volume (pressure) changes. In this case, box volume (pressure) changes result from changes in the volume of the bulb. It is absolutely requisite that the operator in the plethysmograph hold his breath during the act of squeezing the bulb, so as not to alter with his own respiratory efforts the changes in box volume (pressure). The mouth pressure vs. box volume (pressure) tracing thus produced is measured, and the resulting volume calculated, as described in the "Data Reduction" section.

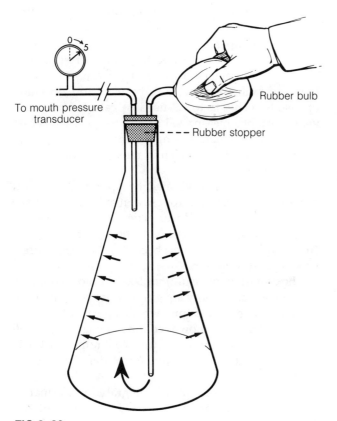

To mouth pressure transducer

Rubber bulb

---- Rubber stopper

FIG 2–20.
Design of isothermal bottle for use in quality assurance testing of plethysmograph. A 3- to 6-L flask is fitted with a stopper with two ports, one of which is connected to a bulb (approximately 100-ml volume), the other of which is connected by tubing to the mouth pressure transducer. The flask is filled with metal wool, which will absorb the heat generated by compression of the gas in the flask when the bulb is compressed, thereby keeping conditions isothermal. The effective volume of the isothermal bottle would be the volume of the flask plus the tubing plus the bulb minus the metal wool.

We have encountered the suggestion that in calculating bottle volumes, the partial pressure of water vapor not be subtracted from barometric pressure as the gas in the bottle is, intuitively at least, not at BTPS. However, as the temperature in the cabinet and therefore the bottle will be raised by the body temperature of the operator, we believe the bottle values should be calculated just as one would a subject's efforts. While no widely accepted standards exist for desirable accuracy of plethysmographs tested in this manner, it seems reasonable to expect a recovered value at least within ±5% of the effective volume of the bottle; the more critical practitioner might expect a recovered value within ±0.05 L, as suggested by the Epidemiology Standardization Project for helium dilution quality assurance.

Procedure
We have already discussed the importance of the subject's being relaxed during end-tidal lung volume determinations, and the role of the practitioner's thoroughly explaining the procedure in eliciting that relaxation. In no method is that relaxation more important than in plethysmography. All the other factors tending to cause anxiety and a concomitant alteration in lung volume are compounded in the case of plethysmography by the uneasiness most subjects feel at being closeted. It is therefore very important for the practitioner performing plethysmography to provide the subject a detailed description of what to expect, and to otherwise make the subject comfortable with the procedure. In particular, the practitioner should clearly explain to the subject the "panting" maneuver that is used (and explained below), and the need to make such panting respiratory efforts against the closed shutter when so instructed. It often helps to have the subject pant with his hand over his mouth to demonstrate and accustom him to the sensation. Furthermore, if the plethysmograph is one in which the door cannot be released from inside the compartment, the subject should be reassured the door will be opened at any point he so requests. Following such preparation, the general procedure for determination of TGV by plethysmography would be as follows.

1. Make the appropriate adjustment if the plethysmograph system provides for electronic correction of the subject's displacement of cabinet volume. This adjustment usually consists of entering the subject's weight. If such electronic correction is not provided, the displacement can be accounted for mathematically, as will be discussed in "Data Reduction."

2. Balance the transducers if necessary. In most plethysmograph systems, it is necessary to balance the transducers just prior to testing. The exact procedure varies, and one should consult the manual for the plethysmograph used. The transducers should be balanced without the subject in the cabinet.

3. Have the subject sit in the cabinet. Ensure that the pneumotachography apparatus is positioned appropriately and the subject is comfortable.

4. Put a mouthpiece on the pneumotachography apparatus; rubber or plastic ones with large flanges are used to minimize the chances of a leak. Give the subject a nose clip, and ensure he knows how to place it properly.

5. With the vent opened, close the cabinet door. It is important to have the vent opened while closing the door to prevent damage to the transducers from the high pressures that may occur.

6. Allow the temperature in the cabinet to equilibrate. After the door is closed, the temperature in the cabinet will gradually rise due to the subject's body heat. It is necessary to wait for the temperature to become relatively stable in order to avoid the effect of changing temperature on the box volume (pressure) during test maneuvers. Temperature changes can be assessed by closing the vent and observing the recorder trace. If the temperature is still rising, the position of the trace will move laterally with each breath. When thermal equilibration is achieved, the end-expiratory point of the trace will become replicable.

7. As the system approaches equilibrium, have the subject insert the mouthpiece, apply the nose clip, and brace his cheeks with his hands in such a way as to prevent his cheeks from expanding during the panting maneuvers. This last precaution is taken to prevent the subject from altering the alveolar pressure propogated to the closed shutter.

8. Encouraging the subject to relax, close the vent and observe the tracing for a stable end-expiratory level. For most plethysmographs presently in use, end expiration is assessed by the position of the box volume (pressure) trace (usually the leftmost point on the X-axis). Some newer computerized systems, as well as some manual systems outfitted with an additional recorder, provide a volume-vs.-time tracing, in which case end expiration can be assessed in the conventional manner.

9. When a stable end-expiratory level is established, close the shutter at end expiration. Many systems provide automatic closure, allowing the operator to activate the shutter at any time during expiration, with closure occurring at the next occurrence of zero flow.

10. When the shutter closes, have the subject pant against the shutter. Pants, in this context, are respiratory excursions that are small (less than 100 ml) and quick (1 to 2 cycles/sec). Record two or three excursions, open the shutter, and have the subject return to normal breathing.

11. Measure the recorded tracing, as illustrated in Figure 2–21. Most plethysmograph systems include a graticule fitted to the face of the oscilloscope screen that allows the operator to align the slope of the tracing with a grid line, and make a direct reading of the angle or tangent of the best-fit line through the tracing. The tracings produced during

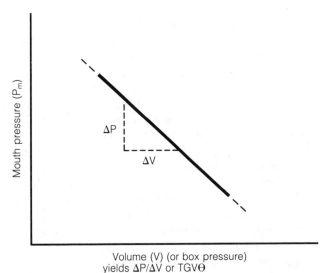

FIG 2–21.
Measurement of mouth pressure vs. box volume (pressure) plot for determination of thoracic gas volume. A line of best fit *(dotted line)* is drawn through the trace, which is usually already fairly linear, and dP/dV calculated. This value is then used as described in the text.

closed-shutter panting are generally closed, linear "loops," through which a line of best fit (slope) is easily imagined. Whereas opened shutter panting for measurement of airway resistance may produce a variety of patterns with pathophysiologic significance, deviations from a linear loop in closed shutter panting is almost invariably due to procedural problems, such as failure to keep the cheeks rigid or the glottis opened.

12. Repeat the procedure several times as necessary to gain reproducible results. With good technique, TGV is highly reproducible in most subjects. It is not uncommon, however, to observe a "settling down" phase in which TGV sequentially decreases on each of the first few maneuvers as the subject overcomes his apprehension and relaxes.

Before leaving our discussion of methodology for plethysmographic determination of lung volumes, one more observation seems necessary. While computerization has come more slowly to the plethysmograph than to many other devices in the armamentarium of pulmonary function equipment, the last couple of years have witnessed the virtual disappearance of the noncomputerized plethysmograph from among those commercially available. The resulting automation, in contrast to the automation that has on balance been such a boon to other types of pulmonary function testing systems, has been largely lamentable. The problems we have encountered with computerized plethysmographs range from intractable sequencing, which makes difficult the testing of subjects who cannot respond quickly or correctly to cues, to poor data reduction algorithms, which produce grossly inaccurate values. Even more than with spirometry or other devices already discussed, the practitioner should be exceedingly critical of the automation component of any plethysmograph system. Particularly if he is involved in evaluating systems for purchase, the practitioner should ensure that an automated plethysmograph has two features of cardinal importance: (1) a manual shutter closure mode, in which the operator can supercede any automatic shutter sequence to which some subjects may be unable to conform, and (2) provision for operator alteration of the line of best fit drawn through loops by the computer.

Data Reduction

The mouth pressure vs. box volume (pressure) (dP/dV) tracing obtained during testing is translated into TGV on the basis of a physical principle (Poisson's law) which holds that in a closed container, changes between pressure and volume of gas are opposite and a function of temperature changes. If the temperature remains constant, pressure and volume are then inversely related (Boyle's law), or

$$P_1V_1 = P_2V_2$$

In applying this principle to plethysmography, three things are known by definition: (1) P_1, the pressure in the lungs at end expiration, is equal to barometric pressure ($P_1 = P_B$); (2) P_2, the pressure in the lungs at the end of a breathing excursion (pant), is equal to the original pressure plus or minus whatever change takes place during the excursion ($P_2 = P_B \pm dP$); and (3) likewise, $V_2 = V_1 \pm dV$. Therefore,

$$P_B \times V_1 = (P_B \pm dP)(V_1 \pm dV)$$

Solving for V_1, which is TGV, and ignoring dP on the left side of the equation, which is conventionally held to be negligible,

$$TGV = P_B \times (dV/dP)$$

Reflecting the calibration factors discussed earlier, the actual working equation for calculating TGV (in milliliters) is

$$TGV = [(P_B - 63) \times BVCF] / [(dP/dV) \times MPCF]$$

where P_B is barometric pressure in cm H_2O, 63 is water vapor pressure (in centimeters of water) BVCF is box volume calibration factor, and MPCF is mouth

pressure calibration factor. Two further adjustments may be necessary depending on the plethysmograph system. First, if the system does not provide correction for the subject's displacement of box volume, a correction factor is calculated as follows, and multiplied times the TGV:

$$(BV - WT/2.36)/BV$$

where BV is the internal volume of the box (in liters) and WT is the subject's weight in pounds. Second, the mechanical dead space of the system from mouthpiece to shutter may be subtracted. No adjustment to BTPS is necessary; the value will be at BTPS as measured.

RESPIRATORY MUSCLE FORCE MEASUREMENTS

The last few years have witnessed a burgeoning interest in respiratory muscle function. One of the simplest and most clinically useful ways to assess that function is measurement of the aggregate force, or pressure, that the respiratory muscles can generate against an occlusion at the mouth. The method often used to make such measurements is to simply record a subject's efforts with a pressure gauge or manometer. While this method is convenient, lending itself readily to bedside determinations, it can, like PEFR measurements, yield misleading information.

The source of error in this case is the role of lung volume in the generation of muscle force. As one might guess, inspiratory force is greatest near RV, and decreases as lung volume moves toward TLC; conversely, expiratory force is greatest near TLC, and decreases as lung volume moves toward RV. Simply having the subject inspire to what is presumed to be TLC and measuring expiratory force, or expire to what is presumed to be RV and measuring inspiratory force, requires two assumptions that should not be made. The first assumption is that the subject actually inspired or expired completely. The ERV, as we have already suggested, is variable even in normal subjects, and both the ERV and IC can be variable in the extreme in the types of subjects for whom respiratory muscle force testing is most often indicated, i.e., subjects with neuromuscular disease and subjects with muscle weakness secondary to chronic obstructive lung disease. The second assumption is that the subject, even with a good ERV, is reaching an RV that occupies the normal quarter to third of total lung volume. Subjects with neuromuscular disease, and certainly those with severe hyperinflation from airway disease, often have increased residual volumes relative to total lung volumes, with the RV/TLC ratio sometimes being as high as 0.75. Obviously, in two subjects with the same actual muscle strength, the measured force in one who, for coincidental reasons such as discoordination or airway closure, is performing the procedure with his lungs still three quarters inflated will be much lower than the other who is able to expire to one-fourth of total lung volume and gain the associated mechanical advantage. As a result, a subject may be misdiagnosed as having muscle dysfunction when, in fact, his muscle force is normal for the lung volume at which it was measured. By extension, even if one is only interested in trends, the measured forces, particularly inspiratory forces, may wax or wane simply as a function of a subject's changing lung volume, while actual muscle strength is unchanged.

Based on these considerations, we strongly discourage the admittedly widespread practice of measuring muscle forces without simultaneous determination of lung volume. Although requiring more elaborate equipment, as well as determination of the FRC (or, preferably, TGV) on each occasion that muscle forces are measured, the technique described below, which measures muscle forces relative to lung volume, may mean the difference between an accurate and a potentially misleading assessment of muscle function. Realizing, however, that in many settings a convenient measurement is preferred to an accurate one, we will also describe the use of the hand-held, or portable, pressure gauge.

Equipment

The hand-held, or portable, pressure gauge should, by most recommendations, have a range of at least -60 to $+100$ cm H_2O. The reason this range is "acceptable" for pressure gauges has always eluded us, both because many subjects exceed those values, and because the same sources often recommend that when a pressure transducer is used (as described below) it have a range of ± 200 to 250 cm H_2O. The gauge is connected to a large-bore three-way (Y or T) valve such that the port to which the subject is connected can be opened to the atmosphere in one position and connected to the gauge in the other position. At some point between the patient port and the gauge, a "controlled leak" should be inserted into the apparatus. This leak, consisting of a tube 1 mm in diameter and 15 mm in length, is

necessary to prevent the subject's generating additional pressure with his facial muscles. The patient port should be fitted with a large flanged rubber mouthpiece; this type of mouthpiece is necessary to help minimize leaks.

The type of apparatus used to measure muscle force and lung volume in simultaneity, is shown in Figure 2–22. This arrangement includes the same sort of valve described above, a pressure transducer with range of ± 200 to 250 cm H_2O and necessary associated signal conditioning electronics, spirometer or pneumotachograph, and two-channel strip recorder. Here, too, a "controlled leak" must be incorporated between the subject port and occlusion.

Systems employing pressure transducers should be calibrated before each test, while pressure gauges should be checked for accuracy at regular intervals of, say, once a month. In both cases, a manometer should be used. In calibrating a transducer-recorder

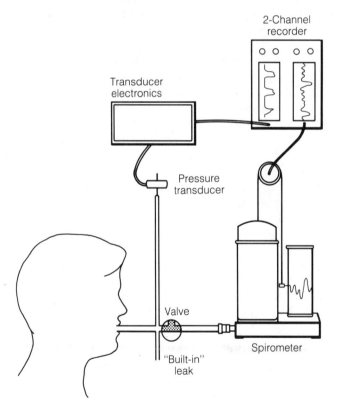

FIG 2–22.
Schematic diagram of typical system used for measuring volume in simultaneity with muscle force. Shown are the valve by which the subject's breathing can be directed into the volume measuring device or occluded, the pressure transducer that will measure the pressures generated against the occlusion, the transducer's electronics, a spirometer (or other volume measuring device with electrical output), and the two-channel recorder to display volume and pressure simultaneously.

system, a pressure of 10 or 20 cm H_2O is applied and the recorder adjusted to the appropriate deflection. One or two higher pressures are then applied to ensure range and linearity. This procedure should be performed for both negative and positive pressures. In a simultaneous volume system, the spirometer or pneumotachograph and volume tracing are calibrated as described in the section on spirometry.

Procedure

There is some debate as to whether muscle forces are more meaningful measured at FRC, or at the volume which should produce the highest value (near TLC for expiratory force, and near RV for inspiratory force). We believe it is useful to do both, a practice that yields four values: maximal expiratory pressure (MEP) at FRC, MEP at TLC, maximal inspiratory pressure (MIP, also termed negative inspiratory force, or NIF) at FRC, and MIP at RV. The following discussion outlines the steps common to all four measures and the steps peculiar to each.

1. Explain the procedure, putting particular emphasis on the need for maximal effort. Much of a subject's maximal muscle force represents reserve that is not used in other pulmonary function maneuvers, so that these measurements require a more concerted effort than is required for any other procedure. It usually helps to make clear to the subject the purpose of the test—to test muscle *strength*—which the subject can relate to what would be required to test the strength of a skeletal muscle.

2. Have the subject sit erect. Muscle forces, like some other measures of respiratory system function, may be occasionally measured with the subject in some other position, either because the subject's movement is limited or to assess the effect of postural changes. If not sitting, the subject's position should be noted on any report or other reference to the results.

3. Ensure the directional valve is turned so the patient port is connected to the opened (atmospheric) port.

4. Have subject insert the mouthpiece, ensuring that flanges are properly placed between the teeth and lips, and breathe normally. Some subjects, particularly those with neuromuscular dysfunction, may not be able to maintain a seal. In such cases, at least two options are available. First, if another person is available to assist with the testing, he can use his fingers to help secure the subject's lips around the mouthpiece. Second, a mask may be substituted

for the mouthpiece, provided the mask is the type that can be pressed securely against the subject's face to form an airtight seal.

MEP at FRC
Our personal practice is to perform these measurements at end inspiration (FRC + tidal volume) rather than at true FRC, because most subjects seem to do better, probably because at end inspiration, one is in an "expiratory mode." The difference in volume is accounted for in calculating the percent of TLC at which the pressure was measured (see "Data Reduction" section).

5. Warn subject that performing expiratory pressure maneuvers may cause his ears to "pop" (similar to what occurs during descent in an airplane), but that the sensation should not deter him from exerting maximal effort.

6. After a few normal breaths to establish an end-expiratory level, close the directional valve at the end of an inspiration, and exhort the subject to push as forcefully as possible against the occlusion.

7. Remind the subject, as he is pushing, to keep his lips sealed tightly around the mouthpiece.

8. Continue the effort for approximately 5 seconds, all the while encouraging the subject to push harder.

9. Open the valve, and have the subject remove mouthpiece.

10. If a gauge is being used, record reading of highest pressure achieved after the inertial overshoot of the pen.

MEP at TLC
11. Following the same general provisions as above, have the subject inspire to TLC, close the valve, and elicit a maximal expiratory effort.

MIP at FRC
12. If necessary, switch the pressure line from the positive gauge or side of the transducer to the negative gauge or side of the transducer.

13. Close valve at end expiration, and have the subject pull as forcefully as possible against the occlusion.

MIP at RV
14. Have the subject expire to RV, close the valve, and elicit a maximal inspiratory effort.

Each of the four measures should be repeated at least three times. In our laboratory, if these three manuevers do not yield reproducible values (defined arbitrarily as ±5% or 5 cm H_2O, whichever is greater, between the two best), additional attempts, up to a total of five, are performed. The subject should be allowed a few minutes of rest between each manuever.

Data Reduction

If a gauge is being used, data reduction consists of simply recording the readings taken directly from the dial. In a simultaneous volume system, the highest pressure generated for each of the four measures is determined from the pressure tracings, and the lung volume at the point the valve was closed is calculated (as FRC plus recorded inspiration, or FRC minus recorded expiration). Some authors suggest that a transient peak pressure occurring at the beginning of an effort is an artifact and should not be used. While the pen on gauges may overshoot due to mechanical inertia, and this overshoot should be ignored, we do not agree that when using a simultaneous volume system, such as we have described, it is necessary to ignore the initial peak value if it is the highest pressure generated. A peak pressure that decays to a slightly lower stable value may reflect the physiologic phenomenon known as *stress relaxation*. Using a gauge, this phenomenon cannot be differentiated in the overshoot of the dial pen, but a properly damped recorder pen will not exhibit such inertial behavior, so that any pressure recorded should be considered legitimate. As further evidence of the legitimacy of such peak initial pressures in a simultaneous volume system, many subjects, as they continue to exert force, will duplicate or even exceed that peak later in the 5-second effort. The FRC or preferably TGV used in these calculations should be one measured at the time the muscle force studies are done.

As discussed in the introduction to this section, the value of and necessity for simultaneous determination of lung volume is to allow correlation of muscle forces with the degree of lung inflation at which they were generated. To do so, the calculated lung volume for each pressure is divided by TLC to find the percent of TLC (%TLC). The predicted pressure can then be determined from the study of Cook et al., which provides normal means and standard deviations for 10% increments of TLC.[6] Although this study used a significantly different methodology, we have found the predicted values to correlate well with those obtained in normal subjects by the simultaneous volume method described herein.

EXPIRED GAS MEASUREMENTS

Many important indices of pulmonary system function require quantification of constituent parts of the alveolar gas mix. The procedures by which such quantification is made may as a group be termed *expired gas measurements*. The full spectrum of such measurements and their applications is enormous, necessitating limitation of the present discussion to those expired gas measurements with the greatest applicability to clinical respiratory therapy, which are those involving respiratory gases. We will concentrate on measurement of expired oxygen, carbon dioxide, and nitrogen. These gases are measured in two expired forms, as required for various applications: *mixed-expired*—the amalgam of gases from an entire expiration, containing, therefore, a mixture of deadspace and alveolar gas; *end-tidal*—the last gas expired during a normal expiration, taken as a measure of alveolar gas.

Equipment

For some applications, merely the concentration of expired gas need be known, while for other applications the volume of expired gas is required. Accordingly, we will examine both the analyzers used to measure the concentration of particular gases, and the devices with which the volume of an expired gas can be determined.

Gas Analyzers

Many types of expired gas analyzers are widely used, two of which can detect a variety of gases, the remainder of which are "dedicated" analyzers designed to detect one particular gas. The two types of analyzers capable of measuring multiple gases are the *mass spectrometer* and the *gas chromatograph*.

A mass spectrometer measures gas concentration by actually "counting" the relative number of ionized molecules of each gas. A sample of the gas to be analyzed is drawn by a vacuum pump into a chamber, where the molecules are bombarded by an electron beam. The positive ions thereby produced are then drawn into a strong magnetic field, which causes the ions to separate according to their charge-to-mass ratios. Each type of ion then follows a different downward trajectory, with the heaviest ion following the outermost, and the lightest ion the innermost trajectory. Collecting plates placed in the paths of these predictable trajectories produce an electrical output proportional to the number of ions of a particular mass (Fig 2–23). The mass spectrometer is capable of measuring, with outstanding stability and extremely fast response time, a wide variety of respiratory and other gases, making it ideal for many applications. The primary limitations of mass spectrometry are more circumstantial than inherent: mass spectrometers are very expensive and many require significant maintenance. Two minor inherent limitations are that mass spectrometry cannot differentiate nitrogen and carbon monoxide, due to their having the same molecular weight, and that the sampled gas cannot be recovered, limiting use of the mass spectrometer in closed circuits.

Gas chromatography separates gases by a process known as selective adsorption, and then measures each gas with one or more of several types of detectors. Selective adsorption employs a carrier gas, such as helium, to transport the sample to be analyzed (mobile phase) through a column of packing material (diatomites for nitrogen and oxygen, and porous polymers for carbon dioxide) that separates the gases according to their molecular size (stationary phase), and then emits, or *elutes*, them in a predictable sequence. The column is often enclosed in a heated chamber or oven to increase the volatility of the gases. The emitted gas is analyzed, most commonly in the gas chromatographs used in respiratory care setting, by means of a thermal conductivity detector. The operation of thermal conductivity analyzers was outlined in the description of the katharometer used in the helium dilution procedure.

In a gas chromatograph, the output of the analyzer rises and then falls as each gas is emitted from the separating columns in sequence, thereby forming a series of peaks, each of which is proportional to the concentration of the corresponding gas. These peaks may be recorded to produce a *chromatogram*. The process of gas analysis by chromatography is illustrated in Figure 2–24. The gas chromatograph is generally capable of measuring any gas that can be separated by selective adsorption with the appropriate adsorbent column, but is limited in its application by at least two factors. First, the chromatograph is designed to measure discrete samples of injected gas, and may require several minutes to quantitate some gases. While certain modifications may enable the gas chromatograph to provide repetitive measurements of these respiratory gases as frequently as every 30 seconds, it clearly cannot be used in applications requiring fast response, such as continuous end-tidal sampling.[39] Second, the chromatograph cannot measure the gas used as a carrier gas if it is also a constituent of the sample. Nitrogen is probably the most often used carrier gas for gas chromatography in general, but can be replaced by helium or by hydrogen. Another consideration in gas chromatography is the need to periodically replace or recondition the column(s), which are generally degraded by moisture and/or carbon dioxide.

More than any other of the descriptions of gas analyzers in this section, the foregoing discussion of gas chromatography is a gross oversimplification of the process. A large body of literature, including periodicals, is devoted specifically to this method of analysis; the interested (and stalwart) reader is directed to any of the many available resources for a more detailed explanation of this complex process.

The widely used dedicated analyzers include one each for nitrogen and carbon dioxide, and three for oxygen. The spectral emission analyzer used for *nitrogen* has already been discussed in the section on lung volume determination by nitrogen washout.

The device commonly used for measurement of *carbon dioxide* is the infrared analyzer, which utilizes the radioabsorptive quality of CO_2. In this process, energy from an infrared source is passed through two parallel cells, the sample cell, and the reference cell, and into two halves of a detector cell which are divided by a thin metal diaphragm located close to an electrically isolated fixed plate (Fig 2–25). The detector cell contains the same gas as that to be analyzed, thereby making the detector specific for that particular gas. The infrared radiation causes the molecules of gas in the two detector cell compartments to vibrate, and increase the pressure within the compartment. As long as the sample cell contains no carbon dioxide, the same amount of infrared energy reaches both halves of the detector cell, keeping the

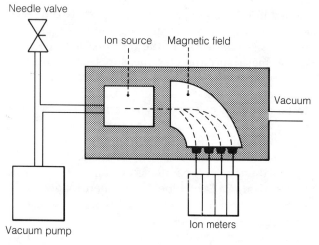

FIG 2–23.
Schematic diagram of a mass spectrometer.

Needle valve

Ion source   Magnetic field

Vacuum

Vacuum pump

Ion meters

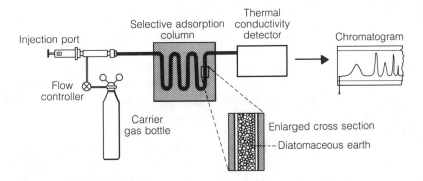

FIG 2–24.
Schematic diagram of a gas chromatograph. The output of the thermal conductivity detector can be displayed to provide a chromatogram, the peaks of which correspond to the concentration of the various gases analyzed.

pressures equal and the diaphragm stationary. When sample gas containing carbon dioxide is brought into the sample cell, the carbon dioxide absorbs radiation, reducing the energy reaching that half of the detector cell. The greater amount of energy reaching the reference side of the detector cell creates a pressure difference which pushes the diaphragm toward the fixed plate, altering the capacitance, and creating an electrical output proportional to the concentration of carbon dioxide in the sample gas. A rotating chopper blade interrupts the infrared energy to create a pulsatile signal.

Infrared carbon dioxide analyzers are affected to one degree or another by moisture in the sample gas, changes in barometric pressure and temperature, vibration, and composition of the atmosphere inside the cabinet housing the detection apparatus. The influence of moisture makes it desirable to dry the sample gas by drawing it through a desiccant prior to analysis. The sensitivity to barometric pressure and temperature requires the analyzer be recalibrated if a significant change in either occurs. Furthermore, the sensitivity to temperature transients

makes it important that the analyzer be turned on a sufficient time prior to use (or left on) to ensure the heat-producing elements (infrared source, chopper motor) are stable. This required warm-up period may be up to 2 hours or longer, depending on the analyzer and the application; the longer the period over which measurements are to be made, the longer the period required for thermal stability. The susceptibility to vibration makes it desirable to mechanically isolate or shock-mount the sampling head by placing it on a padded surface or by suspending it with springs or rubber tubing. The composition of the atmosphere inside the housing of the sampling chamber affects the operation of the analyzer if any of the constituent gases absorb infrared energy. This effect is usually obviated by a mechanical adjustment, and the user should consult the manufacturer's manual as to if, how, and when that adjustment is to be made.

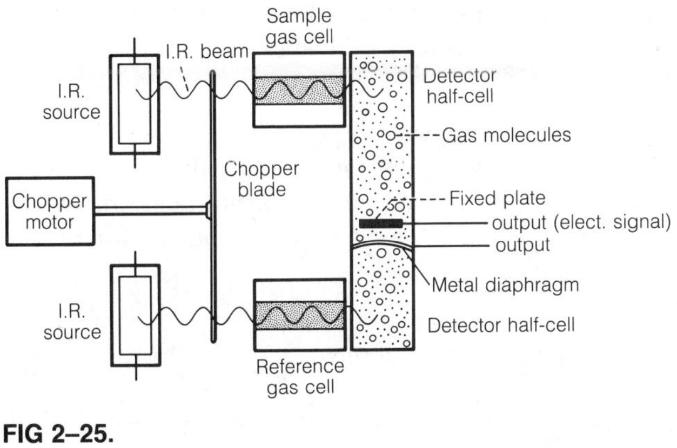

The three types of *oxygen analyzers* in most common use are paramagnetic, polarographic, and thermoconductive. Paramagnetic analyzers exploit the fact that oxygen tends to disrupt a magnetic field, while diamagnetic gases, such as nitrogen, do not. A glass dumbbell-shaped container filled with nitrogen is suspended on a filament in a magnetic field. As sample gas containing oxygen is introduced into the magnetic field, the nitrogen-filled container rotates in proportion to the quantity of oxygen. The rotation of the container is determined in one of several ways to provide an output signal. Most commonly, a light focused on a mirror attached to the glass container is reflected to a calibrated scale. Paramagnetic analyzers are sensitive to moisture, the density of background gases in the sample, and barometric pressure. As a result, sample gas is pulled through a desiccant to dry it prior to entering the magnetic chamber, and the analyzer should be re-

FIG 2–25.
Schematic diagram of an infrared carbon dioxide analyzer.

calibrated when a significant change in barometric pressure occurs. Even with recalibration, however, the accuracy of paramagnetic analyzers may be compromised when used in settings where barometric pressure is significantly different from that at sea level.

The polarographic oxygen analyzers used for expired gas measurements operate in essentially the same fashion as the oxygen electrodes used for blood gas analysis, which are discussed in the section "Blood Gas Measurements. " One difference concerns the response time of the blood gas electrodes, which may be as long as 90 seconds, and therefore unsuitable for many expired gas applications. Certain modifications used by some manufactuerers can effectively reduce the response time of such units to 200 msec.[39] Polarographic analyzers are affected by accumulation of moisture on the sensor, changes in barometric pressure, and increases in the pressure under which the sample gas is analyzed. Therefore, as in the case of infrared and paramagnetic analyzers, the sample gas is usually dried and the analyzer recalibrated if a significant change in barometric pressure occurs. The sensitivity to changes in sample pressure necessitates introduction of the sample at a constant, controlled pressure.

The thermoconductive principle has already been outlined in discussion of the katharometer used for measurement of helium. In this case, oxygen is measured by its thermoconduction relative to nitrogen. As in the case of helium analysis, moisture and carbon dioxide should be removed from the sample gas prior to analysis.

The calibration of expired gas analyzers varies in particulars between types of devices and even between models of a given type. Consequently, the practitioner is referred to the manufacturer's literature for initial calibration procedures. There are, however, certain principles common to the calibration of all gas analyzers used for expired gas measurements. These principles should be considered, whether or not they are mentioned in the manufacturer's literature. *First,* calibration must include actual analysis of gases from an external source and of known concentration. The calibration gas values must be reliable, and should ideally be confirmed by chemical analysis (such as the Scholander technique) of each tank. In settings without ready access to such techniques, the practitioner might consider one of the following: (1) purchasing two tanks of each calibration mixture, one each from two different suppliers (the analyzer's correctly reading one after being calibrated with the other would effectively confirm the accuracy of both); or (2) purchasing one tank of each calibration mixture, having these tanks sent to a laboratory which can provide chemical analysis for confirmation of concentrations, then reserving these tanks to be used solely as calibration standards (meaning analysis of samples from newly purchased tanks would be made following calibration with these reference tanks).

Second, for most of the analyzers described, two calibration points should be checked, one at the lower end and one at the higher end of the range likely to be encountered during the particular measurement to be made (remembering that room air provides a low-end point for CO_2, and a high-end point for O_2 and N_2). The infrared carbon dioxide analyzer, which is alinear or artificially linearized, should be checked with at least one additional intermediate value to allow construction of a linearization table or to check the integrity of the linearization electronics if present. *Third,* all calibration should be made through the exact sampling circuit to be used during testing. As already noted, most of the analyzers are affected by the pressure under which the sample gas is analyzed. As a result, if calibration gas is introduced into the analyzer through a short piece of tubing with little resistance, while sample gas is introduced through more tubing, desiccant, stopcocks, etc., with more resistance and, hence, a bigger pressure drop, the analyzed values will be inaccurate. *Fourth,* calibration tank gases are dry, which is one more reason for desiccating sample gas prior to analysis in most of the dedicated analyzers. In some applications, the gas sample may not be dried, in order to improve the response time of the analyzer (for end-tidal sampling, for example). While not affecting measurements made by some mass spectrometers or gas chromatographs, such measurements of moist sample gas made with dedicated oxygen and carbon dioxide analyzers calibrated with dry gases require mathematical correction for the effect of water vapor (see "Data Reduction" section).

Volume Devices

The volume of expired gas (in the present context) can be measured either continuously or by collection. The particular devices available can be categorized as follows:

Continuous devices
- Integrating flow devices
- Cumulating meters
  Wright respirometer and similar devices
  Dry gas meter

Collection devices
- Tissot spirometer
- Large gas bag (Douglas-type).

Integrating flow devices were described in the section on spirometry measurements, and the reader should review the limitations associated with those devices. The Wright respirometer measures volume by means of vanes which rotate as the expired gas is directed against them and in turn move hands affixed to calibrated dials. It is designed to operate at a continuous flow of 20 L/min, or a reciprocating flow of 7 L/min. At lower or higher flows, its readings of volume may be low or high, respectively. Dry gas meters use a system of valves to alternate gas between two bellows attached to a shaft which is out of phase by 90 degrees, much like a two-cylinder engine. Dry gas meters are sometimes outfitted with a potentiometer to provide an output signal for use with a recorder.

Both the *Tissot spirometer* and the *Douglas-type gas bag* were introduced in our discussion of the traditional method for determining lung volume by nitrogen washout. To reiterate in the present context, Tissot spirometers are large water-sealed spirometers of 50- to 600-L capacity. Tissot spirometers are also sometimes equipped with a potentiometer, but conventionally volume is measured directly as bell movement relative to a scale affixed to the Tissot body. Douglas bags are large gas bags of 50- to 200-L capacity which are pliable and made of materials relatively impermeable to CO_2, such as polyvinyl. Volume is measured after collection is completed by evacuating the bag through or into one of the other devices described.

When a collection device is used, gas concentrations can also be determined by analyzing a small aliquot of the collected gas. In order to measure gas concentrations when one of the continuous volume monitoring devices is used, it is necessary to either collect the gas in a Tissot or Douglas bag placed distal to the volume device, or to place a mixing chamber in series. A mixing chamber is simply a chamber, usually rectangular and made of Plexiglass, with a volume of 5 to 15 L, entry and exit ports, a sampling port, and either baffles or a fan inside the chamber to ensure gas mixing.

Procedure

As already mentioned, expired gas measurements have a tremendous number of applications, including but certainly not limited to:

- Exercise testing
- Indirect calorimetry (metabolic inferences made from analysis of expired gases)
- Dead-space determinations
- Cardiac output (by direct and indirect Fick methods)
- Chemical control of ventilation (ventilatory response to hypercarbia and hypoxia)

A detailed description of most of these procedures is well beyond the scope of the present discussion, and such descriptions are widely available elsewhere. We will focus on a few points of procedure affecting expired gas measurements in general.

1. When end-tidal measurements are made, the sampling should be done very closely to the mouth, as, for example, by connecting the sampling tube from the analyzer to a needle inserted at an angle into the rubber mouthpiece (in which the subject will be breathing) so as to place the end of the needle at the aperture of the mouthpiece.

2. In most cases, including baseline measurements prior to exercise or ventilatory response studies, the subject is assumed to have no volitional component to his breathing. While this assumption is probably never true, it is important that the subject be as relaxed as possible before any measurements are initiated, in order to minimize the effects of voluntary hyperpnea.

3. A number of the variables commonly derived from expired gas measurements are affected by what and when a subject has eaten. For some applications, it may be necessary to arrange the time a measurement is made accordingly, or even to ensure the subject is fasting.

4. For variables of which volume is a component, the value generally used is the volume expired per minute (minute volume or $\dot{V}_E$). Volume should be measured for several minutes, and the total divided by the number of minutes to provide an average; measuring for only 1 minute will often yield spurious values. Accordingly, the time over which volume is collected must be carefully determined.

5. Mechanical deadspace must always be washed out with the subject's expirate before any measurements are made or collection is started. When Douglas bags are used, they should be *completely* evacuated to the point of wadding by use of negative pressure before any expired gas is collected. With all collection (as opposed to flow-through) devices, a tap should be placed between the device inlet and the tubing leading to it. This tap

should first be turned to allow washout of the conducting valves and tubing, and then turned to allow expired gas to enter (timing would begin precisely as the tap is turned). When mixing chambers are used, the chamber as well as all valves and tubing must be purged before sampling begins. That washout has been achieved can be determined by sampling gas from the chamber. The oxygen concentration will fall, and the carbon dioxide concentration will rise; washout is complete when these values become relatively stable.

6. Certain assumptions are made in many applications of expired gas measurements. These assumptions may not be valid in the presence of lung disease or under nonstandard conditions, including such simple factors as an inspired oxygen concentration above 21%. The practitioner should seek to ensure that he understands the assumptions involved in any expired gas measurement, and avoid making the measurement under conditions that invalidate the assumptions.

Data Reduction

The indices that can be derived from expired gas measurements are, like the procedures, too numerous to recount here. Our discussion will address two general considerations and outline the formulae for a handful of the most common calculated indices.

The first general point concerns the condition in which expired gas measurements are reported. When expired volume alone is reported, it is expressed at BTPS. When volume is combined with a gas concentration, the resulting value is conventionally expressed at STPD (for *s*tandard *t*emperature *p*ressure *d*ry). The factor to convert volume from ATPS to STPD is derived as

$$[(P_B - P_{H_2O} \text{ at } T)/760] \times [273/(273 + T)]$$

where P_B is barometric pressure, T is ambient temperature in degrees centigrade, and P_{H_2O} at T is partial pressure of the water vapor at that ambient temperature. A volume at BTPS would first be converted to ATPS, and then to STPD.

The second general point concerns the effect of water vapor on expired gas measurements. As noted above, sample gas is usually dried prior to analysis, but may not be for some applications. When dry gas is used for calibration, and undried gas is sampled, a different STPD (or actually STP) factor is used:

$$(P_B - 760) - [273/(273 + T)]$$

A useful review of the effect of water vapor on expired gas measurements has been provided by Norton and Wilmore.[30]

The calculated expired gas indices most used in respiratory therapy are oxygen uptake ($\dot{V}O_2$), carbon dioxide output, ($\dot{V}CO_2$), respiratory exchange ratio (RER, or R), and physiologic deadspace. *Oxygen uptake* is the difference between the volume of oxygen inspired and the volume of oxygen expired, both volumes of oxygen being equal to total volume multiplied by the fractional concentration of oxygen. Therefore,

$$\dot{V}O_2 = (\dot{V}I \times F_{IO_2}) - (\dot{V}E \times F\bar{E}_{O_2})$$

where $\dot{V}I$ is inspired volume, $\dot{V}E$ is expired volume, F_{IO_2} is the inspired fractional concentration of oxygen and $F\bar{E}_{O_2}$ is the mixed expired fractional concentration of oxygen. Based on this formula, intuition suggests the most accurate measure of $\dot{V}O_2$ would come from actually measuring both $\dot{V}I$ and $\dot{V}E$. In practice, such is not the case. Using two separate volume measuring devices introduces an additional source of error; even small calibration errors of different sign in the two devices can cause large errors in calculated $\dot{V}O_2$. As a result, it is preferable to measure $\dot{V}E$ and then calculate $\dot{V}I$ based on the principle that the volume of expired nitrogen must equal the volume of inspired nitrogen because nitrogen is not consumed or produced. Thus,

$$\dot{V}I \times F_{IN_2} = \dot{V}E \times F\bar{E}_{N_2}$$

or, solving for $\dot{V}I$,

$$\dot{V}I = \dot{V}E \times F\bar{E}_{N_2}/F_{IN_2}$$

Rather than actually measuring nitrogen, necessitating an additional analyzer, nitrogen is taken to be the volume not occupied by oxygen and carbon dioxide (the total of the three fractional concentrations being 1):

$$F\bar{E}_{N_2} = 1 - F_{EO_2} - F_{ECO_2}$$
$$F_{IN_2} = 1 - F_{IO_2}$$

Combining formulas, oxygen uptake is actually calculated as

$$\dot{V}O_2 = \dot{V}E \times STPD \times ([F_{IO_2} \times (1 - F\bar{E}_{O_2} - F\bar{E}_{CO_2})/ 1 - F_{IO_2}] - F\bar{E}_{O_2})$$

While *carbon dioxide output* is determined on the same basic principle as oxygen uptake, the actual calculation is made considerably simpler by the fact inspired CO_2 can be taken to be zero. The formula, then, is

$$\dot{V}CO_2 = \dot{V}E \times STPD \times F\bar{E}_{CO_2}$$

The *respiratory exchange ratio* is the ratio of carbon dioxide output to oxygen uptake, or

$$R = \dot{V}_{CO_2}/\dot{V}_{O_2}$$

The respiratory exchange ratio is to be distinguished from the respiratory quotient (RQ), which is the ratio of carbon dioxide production to oxygen consumption at the cellular level. *The value derived from expired gas measurements is not the respiratory quotient.* Failure to remember this distinction has led to the practice of inferring metabolic status from expired gas measurements in many instances where such inferences are partly or wholly inappropriate.

Physiologic deadspace is directly measured, and usually expressed, as a fraction of the tidal volume (V_D/V_T). This measurement requires a simultaneous blood gas determination, and is calculated as

$$V_D/V_T = (Pa_{CO_2} - P\bar{E}_{CO2})/Pa_{CO2}$$

where Pa_{CO2} and $P\bar{E}_{CO2}$ are the arterial and mixed expired partial pressures of carbon dioxide. The fractional concentration of CO_2 would be converted to a partial pressure as

$$P\bar{E}_{CO2} = (P_B - 47) \times F\bar{E}_{CO2}$$

where P_B is barometric pressure. It is sometimes proposed that end-tidal CO_2 can be substituted for arterial CO_2 to provide a measurement of V_D/V_T without a blood sample. End-tidal CO_2 concentrations, however, are reliable estimates of arterial P_{CO2} only in relatively normal lungs; in subjects with diseased lungs, in whom determination of deadspace is most important, end-tidal CO_2 should not be substituted for Pa_{CO2}.

BLOOD GAS MEASUREMENTS

Of all pulmonary function measures, "blood gases" is the one with which respiratory therapists will be most familiar. The term *blood gases* is loosely used to designate determinations of the tensions of respiratory gases in blood, as well as acid-base indices, and a number of associated measured and derived variables. The major parameters associated with the term "blood gases" are outlined in Table 2–5. While blood gas analysis generally infers in vitro analyses employing invasive techniques, the present discussion will be expanded to include certain newer in vivo analyses employing noninvasive techniques.

TABLE 2–5.

Major "Blood-Gas" Parameters

SYMBOL*	DEFINITION	UNITS†
	Measured	
P_{O_2}	The tension, or partial pressure, of oxygen	mm Hg
P_{CO_2}	The tension, or partial pressure, of carbon dioxide	mm Hg
H^+	Hydrogen ion concentration (very roughly speaking, is the measure of *acid* in considerations of acid-base)	nEq/L
pH	Negative logarithm of H^+ *activity*	("pH units")
$\%HbO_2$	Oxyhemoglobin, or hemoglobin combined with oxygen; represents measured oxygen saturation (S_{O_2})	%
%COHb	Carboxyhemoglobin, or hemoglobin combined with carbon monoxide	%
%MetHb	Methemoglobin, or hemoglobin containing ferric iron	%
	Derived‡	
S_{O_2}	(Calculated) oxygen saturation (saturation of hemoglobin with oxygen)§	%
HCO_3^-	Bicarbonate (the major blood *base*)	mEq/L
BE	Base excess (base deficit): the amount of bicarbonate above or below the normal base buffer level.	mEq/L
Cx_{O_2}	Oxygen content (x representing type of blood; see note below)	vol%
$P(A - a)_{O_2}$	Alveolar-arterial oxygen tension difference; the difference between the level of oxygen in the lungs and the level of oxygen in arterial blood	mm Hg

*These symbols are generally combined with a modifier which designates the source (a for arterial, A for alveolar, v for venous, $\bar{v}$ for mixed venous, c' for end-capillary, etc.) Examples of combined symbols would be Pa_{O2} for arterial oxygen tension, Cv_{O2} for venous oxygen content.
†mm Hg = millimeters of mercury (also termed torr); nEq/L = nanoequivalents per liter; mEq/L = milliequivalents per liter; vol% = volumes percent (milliliters per 100 milliliters).
‡Bicarbonate (standard bicarbonate) and content can also be measured directly, but are more commonly calculated.
§$\%HbO_2$ and S_{O2} are, rightly or wrongly, as in this chapter, often used interchangeably.

Invasive Techniques

Invasive blood gas techniques involve two considerations: collection of the sample and analysis of the sample. The discussions of equipment and procedure will be divided along those lines.

Equipment

The discussion of equipment for blood gas measurements will be divided into that used in obtaining the blood sample, and that used for analyzing the sample.

Sample Collection.—Our format here will differ from previous discussions of equipment in as much as what is described here is more a list of supplies. The following list is intended to give the practitioner a general idea of the items to be assembled in order to perform an arterial puncture; however, the particulars may vary depending on personal preferences of the person obtaining the sample and/or policies of the institution in which the procedure is performed. In general, the following supplies are needed:

1. Hypodermic needle(s). The choice of gauge and length of needle to use may be influenced by a number of considerations. Smaller-gauge (25-gauge) needles are often used for punctures of the radial artery or of any artery that feels small when palpated. Small-gauge needles tend to cause less discomfort to the subject but can restrict the flow of blood into the syringe and are more susceptible to clotting. Conversely, larger-gauge needles (20- to 23-gauge) make collection of the sample easier but are more likely to cause the subject discomfort. By most accounts, the length of needle used is also a function of the site at which the sample is to be taken. Shorter (⅝-in.) needles are commonly used for punctures of radial or other relatively shallowly situated arteries, while longer (1½-in. or longer) ones are used for brachial or femoral punctures. Actually, this distinction is largely artificial in that a ⅝-in. needle is usually long enough for a brachial artery puncture, while no harm is done in using a longer needle for a radial artery puncture. The needle used is one of the items that is really a matter of the sampler's personal preference. One practical consideration worthy of mention is the advantage of using a needle with a clear or transluscent hub (the receptacle into which the syringe goes); such a hub makes it much easier to ascertain when an artery is punctured.

2. Syringe(s). Blood gas samples are most commonly collected in syringes, rather than the evacuated tubes used for collection of blood for other purposes, in order to keep the sampling process anaerobic and the sample at barometric pressure (introducing the blood into a partial vacuum would al-

ter the gas tensions). Historically, glass syringes have been preferred over plastic syringes for two reasons. First, glass syringes more readily fill from arterial pressure, making it more obvious when the artery is punctured, and reducing the need to aspirate. Second, there is some evidence that the respiratory gases, particularly oxygen at high concentrations, may transfer through certain types of plastic syringes. Given the first reason, it probably is advisable for the beginning practitioner to use glass syringes. However, considering that the experienced practitioner will generally be able to identify the moment of puncture as well using a plastic syringe as a glass one, and that a gentle aspirating force does no harm and is sometimes necessary with glass syringes as well, and that the evidence for gas transfer through plastic syringes is controversial (except at high oxygen concentrations, or when there is a long delay between obtaining the sampling and analyzing it), there is really no reason not to use plastic syringes if so desired. It has been suggested that the size of syringe should be the smallest that will hold the amount of blood required for analysis in order to minimize the amount of anticoagulant required to fill the dead space of the needle and syringe, with the resulting dilutional effect (see below).[29] However, the same point is served in simply obtaining a larger sample for any given syringe size. Therefore, the size of syringe used is largely a matter of personal preference, although the practitioner should avoid obtaining a sample that is small relative to the size of the syringe.

If the sample is to be obtained from an in-dwelling catheter (see "Procedure" section), an additional "waste syringe" is required.

3. Anticoagulant. An anticoagulant is introduced into the syringe, usually prior to performing the puncture, to prevent the blood from clotting. A number of anticoagulant agents are available, but some may have a deleterious effect on one or more of the blood constituents to be measured. The agent most commonly used is liquid sodium heparin (1,000 IU/ml). Due to concern about the dilutional effect of introducing a liquid into the blood sample, even in small amounts (see *Procedure* section), some have turned to use of lyophilized (dry) heparin. A number of manufacturers now offer "preheparinized" plastic syringes (some of which are also designed to fill as easily from arterial pressure as would a glass syringe).

4. Rubber plug or syringe cap. After obtaining the sample, the syringe must be sealed by inserting the end of the needle into a rubber plug, or by re-

moving the needle and placing a cap, designed for that purpose, on the end of the syringe.

5. Gauze pad(s) or cotton ball(s). Used to compress the puncture site.

6. Antiseptic solution. The puncture site is treated with a suitable antiseptic solution prior to the puncture. Suitable solutions include isopropyl alcohol, povidone-iodine, and chlorhexidine.

7. Container of ice, or other coolant. Most often, once the sample is obtained and the syringe sealed, it is, for reasons discussed later, placed in ice. Preferably a mixture or "slush" of ice and water should be used. The container should be large enough to allow immersion of the syringe at least to the top of the sample. If available, other coolants capable of quickly lowering the temperature of the sample to between 1° and 5°C may be used.[29]

8. (Optional) Local anesthetic solution, syringe(s) and needle(s). If local anesthetic is to be administered (see *Procedure* section), the practitioner will also need the anesthetic solution (commonly 0.5% to 2% lidocaine), a 1- or 2-ml syringe, and a small hypodermic needle (25- or 26-gauge, 1/2 or 5/8-in. length).

Sample Analysis.—Two types of instrumentation are widely used in obtaining the measured variables listed in the Invasive Techniques section of Table 2–5. First is the blood gas analyzer, which provides analysis of oxygen tension P_{O_2}, carbon dioxide tension P_{CO_2}, and pH. Second is the spectrophotometer, which provides identification and quantification of different forms of hemoglobin. Additionally, instrumentation providing direct measurement of oxygen content is available, but is not so commonly used, and will not be discussed here.

Blood Gas Analyzers.—The typical contemporary blood gas analyzer is actually three discrete measuring devices in one unit; P_{O_2}, P_{CO_2}, and pH are each measured by a different electrode. We will outline the function of each separately. There is really no diversity of equipment to be considered here, as all commercial blood gas analyzers use the same essential instrumentation.

The Oxygen Electrode.—Commonly called the Clark electrode, this device is illustrated in Figure 2–26. The Clark electrode is polarographic, consisting of a silver-silver chloride anode, platinum cathode, and potassium chloride bridge. The anode catalyzes an oxidation reaction in which it attracts anions and

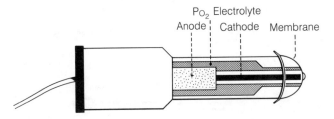

FIG 2–26.
The Clark (oxygen) electrode.

liberates electrons. These electrons flow to the cathode, producing a constant current. When a sample is introduced into the analyzer, oxygen from the blood sample passes through the semipermeable membrane (most commonly made of polypropylene), diffuses through the electrolyte solution in which the electrode is bathed, and migrates to the cathode. There, a polarizing voltage of approximately one-half volt catalyzes a reduction reaction in which electrons are "consumed" by combining with the oxygen and water (in the electrolyte) to form hydroxyl ions. This loss of electrons alters the conductivity of the electrolyte solution, accelerating the flow of electrons between anode and cathode. The resulting change in current between cathode and anode is proportional to the amount of dissolved oxygen in the blood sample. This process is affected by temperature. The presence of the anesthetic agent halothane in analyzed blood also causes erroneous readings of oxygen tension by polarography.

The Carbon Dioxide Electrode.—Also known as the Severinghaus electrode, this device is actually a pH electrode. As shown in Figure 2–27, the electrode is separated from the blood sample by a membrane made of a material (usually silicon) selectively permeable to carbon dioxide. Also, a nylon spacer is placed between the silicon membrane and electrode in order to ensure adequate sodium bicarbonate solution is present in the interstice between membrane and electrode. When a blood sample is introduced into the analyzer, carbon dioxide (in accordance with Henry's law) diffuses across the membrane in proportion to its partial pressure in the sample. The carbon dioxide diffusing into the sodium bicarbonate solution in which the electrode is bathed combines with water to form carbonic acid which in turn forms bicarbonate and hydrogen ions. The change in hydrogen ion concentration thus produced, which is proportional to the amount of carbon dioxide, is measured in the manner described below for pH electrodes. The Severinghaus electrode differs from

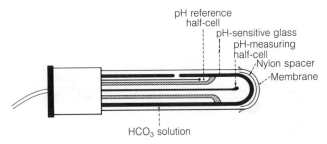

FIG 2–27.
The Severinghaus (carbon dioxide) electrode.

the standard pH electrode in that both half-cells are silver-silver chloride and are contained in one unit.

The pH Electrode.—The pH electrode consists of two half-cells, commonly termed the measuring and reference electrodes, connected by an electrochemical bridge of potassium chloride. Figure 2–28 illustrates this arrangement. The measuring electrode consists of a capillary tube of "pH sensitive" glass (permeable to hydrogen ions) inside a chamber filled with buffer solution of 6.84 pH. The reference cell contains a mercury-mercurous chloride paste known as calomel (the reference half-cell is often referred to as a calomel electrode) which provides a constant reference voltage. When a blood sample is intro-

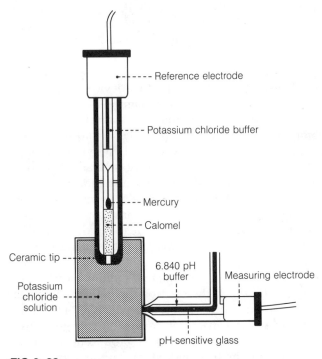

FIG 2–28.
The pH electrode system, showing the measuring and reference electrodes.

duced into the analyzer, part of it enters the capillary tube within the measuring electrode. The sample invokes a voltage across the pH sensitive glass, which is a logarithmic function of the hydrogen ion concentration in the sample, and reflects the difference between the pH of the sample and the 6.84 pH of the measuring electrode buffer. Thus, the change in electrical potential in the circuit composed of measuring electrode, potassium chloride bridge, and reference electrode is a measure of the pH of the introduced sample.

The voltage supplied by the calomel in the reference pH electrode is, like the output of the Clark electrode, affected by temperature. Accordingly, all of the electrodes are commonly enclosed in a constant-temperature water bath or heated block, a practice which also serves other purposes discussed later.

Blood gas analyzers are most often calibrated using gases with known concentrations of oxygen and carbon dioxide, and buffer solutions with known pH. In all three cases, calibration consists of setting a low (or "balance") point and a high (or "slope") point. For the oxygen electrode, the balance point is usually set using 0%, and the slope point 12% to 20%. For the carbon dioxide electrode, the balance point is generally 5%, the slope point 10%. One level of oxygen and one of carbon dioxide are commonly combined in a gas mixture (e.g., 5% CO_2 and 12% O_2, 10% CO_2 and 0% O_2) to reduce the number of tanks involved. The reliability of commercially prepared gases varies considerably, making it advisable to verify the assigned values by some method such as those suggested in the discussion of expired gas measurements. For the pH electrode, the balance point is usually set using a buffer solution with a pH of 6.842, the slope point using one with a pH of 7.384. The accuracy of these buffers should be traceable to National Bureau of Standards (NBS) reference buffers, as are most brands of commercially available pH buffers. If "homemade" buffers are used, these should frequently be checked against NBS referenced buffers.

Most of the currently available blood gas analyzers include circuitry through which the flow of gas into the sample chamber can be controlled; less often they also include a system for infusion of the pH buffers. In many of the newer computerized analyzers, the calibration procedure is completely automated. In a case where introduction of the calibration media is not partly or wholly automated, there are several points to remember. First, the gases should be humidified prior to analysis. Second, the gases should be allowed to flow through the humidifier and analyzer for several minutes before any adjustments are made. Third, the containers of pH buffers should be kept sealed, except when an aliquot is being withdrawn for use in calibration, in order to minimize contamination.

In some settings, calibration of the gas electrodes is performed using tonometered blood rather than gas. Tonometry, of which there are several different methods, is, in the present context, simply the process of exposing a liquid to a flow of gas until the partial pressure of the gas in the liquid is in equilibrium with the source gas. The use of tonometered blood for calibration is preferred by some because of a phenomenon known as the "blood-gas factor." Whether one uses gas or tonometered liquids for calibration, the blood-gas factor is something with which the practitioner should be familiar.

This phenomenon results from the fact that the Clark electrode, as discussed above, consumes oxygen in the process of measuring it, leading to oxygen gradients around the cathode. The gradients so created are different for gas and blood, meaning the recovered values for gas may be higher than those for blood samples even though both have the same partial pressure of oxygen. Thus, calibrating with a gas introduces a certain error into the analysis of blood samples. While the magnitude of the blood gas factor has been reduced in most contemporary analyzers, it is still variously estimated to range from 1.2% to 15% and varies (even within a given analyzer) with a number of factors, most notably the oxygen tension.[2, 16, 24] While some laboratories and computerized analyzers routinely apply a blood-gas factor correction, it is generally agreed that such a correction is of little consequence unless a measured tension is above 100 mm Hg. The blood-gas factor for a particular analyzer would be determined, according to one method, by tonometering blood with a gas containing a precisely determined oxygen concentration, and calculating

$$(P_{O_2}sg - P_{O_2}tb)/P_{O_2}sg$$

where $P_{O_2}sg$ is the partial pressure of oxygen in the source gas, and $P_{O_2}tb$ is the tension of oxygen in the tonometered blood as measured by the analyzer.[36] We prefer to substitute the value actually recovered from introducing the source gas into the analyzer for $P_{O_2}sg$. In either case, this factor would then be multiplied by the gas calibration value, and that amount added to the gas calibration value to derive the number to which the Clark electrode reading is actually set. The blood-gas factor varies in a given analyzer

at different oxygen tensions, making it necessary to determine separate factors for several different ranges of oxygen tensions. The factor may also change with time, and with analyzer maintenance. Thus, at least one source suggests determining the factor daily and whenever the membrane is changed.[23] In some laboratories, the correction is applied to analyzed samples rather than to the calibration setting (see "Data Reduction" section).

The question of the appropriate frequency for calibration of blood gas analyzers requires introduction of the concept of "two-point" versus "one-point" calibration. A full calibration, using two standards for each parameter as described above, is termed a *two-point calibration*. An abbreviated calibration, using one standard for each parameter (usually the high standards for oxygen and pH, and the low for carbon dioxide), is termed a *one-point calibration*. A one-point calibration is made to correct the drift which commonly occurs in blood gas analyzer output over even short periods of time, and to check for analyzer failures, such as a ruptured membrane, which can occur precipitously. A one-point calibration should, by most accounts, be performed prior to *each* sample analysis;[1, 27] at least one source allows it sufficient time to do a single one-point calibration prior to a series of measurements, if several samples are to be analyzed one after another, provided the period of analyses does not exceed 20 minutes.[26] A two-point calibration should be performed at least every 8 hours, while one source suggests one should also be done if the one-point calibration requires readjustment of the P_{O_2} reading by more than 3 mm Hg, or the P_{CO_2} reading by more than 2 mm Hg[26] and another source suggests one should be done after every 50 analyses (or at least every 8 hours).[36] Many computerized analyzers perform one- and/or two-point calibrations automatically at regular intervals.

Quality assurance in blood gas analyzers is usually realized through use of tonometered blood and/or commercially available materials with known values of P_{O_2}, P_{CO_2}, and pH. These commercially available materials utilize a number of different media, including aqueous buffers, emulsified fluorocarbons, hemoglobin solutions, denatured red blood cell solutions, glycerin solutions, etc. Whatever the media, the commercial products usually provide three "levels" which provide values in the low, middle and upper clinical ranges for all three variables. Such "controls" (as they are commonly termed) should be analyzed every 4 to 8 hours, under the same conditions as one would analyze a blood sample. In particular, in analyzers that do not have a preset analysis time (see "Procedure" section), the analysis time used for controls should be the same as that for blood samples. The results of each analysis of a control is compared to the analyzer's historical performance against that control (the three levels for three variables providing nine points for comparison).

This comparison is probably best and most commonly made by means of a Levy-Jennings plot. Such plots (Fig 2–29) display the mean value and standard deviations on the Y-axis and some measure of time (hours, days, shifts) on the X-axis. While the manufacturers of commercial controls generally provide target values and ranges, the mean value and standard deviations should be determined initially, and then recalculated at regular intervals, from the laboratory's own cumulative data. The laboratory's values must fall within the acceptable range provided by the manufacturer, but the range of ±2 SD as calculated from the laboratory's data for each variable should be considerably narrower than the ranges provided by the manufacturer, which are often so wide as to be useless.

In comparing newly recovered control values to Levy-Jennings plots of previous data, the practitioner will be able to detect not only acute failures of the analyzer, but slowly developing malfunctions (e.g., protein contamination) as well, provided he is cognizant of certain patterns. The first pattern is that of a "random error." An unacceptable value is one that lies outside the ±2 standard deviation limits, but by definition 5 of every 100 data points will; the important distinction to be drawn is between an unacceptable point which signals analyzer failure and one that occurs due to chance. When an unacceptable value is recovered, the control is normally run again after the analyzer has been recalibrated. If the second recovered value is within limits, the initial value was a random error; if three recovered values are beyond two standard deviations in the same direction, the analyzer is said to be "out of control,"

and reparation (complete calibration, replacement of membrane, cleaning of electrode, etc.) must be made in accordance with the manufacturer's instructions. Unacceptable points should not be omitted from the record of cumulative data; otherwise, the laboratory's ±2 SD range will gradually become unrealistically narrow. The third pattern is a "shift," which denotes a move of the mean line away from the previous mean line, but still parallel to it. This pattern usually denotes an acute, finite change, which might be something known, such as a membrane change, or something unsuspected, such as a change in analyzer temperature. The fourth pattern is a "trend," which is a gradual, angled divergence of data points from the mean line, which generally denotes an insidious change, such as protein accumulation on an electrode. "Shifts" and "trends" may both result in values that are "out of control," but may also occur within the limits of ±2 SD; even when the values remain within those limits, the occurrence of either pattern should be investigated, as such changes may result in systematic differences in the laboratory's measured values.

An adjunct to the above quality assurance measures is proficiency testing, which consists of running controls, as above, but with the expected recovery values unknown to the laboratory at the time of analysis. The results are sent to the supplier, who later notifies the laboratory of the target values, the performance of all other laboratories participating, and the comparative statistics for the laboratory's own values. Such controls are available from a number of private commercial sources, and participation in such a program by any institution performing blood gas analyses is being required more and more by various regulatory agencies.

Spectrophotometers.—A spectrophotometer consists of a light source that generates one or more particular wavelengths, a cuvette through which the

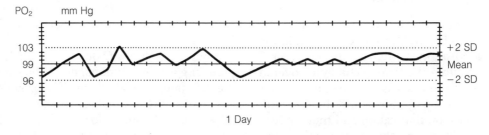

FIG 2–29.
Example of a Levy-Jennings plot of blood-gas quality control data. In this particular example, quality control values for the middle level PO$_2$ control are plotted on a daily basis. Note the mean line, and the lines for ±2 SD.

light is directed, and a photomultiplier which measures the intensity of the light leaving the cuvette. For spectrometers used in blood gas analyses, which are termed *oximeters,* the wavelengths used are those whose vibrational frequencies correspond to various types of hemoglobin, particularly hemoglobin combined with oxygen, or *oxyhemoglobin.* By introducing a blood sample into the cuvette and measuring the absorption of the different wavelengths, the concentration of different forms of hemoglobin can be determined. Simpler spectrophotometers may measure only total hemoglobin and/or oxyhemoglobin, while more sophisticated models may measure one or more of the other forms of hemoglobin, including *carboxy*hemoglobin (combined with carbon monoxide) and *meth*emoglobin (containing ferric iron).

Standard calibration and quality assurance procedures for oximeters are not as well formulated as those for blood gas analyzers. The practitioner should consult the manufacturer's instructions for calibration. There are commercial materials available for quality assurance testing of oximetric values for different types of hemoglobin, but their utility has not been fully established. At the very least, the oximeter should be checked for accuracy of the total hemoglobin measurement by analysis of a sample with a hemoglobin value established by way of a standard technique.

Procedure

As in the case of equipment, the discussion of blood gas procedure will be divided into sample collection and sample analysis.

Sample Collection.—Samples for blood gas analysis are obtained by means of either a "single-stick" arterial puncture or via an in-dwelling catheter.

Arterial Puncture.—While we have consistently stressed the importance of a thorough explanation to the subject prior to commencing all other procedures included in this chapter, our advice regarding arterial punctures is somewhat different. In our experience, a description of what is entailed in an arterial puncture, particularly any allusion to the artery's lying deeper than a vein, may result in unnecessary apprehension; we have found it beneficial in many instances to wait until after the puncture to tell the subject it was an arterial puncture. Of course, the

beginning practitioner, who is less proficient at obtaining the sample quickly, may well want to warn the subject beforehand. If a subject is receiving anticoagulant therapy, the practitioner should confirm with the ordering physician that the puncture is permissible.

1. Select the site of puncture. The two sites most commonly used are the radial artery at the wrist and the brachial artery at the antecubital fossa. Less commonly, the femoral artery below the inguinal ligament is used. Current convention holds the radial artery to be the site of choice, owing to its accessibility, the presence of collateral circulation and presumed greater safety. One author goes so far as to suggest punctures by nonphysicians be limited to the radial artery.[36] We believe this predilection for the radial artery is unjustified. In our experience, brachial artery punctures, when performed by an experienced practitioner, are often less painful (according to subjects who have also had radial punctures, as well as our own observation of subject response) than radial punctures. Furthermore, in the thousands of brachial punctures performed under our supervision, we are unaware of a single incidence of complication. The site used in a given subject, unless proscribed by institutional or other policy, should depend on the practitioner's palpation of the four primary loci (i.e., right and left radial and brachial arteries) to determine which is the most accessible.

2. Cleanse the puncture site with one of the antiseptic solutions discussed earlier, using sterile gauze or cotton to apply it with a circular motion spiraling outward from the intended point of puncture (thereby preventing recontamination).

3. Administer local anesthetic, if necessary. While it might seem, and indeed is often proposed, that local anesthetization is necessary to prevent alteration of blood gas values due to changes in breathing from the pain of the puncture, such has been shown not to be the case.[28] In general, local anesthetic is not necessary, and we recommend its use be reserved for instances in which the subject is particularly apprehensive, or in which the practitioner believes the puncture may be difficult. When it is to be used, the practitioner should determine that the subject does not have a known allergy to the drug. The solution is injected, via a small gauge needle (as discussed above), in approximately equal aliquots into the tissue above the artery and on either side of the artery at the intended point of puncture. The needle is moved to each position by first with-

drawing it nearly to the surface. At each site, the practitioner should pull gently on the plunger prior to injecting the anesthetic in order to ensure the needle is not *in* a blood vessel; if blood is aspirated, the needle must be withdrawn and the procedure resumed with a new needle, syringe, and solution. *Never inject these solutions into a blood vessel.* After withdrawing the needle, rub the area to facilitate absorption, and allow a few minutes for the anesthetic to take effect.

5. Prepare the puncture syringe. If a syringe device containing lyophilized heparin is used, the following steps are unnecessary. Otherwise:

- Attach a needle to the syringe.
- If a multiple-use vial of anticoagulant solution is used, apply isopropyl alcohol, or other antiseptic solution, to the rubber stopper of the vial.
- Draw ½ to 1 ml of solution into the syringe.
- Move the plunger in and out several times to thoroughly coat the interior of the syringe with the anticoagulant.
- If the anticoagulant was taken from a vial with a rubber stopper, remove the needle and replace it with the needle to be used for the punctures. (While the same needle is often used both to withdraw the anticoagulant and to perform the puncture, recommended practice is to use separate ones, as the puncture of the rubber stopper may slightly dull the first needle.)
- Holding the syringe with the needle upward, expel the air; then, with the needle pointing downward, expel the anticoagulant solution through the needle.

This process serves a twofold purpose, both lubricating the syringe and eliminating the air that would otherwise fill the needle and syringe deadspace. However, the liquid anticoagulant itself has a dilutional effect, particularly on carbon dioxide tensions, and the practitioner should be careful to expel all excess solution. Furthermore, reflecting this dilutional effect, it is probably good practice to use the smallest syringe that will contain the desired sample volume. It is of incidental interest that the dilutional effect of solutions such as heparin can be distinguished from that caused by air by the fact dilution with heparin causes little if any change in pH.[4, 14, 38]

6. If the puncture is to be of the radial artery, perform a *modified Allen's test* to demonstrate the presence of collateral circulation in the hand of the wrist to be used. Have the subject form a fist. With both hands, place your fingers, as if taking a pulse, on the radial and ulnar arteries (on opposite sides of the wrist). Apply sufficient pressure to occlude the arteries, and have the subject partially open his hand (which should be blanched). The fingers occluding the ulnar artery are removed while the palm and fingers are observed. The color should return to the palm and fingers within 15 seconds; if not, there is inadequate collateral circulation, and that wrist should not be used for radial puncture.

7. Position the arm appropriately. For radial punctures, the wrist is generally abducted with the palm upward, and the wrist extended. In our experience, placing a rolled towel or something of the sort under the wrist to act as a fulcrum improves the positioning of the artery for puncture. For brachial punctures, the arm is fully extended and rotated until the palpable pulse at the antecubital fossa is maximized. Here too it is sometimes helpful to place a small pillow or rolled towel under the elbow.

8. Palpate the artery and determine the point of puncture. With the hand that will not be holding the syringe, palpate the artery with one or two fingers to determine the size and depth of the artery and the exact point of puncture. Many sources of instruction on arterial punctures suggest palpating with two fingers placed slightly apart, and using the point where the artery passes between them as the puncture target. We have always found it more useful to palpate with one finger or two fingers placed together and aim for the point under the finger(s), with the needle/syringe at an appropriate angle to intersect the artery at its adjudged depth.

9. Perform the puncture. Holding the syringe, most commonly between the thumb and index and middle fingers "as one would hold a dart,"[29] with the bevel of the needle facing upward, penetrate the skin. There is some question as to the best angle at which to enter: one author suggests as small an angle as possible[36] (the syringe being almost parallel to the subject's wrist in the case of radial punctures) in order to make the arterial fenestration oblique and optimize closure when the needle is withdrawn, while another suggests a 45-degree angle;[26] we have generally had the best results using a somewhat greater angle, between 45 and 90 degrees. In theory, the larger the angle, the greater the chance the needle will go completely through the artery, but we have found this consideration to be of little practical import. The angle used will largely be a matter of personal preference; we know of no evidence as to the advantage of any particular angle.

Once the skin is punctured, which should be done quickly, advance the needle slowly toward the targeted point where the artery should lie under or between the finger(s). While advancing the needle, carefully observe the needle hub and syringe for blood flow. As mentioned earlier, use of a needle with a clear or transluscent hub facilitates detection of such blood flow. Ideally, the subject's pulse pressure will cause blood to flow freely into the syringe. With some syringes, or in subjects with low pulse pressure, however, the blood flow may be limited to a small amount entering the needle hub. In any case, once the artery is punctured, the plunger may be *gently* pulled to facilitate filling of the syringe to the desired volume.

In some cases, there will be no blood flow at all when the artery is punctured. Accordingly, if the practitioner feels he has punctured an artery despite the absence of blood flow, he may pull gently on the plunger, which will, not infrequently in such cases, initiate blood flow. Likewise, it is not uncommon to go completely through the artery as the needle is advanced. If the needle is advanced without blood return beyond the point at which the artery should be, the practitioner may slowly withdraw the needle while *intermittently* and *gently* pulling on the plunger. In such cases, many instructional texts suggest the needle be withdrawn near to the surface and advanced again. However, in our experience, the application of *gentle, intermittent* aspirating pressure frequently results in locating the artery as the needle is withdrawn. *It is very important, however, that the pulling on the plunger be gentle and intermittent; the practitioner should never apply strong or continuous apirating force while withdrawing the needle.*

10. Obtain the sample. Once the puncture is effected, collect the desired volume. Although contemporary blood gas analysis instrumentation has significantly reduced the sample volume once required, other factors, including the dilutional effects discussed above and the chance that the sample may have to be analyzed more than once, still make it advisable to collect a relatively large sample, particularly in relation to the size of the syringe when liquid anticoagulant is used (e.g., at least a 2-ml sample when a 3-ml syringe is used, or 3.5 to 4 ml when a 5-ml syringe is used, etc.).

11. Withdraw the needle quickly. Particularly if a glass syringe is used, hold the syringe in such a way as to prevent the plunger from slipping.

12. Compress the puncture site. Once the needle is withdrawn, firm pressure must be applied to the site, using a gauze pad or cotton ball. The length of time pressure should be applied is a source of controversy, with suggestions ranging from as little as 1 minute[26] to as much as 5 minutes.[29] At least one source[36] and our personal experience suggest that the time required is about 2 minutes, longer if the subject is receiving anticoagulant therapy. If the subject is cooperative and able, he may be asked to apply the pressure with his other hand, at least while the practitioner performs the following steps, but the practitioner should be emphatic about the amount of pressure required. Otherwise, many subjects used to venipunctures, will apply inadequate pressure or even believe it sufficient to bend their arms to hold the gauze or cotton in place. After the pressure is removed, the practitioner should observe the site for several minutes for evidence of hematoma. If a hematoma appears to be forming, the practitioner should again apply pressure for several minutes.

13. Ensure the integrity of the sample by:

- Turning the syringe with needle upward (immediately after withdrawing it) and expelling any air bubbles present.
- Sealing the syringe by sticking the needle into a rubber stopper, or by removing the needle and placing a cap on the syringe.
- Rolling the sealed syringe gently between the hands to mix the anticoagulant throughout the sample.

14. Place the sample on ice. Particularly if the sample is not to be analyzed immediately or if it is likely to contain a high oxygen tension, it should be immersed in the ice slush discussed earlier. This action is taken to slow the metabolic activity of cells in the blood sample, a process which would otherwise alter the blood gas values.

Indwelling Catheter.—Indwelling arterial catheters are often installed in subjects from whom multiple samples may be needed, such as those critically ill or from whom samples may be needed when a "single stick" might be difficult, such as during exercise testing. The installation usually includes not only the catheter but also apparatus, sometimes fairly complex, for flushing with anticoagulant solution, collecting samples and/or connecting to monitoring devices. The particular procedure used in obtaining a sample from an indwelling catheter will depend on the configuration of this apparatus. Accordingly, we are limited to providing general guidelines applicable to all such configurations.

1. Prepare the sample syringe as described in step 5 above. For collection from an indwelling catheter, the syringe is used without a needle

2. Aspirate "dead space" contents. In almost all cases, the point at which samples are taken from an indwelling catheter circuit is separated from the actual catheter by a length of tubing which, between sample collections, contains anticoagulant solution. The contents of this conduit must be removed before a blood sample is withdrawn. To do so, a "waste syringe" is connected at the sample collection port, and solution is withdrawn until undiluted blood reaches the syringe. Generally, access to the circuit at the sampling point is controlled by a stopcock, which would be opened for withdrawing solution or blood, and closed for changing syringes or flushing the circuit.

3. Obtain the sample. Connect the sample syringe to the sampling port, and withdraw the desired sample volume.

4. Handle the sample as described in steps 13 and 14 above.

5. Flush the circuit with anticoagulant solution. The anticoagulant solution is commonly in an intravenous infusion bag which is placed in a pressurizing device such as those used for blood transfusions. The pressure in these devices is maintained above systolic blood pressure, allowing the circuit to be flushed as needed or a very slow continuous infusion, sustained to prevent clotting. In most settings, after each sample is taken, the mechanism controlling flow is opened to flush the circuit. The circuit should be flushed only long enough to clear blood from the tubing.

During the entire process of obtaining blood from an indwelling catheter, extreme care must be taken not to introduce air into the circuit or to loosen any connection in the circuit.

Sample Analysis.—The values obtained for various of the blood gas parameters can be significantly affected by mishandling of the sample both prior to analysis (preanalytic errors) and during analysis (analytic errors). In addition to careful sampling technique, as discussed above, the chance of preanalytic errors can be reduced by (1) ensuring any air in the syringe is expelled before the syringe is sealed, (2) promptly placing the sample in the ice slush (or other coolant), and (3) minimizing the time between the sample being drawn and being analyzed. The chance of analytic error is reduced

by use of careful technique. Discussion of analysis technique, like equipment, will be separated into that for blood gas analyzers and that for spectrophotometers.

Blood Gas Analyzers.—The precise series of steps performed to prepare and use an analyzer for blood gas analyses will obviously be different for different analyzers, and the practitioner should follow the manufacturer's instructions. There is, however, a common, *general* procedure.

1. Ensure that the analyzer temperature is at 37°C. As we will discuss again regarding data reduction, the P_{O_2}, P_{CO_2}, and pH of blood all change with changes in temperature. We have already noted that the intrinsic performance of both the pH reference (calomel) and Clark electrodes is also affected by temperature. Both considerations make it imperative the analyzer temperature be closely controlled.

2. Perform a one-point calibration as outlined in the section on quality control and assurance. As the reader will remember, performance of a one-point calibration is recommended prior to each analysis or set of analyses.

3. Thoroughly mix the sample by rolling it between the hands, rotating it vigorously, etc.

4. Introduce the sample into the analyzer. In some analyzers, the blood is aspirated through a probe introduced into the tip of the syringe, while in others the blood is injected. (In at least a couple of older models of blood gas analyzer, both modes are utilized; part of the sample is injected for analysis of gas tensions, while a separate portion is aspirated for determination of pH). If using an aspiration-type analyzer, the operator should be careful to keep the probe well into the blood so as not to inadvertently mix air into the aspirated sample inside the analyzer cuvette. Following aspiration of the sample, immediately expel the air that will have been pulled into the syringe, so as to maintain anaerobic conditions of the sample for repeat analysis. If using an injection-type analyzer, it is generally prudent practice (and specifically recommended by some manufacturers) to use what is termed a *double-injection* or *double-push* technique. With this technique, the operator injects one bolus of blood, and (leaving the syringe in the sample port) waits 15 seconds or so and injects a second bolus. The purpose of this maneuver is to facilitate removal of bubbles within the analyzer cuvette.

5. Take the analyzer readings after a specific time interval. Complete response of the Clark electrode may take several minutes following input of a sample, waiting for which is generally impractical. Common practice is to take readings at a specific interval, such as 60, 90, or 120 seconds, following introduction of the sample. Such a practice introduces consistency into the values derived in any particular laboratory. Many automated analyzers extrapolate the reading to what it would be at full response, thus providing both quick and full response. As intimated earlier, it is important that the same interval be used for samples and quality assurance materials.

6. Repeat the analysis. The sample should be analyzed at least twice. Ideally, in settings with more than one analyzer, the repeat analysis would be on a different analyzer. The values obtained in the two analyses should agree to within ± 3 mm Hg for PO_2 and PCO_2 and to within ± 0.02 units for pH.[26]

Spectrophotometers.—Again, the reader is referred to the manufacturer's instructions for the particular oximeter used. In general, the important points to remember are similar to those for blood gas analyzers: (1) the blood sample must be extremely well-mixed; (2) the temperature of the cuvette must be carefully controlled; and (3) the sample introduced into the cuvette must be free of bubbles. Furthermore, correct analysis by spectrophotometry requires hemolysis of the blood sample by either chemical or mechanical means, which may need to be increased for samples of blood containing aberrant hemoglobin.

Data Reduction

The data reduction associated with blood gas measurements includes adjustments of the primary measurements and calculation of derived parameters. There are two adjustments of the primary measurements to be considered; we have already alluded to both. The first is the blood-gas factor, by which PO_2 measurements are corrected (upward) if the analyzer was calibrated with gas. This factor reflects the difference in the way the Clark electrode measures gas and blood. Most commonly, the adjustment, if made at all, is made in the calibration value to which the electrode is set. It may be preferred, however, to adjust recovered sample values, in which case the factor might only be applied to PO_2 values greater than 100 mm Hg.

The second adjustment to the primary measurements is temperature correction. The primary measurements all vary with changes in temperature as a result of which analyses are usually performed with the sample at 37°C to replicate the temperature in the subject from which it was taken. If, however, the subject is hypo- or hyperthermic, analyzing the sample at 37°C will alter the in vivo values. There is considerable controversy as to whether the in vitro measurements in such cases should be corrected mathematically for the difference in the subject's temperature. Our recommendation is that such corrections not be made for three reasons. First, despite the best attempts to make it clear the results are corrected for temperature, such results will invariably be separated from the fact they are so adjusted, and resultantly misinterpreted. Second, there is little understanding of the meaning of altered values in the presence of dysthermia. Third, comparison of serial analyses becomes problematic if the subject's temperature is changing; reporting all values as measured at 37°C provides a common reference.

While arguing against actually changing the reported values, we do stress the importance of the practitioner's understanding the effect of temperature on blood gas indices. Qualitatively, PO_2 and PCO_2 change directly with temperature, while pH changes inversely (i.e., as temperature rises, PO_2 and PCO_2 are increased, and pH is decreased). Quantitatively, within the clinical range of temperatures and blood gas values, the change is *roughly* 7% in PO_2, 4% to 5% in PCO_2, and 0.013 to 0.015 pH units per degree centigrade of change in temperature. If the practitioner does choose to correct reported values, he will need to use one of the several more exacting formulae or nomograms available.

Most of the derived values in Table 2–5 can be calculated, but in many cases the formulae are so complex as to make actual calculation unrealistic in the clinical setting. In these cases, including common ones such as oxyhemoglobin saturation (SO_2) and bicarbonate (HCO_3), the parameters are derived from tables or nomograms that are widely available. The present discussion will be limited to two parameters that the practitioner should be able to calculate, and for which understanding of the mathematical derivation enhances understanding of the concept. The two parameters are alveolar-arterial oxygen difference and oxygen content.

The *alveolar-arterial oxygen difference*, $P(A-a)O_2$ or $A-aPO_2$, is often termed the *alveolar-arterial oxygen gradient* (it is, however, a simple difference, not a *gradient*). It is a measure in mm Hg of the difference between the oxygen inspired, relative to the level of ventilation, and that which finds its way into the blood. As such, it is probably the most useful single measure of *respiratory* gas exchange. To determine $P(A-a)O_2$, first calculate PAO_2, which introduces a fundamental concept with which all respiratory therapy practitioners should be acquainted, namely, the "ideal alveolar air equation." This equation, which permits estimation of the oxygen tension which should be present on the lung side of the alveolar-capillary interface, holds that

$$PAO_2 = [(PB - 47) \times FIO_2] - (PaCO_2 \times [FIO_2 + (1 - FIO_2)/R])$$

where R is the respiratory exchange ratio, and arterial carbon dioxide ($PaCO_2$) is taken to equal alveolar carbon dioxide. As long as the FIO_2 is around 0.21, the above equation may be simplified to

$$PAO_2 = [(PB - 47) \times FIO_2] - (PaCO_2/R)$$

or, if the respiratory exchange ratio is unknown,

$$(PAO_2 = [(PB - 47) \times FIO_2] - (PaCO_2 \times 1.25)$$

reflecting an assumed value of 0.8 for the respiratory exchange ratio. However, this simplified version is not valid if the respiratory exchange ratio is known to be other than 0.8, or the FIO_2 is significantly different than 0.21. Once PAO_2 is determined, the $P(A-a)O_2$, as the label makes clear, is figured as

$$P(A - a)O_2 = PAO_2 - PaO_2$$

Oxygen content (CO_2) is the total amount of oxygen carried in the blood, in milliliters of O_2 per deciliter of blood, or volume percent. As such, it is calculated by adding the amount of oxygen carried in combination with hemoglobin to that dissolved in the plasma. The amount of combined oxygen is calculated as

$$Hb \times 1.39 \times SO_2$$

where Hb is hemoglobin in grams per deciliter, and 1.39 is the amount of oxygen (in milliliters) that can combine with 1 gm of hemoglobin (this constant is variously given as 1.34 and 1.39, and there appears to be little consensus as to which should be used). The amount of dissolved oxygen is calculated as

$$PO_2 \times 0.0031$$

where 0.0031 is the solubility coefficient for oxygen in blood. Combining the two forms of carriage

$$CO_2 = (Hb \times 1.39 \times SO_2) + (PO_2 \times 0.0031)$$

Noninvasive Techniques

Although blood gas measurements derived from analysis of blood withdrawn from the subject are the "gold standard," such determinations have at least two serious drawbacks. First, they are invasive, with attendant discomfort for the subject and the possibility, however slight, of complication. Second, they are episodic, which is to say they are available only for those specific points in time when a sample was taken. Both considerations have led to the development of certain noninvasive alternatives, which, though limited in application, have proven useful in some settings where obtaining a blood sample is not practical, or where continuous monitoring is desired. While methods for noninvasive determination of both oxygen and carbon dioxide are available, the present discussion will be limited to those for oxygen, which are more established than those for carbon dioxide. We will consider two widely employed modalities for the noninvasive determination of oxygen: (1) the ear oximeter, and (2) the transcutaneous electrode.

Equipment

The ear oximeter and the transcutaneous electrode are variations of devices already discussed: the ear oximeter is a spectrophotometric device, and the transcutaneous electrode is a polarographic device.

Ear Oximeter.—An ear oximeter employs the same operating principle as the oximeter used for in vitro measurements we have already discussed. The path between the light source and the detector is contained in a small unit which fits onto the ear (or, alternatively in some models, on the finger). The light passing through the ear and onto the photomultiplier provides determination of oxyhemoglobin saturation, just as with the standard type of oximeter. The ear is, in effect, the oximeter cuvette. The ear is heated by the device to "arterialize" the blood by means of vasodilation.

Ear oximeters are generally capable of measuring oxyhemoglobin saturation above 60% with an accuracy of approximately ±2%, and have proven utility in a number of applications, including exercise testing and sleep testing. The ear oximeter is most useful when utilized to detect *changes* in saturation over time, and much less acceptable for discrete determinations of saturation; indeed, the practitioner should be judicious in using the ear oximeter for "spot checks."

The convenience of the ear oximeter makes it very attractive for use in a broad spectrum of circumstances, but there are limitations. First, an ear oximeter measures saturation. This obvious fact is emphasized because, at least in our experience, the convenience of the ear oximeter has tended to blur the distinction between oxygen tension and oxyhemoglobin saturation, and led to the substitution of saturation for tension in cases where the two are not interchangeable. Furthermore, the ear oximeter assumes a normal relationship between saturation and tension, a relationship that may well not be normal in some types of subjects likely to be studied with the ear oximeter. It is sometimes suggested, and we concur, that when possible, a blood gas sample should be obtained from any subject on whom an ear oximeter is to be used, the relationship between tension and saturation for that subject established, and ear oximetry values viewed in light of any abnormality in that relationship.

The second limitation of ear oximetry is that a number of factors affect its accuracy by altering light absorption. These factors include increased bilirubin and increased carboxyhemoglobin. A third limitation is the ear oximeter's dependency on local perfusion to the ear. In order for the arterialized capillary blood to reflect arterial oxyhemoglobin saturation levels, the perfusion to the ear must be such as to provide oxygen in excess of that consumed by metabolism. Thus, the ear oximeter will not be accurate in the presence of decreased peripheral perfusion, as might occur with low blood volume or decreased cardiac output. A fourth factor that limits employment of the ear oximeter is its occasional failure in subjects with very dark pigmentation.

Most models of ear oximeter provide for electronic simulation of one or more output values, which is intended to serve as a calibration check. Generally, there is no ready means of adjustment if these simulations are incorrect. The only useful means of quality assurance for an ear oximeter is comparison of its reading to saturation determined on a blood sample taken from a subject who has a stable reading on the ear oximeter at the time the sample is drawn. The two measurements should agree to within ±2%.

Transcutaneous Electrode.—It has long been known that there is respiratory gas exchange through the human skin. By heating the skin (commonly to 43°C) to enhance this gas movement and applying electrodes in such a way as to prevent interference from ambient gases, blood-gas tensions can be quantitated. The transcutaneous oxygen electrode is similar to the Clark electrode used in blood-gas analyzers, with the addition of a heating element and thermistor to control skin temperature.

Transcutaneous oxygen tension ($tcPO_2$) has been shown to correlate fairly well with PaO_2 in general, although the correlation varies markedly for different types of subjects in different clinical circumstances. One excellent monograph on the subject of transcutaneous oxygen measurement reports PaO_2 versus $tcPO_2$ correlation coefficients as high as 0.99 in some applications, but as low as 0.52 in others.[18] Historically, the best correlation has been in neonates and infants (purportedly because of their thinner, more permeable skin). It is sometimes suggested that a discrepancy between PaO_2 and $tcPO_2$, when present, may be clinically significant, as in the detection of early shock.

The transcutaneous electrode, like the ear oximeter, has proven invaluable in certain settings, but there are a number of limiting factors. The accuracy of the transcutaneous electrode is even more susceptible than the ear oximeter to changes in perfusion to the electrode site. It is also affected by thickness of the subject's skin, making it unusable in some adults. Anesthetic agents, halothane in particular, affect the electrode's performance in this context, just as in the case of the Clark electrode used in blood gas analyzers.

Most transcutaneous electrodes can be calibrated by in vitro and/or in vivo means. In vitro calibration usually consists of setting the zero point and a span point, using either gas or liquids. The gases used are commonly 100% nitrogen for the zero point, and room air for the span point. If the transcutaneous monitor is to be used in the likely presence of arterial oxygen tensions below or above the normal clinical range for adult subjects (e.g., neonates or subjects breathing pure oxygen), a gas with an appropriate concentration of oxygen should be substituted for room air, or used as a third calibration point. Ideally, the gases should be humidified, but may be used dry without a clinically significant error.[18] If liquids are used (and their use is not recommended in some transcutaneous electrode systems), a reducing agent (such as $Na_2S_2O_4$) provides the zero point, while a solution tonometered with the appropriate concentration of oxygen provides the span. Whichever approach is used, it is critical that the temperature be maintained during calibration. The manufacturer's literature should be consulted for the specific calibration routine for a particular electrode system.

Calibration of transcutaneous electrodes by in vitro methods is somewhat suspect, particularly when the electrode is to be used in adult subjects, because differences in skin permeability result in a variability of in vivo performance. In vivo calibration is achieved, as with the ear oximeter, by obtaining a blood gas sample, and comparing the results. Any $tcPO_2$-PaO_2 difference thus determined might be used to adjust the transcutaneous electrode reading or, alternatively, to determine a conversion factor, with the actual measure of $tcPO_2$ left alone. If the electrode is located on a limb, the zero point may also be checked in vivo by momentarily inflating a blood pressure cuff on the limb to eliminate perfusion to it.[18]

Procedure

The cardinal points in using either the ear oximeter or transcutaneous electrode are proper preparation of the site and proper attachment of the device.

Ear Oximeter.—Some models of ear oximeter are attached to the antihelix of the pinna, while others are attached to the lobe.

1. Prepare the site. The site should be cleansed with alcohol to remove body oils, which may interfere with the oximeter's performance, and thoroughly dried. The site should then be vigorously rubbed between the operator's fingers to provide an initial increase in perfusion to the spot.

2. Attach the probe. Of the two models of ear oximeter in widespread use, one simply clips onto the ear, while the other is fastened to a support strapped to the head. Particularly in the latter case, it is necessary to secure the cable connecting the ear probe to the unit's electronics in such a way as to prevent its movement from dislodging the probe. In subjects with longer hair, the operator will also want to ensure that no hair strands, which may also interfere with performance, are caught in the ear probe.

3. Wait for arterialization. Wait the length of time specified by the manufacturer or until readings become stable before recording any measurements. (Of course, as discussed earlier, in some subjects with labile peripheral perfusion, the readings may never become completely stable.)

The ear oximeter, which is generally heated to only 41°C, can be worn for hours with no deleterious effect.

Transcutaneous Electrode.—The transcutaneous electrode is far more susceptible to erroneous readings due to improper technique than is the ear oximeter. Accordingly, the practitioner should carefully review the manufacturer's instructions on the use of the device.

1. Choose the site. In the case of the transcutaneous electrode, the first step is to determine the site at which the electrode is to be applied. This choice of site is an important decision because different parts of the integument have different perfusion-to-oxygen consumption relationships, meaning that variably accurate reflections of arterial oxygenation will be obtained depending on the placement of the electrode. In general, the skin at the measurement site should be smooth, hairless (although it can be shaved), thin, located over a large capillary bed, in a convenient position, and devoid of scar tissue, blemishes, abrasions, or other lesions. Suitable sites include the chest (particularly in newborns), the neck by the carotid artery, the inside of the forearm, the inside of the thigh, and, in neonates, the abdomen and back. Other than shaving, if necessary, no skin preparation is necessary or recommended. Indeed, practices sometimes suggested, such as application of vasodilating substances, or "stripping" the skin to remove dead cells by applying and removing adhesive tape repeatedly, have been shown to be unnecessary, harmful, or both.[18] If the subject's skin is moist, cleansing it with alcohol or acetone may improve the chances of the electrode's remaining attached.

2. Apply the electrode. The electrode should be applied according to the instructions of the manufacturer. Normally, an adhesive ring, which provides a good seal between the electrode and the skin, is applied to the electrode body. A drop of distilled water, which improves conductivity between skin and electrode, is placed on the precise spot where the cathode surface of the electrode is to be placed. Once the electrode is in place and readings have stabilized, the integrity of the adhesive seal can be tested by blowing 100% nitrogen around the electrode and noting no change in reading.

3. Secure the electrode, if necessary. If the subject is not horizontal during the period of measurement, it may be necessary to secure the electrode to the subject with tape to prevent the weight of the

electrode from pulling on the adhesive ring and creating breaches in the seal. However, the electrode should not be taped with excessive pressure, which might interfere with local perfusion.

4. Monitor the electrode temperature. Due to the significant effect of changes in electrode temperature on the output of the transcutaneous electrode, it is important to monitor and, if necessary, adjust the electrode temperature.

5. Reposition the electrode periodically. As a result of the electrode temperature required to maintain hyperemia, it is necessary to change the electrode site periodically if the electrode is to be used on a subject for an extended period. While the electrode may remain at one site for as long as 6 hours in a healthy adult, it may be necessary to change it as frequently as every hour in subjects who are suffering shock or hypothermia.[18] The operator should carefully monitor the area surrounding the electrode for redness and move, or at least remove, the electrode should such appear.

Data Reduction

The specific format in which results for either the ear oximeter or the transcutaneous electrode are reported will depend on the application and personal preference. For example, reported values might be readings at specific intervals during exercise testing, readings taken at the time of certain occurrences such as suctioning, or readings batched to reflect the amount of time spent at different values during sleep abnormality testing.

REFERENCES

1. Adams AP, Morgan-Hughes JO, Sykes MK: pH and blood gas analysis, methods of measurement and sources of error using electrode systems. *Anaesthesia* 1967; 22:575–597.
2. Bird BD, Williams J, Whitman JG: The blood gas factor: A comparison of three different oxygen electrodes. *Br J Anaesth* 1974; 46:249–252.
3. Boushey HA, Dawson A: Spirometry and flow-volume curves, in Clausen JL (ed): *Pulmonary Function Guidelines and Controversies.* New York, Academic Press, 1982, pp 61–82.
4. Bradley JG: Errors in the measurement of blood P_{CO_2} due to dilution of the sample with heparin solution. *Br J Anaesth* 1972; 44:231.
5. Burns KL: An evaluation of two instruments for assessing airway flow. *Ann Allergy* 1979; 43:246–249.
6. Cook CD, Mead J, Orzalesi MM: Static volume-pressure characteristics of the respiratory system during maximal efforts. *J Appl Physiol* 1964; 19:1016–1022.
7. Cotes JE: *Lung Function Testing Guidelines and Controversies.* New York, Academic Press, 1982, pp 91–97.
8. Dawson A: Pneumotachography, in Clausen JL (ed): *Pulmonary Function Testing Guidlines and Controversies.* New York, Academic Press, 1982, pp 91–97.
9. Eichenhorn MS, Beauchamp RK, Harper PA, et al: An assessment of three portable peak flow meters. *Chest* 1982; 82:306.
10. Ferris BG: Epidemiology standardization project. *Am Rev Respir Dis* 1978; 118:1–120.
11. Gardner RM, Backer DC, Braemice AM Jr, et al: ATS statement—Snowbird workshop on standardization of spirometry. *Am Rev Respir Dis* 1979; 119:831–838.
12. Gardner RM, Hankinson JL, West JB: Evaluating commercially available spirometers. *Am Rev Respir Dis* 1980; 121:73–82.
13. Hankinson JD, Viola JO: Dynamic BTPS correction factors for spirometric data. *J Appl Physiol* 1983; 55:1354–1360.
14. Hanson JE, Simmons DH: A systematic error in the determination of blood P_{CO_2}. *Am Rev Respir Dis* 1977; 115:1061–1063.
15. Hathirat S, Renzetti AD, Mitchell M: Measurement of the total lung capacity by helium dilution in a constant volume system. *Am Rev Respir Dis* 1970; 102:760.
16. Herring K, et al: Response of the oxygen electrode to various calibration materials (abstract). *Respir Care* 1979; 25:59–60.
17. Hetzel MR, Williams IP, Shakespeare RM: Can patients keep their own peak flow records reliably? *Lancet* 1979; 1:597–599.
18. Huch R, Huch A, Lubbers DW: *Transcutaneous PO_2.* New York, Thieme-Stratton Inc, 1981.
19. Inshkin D, Patel A, Calvarese B, et al: Overestimation of forced expiratory volumes and flowrates measured by volumetric spiratometry when ATPS to BTPS correction is applied. *Am Rev Respir Dis* (abstract). 1981; 123:83.
20. Jackson JM: Peak expiratory flows. *Br Med J* 1961; 1:1750.
21. Jalowayski AA, Dawson A: Measurement of lung volume: The multiple breath nitrogen method, in Clausen JL (ed): *Pulmonary Function Guidelines and Controversies.* New York, Academic Press, 1981, pp 115–127.
22. Joint Committee on Pulmonary Nomenclature: Pulmonary terms and symbols—Report of the ACCP-ATS. *Chest* 1975; 67:583–592.
23. Kanner RE, Morris AH (ed): *Clinical Pulmonary Function Testing: A Manual of Uniform Laboratory Procedures for the Intermountain Area.* Salt Lake City, Intermountain Thoracic Society, 1975.
24. Leary ET, Delaney CJ, Kenny MA: Use of equilibrated blood for internal blood gas quality control. *Clin Chem* 1977; 23:493–503.
25. McPherson SP: *Respiratory Therapy Equipment.* St Louis, CV Mosby Co, 1977.

26. Mohler JG, et al: Blood gases, in Clausen JL (ed): *Pulmonary Function Guidelines and Controversies.* New York, Academic Press, 1982, pp 223–257.

27. Moran RF: External factors influencing blood gas analysis: Quality control revisited. *Am J Med Tech* 1979; 45:1009–1011.

28. Morgan EJ, et al: The effects of unanesthetized arterial puncture on P_{CO_2} and pH. *Am Rev Resp Dis* 1979; 120:795–798.

29. National Committee for Clinical Laboratory Standards: Tentative Guidelines for the Percutaneous Collection of Arterial Blood for Laboratory Analysis. *NCCLS Publication:* Vol 1, No 10, 1979.

30. Norton AC, Wilmore JH: Effects of water vapor on respiratory measurements and calculations. *Analyzer* 1980; 9:6–9.

31. Perks WH, Cole M, Steventon RD, et al: An evaluation of the vitalograph pulmonary monitor. *Br J Dis Chest* 1981; 75:161–164.

32. Perks WH, Tams IP, Thompson DA, et al: An evaluation of the Mini-Wright peak flow meter. *Thorax* 1979; 34:79–81.

33. Pierson DJ, Dick NP, Petty TL: A comparison of spirometric values with subjects in standing and sitting positions. *Chest* 1976; 70:17–20.

34. Ritchie B: A comparison of forced expiratory volume and peak flow in clinical practice. *Lancet* 1962; 2:271.

35. Ruppel G: *Manual of Pulmonary Function Testing,* ed 3. St Louis, CV Mosby Co, 1982.

36. Shapiro BA, Harrison RA, Walton JR: *Clinical Application of Blood Gases,* ed 3. Chicago, Year Book Medical Publishers, 1982.

37. Shephard RJ: Some observations or peak expiratory flow. *Thorax* 1962; 17:39.

38. Sigaard-Andersom O: Sampling and storing of blood for determination of acid-base status. *Scand J Clin Invest* 1961; 13:196–204.

39. Snow M: Instrumentation, in Clausen JL (ed): *Pulmonary Function Testing Guidelines and Controversies.* New York, Academic Press, 1982, pp 27–47.

40. Sobol BJ: Spirometry and forced flow studies in Chusel EL (ed): *The Selective and Comprehensive Testing of Adult Pulmonary Function.* Mount Kisco, NY, Futura Publishing Co, 1983, pp 29–53.

41. Tinker CM: Peak expiratory flows. *Br Med J* 1961; 2:177.

42. Townsend MC: Spirometric forced expiratory volumes measured in the standing versus the sitting posture. *Am Rev Respir Dis* 1984; 130:123–124.

43. Ullah MI, Cuddihy V, Saunders KB, et al: How many blows really make an FEV_1, FVC, or PEFR? *Thorax* 1983; 38:113–118.

44. Zarins LP: Closed circuit helium dilution method of lung volume measurements, in Clausen JL (ed): *Pulmonary Function Guidelines and Controversies.* New York, Academic Press, 1982, pp 129–140.

Interpretation of Patient Assessment Data

Edward P. Didier, M.D.

The nature of physical assessment of patients with respiratory problems and the forms used in recording patient data have been discussed in Chapters 1 and 2. The purpose of this chapter is to describe the process whereby these sometimes seemingly random lists of data are processed into one or more diagnoses in preparation for the final step—development of the respiratory care plan (see Chapter 4). Clearly the topic is too large to be covered comprehensively, and the student will soon see that experience is the best teacher when it comes to knowing what is going on with his patients.

Although most hospitalized patients may be presumed to have some form of disease or disorder, the perceived "illness" of the patient may not appear consistent with the actual or presumed diagnosis. To be aware of this is to be able to successfully treat the patient and not his chart. There is an enormous variability among patients to the perception of and reaction to pain, to the physical consequences of the disease or disorder, to the social and psychological reactions of family and friends and to the various treatment options available. A comprehensive utilitarian concept of the patient's illness includes consideration of his ability to perceive and manage all of these factors as well as to deal with the physical consequences of his disease. It is important that those involved in the care of the patient consider these qualities as well as the "hard" information generated by the diagnostic investigation.

"NORMAL" PATIENT DATA (VALUES)

Biological data are rarely considered as absolute values, but rather as being within or outside of a "normal range." Even this normal range of values should not be construed as having a sharp border, since individual or temporal variation, sampling error, or contamination may result in "abnormal" values in the absence of real disease or disorder and vice versa. Similarly, some patients with chronic disease (to which they have accommodated or for which they have compensated) may show test results that are outside of the biologic norms but represent the patient's "normal" value for the chronic disease state. For example, many patients with chronic obstructive pulmonary disease live with an arterial carbon dioxide tension (Pa_{CO_2}) well above the normal range. They may also have an arterial oxygen tension (Pa_{O_2}) lower than the predicted value. In effect, they have established their own normal values that could be of importance should they ever require ventilatory support for any reason. In this event, the clinician should strive to return this type of patient to *his* range rather than the "normal" normal.

Finally, because of the large number of interrelated variables in biologic systems, it is rare that one single laboratory value is sufficient for a comprehensive diagnosis. Generally, each finding must relate to the others in a predictable manner that will assure the clinician that he is on the right track before recommending a specific course of treatment. Not all patient complaints can be attributed to a single disease or disorder, and diagnostic tests are selected to provide the greatest information at a practical minimum of cost and discomfort. For example, a patient may be unaware that he has arteriosclerotic, cardiovascular, and chronic obstructive pulmonary disease, but is admitted to the hospital for treatment of an incapacitatingly painful hip due to degenerative changes. The history, physical examination, and diagnostic "routine" laboratory work may suggest the presence of the first two disorders, and further investigation may be ordered to direct appropriate and safe management of the hip problem.

In the remainder of this chapter, we will discuss the acquisition, arrangement, and interpretation of patient data on the basis of the individual item as well as the major interrelationships between items. We will confine the examples and illustrations to pulmonary and cardiopulmonary diseases, but the same general principles apply to patients with diseases of other organ systems. Obviously, the discussion in this chapter cannot be encyclopedic because of space limitations. The objective will be to provide the reader with an understanding of the sequential nature of acquiring and interrelating patient data for diagnosis and treatment. This organized approach will help avoid unnecessary procedures and most effectively use resources, and can be applied in almost any situation.

HOSPITAL ADMISSION DATA

When a patient has a significant medical complaint, he usually seeks the advice of a physician, most usually in the physician's office, clinic, or emergency department. The physician may have a variety of laboratory tests and diagnostic procedures available to him, or he may have very few. In the latter case, after listening to the patient, asking questions, and performing an examination, the physician may order laboratory tests, x-rays, and other diagnostic tests from freestanding facilities (capable of performing them) or may refer the patient to the hospital for these procedures if the medical condition of the patient or the complexity of the laboratory procedure warrants this approach.

On admission to the hospital, there is usually an information-gathering routine which is necessary to establish the database described in Chapter 1. When practical, height, weight, and general appearance are noted and recorded by the admitting nurse,

along with a brief history of current medication and drug use, and "vital signs." These usually include temperature, pulse rate, respiratory rate, and blood pressure. In some instances, where local custom dictates, there is also an "admitting" chest x-ray, blood cell count, and urinalysis, although more and more of these "routine" tests are omitted unless specifically ordered by the physician.

The Medical History

The medical history is reported in a section of the hospital chart and may vary from a relatively few words to an encyclopedic presentation of every detail that the patient can recall or which can be extracted from family and previous medical records. The length of the history varies depending on the nature and severity of the illness, the type of institution, the desires of the physician as well as institutional custom. The medical history is necessarily short if the patient is unable (or unwilling) to give one, or if no relatives or other knowledgeable friends or witnesses are available.

The Physical Examination

The physical examination should be thorough and comprehensive. In actual fact, the examination may vary somewhat in completeness. This examination usually progresses from the patient's head to his toes, and all audible, visible, or palpable abnormalities are listed and described. If the chief complaint or the presumed diagnosis is referable to a single organ system or anatomic area, particular scrutiny may be devoted to this locale, but ideally the whole patient is examined with diligence, at least in the first examination. In subsequent visits, only one or two systems, e.g., heart and lungs, may be examined. Physical examination of the chest is discussed in Chapter 1.

HOSPITAL CARE RECORD
Nurses' Notes

Whatever is done for or to the patient is customarily listed sequentially in the nurses' notes, which also may provide information on the mood, attitude, and ability of the patient to cooperate or help himself. If the patient is admitted to an intensive care unit or a coronary care unit, there may be special forms or flow sheets to help keep specific information in an easy to use manner.

Treatment Records

In another section of the hospital chart are tabulated the drugs and medications, fluids, procedures, and other ministrations—usually in chronological order. If appropriate, a running summary of intake and output is kept here. By this means, the physician can conveniently check if all medications are administered as ordered, and continuously assess the nutritional and fluid status of the patient. In many hospitals, respiratory therapy records are found in a separate part of the chart.

Laboratory Reports

Most often, laboratory results, certain radiographic reports, and some special studies are kept in a specific section of the hospital chart. Usually they are presented in chronological order, and frequently arranged in color coded or tab coded groups, so one may efficiently find blood chemistry, hematology, microbiology, urinalysis, and special studies reports.

Results of special studies, such as ultrasound scans, angiography, special electrocardiograms, high-technology imaging, pathologists' reports, pulmonary function tests, and nuclear medicine reports are provided on appropriately designed forms that can be identified at a glance and located easily. Such reports may also include a narrative description of the findings as well as the images, graphs, and tracings generated during the examination.

THE DIAGNOSIS: AN EXAMPLE

In order to better visualize the diagnostic process, let us now consider the case of a hypothetical female patient who is admitted to the hospital for treatment of degenerative arthritis of the hip. For the purpose of illustration, let us assume that she is not aware of any disorder other than her painful hip, which has finally caused her to miss work and seek medical help. Since our patient is fictitious, we will create for her a complex hospital course with enough complications so that we can evolve a reasonable number of diagnostic regimens and a complex data acquisition course.

History and Physical Examination

The admission routine discloses two important facts: blood pressure is 160/100 mm Hg (above the normal range) and the patient has a productive cough, particularly bothersome in the morning.

While she tells the doctor she is in the hospital because of a painful hip, he is about to gain additional important information by questioning. The history reveals the following details: (1) the hip pain has been progressive over the past 5 years; (2) the patient has been a 1 pack/day cigarette smoker for 45 of her 60 years, with occasional bouts of productive coughing and "loud breathing," as well as the morning cough. She has never taken medicine other than aspirin and proprietary medicines and uses no alcohol other than occasional beer. Other than in the hip, she has not been bothered by pains or aches that have caused her to seek medical help. She has never been told that she has high blood pressure.

Her history provides several indications (or clues) that she may have lung disease and possibly cardiovascular disease, so further information will be sought via the physical examination. The positive findings of the initial physical examination are as follows: she has a ruddy complexion with a darker hue during coughing, coarse rhonchi over both lung bases that clear somewhat with cough, and fine wheezes during expiration. The blood pressure is measured several times in both arms while sitting and lying down and is found to be 160/180 mm Hg systolic 100/110 mm Hg diastolic. Heart size is at the upper limit or normal by percussion, murmurs are not heard, and the neck shows no excessive jugular venous engorgement. The remainder of the physical examination is within normal limits except for limitation of motion and pain of the hip. An orthopedic surgeon has thoroughly evaluated this problem and the results of his consultation are on the chart.

Discussion

Both the history and physical examination have indicated the strong possibility of pulmonary and cardiovascular disease. The fact that the patient has a 45 pack-year history (one package of cigarettes a day for 45 years) is enough to cause her doctor to suspect the patient has also developed some of the symptoms of chronic obstructive pulmonary disease, as suggested by coughing and wheezing. The darkening of her complexion during coughing suggests that her oxygen saturation decreases with forced exhalation and she may well be found to have developed an increased hemoglobin concentration in order to increase the oxygen-carrying capacity of her blood. Rhonchi indicate the presence of secretions in the larger airways and support a diagnosis of chronic bronchitis. The wheezes indicate the presence of airway obstruction, but do not quantitate the extent of damage. Blood pressure measurements are taken in upper and lower extremeties and bilaterally to rule out anatomical vascular abnormalities that could be mistaken for generalized systemic disease. The absence of murmurs in the auscultation of the heart suggests the absence of specific valvular dysfunction. The fact that the jugular veins are not engorged and that the liver is not enlarged help to relieve the suspicion of heart failure.

In our hypothetical patient, the physician will pursue the evaluation and diagnosis of the problems in a sequential and coordinated manner, selecting those tests that are most likely to lead to proper diagnostic conclusions. His aim will be to establish a diagnosis conclusively without missing important elements, while avoiding the temptation of ruling in or out every conceivable diagnostic possibility no matter how unlikely. Realizing that each test results in a cost to the patient, he will order the common high-yield procedures, following with others only when indicated.

The Laboratory and X-Ray Studies

Initial tests for our patient's suspected lung condition will include a posteroanterior chest x-ray, with either a stereo pair or a lateral view, arterial blood gases, and simple pulmonary function tests. A sputum specimen will be collected and inspected for bacteria, cells, and possibly for culture studies. The physician may decide to order a blood chemistry profile, since the automated processing makes the 12 (or more) values inexpensive and provides information about several body functions. This profile usually includes sodium, potassium, calcium and phosphorous, total protein, glucose, two or three enzyme levels, bilirubin, uric acid, creatinine, and albumin.

To evaluate the cardiovascular problem, he will order an electrocardiogram and some additional blood chemistry studies, particularly cholesterol and triglycerides. A urinalysis would also be appropriate.

Anteroposterior, lateral, and oblique x-ray studies of the hip and a serum protein electrophoresis have already been done to evaluate the nature of the hip disease.

Results and Interpretation of Preliminary Studies

The patient's chest x-ray shows the following abnormalities: moderate hyperlucency of the lung fields and slight flattening of the diaphragm (possible emphysematous changes), some basilar fibrosis and pleural thickening with slightly enlarged hilar nodes bilaterally (possible chronic bronchitis), and a cardiac shadow moderately larger than normal. Unfortunately, there is also a dense, 2-cm opacity in the lower lobe suspicious of neoplasm (Fig 3–1).

The arterial blood gas determination with the patient breathing room air shows a slight decrease in PaO_2 (65 mm Hg), a normal $PaCO_2$ and pH, but a carboxyhemoglobin level of 8% and a hemoglobin level of 16 gm/dl, with an oxygen saturation of 86%.

Pulmonary function tests show a moderate decrease in forced expiratory flow (FEF) in the flow-volume curve. The forced expiratory volume in 1 second (FEV_1) is 70% of predicted. It is also noted that there is modest improvement when the maneuver is repeated after the administration of bronchodilator. The maximum voluntary ventilation was found to be 51% of the predicted normal (Table 3–1). Examination of the sputum disclosed many necrotic-appearing cells, leukocytes, and many gram-negative bacteria. The chemistry data are within normal limits except for a blood glucose level of 120 mg/dl (normal, 70 to 100 mg/dl) and a creatinine level of 1.5 mg/dl (normal, 0.6 to 0.9 mg/dl).

The electrocardiogram shows only some nonspecific T-wave abnormalities. The nonspecific nature of the T-wave changes does not help in the diagnosis. There are no cardiac rhythm abnormalities. The serum lipid determination, however, shows a cholesterol of 350 mm/dl (normal, <290 mg/dl) and triglycerides of 180 (normal, <140), suggesting the possibility of arteriosclerotic cardiovascular disease.

The hip x-rays confirm the presence of extensive degenerative arthritis of the hip without fracture; normal serum electrophoresis rules out the possibility of myeloma.

Continuing Studies

It is now clear that our patient has three treatable conditions and the possibility of a fourth that could be life-threatening. Priorities compel the physician to evaluate the x-ray density in the right lower lobe. Of the various possible approaches, the one with the least uncertainty and the greatest likelihood of correct diagnosis is flexible fiberoptic bronchoscopy with biopsy or bronchial brushing. This may be done with radiologic guidance (image intensification or fluoroscopy). In our patient, microscopic examination of cells obtained during the procedure disclosed the presence of squamous cell carcinoma. Now the patient must be considered for a thoracic surgical procedure, and yet very little has happened with regard to her painful hip!

TABLE 3–1.

Preoperative Pulmonary Function Test Results*

MEASUREMENT	SYMBOL	PREDICTED NORMAL†	PREBRONCHODILATOR	
			OBSERVED	% PREDICTED
Lung volumes				
Total lung capacity, L	TLC	5.54	6.0	110
Vital capacity, L	VC	3.02	3.43	113
Residual volume, L	RV	2.53	2.57	100
RV/TLC ratio, %	RV/TLC	45.6	43.5	96
Functional residual capacity, L	FRC	2.77	2.74	99
Expiratory reserve volumes L	ERV	0.24	0.87	355
Spirometry				
Forced vital capacity, L	FVC	3.02	3.0	100
Forced expiratory volume in 1 sec, L	FEV_1	2.23	2.11	94
FEV_1/FVC ratio, %	$FEV_{1\%}$	74.0	70.0	
Forced expiratory flow$_{25\%-75\%}$, L/sec	$FEF_{25\%-75\%}$	2.2	1.0	46
Lower limit FEF$_{25\%-75\%}$, L/sec		1.2		
Maximum voluntary ventilation, L/min	MVV	82.0	50.9	62
Ventilation distribution				
Slope phase III, % N_2/L	III	2.0	0.3	

*Mild to moderate obstructive pulmonary disease is present. (See text for details.)
†Sex: F; height: 166.4 cm; arm span: 171.4 cm; weight: 88.6 kg.

X-Ray Imaging

Conventional x-ray images are two-dimensional "shadow pictures" of three-dimensional structures and require experience and training to interpret. The photographic image produced is a negative image developed when x-rays impact on a screen causing the emission of light. A photosensitized film adjacent to the screen is exposed according to the amount of x-ray reaching the screen. As the rays penetrate the patient's body, they are absorbed and scattered to varying degrees by the tissues. A chest x-ray shows the darkest exposure when the rays pass through the least dense tissues—the air-filled lungs. The most dense structures, the calcium-containing bones, prevent the passage of the x-rays so they appear as white or transparent on the film. The other structures absorb the rays depending on their water content, which absorbs more than air but less than bone (Fig 3–1).

Because the x-rays are diverging as they leave the tube, the shadow cast by the object being x-rayed is somewhat larger than the object itself. This could cause mistakes in interpretation. A "standard" chest roentgenogram is made with the patient 6 ft from the x-ray tube, standing (or lying) as close as possible to the film cassette. Sometimes, two exposures are made on two cassettes, the second occurring very briefly after the first, but with the tube being moved a few inches. This technique produces two images made from a slightly different angle so that they may be placed in an apparatus that allows the interpeter to view the right film with his right eye, and the left film with his left eye, thereby producing a stereoscopic image. By this means, the two flat x-rays appear three-dimensional, and abnormalities can be located more precisely. An alternative to the stereoscopic view is the lateral chest roentgenogram, which helps to locate objects in the anteroposterior relationship. The lateral chest x-ray suffers

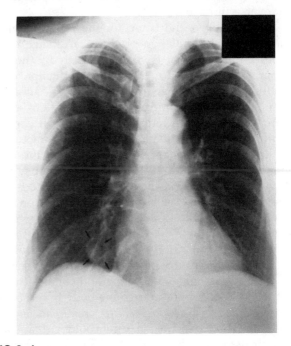

FIG 3–1.

Chest x-ray. Note 2-cm opacity in the lower lobe.

from "blind spots" created by the prominence of the spinal column, heart, and ribs.

By locating the position of the x-ray tube appropriately, x-ray images can be created to minimize the obstruction by skeletal elements of organs under scrutiny. These views are named according to the area targeted (e.g., apical view) or the position of the body with respect to the direction of the rays (e.g., oblique views). The intensity of the radiation is adjusted according to the size of the patient, so that there will be sufficient contrast to distinguish the various structures. Similarly, when the desire is to examine the heart and vasculature of the chest, the contrast can be adjusted so as to emphasize these structures, but the details of the soft tissues are lost.

"Portable" chest x-rays are made by using a movable x-ray apparatus and cassette to examine patients in their hospital beds or in the operating room. There are disadvantages to this technique, the main one being the variability in the distance between the tube and the cassette, and thus in the degree of magnification of the image and the variability in the position of the patient (i.e., sitting, semisitting, recumbent, etc.). There is also poorer resolution of the image, which refers to the minimum size of objects of varying contrast which can be discriminated. Portable chest x-rays are usually done "AP" (anteroposterior), meaning that the beam travels from the front of the chest to the back, where the x-ray plate is placed. Standard chest x-rays are called "PA" (posteroanterior), where the beam passes in the reverse direction.

Fluoroscopy is the name for the x-ray imaging process whereby radiation produces an image on a fluorescent screen that is viewed directly by the examiner. This technique allows the production of a "real-time" image. Image intensification is an electronic technique for processing of this type of x-ray to greatly reduce the radiation exposure. It can be used in the manipulation and reduction of fractures, to guide catheters into specific branches of the pulmonary or systemic vasculature, to guide biopsy forceps to specific sites in the lungs through the bronchoscope, and to visualize the flow of contrast material through the vasculature, the digestive tract, or the airways.

A further dimension in x-ray imaging becomes possible with computer processing of the image signal. Computer-augmented tomography allows the x-ray "dissection" of portions of the body by processing multiple x-ray exposures to create an image much like that available if one could cut a slice through the part being examined. By adjusting con-

trast with the computer program, it is possible to discriminate even various densities of soft tissue from one another, and by adding contrast material to the vasculature or cavity, even greater detail in the image is possible.

Magnetic Resonance Imaging (MRI)

This is a technique whereby even more sophisticated imaging of body contents can be made by the use of sophisticated computers, radiowaves, and the fact that atoms of tissue can be made to resonate proportionally to their specific magnetic properties. The use of this technique is still limited in chest disease.

Angiography

By the injection of radiopaque (contrast) material into arteries, the configuration of the vascular supply to specific organs may be demonstrated radiographically. With radiographic guidance, it is possible to introduce catheters into selected vessels, inject the contrast medium, and obtain x-ray images of an organ or even a portion of an organ. These images cannot only disclose the nature and distribution of the blood supply, but also can show the contour and size of the organ, and discriminate areas with a variance in circulation that might be caused by compression by tumor. Angiography is commonly used in the evaluation of the vasculature of the brain, heart, lung, bowel, kidney, and the aorta and its branches. Cineangiography refers to the recording of the changes as they take place on motion picture film. This technique has been largely replaced by the use of videotape that allows the display of such things as the beating heart and pulsating vessels.

Ultrasound

It is possible to produce images of organs and structures by the use of sound waves directed toward the target by a transducer. The waves are reflected from the target structure depending on its density, and a detector converts the reflected waves to a visible signal on a photographic surface. This technique is used to examine soft tissue structures such as the heart, the intrauterine fetus, abdominal organs, and endocrine glands. There are many other non–x-ray, noninvasive methods of creating images of body structures, but space considerations preclude a description of them all.

Blood Chemistry

There are several thousand laboratory tests available to assist in the evaluation and treatment of disease. By proper selection and use, the doctor can detect biologic abnormalities that may have no specific clinical manifestations, discriminate between similar possible diagnoses, select the most effective treatment regimens, and evaluate the status and involvement of individual organs. We will discuss only the more important tests that have relevance in our case presentation.

With few exceptions, a single blood chemistry value provides little useful information. Electrolyte determinations are a good example of this since they are so complexly related to each other. The automated chemistry group provides concentrations of at least four ions and sometimes as many as seven (Na^+, K^+, Ca^{++}, Cl^-, PO^{--}, Mg^{++}, and HCO_3^-). From these data, considerable information may be gathered regarding the metabolic status, particularly when arterial tensions of oxygen, carbon dioxide, and hydrogen ion (pH) concentration are measured simultaneously. Here one may gain indirect information about interrelated functions of the heart, lungs, liver, and kidney.

The determination of enzyme levels makes it possible to evaluate the type and degree of organ-specific disease, but there are so many different types of enzyme analysis available that discussion here would be tedious.

The glucose level in the blood of normal people varies greatly with dietary intake and activity, so it is important to do the determination after the patient has been fasting for at least 8 hours. The fact that the concentration is elevated does not mean that the patient has diabetes mellitus, but it suggests there is a disorder in glucose metabolism, which should be further investigated.

Protein and albumin in the blood serve as replacement sources for cell protein, as H^+ buffers, as transport media for many substances (protein-binding), for osmotic homeostasis and are vital elements in the immunologic mechanisms. Abnormal levels can be related to liver disease, malnutrition, and some specific diseases of the bone marrow. Protein electrophoresis provides information about the concentration of many different protein elements (important in nutritional assessment) and can detect the presence of abnormal plasma proteins, as are seen in certain deficiencies.

Arterial Blood Gas Analyses

With the development of automated electrodes, analysis of O_2 and CO_2 tension and pH (hydrogen ion concentration) has become a reasonably simple procedure. The tension of gas in arterial blood changes rapidly under a variety of conditions, so the conditions at the time of sampling must be recorded in order to make interpretation possible. The results must be considered as reflecting the status of gas exchange and hydrogen ion concentration only at the particular time of sampling. Some values, such as base excess/deficit and HCO_3^- are derived rather than measured, and reflect chronic or longer-standing adjustments of the buffer mechanism. Oxygen saturation is usually measured and can reflect abnormalities in hemoglobin (such as carboxyhemoglobin in smokers and methemoglobin caused by some drugs).

Electrocardiogram

The ECG is a recording or display of the electrical activity of the heart. It is widely used, thoroughly studied, and relatively inexpensive. Although of unquestionable value in cardiology, it is easy to overlook its limitations. Like most other clinical assessment procedures, it is most useful when used with other modalities.

The ECG is the gold standard for evaluating rhythm disturbances of the heart and the almost infinite number of things that can affect the heartbeat. It can also provide information on the electrical changes related to abnormalities, such as hypertrophy, ischemia, and infarction. Variations in electrocardiographic technique have been developed to address problems beyond the capability of the single resting ECG. For example, an exercise ECG provides information about cardiac reserve (stress testing), and continuous long-term ambulatory monitoring (Holter monitor) is used for the recognition of infrequent or unusual arrhythmias.

Bronchoscopy

Visual inspection of the airways is made possible by use of the bronchoscope. There are two general types—rigid and flexible. The use of the rigid bronchoscope has been greatly reduced by the advancing fiberoptic technology, but there are a few instances when it is the method of choice: i.e., removal of large objects from the airway, obtaining large biopsies, and in dealing with brisk hemorrhage. The fiberoptic bronchoscope is small in diameter, flexible, and has a steerable tip that can be maneuvered into fourth- or fifth-order bronchi for examination or biopsy. Also, by use of brushes and forceps through the aspiration channel, biopsy and instrumentation can be accomplished. A recent adaptation of laser technology has made possible the removal of certain airway tumors by dessication.

CLINICAL USE OF PULMONARY FUNCTION TESTING

Outside of the research laboratory, pulmonary function tests are useful in: (1) identifying and classifying certain types of lung disease, (2) evaluating the effectiveness of treatment, (3) documenting the progress of pulmonary disease, (4) providing a yardstick for compensating the disabled, and (5) assessing risk factors prior to surgery.

In Chapter 2, the technology of pulmonary function testing (PFT) devices is described, along with detailed descriptions of the technique of performing the tests. In order for pulmonary function tests to be useful, there must be assurance that they have been properly performed on accurate, well-calibrated equipment. Obviously, if the diagnostic values are not reproducible or are otherwise spurious, therapeutic errors will be possible. Let us now consider each of the above items separately.

Identifying and Classifying Lung Disease

Pulmonary function tests may identify airways disease, respiratory pump (chest wall and diaphragm) abnormalities, and abnormalities in the pulmonary parenchyma (tissue) itself. No single test can do it all, yet the clinician must not be extravagant in ordering more information than is necessary, since each determination results in a charge that must be paid by someone.

The measurement of gas flow and lung volumes makes up the bulk of PFTs in general use. This is accomplished by spirometry or flow volume techniques (using pneumotachometry). The data provided allows the clinician to characterize deviations from normal as either restrictive or obstructive.

Restrictive disease includes disorders of lung volumes caused by chest wall deformity, neuromuscular disease, or structural change in lung tissue (fibrosis, pneumonia). In these conditions, lung volumes are reduced (restricted).

Obstructive pulmonary disease relates to airway abnormality such as is seen in asthma, emphysema, bronchitis, and chondromalacia (softening of the tracheal cartilage). In these disorders, gas flow is reduced (obstructed), particularly during expiration. In many instances of pulmonary dysfunction, there are elements of both restrictive and obstructive pathology, requiring a certain degree of elegance in the interpretation of the PFT to quantitate the relative importance of each. An example of this would be the coexistence of pneumonia (a restrictive disorder) with chronic bronchitis (an obstructive one).

Unfortunately, the entire lung volume cannot be measured with "simple" equipment. The residual volume (RV) is the volume of gas remaining in the lung after a maximal expiration. One must measure this residual volume (RV) to determine total lung capacity (TLC). The three techniques used most commonly to measure this volume are (in increasing order of complexity): (1) the open-circuit nitrogen washout, (2) the closed circuit helium dilution, and (3) whole-body plethysmograph. It is usually important to include the measurement of RV, particularly with obstructive lung disease, since, as a result of airway obstruction during expiration (due to structural changes in the lung tissue), the lung tends to become "hyperinflated" and there is a concomitant disproportionate increase in RV. One indication of a significant degree of obstructive lung disease is an RV/TLC ratio of greater than 0.45 (or if expressed in RV/TLC percent, greater than 45%).

The early recognition of lung disease has long been a clinical objective. As yet, there is no simple, inexpensive, and expedient means of doing this. As with most biologic testing, PFT results are interpreted on the basis of acceptable "normal range" values, based on the results of thousands of tests performed on a presumably "normal" population. These "normal" values subtend a broad range, and even though they are "adjusted" for body size (height and/or arm span), there is sufficient latitude to preclude the early recognition of lung disease in any individual. It has been found, for instance, that a habitual cigarette smoker will not notice symptoms of obstructive disease until his FEF values are down to 40% of normal. If this individual performed this test in the range of "high normal" or "supernormal" prior to taking up smoking, he could undergo a serious amount of lung damage before degrading his flow capability to the "low normal" prediction. It is unfortunate that every potential victim of lung disease cannot provide his own "normal value" of function before the disease process begins.

Since we all spend most of our lives breathing

quietly at rest, we may not be aware of degradation of our pulmonary function until we are stressed. Most PFTs are designed to evaluate function at the limits of performance and are so named; i.e., maximum voluntary ventilation (MVV), maximum mid-expiratory flow (MMEF), peak (expiratory) flow (PF), and maximum inspiratory flow (P_{Imax}). Conditioned athletes may extend their performance well beyond the predicted "normal range," while ordinary sedentary people may barely reach the "low normal." Looked at from this vantage, this type of PFT may be considered as a measure of one's pulmonary "reserve."

There are some types of lung disease that do not result in easily measurable decrements in either flow or volume, and that may coexist with unremarkable "standard" PFTs. Tests that assess the distribution of lung gas can help identify these variations. The most common is called the single breath nitrogen elimination test. It is accomplished by having the subject inhale maximally O_2 (from RV to TLC), and then breathe into a spirometer at a constant rate through an N_2 meter. When N_2 concentration is plotted on the ordinate and volume on the abscissa, a characteristic curve is generated from which much information can be derived (Fig 3–2). First, it is possible to measure the anatomic deadspace, which is the volume at the midpoint of phase II. Second, the homogeneity of gas distribution is indicated by the slope of phase III, the steeper slope indicating uneven mixing of the inspired gas. The third value that can be determined is the closing volume (CV), which represents the point at which a significant number of airways begin to close. As expected, reproductivity of this test depends on proper instruction and performance of the patient. He must take in a full breath of O_2 from RV to TLC, and he must breathe it out at a constant rate through the N_2 meter into the spirometer. If the patient cannot do this, the test is without value.

It is rare that the clinical management of pulmonary disease requires the use of whole-body plethysmographic studies of pulmonary function. Most use of this type of equipment is related to clinical or basic research. The equipment is complex, expensive, and subject to exotic and difficult-to-recognize malfunctions. In addition, its size and complexity present a threat to the patient and a challenge of his ability to cooperate and follow directions. It cannot be used effectively in very sick patients.

Another method of assessing gas distribution is accomplished by having the patient inhale a radio-

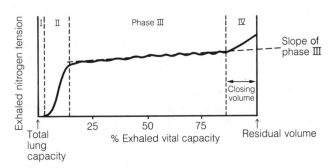

FIG 3–2.
Single-breath nitrogen elimination test.

active gas, usually xenon 133, and subsequently generating a "picture" of the lung with the inhaled gas by gamma-ray–detecting cameras. This method is described at the end of this chapter.

There are numerous additional pulmonary function tests that assess gas exchange and pulmonary reserve indirectly, many of which are thoroughly reviewed in Chapter 2. Some of the simpler "screening" tests that are not complex require minimal special equipment, and can direct the further investigation of whatever pathology of therapeutic course appears appropriate. One commonly used test is the so-called "match test." Here, a lighted paper match is held 6 in. from the patient's open mouth. He is asked to blow the match out without pursing his lips. Failure to accomplish this task indicates a significant degradation of the patient's ability to generate expiratory gas flow.

Another technique is to accompany the patient up a flight of stairs, noting the ease with which he accomplishes the climb, and the degree of shortness of breath that it generates. These simple tests (which cost nearly nothing) can be very useful to the experienced clinician.

Evaluation of Effectiveness of Treatment

It is not uncommon to perform routine spirometry or a pneumotachograph study (flow-volume curve) and follow in a short interval by repeating the study after the administration of an aerosolized bronchodilator. This approach accomplishes two things: (1) it indicates an element of reversible obstructive airway disease if there is a substantial improvement in flow after bronchodilator, and (2) it occasionally indicates an overuse of bronchodilator if there is a decrement in flow.

In other instances, change in PFT results may suggest the efficiency (or otherwise) of medical treatment. The effectiveness of conservative or surgical correction of kyphoscoliosis may be demonstrated by PFTs. The effective management of heart failure is also usually accompanied by improved pulmonary performance, and the severity and/or responsiveness to therapy of neuromuscular disease is easily demonstrated by changes in serial PFT. An interesting application of spirometry is in demonstrating the adequacy of pain relief by various methods in post-surgical patients.

Documenting the Progress of Pulmonary Disease

PFT is sometimes used to document the progress of disease, e.g., panacinar emphysema, pulmonary fibrosis, Guillain-Barré disease, or acute asthma, or to evaluate the potentially toxic side effects of drug therapy. An example of the latter is in the use of the anticancer agent bleomycin, which is known to cause interstitial pulmonary fibrosis in certain patients. Early recognition of this complication can result in the adjusting of dosage or using an alternative form of treatment.

Although spirometry and flow volume curves are useful for this purpose, many clinicians prefer a diffusion test. There are several versions of diffusion tests, most of which use small amounts of carbon monoxide as a trace gas to measure the rate of diffusion across the alveolar membrane. The advantage of using carbon monoxide as the indicator gas is that it is tightly bound by hemoglobin, and therefore makes a "one-way trip" from the lungs into the blood. There are two varieties of the test; one is called the "single breath" test, the other is called "steady state" test. Neither of them allows enough carbon monoxide into the blood to do any damage, and both are capable of indicating a "diffusion" barrier to gas transport if one exists.

Another useful value having to do with pulmonary performance is "compliance." This value is a measure of the ease of distensibility of the lung, and it is sometimes measured for both the lung and for the chest wall. Unfortunately, this requires obtaining a reading of the intrapleural pressure, which is not easily done. One method involves the insertion of a catheter into the pleural space, but such an invasive procedure is hardly ever justified for clinical use. The usual method is the use of an esophageal balloon, the internal pressure of which, if properly situated and adjusted, is equivalent to intrapleural pressure. This is an uncomfortable procedure, poorly tolerated by most people and, therefore, it is rarely performed outside the research laboratory.

Total static respiratory system compliance can be measured without an esophageal balloon by using a spirometer, an interrupter to stop flow at various lung volumes, and a pressure transducer to measure airway pressure at these various volumes. This technique does not allow the separation of the two components of compliance (chest wall and lung), but is useful in some situations, particularly when patients are being mechanically ventilated.

Disability Compensation

A great stimulus to the development and standardization of pulmonary function tests resulted from the recognition of the relationship between mining operations and pulmonary disease. The prevalence of black lung disease among coal miners, and various other types of pneumoconiosis among miners of other substances, called for a reproducible means of quantitating the extent of disease. This type of exposure can lead to a restrictive type of lung disease which is progressive, ultimately resulting in severe limitation of activity, occasionally malignant change, and death.

Other industrial exposures have subsequently resulted in the recognition of the relationship between presence of toxins in the work place and systemic illnesses in a large variety of environments. This, of course, has led to the promulgation of guidelines, laws, and standards regulating the minimal tolerance of such exposures, the mandatory control and safety measures, and even changes in methods of production and procedures in the workplace. Current practice dictates that company owners become responsible for both medical costs and maintenance of those affected due to toxic environment in the work place. This whole field has come to be known as disability compensation, a most contentious area that has provided career opportunities for countless lawyers and courtroom personnel.

In actual fact, "disability" has taken on a legalistic meaning and cannot really be determined by pulmonary function testing or any other single modality. PFTs can quantitate the degree of impairment of pulmonary performance, but they represent only one of many factors that go into the determination of disability. For example, a given decrement in pulmonary function might represent total inability of a construction worker to perform his job, while the same decrement would not interfere with the performance of a dispatcher. In actual fact, many elements are considered in the attempt to quantitate disability, including physical findings (range of motion, hearing loss, visual impairment, stress-related disease, etc.), x-ray findings, psychological testing, pulmonary function testing, and even aptitude testing.

Assessing Risk Factors Prior to Surgery

A means of identifying those patients who were most likely to suffer pulmonary complications following anesthesia and surgery would obviously be desirable. The hope that pulmonary function tests would completely provide this means has not been realized. It is generally accepted that all patients accept some risk of pulmonary complications after anesthesia and surgery, but there would be great savings in resources and effort if the individuals who will have problems could be identified preoperatively.

Factors known to increase the risk of anesthesia and surgery include the presence of acute or chronic lung disease, cigarette smoking, old age, surgical procedures of the upper abdomen or thorax, obesity, and surgical procedures that last more than 3 hours. In the face of any of these factors, abnormal pulmonary function results should alert the medical, nursing, and respiratory therapy staff to take extra precautions, such as ensuring preoperative and postoperative bronchial hygiene. The depressant effects of anesthetic agents, the use of narcotics to control postoperative pain, the loss of the cough reflex, and ciliary action of respiratory epithelium, all work together to increase the likelihood of retained secretions, closed airways, and atelectasis.

Another objective of the thoracic surgeon is to be able to anticipate accurately the effect that a proposed lung resection will have on the patient's pulmonary reserve. For example, if it appeared that a pneumonectomy would be required to treat a cancer of the lung, it would be desirable to know with some certainty that the remaining lung would be sufficient to the patient's need. Unfortunately, PFTs alone have not satisfied that objective, probably because there are so many variables in motivation as well as function that cannot adequately be measured.

Rarely is the decision to operate (or not operate) based on PFTs alone, although the tests are often ordered preoperatively with this objective at least in mind. Toward this end, some investigators have attempted to temporarily occlude the airway and blood supply to the affected lung simultaneously to see how much decrement in respiratory function would result. This technique has had poor correlation with the postoperative results and is no longer widely used.

There is general agreement that the medical history, particularly the history of previous surgical procedures, is very helpful in assessing risk, and that presence or absence of the above-mentioned risk factors is very important. This does not imply that PFTs have no place in this assessment, rather that they provide one type of information that must be used cautiously and in concert with every other source of evaluation in the decisions regarding surgery.

Therapeutic Action: An Example

A Decision to Operate

The previously described patient has now been evaluated and been found to have the following disorders: moderate hypertension, with the increased risk factors of elevated cholesterol and triglycerides; moderate chronic bronchitis, obstructive airway disease; degenerative arthritis of the hip, and squamous cell carcinoma of the right lung. The modest elevation of the serum glucose level does not suggest diabetes mellitus in the absence of symptoms, and can be managed by proper diet.

At surgery, the patient was administered a general anesthesia, and mediastinoscopy was done. This was accomplished by inserting a mediastinoscope through a small incision in the suprasternal notch into the superior mediastinum and examining the lymph nodes in the pretracheal, subcarinal, and hilar areas. If any appeared suspicious of being involved with cancer, a biopsy would be done for examination by a pathologist.

The nodes appeared uninvolved, so the surgeon proceeded to thoracotomy and lower lobectomy under general endotracheal anesthesia. Postoperatively, the patient failed to ventilate adequately, so the endotracheal tube was left in place, and mechanical ventilation was instituted. Through an arterial catheter, periodic arterial blood samples were taken and O_2, CO_2 tension, and pH determination were done. Normal range tensions of O_2 and CO_2 were attainable with an inspired O_2 fraction ($F_{I_{O_2}}$) of 0.4 with a minute ventilation of 9 L at a frequency of 10 cycles/minute. The peak airway pressure for a tidal volume of 900 ml was 43 cm H_2O, but during end-inspiratory pause, was 28 cm H_2O, and the endotracheal tube had to be suctioned frequently due to bronchial secretions. Inspiratory force measurements ($P_{I_{max}}$ ranged between -15 and -20 cm H_2O), suggested that the patient had inadequate respiratory muscle strength to sustain ventilation without assistance. There was only a small air leak in the chest tube drainage.

On auscultation of the chest, expiratory wheezes were heard diffusely with some coarse rhonchi at the lung bases. Therefore, chest physical therapy and periodic use of an aerosolized sympathomimetic bronchodilator was ordered. After the first bronchodilator treatment, the peak airway pressure was found to be 25 cm H_2O for a tidal volume of 900 ml.

The next morning, with the same ventilator settings, the arterial oxygen tension had increased to 200 mm Hg, with carbon dioxide tension of 40 mm Hg. The airway secretions had decreased considerably in amount. A specimen from the airways was aspirated into a sterile collection bottle and sent to the laboratory for culture. A portable chest x-ray showed the chest tubes to be properly located; there was no pneumothorax and the lungs were well expanded. Inspiratory force measurements were found to be in the range of -40 to -60 cm H_2O, so mechanical ventilation was discontinued, the endotracheal tube was connected to a T-piece, and administration of 40% O_2 via an all-purpose nebulizer was started. After an hour, arterial blood gas analysis confirmed adequate gas exchange and the endotracheal tube was removed. The sputum culture previously sent to the microbiology laboratory was reported to contain *Pseudomonas aeruginosa*. The patient was continued on the cephalosporin antibiotic, which had been started at the time of surgery, and chest physical therapy was continued.

Chest tubes were clamped and subsequently removed on the third postoperative day, and ambulation was started. Chest physical therapy was discontinued, but bronchodilator by aerosol was continued and oral theophylline and a thiazide diuretic were ordered on a daily basis. After counseling regarding a low-sodium, low-fat, low-cholesterol diet and smoking cessation were completed, the patient was sent home to recuperate.

Discussion

Because the thoracic tumor could possibly be responsible for the enlarged hilar nodes, study of this problem before opening the chest cavity seemed appropriate, since, if the nodes were involved, the malignancy would be considered inoperable and alternative means of treatment (such as radiation or chemotherapy) would be sought. Mediastinoscopy and computer-augmented tomography could have been used. The latter can only provide an image, not a histologic diagnosis, while mediastinoscopy can result in a tissue specimen for pathologic examina-

tion. Thus, mediastinoscopy was the procedure of choice.

Despite great advances in surgical technology and anesthesia, any surgical process is inherently stressful, with many metabolic, enzymatic, and humoral changes occurring simultaneously. Unexpected complications can arise out of the body's inability to cope with minor assaults on its homeostasis. Except in the case of infection or technical problems at surgery, rarely is it possible to identify a specific cause or remedy for those stress-related problems, so we treat empirically. For example, in this case, the patient did not ventilate adequately after an uncomplicated pulmonary resection. There was no obvious reason, such as residual anesthesia effect, too much muscle relaxant, too much pain medication, too much fluid or blood transfusion, or a sudden severe change in cardiac or pulmonary performance, so the choice was made to institute mechanical ventilation and await further clues as to the cause. At this time, one could expend effort and resources trying to identify a cause for the patient's failure to ventilate adequately. The inspiratory force measurement suggested a weakness of respiratory muscles, since it was found to be below the normal range.

When assessing arterial blood gases, one must know what inspired oxygen tension the patient is breathing. When one finds a "normal" O_2 tension with the patient receiving a 40% O_2 mixture, there is cause for concern, since the patient is only achieving the same tension of O_2 in arterial blood as a "normal" person achieves while breathing 21% O_2 (air). It was obvious that our patient had a problem that prevented normal oxygenation of arterial blood (see below).

Assessment of peak airway (ventilator) pressure and pressure during an end-expiratory pause gives a reasonable estimate of pulmonary resistance and compliance. Measured by this means, lung compliance (volume/pause pressure) provides a clue to a number of conditions, including fluid overload, airway obstruction by secretions, and insufficient control of the pleural space (e.g., blocked chest tube with pneumothorax or hemothorax). Airway obstruction may be revealed by finding an increase in airway resistance.

Sputum cultures are often obtained casually in the mistaken belief that one can recognize the development of pneumonia if the culture is positive. In actual fact, there is a poor relationship between culture results and significant pulmonary infection. A properly fixed and stained smear of sputum can indicate whether or not the sputum sample is representative of deep lung secretions, by the number and appearance of the epithelial, squamous, and other identifiable cells, and whether or not they are of microbiologic significance. The diagnosis of pneumonia, however, can be made with assurance only when several signs and symptoms occur simultaneously, including x-ray evidence, fever, positive culture, cough, and, often, positive blood culture. In the presence of x-ray findings but insufficient collaborative evidence of pneumonia, the clinician will often refer to the entity as "pneumonitis," which is usually interpreted to mean that "if it gets any worse, it might become pneumonia."

Getting patients "off the ventilator" has generated much literature and many suggested protocols. Weaning can be a challenge under some circumstances, particularly when ventilator use has been prolonged. It is clear that successful weaning in some instances requires a multifaceted approach, which is best summarized in Figure 3–3. When a patient is able to breathe adequately, she is easy to wean, as in our case.

Chest physical therapy was seen to be helpful in mobilizing our patient's secretions. The following guidelines to the use of chest physical therapy are applicable in many situations, and help to identify the level of treatment as well as the person responsible (Table 3–2). The most convincing evidence that a program of chest physical therapy is effective comes from the rapid resolution of fever and improvement in chest x-ray abnormalities.

Case Report

After 6 weeks of recovery and rehabilitation, our patient was ready for hip surgery. This hospital ad-

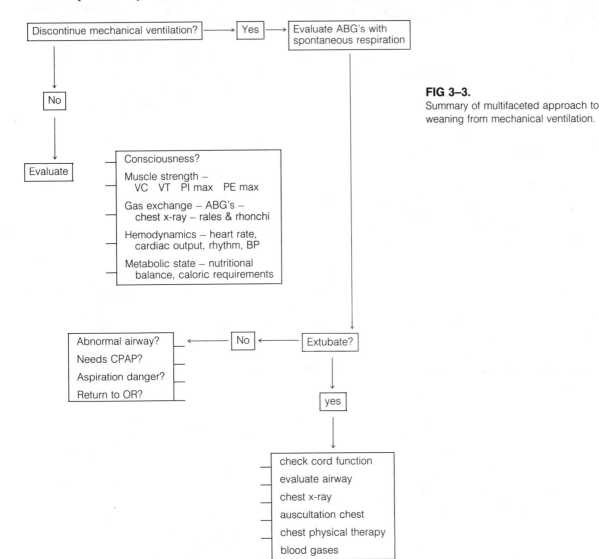

FIG 3–3.
Summary of multifaceted approach to weaning from mechanical ventilation.

TABLE 3–2.

Guidelines for the Use of Chest Physical Therapy

Chest Physical Therapy I

Hospital nursing will remain responsible for delivering chest physical therapy I. Ordering of chest physical therapy I may be a part of standing postoperative orders, may be a part of standing nursing care plans, or may be a decision between the primary physician and the nursing staff as to what measures may be taken by the nursing staff to promote pulmonary hygiene. Standing orders, physician's order sheets, or nursing care plan written orders for chest physical therapy I should give the nurse some guidance as to how long this should continue, such as "turn from side to side," "encourage deep breathing with the use of incentive device," and "cough patient every hour for the first 24 hours, and then every 4 hours until the patient is up and about."

Chest physical therapy I or nursing care measures to promote bronchial hygiene include

1. Frequent position changes/nursing from side to side.
2. Encouraging periodic deep breathing; incentive devices may be indicated here.
3. Instructing patients in proper cough technique and encouragement of periodic coughing.
4. Chest clapping/vibration with or without the use of mechanical chest percussors.
5. Aspiration of secretions from the tracheobronchial tree when endotracheal and tracheotomy tubes are in place.

Some indications for chest physical therapy I would be:

1. Patients on strict bedrest.
2. Postsurgical, particularly thoracic and upper abdominal surgery.
3. After general anesthesia.
4. As a part of pulmonary prep.
5. Patients in coma due to stroke, drug overdose, liver failure, diabetic coma, etc.

Chest Physical Therapy II

Physicians should state the indications (as listed below), the specific area of the lung to be worked on, and the number of days treatments are to be continued. It is seldom necessary for chest physical therapy II procedures to be done more than once on every shift, three times a day, or for more than 3 days.

Chest physical therapy II involves

1. Specific segmental drainage of the lung, which usually requires posturing for gravity assist.
2. Specific chest wall manipulation techniques.
3. Stimulation of forced spontaneous cough.
4. Direct tracheal suctioning for secretion removal when there is no endotracheal tube/tracheotomy tube in place, often referred to as nasotracheal suctioning.
5. Use of methods to promote lung expansion.
6. Use of bronchodilators to promote pulmonary hygiene when administered as an aerosol.

The indications for chest physical therapy II to promote bronchial hygiene are

1. Secretion retention as a result of failure of preventive measures for patients who have cystic fibrosis or severe chronic obstructive pulmonary disease and who have chronic secretion retention, atelectasis, and infection.
2. Severe chronic bronchitis with excessive airway secretion associated with surgery.
3. Resolving status asthmaticus.

4. The uncooperative patient who has excessive airway secretion and no endotracheal tube in place.
5. Patients with absent cough reflex who cannot expel pulmonary secretions.
6. Secretion retention associated with bronchospasm.
7. Patients with weakened respiratory musculature.

The primary physician remains responsible for ordering procedures for his patient, and this procedure policy of delivering chest physical therapy is in no way meant to restrict the nursing staff or the medical staff care of patients.

mission was similar to the previous one, but there were no surprises. Her admission workup showed the hypertension to be under good control and her chronic bronchitis to be greatly improved. She had been using occasional aerosolized bronchodilators and oral theophylline. Most importantly, she had stopped smoking. In addition, she had followed a low-cholesterol diet and taken a thiazide diuretic daily.

Her physician decided that a repeated chest x-ray, pulmonary function tests, protein electrophoresis, and some hematologic clotting studies were indicated. The anesthesiologist asked for arterial blood gases and a chemistry group prior to surgery. The patient also had blood cross-matched for surgery.

Discussion

Since the patient has ceased smoking cigarettes for over 7 weeks, her bronchitis should be considerably improved. Emphysematous changes, however, are not entirely reversible and one can expect some evidence of persistent obstructive airway disease. Protein electrophoresis was ordered again to rule out systemic disease that might be associated with the hip problem and to make sure that total protein was sufficient for wound healing. The blood and clotting studies were required to avoid unnecessary blood loss during a surgical procedure where transfusion is usually necessary. There are many coagulation tests available, but in the absence of a history of bleeding problems, a few screening tests are adequate. Prothrombin time, platelet count, and bleeding time are usually sufficient. By no means will normal results in these tests guarantee adequate hemostasis, since the clotting mechanism is complex and changeable, but one can avoid problems more easily than one can correct them.

The anesthesiologist was concerned about the patient's ability to exchange oxygen and carbon dioxide as well as hydrogen ion homeostatis (acid/base status). As mentioned previously, O_2, CO_2 tensions, and pH of arterial blood, along with ion concentrations from the chemistry group, provide a large amount of information for a small investment. He was concerned because of the experience after the last anesthetic procedure, where the patient required prolonged postoperative mechanical ventilation for no obvious reason.

Surgery

Our patient was scheduled for total hip arthroplasty under general anesthesia (regional anesthesia such as spinal or epidural block technique could also have been selected, the decision being based on the desires of the patient and surgeon as well as the physical and mental status of the patient). The procedure went well and the patient was given three units of cross-matched blood to replace that which was lost. She was started on a broad-spectrum antibiotic during surgery and returned to her room in stable condition.

Small doses of morphine sulfate were administered to help ease the pain from the surgical incision. Intravenous fluids were continued and urine output was measured continuously. The patient was encouraged to take deep breaths and was turned from side to side every 2 hours. She was given 40% O_2 through a nonheated, all-purpose nebulizer after complaining of a sore throat. A small dose of crystalline warfarin sodium (Coumadin) was administered prophylactically to lessen the risk of thromboembolism, and the patient was allowed sips of water. The next morning, she was allowed light liquids for breakfast. Pain medication was not necessary until late in the morning when she was allowed to sit in a chair. During the day, she progressed to a full diet, the urinary catheter and intravenous lines were removed, and physical therapy for hip motion was started. A chest x-ray showed no new pathologic findings.

Discussion

Postoperative pain can be a problem for patients with lung disease (or with many other disorders), since many of the pain relievers are also respiratory depressants. It is frequently necessary to compromise on pain relief to avoid serious depression of important functions. There is no good way to quantitate pain other than to listen to what the patient says, and there is an enormous variability in a person's pain tolerance. Good nursing procedures and personal encouragement do much to help the pa-

tient through the postoperative period with the least amount of depressant medication.

Another concern in the surgical patient is fluid balance, since the oral intake of fluid usually is restricted for at least a day (and sometimes much longer), and there may be greatly increased insensible loss. Blood loss at surgery further complicates the management by causing shifts from intra- and extracellular compartments. An important means of assessing the fluid status is the continuous measurement of urine output, body weight, and the tension gradient of oxygen between the alveolar gas and arterial blood (the $A-a$ O_2 gradient). Alveolar O_2 tension is difficult to measure directly, so when the patient is breathing air, it is calculated by using the simplified alveolar gas equation:

$$P_{AO_2} = P_{IO_2} - (P_{ACO_2}) \, (1.2)$$

where P_{IO_2} is the inspired O_2 tension, P_{ACO_2} is assumed to be identical to P_{aCO_2} (which is measured), and 1.2 is the reciprocal of the assumed respiratory quotient ($\dot{V}_{CO_2}/\dot{V}_{O_2}$). Thus, by deriving the F_{IO_2} or P_{IO_2}, and doing arterial blood gas analysis one may determine $A-a$ O_2 gradient. This is a convenient way for the clinician to estimate right-to-left shunting of blood in the gas exchange areas of the lung. Complex or precise derivations of the degree of shunting are not needed in the clinical situation. Oxygen administration in this patient was ordered to relieve mild hypoxia, and to deliver nebulized water to the areas irritated by the endotracheal tube. On the basis of prompt awakening from anesthesia, absence of clinical signs of distress and general rapid progress, arterial blood gas analyses were not needed to manage the patient, even though she had some obstructive lung disease.

Crystalline warfarin sodium is a substance that interferes with blood coagulation in a dose-related manner, and is used here to help prevent the formation of blood clots in the lower extremity. In patients immobilized in bed after pelvic or hip surgery and certain other conditions, there is an increased risk of this happening, which in turn increases the risk of a clot breaking away and being carried to the lungs as a pulmonary embolus.

Whenever possible, in the postsurgical patient, natural processes should not be interrupted, or at least be allowed to return to function as soon as possible. When oral alimentation is possible, it is much preferable to the intravenous route, and usually accomplishes a much more satisfactory fluid balance than can be achieved by even the most elegantly controlled artificial means. Similarly, the prevention of pulmonary embolism and other respiratory complications, return of bowel and bladder function, muscle tone and balance, and even a better mental attitude seem to progress more satisfactorily when the patient can return to normal activity. Early ambulation is the usual objective in the surgical patient, and fortunately, total hip replacement usually allows this.

Complication

After four days of satisfactory progress, the patient returned from a physical medicine exercise session complaining of severe shortness of breath. Examination disclosed the following: temperature, 37.5°C; pulse rate, 120 beats/min; blood pressure, 140/88 mm Hg (both arms); respirations, 28/min; auscultation, moderate expiratory wheezing (lungs), rapid heart rate, no murmurs (heart); chest x-ray, no change; arterial blood gases (breathing air), Pa_{O_2}, 48 mm Hg, Pa_{CO_2}, 30 mm Hg, pH, 7.49, HCO_3^-, 22 mEq/L, base excess (BE) +2 mEq/L, and hemoglobin, 15.2 gm/dl; and ECG, sinus tachycardia and nonspecific T-wave changes.

The presumptive diagnosis was pulmonary embolism, although examination of the lower extremities disclosed no tenderness in the legs. The problem was to confirm the diagnosis and institute therapy. Among the options considered were ventilation perfusion scan with radioactive tracers, right ventricular-pulmonary artery, flow-directed catheterization (Swan-Ganz), and pulmonary angiography.

Meanwhile, the patient was given O_2 by nasal cannula, 4-L/min flow, which failed to relieve her shortness of breath. Because of the discomfort, morphine sulfate was given and an intravenous infusion of lactated Ringer's solution was started.

After a half hour, the patient was more comfortable. Arterial blood gas determination was repeated and showed the following (4 L O_2 nasal cannula): Pa_{O_2}, 125 mm Hg; Pa_{CO_2}, 32 mm Hg; and pH, 7.47.

The patient was scheduled for pulmonary angiography. Under x-ray guidance, an angiography catheter was advanced through an antecubital vein into the pulmonary artery. While the catheter was in the right ventricle, pressure measurements were made. The right ventricular pressure was found to be 26 mm Hg. Two injections of contrast medium were made, one in the right pulmonary artery, one in the left, and multiple films were made. Multiple abrupt small-vessel occlusions were shown in the left lower lobe and the right upper lobe. There was no large-vessel filling defect.

Heparin (10,000 units) was administered and continued at the rate of 1,000 units/hour. The dose of crystalline warfarin sodium was increased and the patient gradually improved symptomatically, which was also evidenced by arterial blood gas analyses. The remainder of the hospital stay was without incident, and the patient was discharged on daily anticoagulant therapy.

Discussion

Pulmonary embolism (PE) is a possibility with almost any surgical procedure, but is somewhat more likely with pelvic, hip, and lower abdominal procedures. Low-dose anticoagulant therapy has been used as a preventive measure for many years. Apparently the true incidence of pulmonary embolism is higher than has been reported, since unexpected emboli are not infrequently found at autopsy.

The severity of the symptoms of PE are related to the size and frequency of the emboli and can vary from no symptoms at all to sudden collapse and death. No single symptom is unvarying or specific, but almost all patients have dyspnea and tachypnea. Other manifestations may include chest pain, cough, hemoptysis, and bronchospasm. Tachycardia is less frequent. The chest x-ray usually shows no change early, but in the case of large emboli, peripheral infiltrates may develop, and if lung infarction occurs, there is sometimes evidence of cavitation. There may be chest wall pain from the pleural irritation and occasionally, evidence of hypoxemia. Note that nasal O_2 restored arterial tension to a safe level, but did not relieve the dyspnea. The feeling of not getting enough air probably arises from some mechanism in the lung other than O_2 desaturation.

The ECG usually shows some nonspecific findings, such as ST- and T-wave changes, as in our patient. Evidence of right ventricular failure appears on the ECG only when the PE is very large and pulmonary artery pressures are severely elevated. There are no specific enzyme or other blood tests that help with the diagnosis.

The presence of pulmonary emboli needs to be established with some certainty, since the treatment is anticoagulation for several months, which carries a certain amount of risk (e.g., gastrointestinal bleeding, stroke, etc.). Some have tried "segmental" or "mini" angiograms by injecting x-ray contrast medium through a wedge Swan-Ganz catheter. A negative finding here does not rule out embolism, however, since only a small portion of the lung is seen.

Another widely used method for diagnosing PE is the ventilation-perfusion scan. The perfusion scan is done by injecting serum albumin labeled with technetium 99m into a peripheral vein. Radiation from this isotope is detected by a gamma camera and displayed via a cathode-ray tube, thus providing a "picture" of the lung perfusion. The ventilation scan is accomplished by the patient inhaling through a closed system a radioactive gas (usually xenon 133) and similarly recording the picture of the "washin" and "washout." By comparing the images of the two scans, the experienced consultant can estimate the probability of PE. The method is unreliable in patients with obstructive lung disease, and was therefore not selected in our patient.

The "gold standard" of diagnosis is a pulmonary angiogram, accomplished as described in the case report. Except in cases in which the pulmonary artery pressure is severely elevated, it is quite safe, and since many different views of the chest may be obtained with the "dye" in the pulmonary vasculature, the yield established in the patient, and the risk of continued anticoagulant therapy was justified.

Summary

We have followed an imaginary patient through two hospital admissions for two quite different diseases. During the course of the first hospital admission, she was diagnosed and treated for a disorder entirely different from her chief complaint. We followed the sequential approach in gathering information about the patient and her disease, and learned how the selection process is carried out for diagnostic tests. We identified some of the problems in dealing with biologic data, and gained some insight regarding the most efficient way to expend diagnostic and therapeutic resources.

SUGGESTED READING

Conrad SA, Kinasewitz GT, George RB: *Pulmonary Function Testing.* New York, Churchill Livingstone, Inc, 1984.

Des Jardins T: *Clinical Manifestations of Respiratory Disease.* Chicago, Year Book Medical Publishers, 1984.

Glauser FL: *Signs and Symptoms in Pulmonary Medicine.* Philadelphia, JB Lippincott, Co, 1983.

Harman E, Lillington G: Pulmonary risk factors in surgery. *Med Clin North Am* 1979; 6:1289–1297.

Marini JJ: *Respiratory Medicine and Intensive Care for the House Officer.* Baltimore, Williams & Wilkins Co, 1981.

Tilkian SM, Conover MB, Tilkian AG: *Clinical Implications of Laboratory Tests,* ed 3. St Louis, CV Mosby Co, 1983.

4

The Respiratory Care Plan

Thomas A. Barnes, Ed.D., R.R.T.

EVALUATION OF CLINICAL DATA

The Patient's Chart

The patient's chart is the legal record of all care provided by the health care team. It is a logical starting point for a review of information and clinical data regarding the patient's pathophysiological state. The "chart" is divided into several sections described in Chapters 1 and 3. The chart should be read in a specific sequence starting with the data sheet found immediately inside the front cover. The data sheet usually provides the admitting diagnosis, names of admitting and attending physicians, ID number, age, occupation, religion, and race, which establishes the patient's identity and the reasons for his hospitalization.

The next section reviewed should be the "physician progress notes" starting with the note written by the physician who completed a physical examination and history on the day of admission. A review of the pertinent findings on the day of admission should provide a detailed explanation of the patient's symptoms, physical findings, the diagnosis, and the initial plan for treatment. In some cases, a series of diagnostic tests may be required before a treatment plan can be developed. Since the progress note section may be long if a patient has been hospitalized for several days, it makes sense to review the rest of this section by starting with the most recent entry and working backward until enough information is gathered. If time is available, it is usually a good idea to quickly review the entire section, looking for major surgical or medical interventions

and the results of major diagnostic tests. Physician progress notes should be reviewed in this much detail only the first time the patient is treated by a respiratory therapist, since a great deal of this information is routinely communicated during shift reports and rounds with attending physicians. However, the physician's progress notes usually include comments regarding the patient's response to medical and surgical treatments that will need to be considered when determining the appropriateness of the respiratory care plan. Also, improvement or deterioration in the patient's overall condition usually will be summarized in the "physician progress notes."

Next, the "physician orders" section should be reviewed to note the prescribed respiratory care and the names of the ordering physician(s). The order sheet should be read starting with the last entry since treatments frequently are discontinued or modified to include different medications, dosages, and parameters. Some hospitals maintain a separate "order book" where prescribed treatments and medications are filed by patient name. Caution should be taken to ensure that handwritten orders are interpreted correctly. Items that are difficult to read or not understood should be confirmed by contacting the attending physician directly. Standards of the Joint Commission on Accreditation of Hospitals (JCAH) recommend that the physician's order for respiratory therapy should specify:

1. Type of treatment.
2. Frequency of treatment.

3. Duration of treatment.
4. Type and dose of medication.
5. Type of diluent and oxygen concentration as appropriate.

Although the JCAH standards for physician orders for respiratory care recommend including "duration of treatment," most practitioners find that specifying a fixed amount of time causes problems. For example, to order a medication nebulizer treatment for 15 minutes would not make sense if the time necessary to nebulize the solution requires more or less time than specified. JCAH guidelines require that a record of physician orders for respiratory care and related respiratory therapy evaluation reports be maintained in the respiratory care department's files and in the patient's chart (medical record). Some respiratory care services require physicians to complete a requisition on which various parts of the order must be specified. Requisitions of this type have specific sections for commonly used modalities of respiratory care. A requisition developed by Loyola University Medical Center (Fig 4–1) has sections that include places for a physician to specify the parameters of the treatment, and also has places for recording (by checking boxes) the indications for and objectives of therapy. Prior to reorder or after 72 hours, the physician using a requisition of this type may be asked to complete a brief retrospective evaluation. If the respiratory care is to be discontinued, the physician would place check marks next to the areas of improvement and check the "objectives achieved—D/C therapy" box. If therapeutic objectives are not achieved, several changes in the order may require a new requisition to be completed. A new requisition would normally be completed for subsequent retrospective evaluations. Orders for respiratory care that are not renewed within 72 hours are usually automatically terminated according to standing protocols.

Most charts have a "treatment section" where "respiratory care procedure notes" and "respiratory care evaluation reports" are filed. Some respiratory care services have designed special forms, which include lists of indications and therapeutic objectives for treatments and oxygen therapy. A form used at Duke University Medical Center includes boxes that can be checked to indicate: (1) if oxygen is "in use," (2) equipment is changed, or (3) the indications and objectives for the procedure and/or oxygen being administered (Fig 4–2). This form has a place for notes regarding the outcomes of each procedure and allows a great amount of information to be recorded in a relatively small space. The use of boxes that can be checked to record indications and objectives of respiratory care provide a useful and efficient way to assure that treatment goals are always in mind.

Loma Linda Medical Center has developed a series of forms for recording a multitude of information about the administration of respiratory care that includes lists of descriptors (Fig 4–3). The respiratory care practitioner using this form writes alphanumeric codes into several labeled boxes on the form that are divided into sections for "pre-," "during," and "post-" treatment entries. This form allows a respiratory care department to generate standardized computer reports that profile various aspects of the respiratory care being administered. The form facilitates retrospective studies on the degree to which therapeutic objectives are achieved since breath sounds, vital signs, and other clinical data are recorded before, during, and after the treatment using standardized descriptors.

Another example of a "procedure note" form that attempts to standardize entries into the medical record is "ventilator flow sheets" (Fig 4–4). Flowsheets are used to record changes in ventilation parameters, physiologic data about the patient (e.g., blood gas studies and pulmonary compliance), and periodic checks of the life support system. Ventilator flow sheets are usually kept at the bedside to facilitate frequent entries but eventually are filed in the patient's chart and become part of the permanent medical record.

Several respiratory care services have policies that require all orders for therapy to be evaluated initially and at 72-hour intervals. Accordingly, special forms for placing "bronchial hygiene" evaluations into the medical record have been developed. A form for this purpose may be divided into sections for diagnosis, data, physical assessment, and recommendations for a bronchial hygiene plan (Fig 4–5).[10] Forms of this type often include a special section for designating a priority level for receiving respiratory care.

The "respiratory care procedure" section of the chart where the forms discussed above are usually filed provides the following information:

1. Names of the practitioners who have provided respiratory care.
2. Type of respiratory care being administered.
3. Frequency of treatment.
4. Date, indications, time, and duration of the therapy administered.

56293

PREMIER

PLEASE STATE
DIAGNOSIS RELATING TO THERAPY:_____

_____

_____ _____
DATE   PHYSICIAN

- RETROSPECTIVE EVALUATION TO BE COMPLETED BY PHYSICIAN AFTER 72 HRS. AND PRIOR TO REORDER. ⟶
- UNLESS DURATION IS SPECIFIED, TREATMENTS WILL BE GIVEN FOR 24 HRS. ALL ORDERS TERMINATE AFTER 72 HRS.
- INDICATIONS AND OBJECTIVES TO BE COMPLETED BY PHYSICIAN **BEFORE** THERAPY IS INITIATED.

UNIT CLERK _____ TIME CALLED_____

THERAPIST _____ TIME REC'D._____

PHYSICIAN'S RETROSPECTIVE EVALUATION
[TO BE PERFORMED EVERY 72 HRS.]
☐ OBJECTIVES ACHIEVED — D/C THERAPY
☐ OBJECTIVES NOT ACHIEVED — RENEW AS FOLLOWS:

_____ _____
PHYSICIAN   DATE

TREATMENTS

INCENTIVE SPIROMETRY [check one]
☐ **PROPHYLACTIC** -Prevent post-op complications
  [circle indication] a. upper abdominal surgery
                     b. thoracic surgery
                     c. documented acute or chronic lung disease
Frequency: **Only one pre & post-op instruction**

☐ **THERAPEUTIC** - Treatment of **documented** acute pulmonary disease (atelectasis segmental or greater).
Frequency of Therapist Supervision:
☐ BID ☐ TID ☐ Other _____

IPPB [check indication]
☐ Atelectasis unresponsive to simpler therapy
☐ Inspiratory capacity less than 1 liter
☐ Ineffective cough mechanism
☐ Severe hypoventilation/avoid mechanical vent.
☐ **STANDING ORDER:** ☐ **CHANGE STANDING**
Frequency: QID   **ORDER TO:** _____
Duration of 24 Hrs.
O_2 Conc.: At pt's FIO_2 _____
Pressure: 20-25 cmH_2O _____

ADMINISTER WITH: [check one]
☐ Normal Saline ☐ Medication (See meds section)

NEBULIZATION THERAPY
☐ MEDICATION NEBULIZER
☐ ULTRASONIC NEBULIZER
☐ SPUTUM INDUCTION: AFB:_____ CYTOLOGY_____
                 PYOGENS:_____ FUNGUS_____
THERAPY OBJECTIVES
☐ Hydration of dried, retained secretions
☐ Administration of pharmacological agent

Frequency:_____ Duration:_____
Length of Tx _____ min.
O_2 Conc. _____ %
ADMINISTER WITH: [check one]
☐ Saline ☐ Medication (See meds section)

MEDICATIONS
☐ METAPROTERENOL (Alupent, 5% Sol.)
☐ ISOETHARINE (Bronkosol, 1% Sol.)
☐ ATROPINE SULFATE (1.0mg/ml)
☐ ACETYLCYSTEINE (Mucomyst, 20% Sol.)
☐ RACEMIC EPINEPHRINE (Vaponephrine, 2.25% Sol.)
☐ CROMOLYN SODIUM (Intal 20mg/2ml H_2O)
☐ OTHER _____
                specify
DOSE: _____ TO _____
    quantity of drug   quantity of dilutent

260649-5

HUMIDITY / OXYGEN

OXYGEN THERAPY
THERAPY OBJECTIVES
☐ Decrease work of breathing
☐ Decrease myocardial work
☐ Treat hypoxia
DEVICE
☐ NASAL CANNULA _____ 1/min.
☐ SIMPLE MASK (35-55%) _____ 1/min.
☐ VENTI MASK .24 .26 .28 .30 .35 .40 .50
☐ MASK WITH RESERVOIR (60-90%)
☐ CPAP MASK (30-100%) _____ %
  5.0cmH_2O 7.5cmH_2O 10.0 cmH_2O 12.5 cmH_2O

HIGH HUMIDITY OXYGEN
☐ AEROSOL (28-100%) FIO_2 _____ %
  _____ Aerosol Mask   _____ Face Tent
  _____ T-Piece   _____ Tracheostomy Collar
NOTE: AEROSOL MASK AND T-PIECE SET UPS WILL BE ANALYZED IF THE ORDERED FIO_2 IS GREATER THAN .40. FOR SYSTEMS ≤ .40 INDICATE IF SYSTEM IS TO BE ANALYZED. ☐ YES

  HEAD HOOD AND CROUP TENT SET UPS ARE ALWAYS ANALYZED.
☐ HEAD HOOD FIO_2 _____ %
☐ CROUP TENT FIO_2 _____ %

DIAGNOSTIC

☐ CARDIAC OUTPUT
☐ HEMODYNAMIC PROFILE

OTHER _____
                 SPECIFY

☐ PRE-OP PULMONARY SCREENING (FEV_1/FVC)
  _____ History of smoking
  _____ Occupational exposure
  _____ Pulmonary signs and symptoms
  _____ Other _____

☐ RESPIRATORY PARAMETERS
  _____ Vt/Vc/NIF   Frequency:_____
  _____ Peak Expiratory Flow

☐ ARTERIAL OXIMETER (non-invasive)
  Duration: 1   2   3   days

☐ MIXED VENOUS OXIMETER (invasive)

☐ RESPIRATORY CONSULTATION

MED. RECORD NO.   •   BIRTH DATE   SEX

PATIENT NAME

ADDRESS   ROOM

Loyola University Medical Center
RESPIRATORY THERAPY REQUISITION

CHART

FIG 4–1.

Examples of forms designed for ordering respiratory therapy (above) and bronchial hygiene therapy (facing page). Top of the form must be signed and dated by ordering physician. Physician must specify the type of respiratory therapy including frequency, duration, type and dose of medication, type of diluent and oxygen concentration. Indications and therapeutic objectives must be checked off. Diagnostic section included for evaluation of therapeutic goals. Specific section for physician's retrospective evaluation to be performed every 72 hours. (Courtesy of Loyola University Medical Center.) *(Continued.)*

58873

PREMIER FORMS

PLEASE STATE DIAGNOSIS RELATING TO THERAPY: _____

UNIT CLERK _____ TIME CALLED _____

THERAPIST _____ TIME REC'D _____

_____ DATE _____ _____ PHYSICIAN

BRONCHIAL HYGIENE THERAPY

TREATMENTS	INDICATION	PHYSICIAN ORDER
	☐ Post-op. Upper abdominal/thoracic surgery. ☐ Post-op. Documented chronic lung disease.	Incentive spirometry. Patient instruction X 2 with cough instruction.
	☐ Documented (by CXR) atelectasis; segmental or greater. ☐ Muscular weakness with ineffective cough and related secretions.	For patients with VC ≥ 10ml/kg: Therapist supervised incentive spirometry with cough instruction BID X 72 hours. For patients with VC<10ml/kg. IPPB wth cough instructions TID X 72 hours.
	☐ Obstructive airway disease (asthma, bronchitis, emphysema, bronchiolitis, BPD) ☐ Impaired mucociliary clearance (pneumonia, cystic fibrosis, COPD, bronchiectasis) ☐ Upper airway edema/obstruction (tracheolaryngeal bronchitis, croup, post extubation edema). ☐ Abnormal, copious secretions that do not clear with cough (bronchiectasis, cystic fibrosis, lung abcess, resolving pneumonia).	Respiratory Therapist to evaluate for QID and prn x72ᵒ medication nebulizer treatments or QID and prn x _____ days metered dose inhaler treatments with spacer. Respiratory Therapy to deliver **all** nebulizer therapy and MDI therapy to patients with artificial airways. Respiratory Therapist and Registered Nurse to instruct all patients with intact upper airways on MDI use for first administration; nursing to monitor patient self-administration of MDI therafter QID and prn. MDI to be kept at patient bedside. **ORDER MEDICATION BELOW.**

Requests for bronchial hygiene protocols other than those outlined above must be approved by the Medical Director of Respiratory Care or his designate. Specify requested bronchial hygiene protocol/physicians order: _____

Specify indication of requested bronchial hygiene protocol: _____

MEDICATIONS	STANDARD ADULT DOSAGE	PREFERRED ALTERNATE DOSAGE
☐ Metaproterenol (Alupent)	0.6% 2.5ml. by nebulizer, or 2 puffs (0.65mg. each) by MDI	
☐ Albuterol (Proventil) (Ventolin)	2.5mg. in 3cc by nebulizer, or 2 puffs (90 mcg. each) by MDI	
☐ Ipratropium bromide (Atrovent)	3 puffs (18mcg. each) by MDI	
☐ Terbutaline (Breathaire)	2 puffs (0.2mg. each) by MDI	
☐ Acetylcysteine (Mucomyst)	20% 4ml. with 0.3ml. Alupent 5% by nebulizer	
☐ Cromolyn Sodium (Intal)	20mg. in 2ml. H₂O for neb. or 2 puffs (800mcg. each) by MDI	
☐ Racemic Epinephrine (Vaponephrine)	2.25% 0.5ml. in 3ml. normal saline by nebulizer	
☐ Other		

EVALUATION DATE: _____ TIME: _____ Patient can perform MDI ☐ yes ☐ no   Intact upper airway ☐ yes ☐ no
VC= _____ ml. Peak flow pre-neb tx= _____ post neb tx= _____ Peak flow pre-MDI tx= _____ post MDI tx= _____
Plan: _____

_____ Therapist: _____

RE-EVALUATION DATE: _____ TIME: _____ Patient can perform MDI ☐ yes ☐ no   Intact upper airway ☐ yes ☐ no
VC= _____ ml. Peak flow pre-neb tx= _____ post neb tx= _____ Peak flow pre-MDI tx= _____ post MDI tx= _____
Plan: _____

_____ Therapist: _____

OXYGEN THERAPY
THERAPY OBJECTIVES
☐ Decrease work of breathing   ☐ Treat hypoxia
☐ Decrease myocardial work   ☐ Post-operative period
DEVICE
☐ NASAL CANNULA _____ 1/min.
☐ VENTIMASK   .24   .26   .28   .30   .35   .40   .50
☐ SIMPLE MASK (35-55%) 5LPM 6LPM 7LPM 8LPM 9LPM 10LPM
☐ MASK WITH RESERVOIR (60-90%)
☐ CPAP (30-100%) ___ %
   5.0cmH₂O   7.5cmH₂O   10.0 cmH₂O   12.5 cmH₂O

HIGH HUMIDITY OXYGEN
☐ AEROSOL (28-100%) FIO₂ ___%
_____ Aerosol Mask   _____ Face Tent
_____ T-Piece   _____ Tracheostomy Collar
NOTE: AEROSOL MASK AND T-PIECE SET UPS WILL BE ANALYZED IF THE ORDERED FIO₂ IS GREATER THAN .40. FOR SYSTEMS ≤ .40 INDICATE IF SYSTEM IS TO BE ANALYZED. ☐ YES HEAD HOOD AND CROUP TENT SET UPS ARE ALWAYS ANALYZED.
☐ HEAD HOOD   FIO₂ _____ %
☐ CROUP TENT   FIO₂ _____ %

CARDIO/RESPIRATORY MONITORING
☐ CARDIAC OUTPUT   ☐ OTHER _____
☐ HEMODYNAMIC PROFILE
☐ PRE-OP PULMONARY SCREENING (Fev1, FVC, peak flow)
   ☐ History of smoking   ☐ Age>70 yrs.
   ☐ Occupational exposure   ☐ Obesity
   ☐ Pulmonary signs/symptons   ☐ Other _____
☐ SPUTUM INDUCTION QD   X1   X2   X3
☐ RESPIRATORY PARAMETERS
   ☐ Vt/Vc/NIF ☐ Peak Expiratory Flow   Frequency: _____
☐ ARTERIAL OXIMETER - Intermittent Checks
   Frequency: XI   BID   TID   Other _____
☐ ARTERIAL OXIMETER - Continous Monitor
   Duration: 1   2   3   days
☐ TRANSCUTANEOUS OXYGEN MONITOR
☐ TRANSCUTANEOUS CARBON DIOXIDE MONITOR
☐ MIXED VENOUS OXIMETER (Invasive)
☐ EXHALED CO2 MONITOR Duration: 1   2   3   days
☐ METABOLIC STUDY (VO₂, VCO₂ RQ)
☐ DEADSPACE STUDY (VD/VT %)
☐ RESPIRATORY CARE EVALUATION HOME CARE

260649-6 REV. 6/87

MED. RECORD NO. _____ BIRTH DATE _____ SEX _____

PATIENT NAME _____

ADDRESS _____ ROOM _____

Ⓛ Loyola University Medical Center
RESPIRATORY THERAPY REQUISITION

CHART

FIG 4–1. (Cont.)

5. The indications and therapeutic objective for each mode of therapy.
6. Subjective information received from the patient regarding the effectiveness of the therapy.
7. Objective information regarding effects of therapy such as adverse reactions or changes in heart rate, respiratory rate before, during, and after therapy, breath sounds, cough, sputum, and arterial blood gas results.
8. Assessment of the degree to which therapeutic objectives are being accomplished.
9. Plans for modifying, adding, or discontinuing modes or frequency of therapy, procedures, or equipment.

DUKE UNIVERSITY MEDICAL CENTER
RESPIRATORY CARE PROCEDURE NOTE

Procedure:	Device:
Frequency:	FIO$_2$ Flowrate
Medication:	Other: Initials:

Indications	Therapeutic Objectives
O$_2$ Treatment	O$_2$ Treatment
☐ ☐ Hypoxia	☐ ☐ Improve Tissue Oxygenation
☐ ☐ Artificial Airway	☐ ☐ Humidify Airway
☐ ☐ Thick Retained Secretions	☐ ☐ Mobilize/Remove Secretions
☐ ☐ Bronchospasm	☐ ☐ Bronchodilation/Improve Ventilation
☐ ☐ Atelectasis	☐ ☐ Reinflate Atelectatic Lung Areas
☐ ☐ Stridor	☐ ☐ Relieve Stridor/Improve Ventilation
☐ ☐ Post Extubation	☐ ☐ Relieve Laryngeal Edema
☐ ☐ Other: _____	☐ ☐ Other: _____

Date: Time:	Date: Time:
Oxygen In Use ☐ Stand-By ☐	Oxygen In Use ☐ Stand-By ☐
Equipment Change: Oxygen ☐	Equipment Change: Oxygen ☐
Other ☐ _____	Other ☐ _____
Note:	Note:

Summary:_____
_____ Initials:_____

Date: Time:	Date: Time:
Oxygen In Use ☐ Stand-By ☐	Oxygen In Use ☐ Stand-By ☐
Equipment Change: Oxygen ☐	Equipment Change: Oxygen ☐
Other ☐ _____	Other ☐ _____
Note:	Note:

Summary:_____
_____ Initials:_____

Date: Time:	Date: Time:
Oxygen In Use ☐ Stand-By ☐	Oxygen In Use ☐ Stand-By ☐
Equipment Change: Oxygen ☐	Equipment Change: Oxygen ☐
Other ☐ _____	Other ☐ _____
Note:	Note:

Summary:_____
_____ Initials:_____

Date: Time:	Date: Time:
Oxygen In Use ☐ Stand-By ☐	Oxygen In Use ☐ Stand-By ☐
Equipment Change: Oxygen ☐	Equipment Change: Oxygen ☐
Other ☐ _____	Other ☐ _____
Note:	Note:

Summary:_____
_____ Initials:_____

FIG 4–2.

Example of a form designed to record information about respiratory care procedures in the medical record. Note the special section for recording the "indications" and "therapeutic objectives" for treatments and O$_2$ therapy. Also, a place to indicate equipment changes, treatment notes and a shift summary statement is provided. (Courtesy of Respiratory Care Service, Duke University Medical Center.)

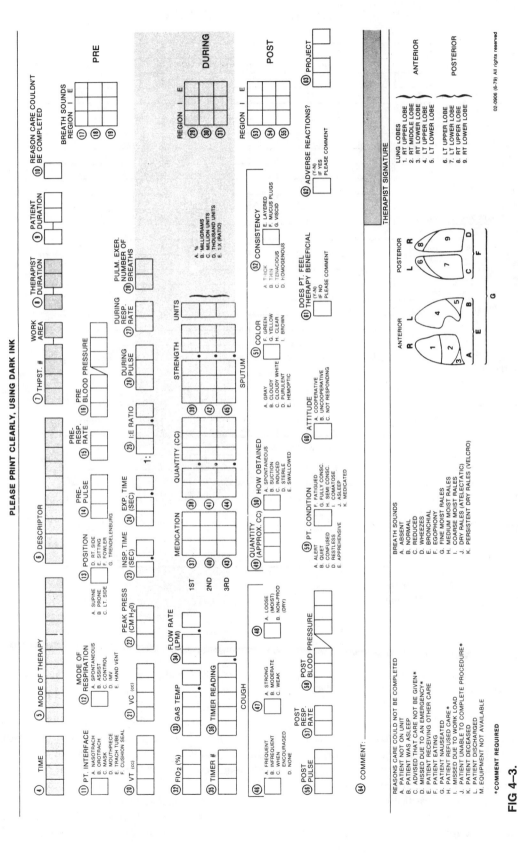

FIG 4–3.

Example of a form designed to record information related to administration of respiratory treatments. Note the separate sections for "pretreatment," "during treatment," and "posttreatment" information. The bottom of the form provides an alphanumeric notation system for describing breath sounds. (Courtesy of Department of Respiratory Care, Loma Linda University Medical Center.)

WASHINGTON HOSPITAL CENTER

DATE/TIME												
SIGNATURE												
MODE OF VENTILATOR												
FIO2												
PEEP (cmH20)												
RATE SETTING (VENTILATOR)												
RATE (TOTAL PATIENT)												
TIDAL VOLUME SET (LITERS)												
TIDAL VOLUME EXH (LITERS)												
MINUTE VENT (L/MIN)												
I:E RATIO												
PEAK FLOW RATE (L/MIN)												
PEAK AIRWAY PRESS (cmH20)												
NORMAL PRESS LIMIT (cmH20)												
SENSITIVITY (cmH20)												
SIGH VOL (LITERS)												
SIGH AIRWAY PRESS (cmH20)												
SIGH PRESS LIMIT (cmH20)												
SIGH RATE (MULTIPLE)												
TEMP OF CIRCUIT												
MASS SPEC TRAP CLEAN												
ET/TRACH TUBE PLACEMENT												
CUFF PRESSURE												
ALARMS												
Pe CO2												
A–a D CO2												

WEANING PARAMETERS

RESPIRATORY RATE												
VT												
MINUTE VENTILATION												
VITAL CAPACITY												
INSPIRATORY FORCE												
MISCELLANEOUS												

**RESPIRATORY THERAPY
ADULT VENTILATOR REPORT**

FORM 814   D-300   5/82

FIG 4–4.
Example of a ventilator flowsheet where data related to therapeutic objectives is recorded at frequent intervals (usually every 2 hours). (Courtesy of the Department of Respiratory Care, The Washington Hospital Center.)

After having reviewed the data sheet, progress notes, physician's orders, clinical records, and treatment sections of the chart, the injury or disease being treated should be clearly in mind. However, the degree of dysfunction may require further investigation such as a review of radiology reports that are usually filed in a separate diagnostic section of the chart. The radiology reports may be enhanced by actually viewing the chest x-ray to gather additional information (Table 4–1). Also, blood gas studies and other pertinent laboratory studies may need to be reviewed to establish baseline or trend data (Table 4–2).

The respiratory care practitioner should discuss with other members of the health care team the patient's treatment plan, and their opinions should be

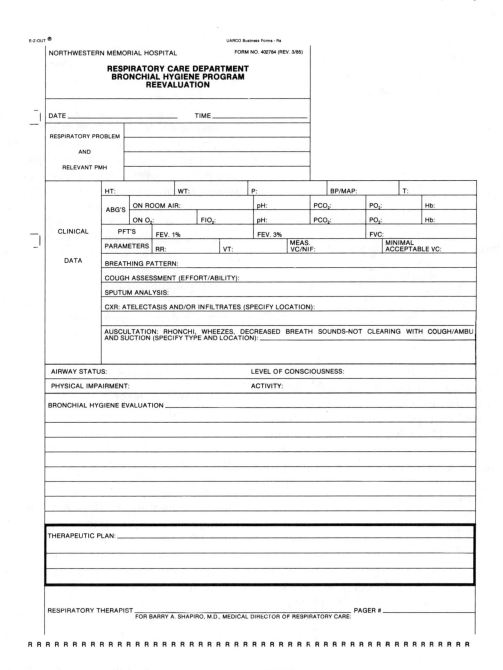

E-Z-OUT ®

UARCO Business Forms - Ra

NORTHWESTERN MEMORIAL HOSPITAL

FORM NO. 402784 (REV. 3/85)

**RESPIRATORY CARE DEPARTMENT
BRONCHIAL HYGIENE PROGRAM
REEVALUATION**

DATE _____   TIME _____

RESPIRATORY PROBLEM

AND

RELEVANT PMH

CLINICAL

DATA

HT: WT: P: BP/MAP: T:

ABG'S | ON ROOM AIR: pH: PCO₂: PO₂: Hb:

ON O₂: FIO₂: pH: PCO₂: PO₂: Hb:

PFT'S | FEV. 1%   FEV. 3%   FVC:

PARAMETERS | RR: VT: MEAS. VC/NIF: MINIMAL ACCEPTABLE VC:

BREATHING PATTERN:

COUGH ASSESSMENT (EFFORT/ABILITY):

SPUTUM ANALYSIS:

CXR: ATELECTASIS AND/OR INFILTRATES (SPECIFY LOCATION):

AUSCULTATION: RHONCHI, WHEEZES, DECREASED BREATH SOUNDS-NOT CLEARING WITH COUGH/AMBU AND SUCTION (SPECIFY TYPE AND LOCATION): _____

AIRWAY STATUS: LEVEL OF CONSCIOUSNESS:

PHYSICAL IMPAIRMENT: ACTIVITY:

BRONCHIAL HYGIENE EVALUATION

THERAPEUTIC PLAN:

RESPIRATORY THERAPIST _____ PAGER # _____
FOR BARRY A. SHAPIRO, M.D., MEDICAL DIRECTOR OF RESPIRATORY CARE:

MEDICAL RECORDS

FIG 4–5.
Example of a form designed to place in the medical record the results of a bronchial hygiene evaluation completed by respiratory therapists. Note the specific sections for diagnosis, clinical data, physical assessment, and for the bronchial hygiene plan. Note the narrative format. (Courtesy of the Respiratory Therapy Department, Northwestern Memorial Hospital.)

solicited at every opportunity. Especially important sources of information are family members and practitioners who see the patient frequently such as house staff (interns and residents), registered nurses, and respiratory therapists who have recently treated the patient. Often the results of recent laboratory or diagnostic tests may have just been received and not posted on the chart. Accordingly, good communication skills are critical to gathering current information and data about the patient. The data listed in Table 4–3 should have been reviewed after reading pertinent sections of the chart and dis-

TABLE 4–1.

Data Available From Chest X-Ray

Presence of, or changes in, consolidation and/or atelectasis
Presence of, or changes in, pneumothorax or subcutaneous
    emphysema
Position of endotracheal or tracheostomy tube
Position of chest tubes
Position of intravascular catheters
Position of, or change in, hemidiaphragms
Position of, or change in, mediastinum
Position and presence of foreign bodies
Presence of, or changes in, hyperinflation
Presence of, or changes in, pleural fluid
Presence of, or changes in, pulmonary edema
Presence of cardiac enlargement
Presence of enlargement or dilation of pulmonary arteries
Presence of pulmonary carcinoma
Presence of bronchial thickening or dilation
Presence of areas of increased density
Presence of fibrotic markings
Presence of thickened diaphragmatic pleura

cussing the patient with other members of the team.

If important clinical data is not available in the medical record, the respiratory care practitioner should recommend that additional data be collected. In some cases, that will involve asking the attending physician to prescribe a specific diagnostic test (see Chapters 2 and 3). In other instances, standing protocols will suggest additional data to be gathered and recorded in the medical record.[2, 4, 8, 10]

Observation of the Patient

The patient should be observed to assess his level of consciousness, orientation to time and place, emotional state, and ability to cooperate. During the initial interview and inspection you should intro-

TABLE 4–2.

Pertinent Diagnostic Data

Blood gas studies
Sputum culture and sensitivity
Chest x-ray
Electrolytes and other blood chemistries
ECG
Spirometry before and/or after bronchodilator
Dead space/tidal volume ratio (V_D/V_T)
Maximum voluntary ventilation (MVV)
Shunt fraction ($\dot{Q}_S/\dot{Q}_T$)
Urinalysis
Angiogram

duce yourself and explain the prescribed respiratory care plan so the patient knows who you are and what to expect. Subjective information that cannot be observed, such as dyspnea, must be solicited directly from the patient. However, if a patient is orthopneic (has to sit up to breathe) dyspnea should be suspected. If the patient tells you he is "short of breath," the subjective complaint should be recorded and a search for more objective data begun. The patient's overall respiratory status should be assessed by observing the items listed in Table 4–4. Remember the cliché, "a picture is worth a thousand words," and use your eyes (and ears) to assess both the obvious and subtle information the patient gives you directly. For example, the ventilatory pattern and accessory muscle activity will indicate how easily the patient can breathe and how much work is expended in the process (in Chapter 1, the procedures for doing a comprehensive respiratory physical examination are discussed).

Additional Pertinent Data

The overall respiratory status of the patient can be assessed further by palpation, percussion, and auscultation (Table 4–5). The techniques for using a stethoscope, your hands, and ears in obtaining this information are discussed in Chapters 1 and 3. The amount of dysfunction will vary considerably from patient to patient, and additional tests to gather other pertinent information may be required. Many of these tests can be done at the bedside, and others must be done in a laboratory. Sophisticated pulmonary function tests to determine diffusion capacity, maximum oxygen intake, and functional residual capacity will require the patient to be transported to the pulmonary laboratory. The respiratory care practitioner will have to evaluate the results of these tests to quantify the extent of the pulmonary dysfunction.

The development of a respiratory care plan may require recommending that additional diagnostic data be obtained in order to further quantify the extent of injury or dysfunction. The number and types of tests done will vary according to the injury and severity of illness encountered. A premium is usually given to tests and procedures that can be done quickly with little chance of injury or complications. The respiratory care practitioner will need to establish the level of dysfunction and therapeutic goals, and verify that all components of the respiratory care plan are appropriate.

TABLE 4–3.

Data Available in Patient Record

LOCATION IN CHART	TYPE OF INFORMATION	PERTINENT DATA
Patient data sheet	Database obtained at admission	Occupation, age, race; admission date; admitting physician; attending physician
Physician orders section	Specific diagnostic studies, treatments and medications	Admission orders; current orders; standing orders
Clinical records section	Shift-to-shift description of patient activities	Vital signs; nursing observations; subjective complaints; patient ambulation; sleep patterns; weight changes; amount and character of pleural drainage
Intake/output section	Record of fluid intake and output	Hourly record in ICU, every 8 hr outside ICU
Medication section	Oral and parenteral medications	Discontinued medications; current medications
Physician reports section	Patient history; physical examination; consultation reports	Primary diagnosis; secondary diagnoses; admitting physical examination; current physical examination; progress notes; comments on laboratory results
Respiratory therapy/physical therapy section	Documentation of respiratory and physical therapy evaluation reports	Respiratory care procedure notes; physical therapy procedure notes; results of ventilatory monitoring; results of pulmonary function tests; results of hemodynamic monitoring; recommendations for modifying respiratory care
Clinical laboratory section	Tests done in the clinical laboratory	Electrolytes; hemoglobin; white blood cell count; blood chemistry analyses; blood gas analyses; sputum culture; Gram's stain results
Radiology, nuclear medicine sections	Radiologic studies; nuclear medicine studies	Chest x-rays; computed tomography; angiography
ECG/EEG section	Cardiology and EEG studies	Electrocardiograms

TABLE 4–4.

Data Available by Inspection

State of consciousness
Chest configuration (shape)
Accessory muscle activity
Asymmetrical chest movement
Intercostal and/or sternal retractions
Breathing pattern
Cyanosis
Flushing
Diaphoresis
Peripheral edema
Clubbing of fingers
Muscle wasting
Venous distention
Capillary refill
Character of cough
Amount and character of sputum

IDENTIFYING CARDIORESPIRATORY DISORDERS

Quantification of Illness

The review and interpretation of data should allow the respiratory care practitioner to quantify the extent of injury or dysfunction. The time available will sometimes limit the review and interpretation of the data. For example, in treating a crushed chest injury in the emergency room, there may not be time initially to confirm a tension pneumothorax by taking an x-ray. However, the experienced practitioner looks for several pieces of data to form a pattern of dysfunction rather than relying on a single test or diagnostic procedure. Even in emergency situations, such as a spontaneous tension pneumothorax, there are usually several clinical signs that indicate the type and severity of the dysfunction and

TABLE 4–5.

Data Available by Auscultation, Palpation, and Percussion

AUSCULTATION	PALPATION	PERCUSSION
Bilateral normal breath sounds	Pulse (rate, rhythm, force)	Diaphragmatic excursion
Increased, decreased, absent, or unequal breath sounds	Asymmetrical chest movement	Areas of altered resonance
Rales (fine, medium, dry, coarse)	Secretions in the airway (palpable rhonchi)	
Rubs (friction, pleural, pericardial)	Tactile fremitus	
Wheezes (high-pitched, diminishing, sonorous)	Tracheal deviation	
Stridor	Crepitation	
Heart sounds	Tenderness	

point to the appropriate emergency treatment. For example, the sudden development of moderate or severe hypoxemia in conjunction with other clinical signs, e.g., absence of breath sounds and chest movement on the affected side, mediastinal (tracheal shift) away from the affected side, would require immediate action on the part of the respiratory care practitioner. If the patient is being mechanically ventilated, a switch to a manual resuscitator and 100% O_2 would be indicated. A chest tube may have to be placed immediately if the tension pneumothorax is massive and involves the collapse of an entire lung. A delay in placing the chest tube may require that a large bore needle be inserted through the intracostal muscles to decompress the pleural space. After the emergency care is rendered and the patient stabilized, a comprehensive treatment plan composed of diagnostic studies and additional modalities of care can be developed.

Establishing specific goals for the return of the patient to normal cardiopulmonary function requires a knowledge of how far away the patient is from his normal baseline values. For example, evaluation of a

patient's oxygenation state would require information on (1) metabolic rate, e.g., higher oxygen consumption due to fever, shivering, or major tissue trauma, (2) level of arterial hypoxemia, (3) hemoglobin concentration, (4) adequacy of tissue oxygenation, and (5) amount of cardiac compensation, e.g., heart rate, blood pressure, urine output. A review of clinical data should allow an impression of "inadequate oxygenation," for example, to be defined quantitatively, so that specific therapeutic objectives can be established. Individual components of the respiratory care plan should address the overall goal of restoring oxygenation to the patient's normal baseline values. The level of dysfunction and therapeutic goals can be quantified as shown in Table 4–6.

Variance From Baseline

A knowledge of the normal baseline values for all of the clinical data reviewed and the implications of variance from normal is important. The selection of components for the respiratory care plan in many situations will be related to the severity of the dys-

TABLE 4–6.

Quantification of Inadequate Tissue Oxygenation*

PHYSIOLOGIC VARIABLE	OBSERVED VALUE	BASELINE VALUE	OBJECTIVES SHORT-TERM	LONG-TERM
Pao_2, mm Hg	45	90	>60	>80
$P\bar{v}o_2$, mm Hg	20	40	>35	40
$Ca\text{-}C\bar{v}o_2$, vol%	6.5	4.5	<6.0	<5.0
Cardiac output, L/min	10	6	<8.5	<7
Heart rate, beats/min	140	75	<120	<100
Hemoglobin, gm/dl	8	14	>12	14
Respiratory rate	35	12	<30	<20

*Therapeutic goal: Restore tissue oxygenation to baseline values.

function. The degree of abnormality (how far physiologic parameters are from the patient's normal baseline values) often provides justification for selecting a particular modality of care.[2, 4, 8, 10]

A comprehensive respiratory care plan will often include indications for each modality of care based on the degree or severity of illness. For example, a decision not to recommend mechanical ventilation might be based on the data presented in Table 4–7. The decision not to ventilate centers around a knowledge of the patient's "normal" baseline values which are substantially higher because of chronic obstructive lung disease. A knowledge of the patient's baseline Pa_{CO_2} eliminates hypercarbia as an acute problem and leads to a recommendation to improve oxygenation by using low-flow oxygen therapy alone.

Secondary Diagnoses

Quite often other dysfunctions are discovered that are far more severe than the original reason for hospitalizing the patient (see Chapter 3). A secondary problem may occur as a complication of the original trauma or problem. For example, a patient may be hospitalized for a fresh water near-drowning incident which may be complicated by the hemolysis of red cells, aspiration pneumonitis, cardiac failure, or head trauma. The respiratory care practitioner needs to be aware of the potential for dysfunction in other organ systems. Especially important is the impact these other problems have on the respiratory disturbances that are being treated.

COMPONENTS OF THE RESPIRATORY CARE PLAN

Therapeutic Objectives

A familiar cliché, "You won't know when you have arrived if you don't know where you're going," is applicable to respiratory care. Clear, concise, and measurable objectives should be identified for each therapeutic goal and included in a comprehensive respiratory care plan. Each component of the care plan should have specific therapeutic objectives related to restoration of normal pulmonary function (Table 4–8). For example, if mechanical ventilation is used to provide adequate ventilation, one of the primary objectives will be to keep the Pa_{CO_2} between ±5 mm Hg of the patient's normal baseline value. There will be other secondary (procedural) objectives such as using the appropriate ventilation parameters, delivering tidal volumes in the range of 10 to 15 ml/kg ideal body weight, and maintenance of spontaneous breathing at a level less than 30 breaths/minute. However, each procedure or treatment should have specific measurable primary objectives related to restoring normal pulmonary function.

Timelines for Evaluating Therapy

Although difficult to do, timelines should be established for evaluating therapeutic objectives. The use of timelines serves many purposes, including:

1. Clarifying the physiologic parameters to be monitored.
2. Establishing a regular schedule for evaluating the level of pulmonary dysfunction.
3. Allowing for timely modification of the respiratory care being provided.
4. Facilitating decisions, such as when treatments and modalities of care should be discontinued.

The need for timelines for evaluating respiratory care is especially important for patients receiving mechanical ventilation. A wealth of information should already be available since these patients are normally monitored extensively around the clock. The pattern of ventilation established for the patient initially may need many modifications during

TABLE 4–7.

Comparison of Baseline and Actual Clinical Data for a Patient With Chronic Obstructive Lung Disease

TYPE OF DATA	OBSERVED VALUE	BASELINE VALUE	BASELINE VARIANCE
Pa_{CO_2}, mm Hg	60	55	+5
Pa_{O_2}, mm Hg	35	50	−15
pH	7.35	7.40	−0.05
Base excess	+10	+10	0
Spontaneous respiratory rate	32	18	+14

TABLE 4–8.

Matching Treatment Indications to Therapeutic Objectives*

TREATMENT INDICATIONS	THERAPEUTIC OBJECTIVES
Hypoxia	Improve tissue oxygenation
Artificial airway	Reverse humidity deficit
Thick retained secretions	Mobilize and remove secretions
Bronchospasm	Bronchodilation/improve ventilation
Atelectasis	Reinflate atelectatic lung areas
Stridor	Relieve stridor/improve ventilation
Laryngeal edema (postextubation)	Relieve laryngeal edema

*Modified from *Procedure Manual: Respiratory Care Procedure Note.* Durham, NC, Duke University Medical Center, 1984.

the first 4 hours, and frequently thereafter. The therapeutic plan should state at what interval the ventilation parameters should be evaluated and the criteria for changing the level of support provided.

Contraindications and Hazards

The treatments and procedures needed to care for seriously ill or traumatized patients have certain risks. The hazards not only can be found with complicated life support equipment such as ventilators but also with simple oxygen therapy devices. The hazards must be clearly understood and plans made to monitor a potential problem. A good example is the need to monitor the temperature of inspired gases during mechanical ventilation. The hazard is reduced if the temperature is checked at frequent predetermined intervals. A ventilator flow sheet at the bedside, which lists the data that will be recorded at frequent intervals, represents a plan for dealing with potential hazards (see Fig 4–4). Contraindications for certain procedures may not present a problem initially, but subsequent changes in the patient's condition may require that the respiratory care plan be modified. For example, if shock develops, the PEEP level may no longer be optimal, but contraindicated. Accordingly, the quick removal of PEEP would be dependent on the practitioner knowing that hypotension was a contraindication and frequent monitoring of the patient's blood pressure was required. Another example would be the development of cardiac arrythmias by a patient receiving a medication nebulizer treatment. A knowledge of the contraindications and side effects of bronchodilators, e.g., cardiac arrythmias, is fundamental to recommending a lower dose, if necessary.

Monitoring Effectiveness

A comprehensive respiratory care plan will identify the data that should be collected to evaluate the effectiveness of the therapy being administered. Many respiratory care departments have quality assurance programs that monitor the care being given to a specific group of patients. These programs monitor how well practitioners meet specific criteria including proper completion of flow sheets and respiratory care procedure notes (Fig 4–6). The focus should be on collecting, at predetermined intervals, data that allow the therapist to assess the patient's response to respiratory care. The data to be collected will vary according to the therapy being administered. However, procedure manuals should include protocols and special forms for each modality of care that indicate the assessment data that should be collected to evaluate progress toward clearly delineated therapeutic goals. The data collected should be analyzed to evaluate the effectiveness of the therapeutic plan and placed in the chart.[1, 4, 8, 10] The relative effectiveness of different types of treatment should be compared in order to find the most economic regimen, e.g., shorter postoperative stay and fewer clinical complications.[3, 5, 6]

Modifying Therapeutic Goals

Therapeutic goals often have to be modified because of complications or contraindications that were identified after the original treatment plan was begun. The practitioner should realize that the initial respiratory care plan may need to be modified and new therapeutic objectives developed if significant changes in the patient's condition occur. The recommendation may be to terminate a particular treatment and to start another or to only modify the tech-

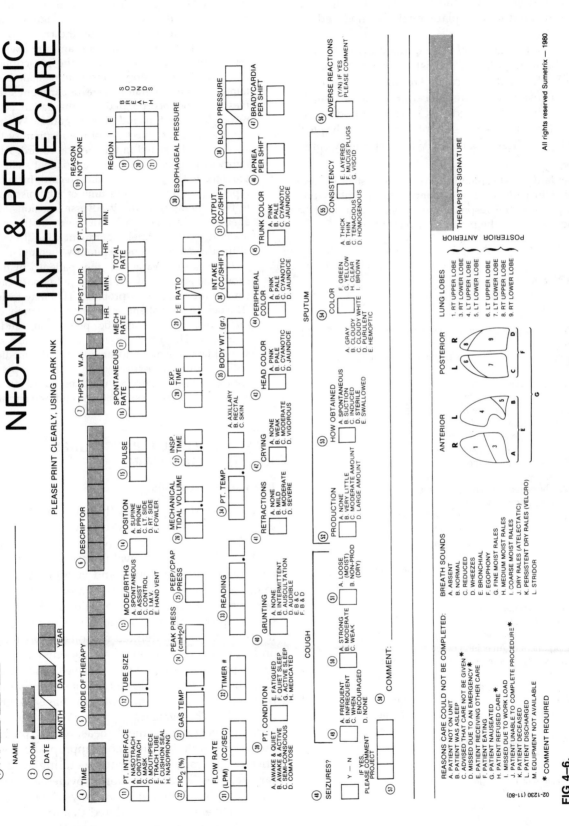

FIG 4–6.
Example of a form designed to collect specific information in several different categories related to neonatal and pediatric respiratory intensive care. Note the descriptors supplied to ensure consistent standard entries into the medical record. (Courtesy of Loma Linda University Medical Center.)

nique for administering the treatment. Examples of the way respiratory care plans might be modified are given in Table 4–9.

One of the goals of a respiratory care service should be to maintain a consistent standard for entries into the medical record. The protocol for completing a respiratory care procedure note is usually based on the widely used "S-O-A-P" method—Subjective—Objective—Assessment—Plan (see Chapters 1 and 17) and JCAH standard V for respiratory care[1]:

> Standard V.—Respiratory care services shall be provided to patients in accordance with a written prescription of the responsible physician, and shall be documented in the patient's medical record.

TABLE 4–9.

Examples of Modifications in Respiratory Care

IPPB
  Adjust sensitivity, flow, volume, and/or pressure
  Adjust F_{IO_2}
  Change patient-machine interface (mouthpiece, mask, orotracheal, etc.)
Incentive Breathing Devices
  Change type of equipment
  Increase or decrease incentive goals
Aerosol Therapy
  Change type of equipment
  Change concentration of medication
  Change dosage of medication
  Adjust temperature of the liquid media
  Modify patient breathing patterns
  Change aerosol output
Oxygen Therapy and Other Gas Therapy
  Change mode of administration
  Adjust flow and concentration
  Adjust gas concentration
Chest Physiotherapy (Bronchopulmonary Drainage)
  Alter position of patient
  Alter duration of treatment
  Alter equipment used
  Alter techniques
  Coordinate sequences of therapies
Management of Artificial Airways
  Change type of humidification equipment
  Initiate suctioning
  Inflate and deflate the cuff
  Alter endotracheal or tracheostomy tube position
  Change endotracheal or tracheostomy tube
  Recommend extubation
Continuous Mechanical Ventilation
  Adjust ventilator settings
  Change patient breathing circuitry
  Adjust alarm settings
  Institute weaning
  Change weaning procedures
  Change type of ventilator

Interpretation.—The prescription for respiratory care shall specify the type, frequency, and duration of treatment, and, as appropriate, the type and dose of medication, the type of diluent, and the oxygen concentration. A written record of the prescription and any related respiratory consultation shall be maintained in the respiratory care department's/service's files, shall be incorporated into the patient's medical record, and shall include the diagnosis. When feasible, the goals or objectives of the respiratory therapy should also be stated in the medical record. All respiratory care services provided to a patient shall be documented in the patient's medical record, including the type of therapy, date and time of administration, effects of therapy, and any adverse reactions. The responsible physician shall document in the patient's medical record a timely, pertinent clinical evaluation of the overall results of respiratory therapy.

Prior to discharge of the patient, instructions should be given in all aspects of pulmonary care relevant to the respiratory problem. This may include instruction to the patient or the patient's family on postural drainage, therapeutic percussion, and other measures. The need for long-term oxygen therapy should be adequately documented in the medical records of patients discharged on such therapy. When appropriate, such need should be based on arterial blood gas analysis results at rest and/or exercise.

EVALUATION OF PRESCRIBED RESPIRATORY CARE

Evaluation Programs

Registered respiratory therapists who have the appropriate experience and education are capable of evaluating patients who have respiratory care prescribed. The therapist evaluator works within specific guidelines developed and is supervised by the medical director. Many respiratory care services have established a special cadre of therapist evaluators, respiratory care clinicians, or clinical coordinators who have well-defined responsibilities for initial and ongoing evaluation of all patients with orders for respiratory care services. Formal evaluation systems have been established primarily for bronchial hygiene to establish which patients have the greatest need.[4, 9, 10] The evaluation process is a quality assurance and cost containment measure that provides a means of rendering the most appropriate and cost effective therapy to patients requiring respiratory care services. The evaluation provides a means for making recommendations to physicians regarding the effectiveness of the ordered therapy. If the therapist evaluator is not in agreement with the prescription and would like to make a recommendation, the patient's physician must be contacted and the problem discussed. The final order, if changed from the original order, must be written in the chart and signed by the patient's physician.[1] The evaluation should be completed to include diagnosis, indications, therapeutic objectives, vital signs, breath sounds, and appropriate equipment.

Some hospitals have established a priority rating schedule which assigns points dependent on:

1. Whether the therapy is indicated or not (0 or 5 points).
2. Patient cooperation ($+1$ or -1 points).
3. Patient response to therapy ($+2$ to -1 points).
4. Whether clinical data supports indications for therapy ($+1$ point each).[4]

The points for each criterion are then added together to determine a patient priority rating. The criteria for points used to arrive at a patient priority rating are communicated to the physician by placing a sticker (Fig 4–7) in the respiratory therapy progress notes. The priority rating classification impacts the delivery of care as follows:

Priority 1 (>10).—Therapy that will be delivered regardless of respiratory therapy staffing levels.

Priority 2 (7–9).—Therapy that has proven beneficial to the patient. Therapy will be provided when staffing levels permit.

Priority 3 (<6).—Therapy that will be withheld after 24 hrs unless further documentation for need of therapy is provided in chart.

Most respiratory care services have policies approved by their medical staff that call for an auto-matic stop of the respiratory care order after three days unless reordered within 24 hours. A label (Fig 4–8) to remind the physician to reorder is placed on the physician order sheet in the chart. Some respiratory care services routinely reevaluate all patients within 48 to 72 hours of the last evaluation or reevaluation.[4, 9, 10]

Appropriateness of Prescribed Treatment

Respiratory therapists should evaluate orders for respiratory care to ensure that therapeutic objectives can be accomplished. This requires that the therapist know the indications and objectives for various modalities of respiratory care. Often the respiratory care clinician finds that the indications for several different modalities for respiratory care are present. A decision to integrate two or more types of treatment may allow a therapeutic objective to be completed sooner. Table 4–10 shows how indications for respiratory care overlap and may require more than one approach to reach a specific therapeutic objective. If an order for respiratory care does not relate to a specific therapeutic goal, it should be discontinued so that limited resources are not wasted. Also, when therapeutic goals are reached and indications for certain modalities of respiratory care no longer exist, the treatment plan should be discontinued or modified. Chapters 5 to 11 deal specifically with the scientific basis of therapeutic objectives for major areas of respiratory care.

Potential Adverse Reactions

There are specific circumstances in which a respiratory care modality will suddenly become hazard-

---

Respiratory Care Services
Patient Care Evaluation of Respiratory Therapy

Patient _____ has been evaluated for the prescribed therapy _____
according to the Respiratory Therapy priority rating protocol (RT #1).

Is Therapy Indicated: ☐ Yes ☐ No
Patient Cooperation: ☐ Cooperative ☐ Uncooperative
Patient Response to Therapy: ☐ Severe Adverse Reaction—requires immediate discontinuation until physician notified
☐ Adverse Reaction—not severe enough for discontinuance
☐ No Response
☐ Some Improvement
☐ Very Noticeable Improvement

Clinical Data: _____
_____

This patient has a _____ rating for prescribed therapy according to the Respiratory Therapy priority rating system.
Clinical Coordinator: _____ Date/Time: _____
120684

FIG 4–7.
Example of a sticker placed in the respiratory therapy progress notes of the patient's chart to notify a physician of his patient's priority score for receiving respiratory care. (Courtesy of the Respiratory Care Service, University of Nebraska Medical Center.)

**Respiratory Therapy Department
Evaluation of Respiratory Therapy**

Date/Time: _____ Your Patient _____

has been receiving _____ Therapy for

the past _____ days.

☐ DC Therapy ☐ Renew Therapy ☐ Change to _____

Please indicate reason for continued therapy:

_____

_____

_____

_____

_____

**Automatic Stop after 24 hours if not reordered.

RT-3 (10/86)   Physician _____

FIG 4–8.
Example of a sticker placed in the physician's order section of the patient's chart to remind him to reorder respiratory care. Note the section for indicating the therapeutic objective. (Courtesy of the Respiratory Care Service, University of Nebraska Medical Center.)

ous and contraindicated. A sudden change in the patient's condition may require immediate termination of the treatment. The classic example is the patient who receives IPPB and develops a tension pneumothorax 5 minutes into the treatment. Being aware of the potential side effects, hazards and contraindications of each modality of respiratory care allow the therapist to constantly be on guard for the signs and symptoms of an adverse reaction. The patient's chart should always be checked for a change in status or recent episode of an adverse response to treatment. Good communication skills are essential since last minute changes in a patient's condition may not be recorded on the chart. This information should always be solicited from other members of the health care team before beginning the treatment.

Clarifying Orders

An incomplete or incorrectly written order for respiratory care becomes the responsibility of the respiratory therapist to clarify. Accordingly, the therapist should ensure that the medical record states correctly and the health care team understands the specifics of the respiratory care being administered. Most respiratory care services have protocols (see Fig 4–1) that require physician prescriptions to include a minimum and critical amount of information. In some cases (such as oxygen therapy via a nasal cannula) only the oxygen flow rate may be needed along with a minimal number of therapeutic objectives. Problems requiring several modalities of respiratory care to be administered concurrently will require a more comprehensive prescription. The advances in technology related to mechanical ventilation require a dialogue to occur between therapist and physician regarding the various modes of ventilation, ventilatory parameters, and methods for weaning. Extensive S-O-A-P notes on the respiratory care treatment section of the chart, use of therapist consultations, and good communication with the attending physician to assure his full understanding of the progress being made should help to clarify the therapeutic objectives. Finally, JCAH guidelines for quality assurance require therapeutic outcomes to be identified at the time respiratory care is ordered.[1]

In summary, a respiratory care plan is central to the team's effort to restore normal pulmonary function. The plan should be developed by: (1) identifying and quantifying levels of dysfunction, (2) describing desired therapeutic outcomes, (3) selecting the appropriate respiratory care to be administered,

TABLE 4–10.

Relating Indications for Respiratory Care to Therapeutic Outcomes

INDICATIONS	THERAPEUTIC OUTCOMES EXPECTED	RESPIRATORY CARE MODALITIES
Dried-retained secretions with weak unproductive cough	Hydrate dried-retained secretions; mobilize/remove secretions; promote expectoration; restore the mucus "blanket"	Aerosol therapy; chest physical therapy IPPB; bronchoscopy; nasotracheal suctioning
Atelectasis	Reinflate atelectatic lung areas; improve distribution of ventilation	IPPB; incentive spirometry; chest physical therapy
Artificial airway	Humidify airway	Aerosol/humidity therapy; airway care
Bronchospasm	Improve ventilation; bronchodilation	Aerosol therapy; IPPB
Hypoxia	Improve tissue oxygenation	Incentive spirometry; oxygen therapy; IPPB; chest physiotherapy
Extubation	Relieve laryngeal edema	Aerosol therapy; airway care
Stridor	Relieve stridor; improve ventilation	Aerosol therapy; IPPB

(4) specifying a means and schedule for ongoing evaluation of the expected therapeutic outcomes, and (5) documenting the therapeutic outcomes in the medical record. The respiratory care plan, if carefully designed and followed, should result in high-quality, cost-effective, safe respiratory care.

REFERENCES

1. *Accreditation Manual for Hospitals: Respiratory Care Services.* Chicago, Joint Commission on Accreditation of Hospitals, 1983.
2. *Blue Cross and Blue Shield Association Medical Necessity Guidelines: Respiratory (Inpatient).* Chicago, Blue Cross and Blue Shield Association, September 1982.
3. Celli BR, Rodriguez KS, Snider GL: A controlled trial of intermittent positive pressure breathing, incentive spirometry, and deep breathing exercises in preventing pulmonary complications after abdominal surgery. *Am Rev Respir Dis* 1984; 130:12–15.
4. Cutler BF, Hurlbert BJ: Bronchial hygiene evaluation system improves hospital's efficiency. *AARTimes* 1984; 8:34–36.
5. Ford GT, Guenter CA: Toward prevention of postoperative pulmonary complications. *Am Rev Respir Dis* 1984; 130:4–5.
6. Jung R, et al: Comparison of three methods of respiratory care following upper abdominal surgery. *Chest* 1980; 78:31–35.
7. *Procedure Manual: Respiratory Care Procedure Note: Form M4202.* Durham, NC, Duke University Medical Center, 1984.
8. Smoker JM, et al: A protocol to assess oxygen therapy. *Respir Care* 1986; 31:35–39.
9. Walton JE, Shapiro BA: Appropriate utilization of bronchial hygiene therapy. *QRB* 1981, pp 21–25.
10. Walton JR, Shapiro BA, Harrison CH: Review of a bronchial hygiene evaluation program. *Respir Care* 1983; 28:174–179.

SECTION II

Therapeutic and Emergency Modalities

5

Oxygen and Mixed Gas Therapy

John W. Youtsey, Ph.D., R.R.T.

The use of oxygen has long been proved to be highly beneficial in the treatment of arterial hypoxemia.[2, 4, 13] As such, oxygen as a medical gas must be considered a drug and treated accordingly. In the early 1920s, Dr. Alvin Barach reported the use of oxygen in the treatment of lobar pneumonia.[3] Since that time, oxygen use in patient care has been influenced as much by medical intuition as by scientific fact. As a result, there has been a lack of agreement among physicians and among respiratory care practitioners as to the indications for oxygen therapy and the most appropriate methods of oxygen delivery. This situation has led to considerable variation in the standards of patient care. In the past 10 years, however, this situation has begun to change significantly. Major advances have occurred in our understanding of oxygen therapy both from a clinical perspective and as well as from a scientific basis. We now have sound clinical studies to better evaluate the benefits of short-term (acute) and long-term (chronic) oxygen therapy. Our understanding of the pathophysiology of hypoxia permits a more logical and consistent approach to oxygen therapy. Studies on the development and progression of oxygen toxicity enables physicians and therapists to identify and control many of the hazards associated with oxygen therapy.

The scientific basis of most oxygen therapy in clinical practice today is based on our understanding of three primary factors:

1. The physiology of oxygen transport in the body.
2. The pathophysiology of hypoxia.
3. Clinical experience in treating hypoxia with oxygen therapy.

Before one can fully appreciate the use of oxygen in clinical respiratory care, it is necessary to understand how oxygen is transported in the body, how normal oxygen concentrations are maintained in the blood, and the physiologic effects of too little oxygen on the cells. It is beyond the scope of this chapter to provide a detailed physiologic explanation of these phenomena; therefore, the discussion of each of these areas will be limited to the information necessary to provide a foundation for the clinical use of oxygen as a pharmacologic agent.

OXYGEN TRANSPORT

Oxygen is transported from the alveolus to the cells of the body in two forms (Table 5–1):

1. *Dissolved oxygen,* oxygen that is dissolved in the blood plasma.
2. *Combined oxygen,* oxygen that is physically bound to the hemoglobin molecule in the red blood cell.

Dissolved Oxygen

The concentration of oxygen (partial pressure) is greater in the alveolus than in the blood perfusing that alveolus. The oxygen molecules diffuse from the alveolus into the pulmonary blood (Fig 5–1). This process will occur as long as the partial pressure of oxygen in the alveolus is greater than that in the pulmonary blood. The oxygen molecules dissolve in the plasma as they enter the pulmonary blood. The amount of oxygen that dissolves in the plasma is dependent upon the solubility of oxygen (solubility

TABLE 5–1.

Relative Amounts of Oxygen Transported by Hemoglobin and Dissolved in Plasma

P_{O_2}	HEMOGLOBIN SATURATION, %	O_2 CONTENT, VOL%*	O_2 DISSOLVED, VOL%
20	35	7.0	0.06
30	58	11.7	0.09
40	75	15.1	0.12
50	84	16.9	0.15
60	90	18.1	0.18
70	93	18.7	0.21
80	95	19.1	0.24
90	97	19.5	0.27
100	98	19.7	0.30

*Based on hemoglobin, 15 gm%; pH, 7.40; and 1 gm of hemoglobin carrying 1.34 ml of O_2.

coefficient) and the partial pressure of oxygen. At 1 atmosphere (760 mm Hg), the solubility coefficient for oxygen is 0.023 ml of oxygen/ml plasma.[1] It is standard practice to use the term volume percent (vol%) which means milliliters of gas per 100 ml of plasma. As a result, the 0.023 ml oxygen/ml plasma converts to 2.3 ml oxygen/100 ml plasma or 2.3 vol% of dissolved oxygen.

For every 760 mm Hg pressure, 2.3 vol% of oxygen is dissolved in the plasma. This is a linear re-lationship between the barometric pressure and the volume percent of oxygen dissolved. If one divides 2.3 vol% by 760, then one can determine the amount of oxygen dissolved for each mm Hg pressure increment:

$$\frac{2.3 \text{ vol\%}}{760 \text{ mm Hg}} = 0.003 \text{ vol\%/mm Hg}$$

This relationship can be utilized to determine the amount of oxygen dissolved at any given partial pressure of oxygen using the following formula:

$$\text{vol\%} = P_{O_2} \times 0.003$$

Figure 5–2 shows this relationship graphically. At a normal arterial blood gas of 80 to 100 mm Hg, the corresponding amounts of oxygen dissolved in the plasma would be 0.24 vol% (80 × 0.003) to 0.30 vol% (100 × 0.003). Even placing a patient on 100% oxygen at sea level, the total amount of oxygen dissolved in the plasma would be only 2.02 vol%. The calculation for this maximum dissolved oxygen is as follows:

```
  760 mm Hg = barometric pressure
-  47 mm Hg = water vapor pressure in alveoli
  713 mm Hg
-  40 mm Hg = alveolar P_CO2
  673 mm Hg
  673 × 0.003 = 2.02 vol%
```

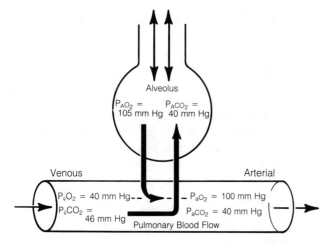

FIG 5–1.

Gas exchange at the alveolus. Gases diffuse in response to a concentration or pressure gradient (partial pressure). Oxygen moves from the alveolus to the pulmonary blood in response to this partial pressure gradient. Simultaneously, carbon dioxide moves from the pulmonary blood (where the partial pressure of CO_2 is greater) into the alveolus. The partial pressure of gases in the alveoli remain relatively stable due to alveolar ventilation (The values are approximate at 1 atmosphere of pressure).

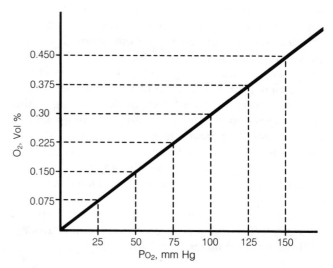

FIG 5–2.

The linear relationship between the amount of dissolved oxygen in plasma and the corresponding partial pressure of oxygen; 0.3 vol% of oxygen dissolved in the plasma will exert an oxygen partial pressure (P_{O_2}) of 100 mm Hg.

Combined Oxygen

Under normal barometric conditions, not enough oxygen can be carried while dissolved in the plasma to meet the tissue demands. The majority of oxygen is carried through the body physically combined with the hemoglobin molecule. The hemoglobin molecule is a protein found in the red blood cell. One gram of hemoglobin is capable of carrying 1.34 ml of oxygen.[27, 30, 32] Normal hemoglobin concentration is 16 gm% (gm per 100 ml blood) for men and 14 gm% for women.[35] A hemoglobin of 15 gm% is generally used as a standard normal value. If one assumes a normal hemoglobin value of 15 gm% and a capacity of 1.34, then the total amount of oxygen that can be bound to hemoglobin is:

$$1.34 \text{ ml} \times 15 \text{ gm/dl} = 20.1 \text{ vol\%}$$

This value assumes 100% saturation of hemoglobin with oxygen. Generally, one will not observe 100% saturation at a normal $F_{I_{O_2}} = 0.21$.

Oxyhemoglobin Dissociation Curve

The ability of oxygen to chemically combine with hemoglobin and form oxyhemoglobin follows a predictable reaction:

$$Hb + O_2 \rightleftarrows HbO_2$$

This reaction has three characteristics that are clinically important. First, the reaction can move in both directions. When the reaction moves to the right ($Hb + O_2 \rightleftarrows HbO_2$), the hemoglobin molecule binds with oxygen. This is the directon observed in the lung. When the reaction moves to the left ($Hb + O_2 \leftrightharpoons HbO_2$), oxygen is being released from the oxyhemoglobin molecule. This is the direction observed at the tissue level. Second, a given hemoglobin molecule is able to combine with more than one molecule of oxygen. This gives rise to the concept of saturation of hemoglobin. Third, the percent saturation of the hemoglobin molecule is dependent upon the partial pressure of oxygen in the blood (P_{O_2}). In other words, the dissolved oxygen in the plasma (the measured P_{O_2}) is the driving force moving the oxygen molecules into the red blood cell and forming oxyhemoglobin. This relationship between the partial pressure of oxygen (P_{O_2}) and the percent saturation (S_{O_2}) is expressed graphically as the oxyhemoglobin dissociation curve (Fig 5–3). It is clearly evident that the ability of hemoglobin to carry oxygen

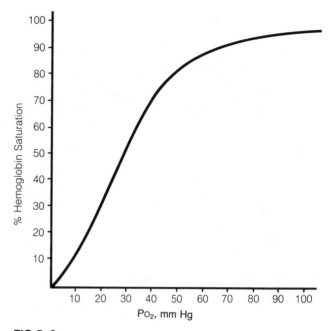

FIG 5–3.
Oxyhemoglobin dissociation curve. The curve describes the affinity of hemoglobin for oxygen. This curve is representative of the relationship between hemoglobin and O_2 when the pH is 7.40 and temperature is 37° C. The curve will shift to the right or left when the pH or P_{CO_2} and/or temperature is changed.

is very much different than that of the blood plasma (see Table 5–1).

The oxyhemoglobin dissociation curve is a dynamic curve in that it will shift to the left or right under certain circumstances (Fig 5–4). The curve will shift to the left when the blood is alkalotic. This increases the affinity for hemoglobin to the oxygen molecules. As a result, less oxygen will be made available to the tissues. On the other hand, the curve will shift to the right when the blood is acidotic. This results in a decrease in the affinity of hemoglobin for oxygen; and therefore, more oxygen will be made available to the tissues.

Increasing temperatures above 38° C will cause a shift to the right and make more oxygen available to the tissues. Lowering temperatures will have the opposite effect on the curve. The relationship between temperature and pH (P_{CO_2}) is very important in understanding the oxyhemoglobin dissociation curve. For example, when a patient has a fever, the elevated temperature is the result of increased metabolic activity in the tissues. These active tissues will have a higher P_{CO_2} and low pH. The end result of (1) increased temperature, (2) increased P_{CO_2}, and (3) lower pH is a shift in the oxyhemoglobin disso-

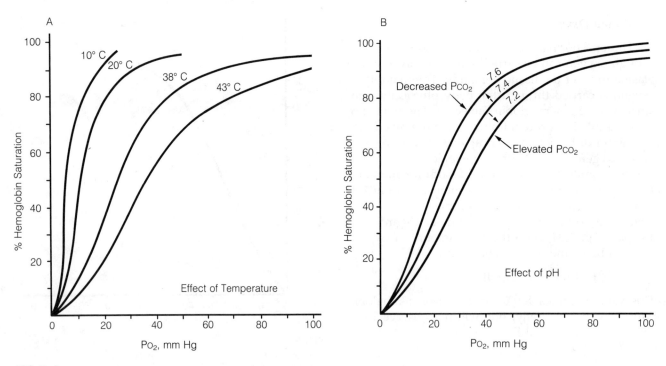

FIG 5–4.
The influence of temperature on the oxyhemoglobin dissociation curve **(A)** and that of pH (and related PCO_2) on the curve **(B)**.

ciation curve to the right, thus making more oxygen available to these active cells. This shift in the curve will make it slightly more difficult for the blood to pick up oxygen in the lung; however, the increased delivery of oxygen to the tissues in this circumstance may be clinically more important.[14]

It is important to be able to differentiate between oxygen content and oxygen capacity; and furthermore, to be able to relate oxygen content and PaO_2. A further elaboration of the oxyhemoglobin dissociation curve will help. The oxygen capacity is defined as the "maximum" amount of oxygen that can combine with hemoglobin and also includes the amount of oxygen dissolved in the plasma at a given PO_2. Oxygen capacity assumes 100% saturation of hemoglobin.

The oxygen content, on the other hand, is defined as the "actual" amount of oxygen combined with hemoglobin and dissolved in the plasma. An example will help to clarify the difference between the two.

Given: PaO_2 = 100 mm Hg
$\quad\quad SaO_2$ = 95%
$\quad\quad Hb$ = 15 gm%
Oxygen
$\quad$capacity = $(1.34 \times Hb) + (PaO_2 \times 0.003)$
$\quad\quad\quad = (1.34 \times 15) + (100 \times 0.003)$

$\quad\quad\quad = 20.1 + 0.3$
$\quad\quad\quad = 20.4$ vol%
Oxygen
$\quad$content = $(1.34 \times Hb \times SaO_2) + (PaO_2 \times 0.003)$
$\quad\quad\quad = (1.34 \times 15 \times .95) + (100 \times 0.003)$
$\quad\quad\quad = (20.1 \times .95) + (0.3)$
$\quad\quad\quad = 19.1 + 0.3$
$\quad\quad\quad = 19.4$ vol%

Clinically it is important to understand the importance of oxygen pressure vs. oxygen content. The oxygen pressure (PO_2) or tension is responsible for the diffusion of oxygen across cell membranes and into the cells. The oxygen content, on the other hand, determines the amount of oxygen that will be available to move across these membranes. Figure 5–5 shows the relationship between the oxygen content, oxygen pressure or tension, and the percent saturation (SO_2) on the oxyhemoglobin dissociation curve. The oxygen content is not only dependent upon the PO_2 and SO_2 as shown in Figure 5–5, but also on the amount of available hemoglobin. If an individual is anemic with a hemoglobin level of 10 gm% (vs. the 15 gm%), a PaO_2 of 70 mm Hg and a SaO_2 of 93%, the oxygen content will now be 12.5 vol% instead of the 18.7 vol% observed when the hemoglobin is 15 gm%. Likewise, if a patient were polycythemic with a hemoglobin of 20 gm%; PaO_2,

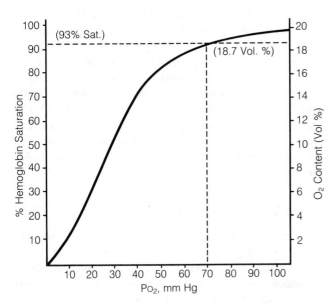

FIG 5–5.
Oxyhemoglobin dissociation curve describing the relationship between oxygen tension and oxygen content. When the P_{O_2} is 70 mm Hg, the percent hemoglobin saturation is 93%, and the O_2 content is 18.7 vol%.

70 mm Hg; and percent hemoglobin saturation, 93%; the oxygen content would be 24.9 gm%. Clinically, therefore, it is possible for the oxygen tension and the percent saturation to remain unchanged, and yet the amount of oxygen available (oxygen content) would vary with the hemoglobin level (Fig 5–6). For this reason, a Pa_{O_2} value is not adequate to determine the available oxygen in a patient. It is necessary to measure both the hemoglobin level and the Pa_{O_2}. In this way, the driving pressure necessary for oxygen movement as well as the amount available are known.

Clinical Significance of Oxyhemoglobin Dissociation Curve

Based on the discussion of the transport of oxygen by hemoglobin and the transport of oxygen dissolved in plasma, several clinically useful observations can be made:

1. At a normal Pa_{O_2} (80 to 100 mm Hg), the arterial blood is approximately 97% saturated with oxygen. Given an adequate hemoglobin, increasing the saturation to 100% by elevating the inspired oxygen concentration will not provide a significant increase

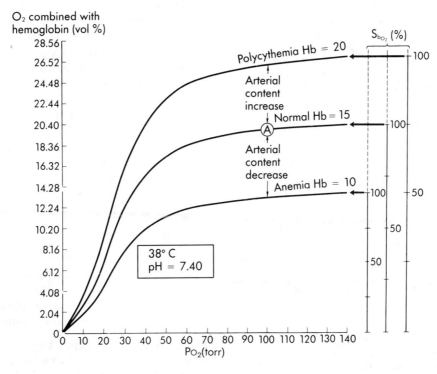

FIG 5–6.
Oxyhemoglobin dissociation curve in anemia and polycythemia. (From Slonim NB, Hamilton LH: *Respiratory Physiology*, ed 4. St Louis, CV Mosby Co, 1981. Used with permission.)

in the amount of oxygen available to the cells; therefore, the higher levels of PaO_2 do not contribute to oxygen transport.

2. There is very little change in the oxygen content between tensions of 70 and 100 mm Hg. At a PaO_2 of 70 mm Hg, the saturation is 93% and the oxygen content is 18.7 vol%. At a PaO_2 of 100 mm Hg, the saturation is 97% and the oxygen content is 19.5 vol%. If a respiratory patient has a normal hemoglobin level, one must evaluate the benefit versus the potential risk of attempting to increase the PaO_2 significantly above 70 mm Hg through the use of supplemental oxygen therapy.

3. The oxyhemoglobin dissociation curve is S-shaped. This means that the curve not only has a flattened portion at the top and bottom, but also a steep part to the curve. Although the 30 mm Hg decrease in PaO_2 had very little effect on the curve between the PaO_2 of 70 and 100 mm Hg; the same 30 mm Hg decrease between the PaO_2 of 70 and 30 mm Hg has a drastic effect on the oxygen content (Fig 5–7). As the PaO_2 falls below 70 mm Hg, major changes in percent Hb saturation can occur with relatively small changes in the PaO_2.

4. The oxyhemoglobin dissociation curve is a dynamic curve in that it changes with the pH, PCO_2, and temperature. One way to monitor shifts in the curve is through the observation of changes in the P_{50}. The P_{50} is the partial pressure of oxygen at which 50% of the hemoglobin is saturated. Normal P_{50} is 27 mm Hg. Increases in the P_{50} (P_{50} above 27 mm Hg) indicate a shift to the right of curve and thus, a decrease in the affinity of hemoglobin for oxygen. Likewise, a decrease in the P_{50} (P_{50} below 27 mm Hg) indicates a shift in the curve to the left and an increase in the affinity of hemoglobin for oxygen.

Mixed Venous Oxygen Content

The oxygen saturation of the mixed venous blood ($S\bar{v}O_2$) provides the best clinical measure for the delivery of oxygen to the local areas and consumption of oxygen by the tissues. The oxygen content of arterial blood (CaO_2) determines the amount of oxygen available to be delivered to the tissues. The oxygen content of the mixed venous blood ($C\bar{v}O_2$) indicates the amount of oxygen left in the blood after leaving the tissues. The difference between the arterial oxygen content and the mixed venous oxygen content is called the arterial-venous oxygen content difference ($CaO_2 - C\bar{v}O_2$) and provides a measure for the amount of oxygen utilized by the body in a given period of time.

The mixed venous oxygen content is accurately measured in blood sampled from the pulmonary artery. Normal arterial oxygen content is approximately 19.8 vol% and the normal mixed venous oxygen content is 14.8 vol% resulting in an arterial–mixed venous oxygen content difference of 5 vol%. This means that when the physiologic parameters (pH, temperature, cardiac output) are normal, the body extracts 5 ml of oxygen from every 100 ml of blood perfusing through the tissues. Assume a cardiac output (CO) of 5,000 ml/min (5 L/min) and an extraction rate of 5 ml/100 ml of blood, the normal oxygen consumption of the body is:

Oxygen consumption

$$= (CaO_2 - C\bar{v}O_2) \times \text{cardiac output}$$
$$= 5 \text{ ml/100 ml} \times 5,000 \text{ ml/min}$$
$$= 5 \text{ ml} \times (5,000 \text{ ml/100 ml})/\text{min}$$
$$= 250 \text{ ml/min}$$

When the cardiac output falls or metabolism is elevated, the tissues will extract even greater amounts of oxygen and the arterial–mixed venous oxygen content difference will increase.

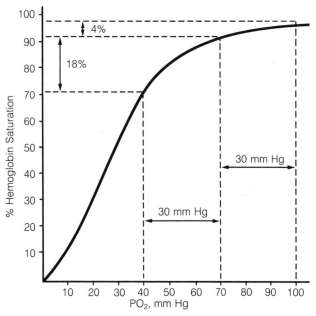

FIG 5–7.
The effect of the steep portion of the oxyhemoglobin dissociation curve on equal changes in the PaO_2 and resultant percent hemoglobin saturation. Between PaO_2 of 70 to 100 mm Hg, the change in percent hemoglobin saturation is 4%. Between PaO_2 of 40 to 70 mm Hg, the change in percent hemoglobin saturation is 18%.

Total Oxygen Availability

The delivery of oxygen to the tissues is dependent upon several factors including:

1. An adequate amount of hemoglobin in the blood.
2. Normal functioning hemoglobin.
3. Adequate saturation of the hemoglobin.
4. An adequate PaO_2 to facilitate diffusion and hemoglobin saturation.
5. Appropriate temperature, pH, and 2,3-diphosoglycerate (2,3-DPG) levels.
6. An adequate cardiac output.

Oxygen transport is defined as the product of the cardiac output and the arterial oxygen content (CaO_2):

$$\text{Oxygen transport} = CO \times CaO_2$$
$$= 5{,}000 \text{ ml/min} \times 19.8 \text{ ml/100 ml}$$
$$= 990 \text{ ml/min}$$

Since the tissues normally extract approximately 250 ml/min of oxygen from the 990 ml/min available (with a normal cardiac output), a significant safety buffer exists. When the cardiac output decreases, the tissues respond by increasing oxygen extraction from the blood.

A decrease in those parameters that monitor the oxygen status of mixed venous blood ($P\bar{v}O_2$, $C\bar{v}O_2$, and $S\bar{v}O_2$) suggests a reduced blood flow through the capillary beds secondary to a fall in the cardiac output. However, severe anemia and increased oxygen consumption can also cause a decrease in these parameters.[26]

A gross measure of cardiac output, based on the *Fick principle,* can be calculated at the bedside if the $CaO_2 - C\bar{v}O_2$ (arterial-venous content difference) is known using the following formula:

$$\text{Given: } O_2 \text{ consumption} = 250 \text{ ml/min}$$
$$CaO_2 - C\bar{v}O_2 = 5 \text{ vol}\%$$

$$CO = \frac{\text{oxygen consumption}}{CaO_2 - C\bar{v}O_2}$$

$$= \frac{250 \text{ ml/min}}{5 \text{ ml/100 ml}}$$

$$= \frac{250 \text{ ml/min}}{5 \text{ ml}} \times 100 \text{ ml}$$

$$= 5{,}000 \text{ ml or } 5 \text{ L/min}$$

Thus far, the emphasis has been on the delivery of oxygen at the tissues. Oxygen availability at the pulmonary or alveolar level is dependent on several factors including:

1. F_{IO_2} of inspired gas.
2. Alveolar ventilation.
3. $\dot{V}/\dot{Q}$ ratio or match.
4. Diffusion of gas across the alveolar capillary membrane.

PATHOLOGY OF HYPOXIA

Hypoxia is defined as that state where there is an inadequate supply of oxygen at the tissue or cellular level for normal cellular functions. Since clinically it is not practical to measure oxygen at the tissue or cellular level, the term hypoxemia is used interchangeably with hypoxia. Hypoxemia means a decreased amount of oxygen in the blood and is observed through reduced oxygen values: PaO_2, CaO_2, and/or SaO_2. States of hypoxemia generally imply hypoxia at the cellular level; however, there are instances where oxygen blood gas values may appear normal and yet cellular hypoxia may exist. For example, in severe cases of anemia, the PaO_2 and SaO_2 may be normal and because of the low hemoglobin level, tissue hypoxia may exist. In this instance, one must also evaluate the CaO_2 in order to have a complete picture of the oxygen status of the patient. Likewise, with patients in hypotensive states, the PaO_2 may appear normal and yet because of poor tissue perfusion, the cells may suffer from hypoxia. In this case, a $P\bar{v}O_2$ and $S\bar{v}O_2$ would be useful in identifying the cellular hypoxia.

For these reasons, it is clinically useful to characterize or classify types of hypoxia. There are four categories of hypoxia:

1. *Anoxic (hypoxic) hypoxia* refers to hypoxia secondary to a problem in gas exchange (oxygenation) in the lung. This may be due to an abnormal ventilation-perfusion match ($\dot{V}/\dot{Q}$) in the lung, a decrease in the F_{IO_2} or PAO_2, or an alteration in the alveolar-capillary membrane due to interstitial fluid or fibrosis.

2. *Anemic hypoxia* refers to hypoxia secondary to a reduced oxygen-carrying capacity in the blood. This may be due to severe blood loss, reduction in red blood cell production, carbon monoxide poisoning, or abnormal hemoglobin disease.

3. *Circulatory (stagnant) hypoxia* refers to hypoxia

secondary to a reduced blood flow in the body. This is generally due to a decrease in cardiac output as a result of congestive heart failure, cardiac arrest, and shock.

4. *Histotoxic hypoxia* refers to hypoxia secondary to the inability of the cells to utilize oxygen. This may be due to cyanide poisoning where cellular respiration is inhibited.

Of the four categories of hypoxia listed above, only the conditions of hypoxia described in anoxic (hypoxic) hypoxia respond significantly to basic modes of oxygen therapy. For example, in anemic hypoxia, the use of supplemental oxygen will increase both the PaO_2 and SaO_2; however, since the oxygen-carrying capacity is low, the tissues will not receive the needed additional oxygen. At best, supplemental oxygen administration will help only in borderline situations and would be only a temporary measure.

In cyanide poisoning, the use of oxygen may be only marginally beneficial. The initial therapy would be the administration of sodium nitrite or sodium thiosulfate. These drugs convert hemoglobin to methemoglobin which then binds with the cyanide to form a stable cyanomethemoglobin. This then allows for normal oxygen utilization in the cell. Also, the use of hyperbaric oxygen can be beneficial in the treatment of cyanide poisoning;[7] however, hyperbaric oxygen therapy is considered an adjunct to the standard medical treatment. Table 5–2 shows the effect of the types of hypoxia on the PaO_2, SaO_2, and $S\overline{v}O_2$.

Effects of Hypoxia

It is often difficult to separate the physiologic effects of hypoxia from those of the disease or disorder causing the hypoxia. Cellular hypoxia will occur when the demand for oxygen cannot be met by the blood perfusing the tissues. As stated previously, hypoxia can be due to any factor that reduces the PaO_2, reduces oxygen transport in the body, and/or interferes with oxygen utilization in the cells. Regardless of the cause, hypoxia impairs the mitochon-drial function in the cells. This alters normal oxidative metabolism. Toxic metabolites accumulate, resulting in cellular damage and, if not corrected, necrosis and cellular death. The clinical signs and symptoms observed in patients are caused by these malfunctioning hypoxic cells.

Brain function is compromised by hypoxemia in advance of other vital organs. In acute situations in which the PaO_2 is approximately 50 to 55 mm Hg, short-term memory may be altered. In addition, euphoria and impairment of judgment may occur. At PaO_2 of 30 mm Hg, loss of consciousness is observed.[13] As the PaO_2 falls or worsens between 55 and 30 mm Hg, cognitive and motor functions deteriorate.[2, 13]

Hypoxia stimulates the rate and depth of ventilation through the aortic and carotid body chemoreceptors. Initially, acute hypoxia will stimulate cardiac rate; however, with worsening hypoxia, the heart rate will slow. Cardiac arrest may also occur in acute hypoxia. As the PaO_2 falls below 30 mm Hg and the saturation level below 50%, circulatory failure and shock will occur. Vasoconstriction and bronchoconstriction occur in the lung as the PaO_2 decreases.[13]

In chronic hypoxic states, the body's physiology will show adaptation to the lack of oxygen and establish compensatory mechanisms. For example, at PaO_2 below 55 mm Hg, the ventilatory drive will increase. This will result in creating a state of hypocapnea which then permits an elevation of the PAO_2 and PaO_2, respectively. In addition, the red blood cell levels of 2,3 DPG will increase shifting the oxyhemoglobin dissociation curve to the right, thus favoring release of oxygen to the tissues. The increased secretions of erythropoietin will stimulate the production of increased numbers of red blood cells by the bone marrow. This results in a greater oxygen-carrying capacity.

Causes of Hypoxia

The most common causes of hypoxia encountered by the respiratory care practitioner fall into the

TABLE 5–2.

The Effect of the Four Categories of Hypoxia on PaO_2, SaO_2, and $S\overline{v}O_2$.

CATEGORY	PaO_2	SaO_2	$S\overline{v}O_2$
Anoxic (hypoxic) hypoxia	Decreased	Decreased	Decreased
Anemic hypoxia	Normal	Normal	Decreased
Circulatory (stagnant) hypoxia	Decreased	Decreased	Decreased
Histotoxic hypoxia	Normal	Normal	Increased

first category of hypoxia: anoxic (hypoxic) hypoxia. Within this class, the hypoxia falls into three physiologic mechanisms: (1) hypoventilation, (2) ventilation/perfusion mismatch, and (3) right-to-left shunt.

Hypoventilation

Hypoventilation can be the result of either a reduction in the alveolar ventilation or due to an increase in the physiologic dead space. In either case, the end result is an increase in the alveolar carbon dioxide tension (PA_{CO_2}). As the PA_{CO_2} increases, the alveolar oxygen is displaced, and the PaO_2 will fall (Fig 5–8). One can see from Figure 5–8 that hypoventilation at room air results in hypoxemia and hypocapnea. If the hypoventilation is the only cause for the hypoxemia, an increase in the FI_{O_2} through supplemental oxygen administration will correct the

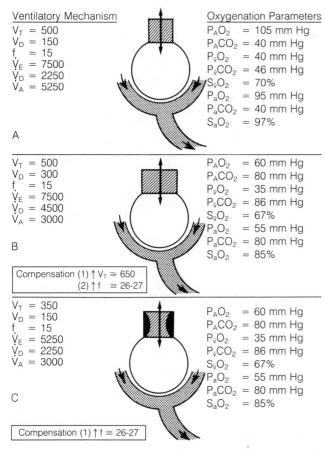

PaO_2 and thus the PaO_2. Although oxygen therapy is warranted in this situation, oxygen administration will not correct the hypercarbia (increase in Pa_{CO_2}). Mechanical ventilation may be required in this instance to correct the high Pa_{CO_2}. In simple hypoventilation, the hypoxemia is dependent upon the PA_{CO_2}. Such uncomplicated cases of hypoventilation would include such problems as drug overdose, muscular paralysis, and neuromuscular disease. In these instances, once the Pa_{CO_2} is corrected, generally the supplemental oxygen can be removed and the PaO_2 (and subsequently, the PaO_2) will return to normal limits.

Ventilation-Perfusion Mismatch

The ventilation-perfusion mismatch is the most common clinical cause of arterial hypoxemia.[25] In theory there should be a uniform distribution of ventilation throughout the lungs that is matched with an equally uniform perfusion of these ventilated alveoli. In reality, however, this is not true. Inspired gas and pulmonary blood flow are unevenly distributed. As a result of this uneven distribution of ventilation and perfusion, regional (and local) differences in the $\dot{V}/\dot{Q}$ ratio (match) exist throughout the lung. Pulmonary disorders, which can affect ventilation, perfusion, or both, tend to exaggerate the $\dot{V}/\dot{Q}$ inequality.

It is helpful to think of $\dot{V}/\dot{Q}$ ratios as a continuum. At one end of the continuum, there is ventilation but no perfusion ($\dot{V}/\dot{Q} = \dot{V}/\dot{0}$). Ventilation without perfusion is called dead space. At the other end of this continuum, there is perfusion but no ventilation ($\dot{V}/\dot{Q} = 0/\dot{Q}$). Perfusion but no ventilation is called a shunt. Along this entire continuum, there is a wide array of $\dot{V}/\dot{Q}$ mismatches possible (Fig 5–9). In true dead space and shunt units, there is not the opportunity for gas to exchange between the alveoli and the pulmonary capillary. In these extreme situations, oxygen therapy will be of little, if any, value. Fortunately, most disorders create $\dot{V}/\dot{Q}$ ratios that fall in between these extremes of dead space and shunt. In these clinical situations where hypoxemia is due primarily to a $\dot{V}/\dot{Q}$ abnormality, oxygen therapy can be very beneficial. Table 5–3 provides a list of diseases or disorders that can be classified as dead space–producing or shunt-producing.

Dead space–producing disorders alone produce little hypoxia. These disorders have their major clinical effect on the alveolar and arterial carbon dioxide level. Shunts, on the other hand, have major impact

FIG 5–8.
Effect of hypoventilation oxygenation values. **(A)**, normal. **(B)**, hypoventilation due to an increase in physiologic dead space. **(C)**, hypoventilation due to a decrease in alveolar ventilation. To compensate for the increase in dead space **(B)**, one must either increase the tidal volume (V_T), or the frequency (f). To compensate for the low alveolar ventilation **(C)**, increase the frequency (f).

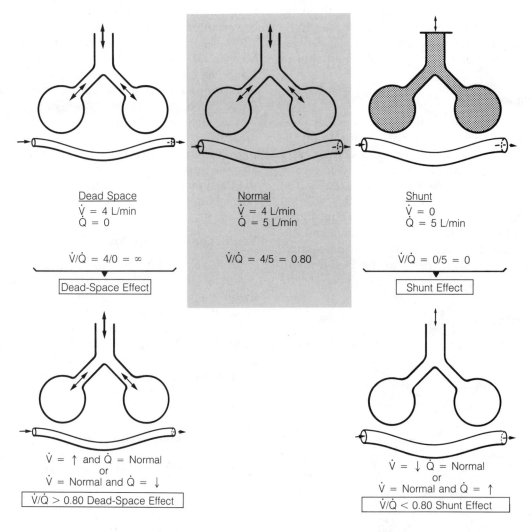

FIG 5–9.
The continuum of $\dot{V}/\dot{Q}$ ratios from dead space to shunt. Total shunt and total dead space are theoretical absolutes and not observed clinically. Pulmonary diseases and disorders create conditions that resemble dead space or shunt and thus are said to create a "dead-space effect" or a "shunt effect."

on oxygenation. Certain types of shunts lead to severe hypoxemia that cannot be corrected with oxygen therapy, while other shunt producing disorders do respond to oxygen therapy (Table 5–4). Obviously, the effect of oxygen therapy on hypoxemia resulting from $\dot{V}/\dot{Q}$ abnormalities is not clear. The lung (particularly the abnormal or diseased lung) is made up of many $\dot{V}/\dot{Q}$ ratios representing the status of various lung regions. The overall state of the lung is dependent upon all the local situations. Clinically, we can only see this net effect or end result. In any pathology, it is most likely that many degrees of both dead space and shunt exist simultaneously. For example, a patient with severe chronic obstructive pulmonary disease (COPD) will have dead space due to the destruction of the alveoli and shunt·secondary to inflammation, partial obstruction, and infection.

Shunt

Clinically, it is important to differentiate between hypoxemia that is due to hypoventilation and $\dot{V}/\dot{Q}$ mismatch (venous admixture) and hypoxemia that is the result of a true shunt situation. In shunt situations, since the alveoli are not in contact with the atmosphere, no amount of oxygen will reach the pulmonary capillaries. This principle is the basis for differentiating hypoxemia due to shunts and venous admixture.[32] A simple alveolar-arterial gradient procedure, a technique that has the patient breathe 100% oxygen for 15 to 20 minutes, is used to esti-

TABLE 5–3.

Dead-Space–Producing and Shunt-Producing Diseases and Disorders

DEAD-SPACE PRODUCING	SHUNT PRODUCING
Acute pulmonary embolus	Acute atelectasis
Decreased cardiac output	Pulmonary edema
Acute pulmonary hypertension	Congenital heart disease
Emphysema	Vascular lung disease
Positive pressure ventilation	Pulmonary tumors
Positive end-expiratory pressure	Intrapulmonary fistula
Anesthesia	Partial airway obstruction
Sedation	Pulmonary fibrosis (diffusion defect)
Central nervous system abnormality	Pneumothorax
Increased work of breathing	Pneumonia

mate the degree of right-to-left shunt. After 20 minutes of breathing 100% O_2, an arterial blood sample is drawn. If the Pa_{O_2} is greater than 550 mm Hg, the hypoxemia was the result of simple hypoventilation or venous admixture ($\dot{V}/\dot{Q}$ mismatch):

When $F_{I_{O_2}} = 1.0$

$P_{A_{O_2}} = P_B - P_{H_2O} - P_{A_{CO_2}}$

$P_{A_{O_2}} = 760$ mm Hg $- 47$ mm Hg $-$

40 mm Hg

$P_{A_{O_2}} = 673$ mm Hg.

The normal anatomical shunt of 3% to 5% allows for a 100 to 125 mm Hg A $-$ a gradient at an $F_{I_{O_2}} = 1.0$.

$P_{A_{O_2}} - (A-a$ gradient$) =$ expected Pa_{O_2}
$673 - (100-125) =$ expected Pa_{O_2} of 548 to 573

If the Pa_{O_2} was less than 550 mm Hg, or if the A $-$ a gradient is beyond the clinically acceptable range of 100 to 125 mm Hg ($F_{I_{O_2}} = 1.0$), then a clinically significant shunt is present. Table 5–5 provides estimates of shunts based on $F_{I_{O_2}}$ and Pa_{O_2}.

CLINICAL EVIDENCE FOR OXYGEN THERAPY

In 1922, Barach reported the use of oxygen in the treatment of lobar pneumonia.[3] Barach observed that "oxygen therapy in suitable cases relieves difficult breathing, restores strength, and helps reduce the swelling in the patient's legs and back."[23] Barach used oxygen in many clinical situations. These early clinical observations by Barach and others created an interest in studying the impact of oxygen therapy in patient care. From that time, the medical literature has continued to demonstrate research case studies and potential uses for oxygen therapy and medical gas therapy. In 1984, the American College of Chest Physicians–National Heart, Lung, and Blood Institute (ACCP-NHLBI) National Conference on Oxygen Therapy made the following observations: "The rationale for oxygen therapy in acute pulmonary conditions is based on extensive clinical experience that untreated hypoxemia often progresses to tissue hy-

TABLE 5–4.

Shunt Disorders That Do and Do Not Respond to Oxygen Therapy

Shunt disorders not corrected by oxygen therapy*
  Atelectasis
  Pulmonary edema
  Pneumonia
  Pneumothorax
Shunt disorders that respond to oxygen therapy
  Hypoventilation
  Pulmonary fibrosis
  Partial airway obstruction
  Venous admixture (shunt effect)

*Oxygen therapy defined as the administration of supplemental oxygen at ambient conditions (excludes continuous positive-airway pressure as a form of oxygen therapy).

TABLE 5–5.

Shunt Estimates Based on $F_{I_{O_2}}$ and Pa_{O_2}*†

	Pa_{O_2}, mm Hg						
	SHUNT ESTIMATES						
$F_{I_{O_2}}$	5%	10%	15%	20%	28%	30%	50%
0.21	95	80	65	60	55	50	42
0.35	150	110	85	65	57	52	45
0.40	185	180	90	70	65	60	47
0.60	315	235	160	105	75	65	52
0.80	460	360	265	180	110	70	55
1.00	573	475	400	290	170	100	60

*Modified from Braun HA, Cheney FW, Loehnen CP: *Introduction to Respiratory Physiology*, ed 2. Boston, Little, Brown & Co, 1980.
†Patient criteria: hemoglobin, >10 gm%; Pa_{CO_2}, 25 to 40 mm Hg; $Ca_{O_2} - C\bar{v}_{O_2} = 5$ vol%; Normals, 5% shunt.

poxia with its grave, frequently irreversible effects on vital organ function . . . . When hypoxemia is corrected in individuals who are hemodynamically intact, tissue hypoxia can be prevented or corrected."[13]

Oxygen therapy has been used successfully in the treatment of numerous pulmonary and nonpulmonary disorders, including acute hypoxemia, acute myocardial infarction, hemoglobinopathy, postoperative oxygen therapy, COPD, dyspnea, and angina pectoris. Oxygen therapy has a sound clinical basis in past and present clinical experience.

GOALS OF OXYGEN THERAPY

In the very broadest sense, oxygen is used to treat or prevent hypoxia. To achieve this goal, supplemental oxygen must be given in sufficient dosage to appropriate patients. Oxygen therapy should supply the needed amounts of oxygen to the tissues so that normal metabolism and cellular function can be maintained. In conditions of hypoxia due to inadequate oxygenation to either normal or abnormal lungs, oxygen therapy is basic and relatively easy to achieve at no significant risk to the patient. But in other situations, such as cardiac failure, cyanide poisoning, or anemic hypoxia, oxygen therapy can become complex and present risk to the patient. For this reason, it is important to expand the goal of oxygen therapy (1) to include the prevention or reduction of physiologic compensatory mechanisms secondary to hypoxia, and (2) to provide adequate amounts of oxygen to the tissues without initiating the adverse effects of oxygen toxicity or oxygen induced hypoventilation.

These goals become clinically significant when one realizes that the primary or direct effects of breathing supplemental oxygen are to[30]: (1) increase the P_{AO_2} (alveolar P_{O_2}), (2) decrease the work of breathing, and (3) decrease the work of the myocardium. If the clinical status of a patient will not be improved by one or more of these direct effects, then the use of supplemental oxygen in this situation should be questioned (Table 5–6).

INDICATIONS FOR OXYGEN THERAPY

Historically, there has been a general lack of agreement on the absolute blood gas values for defining when a state of hypoxemia exists in a patient. No single factor should be used as the criterion for

TABLE 5–6.

Goals of Oxygen Therapy Related to Direct Effects of Supplemental Oxygen

Goals of oxygen therapy
  1. To treat or prevent hypoxia.
  2. To prevent or reduce physiologic compensatory mechanisms secondary to hypoxia.
  3. To provide adequate amounts of oxygen to the tissues without initiating the adverse effects of oxygen toxicity or oxygen-induced hypoventilation.
Direct effects of supplemental oxygen
  1. To increase the P_{AO_2}.
  2. To decrease the work of breathing.
  3. To decrease the work of the myocardium.
Clinical question
  Will one or more of the direct effects of oxygen administration achieve any one or more of the goals of oxygen therapy?
  1. Yes—oxygen therapy should be considered.
  2. No—oxygen therapy should be questioned.

hypoxemia. The indications for oxygen therapy will be different in acute (short-term) and chronic (long-term) situations. In both cases, one must look at several factors:

1. Pa_{O_2} (arterial P_{O_2}).
2. Sa_{O_2} (hemoglobin saturation).
3. Cardiovascular status.
4. Work of breathing.
5. Oxygen transport.

Acute Oxygen Therapy

Oxygen therapy is warranted in acute clinical situations where the Pa_{O_2} is less than 60 mm Hg or the Sa_{O_2} is below 90% saturation.[13] Remember that at a Pa_{O_2} of 60 to 70 mm Hg represents the "dangerous" point on the oxyhemoglobin dissociation curve at which further decreases in the Pa_{O_2} (even small decreases) will result in large decreases in the saturation level (see Fig 5–7). Further declines in the Pa_{O_2} will result in the inability of the blood to carry oxygen. It is generally assumed that tissue hypoxia exists at blood gas levels below these values. In addition to evaluating the blood gas values, the patient should be evaluated for the presence of any compensatory response to hypoxia such as increase in the pulse or respiratory rate. The pH, Pa_{CO_2}, and body temperature should be evaluated since all will affect the oxygen transport via their effect on the oxyhemoglobin dissociation curve. This information should be evaluated against the clinical situation at hand. For example, is the patient conscious? Is the patient coherent or disoriented? Is the patient restless? These types of clinical observations must be made. Also, it is important to know if there has been a sudden onset of the signs and symptoms or whether they have occurred gradually over several hours or days. Finally, in some clinical situations, it is appropriate to begin short-term oxygen therapy without laboratory documentation. It is reasonable to expect that patients in shock from severe injury (hemorrhagic shock), an allergic reaction (anaphylactic shock), or patients with an acute myocardial infarction are at high risk for experiencing severe hypoxia. In these cases, supplemental oxygen therapy would be indicated. If these conditions persist for longer than 1 to 2 hours, then blood gases are indicated to determine if oxygen therapy should be continued or modified. Table 5–7 provides a listing for the indications for acute oxygen therapy.

Long-Term Oxygen Therapy

Long-term oxygen therapy is indicated for patients when the following conditions and criteria are present:

1. An accurate and current diagnosis exists.
2. Significant hypoxemia is present.
3. The patient has recovered from any acute medical problems or exacerbations.

TABLE 5–7.

Indications for Acute Oxygen Therapy

1. Blood gas values: (F_{IO_2} = 0.21)
   PaO_2 <60 mm Hg
   SaO_2 <90%
2. Clinical signs and symptoms
   Mild-moderate hypoxia
   Tachycardia
   Tachypnea
   Cyanosis
   Hypertension
   Restlessness
   Dyspnea
   Disorientation
3. Clinical signs and symptoms
   Moderate-severe hypoxia
   Cardiac arrhythmias
   Labored breathing
   Slow bounding pulse
   Lethargy
   Coma
4. High-risk patients
   Myocardial infarction
   Hemorrhagic shock
   Anaphylactic shock
   Burn patients

4. The patient is in stable condition.
5. Clinical trials of oxygen therapy demonstrate that supplemental oxygen provides overall clinical benefit.

In addition to the above criteria, other indications for oxygen therapy may include:[12, 13, 15, 29]

1. The presence of significant cardiac arrhythmias in patients with mild chronic hypoxemia.
2. Patients in chronic left ventricular failure (congestive heart failure).
3. Significant hypoxemia (PaO_2 less than 55 mm Hg) lactic acidosis, and/or cardiac arrhythmias as a result of exercise.
4. Polycythemia associated with hypoxemia.
5. Cor pulmonale.

Long-term oxygen therapy should also be considered for those patients with advanced COPD who are in a state of chronic respiratory failure with severe hypoxemia, with or without hypercapnea. These patients would be evaluated for continuous oxygen therapy if the PaO_2 is below 55 mm Hg, if they show signs and symptoms of cor pulmonale, or if they show compensatory polycythemia with a PaO_2 below 60 mm Hg.

Hypoxic Drive

The relationship between hypoxia and hypercarbia as stimuli for ventilation is both complex and unclear. As pulmonary disease progresses, arterial hypoxemia precedes hypercapnea. It is the hypercapnea, however, that initially determines the ventilatory drive. In COPD, there comes a point where the ventilatory drive has very little effect on the Pa_{CO_2}. At low or normal Pa_{CO_2} levels, the ventilatory response to hypoxia is inhibited. At elevated Pa_{CO_2} levels, the ventilatory response is more sensitive to hypoxia than to hypercarbia. Here, it is the lack of oxygen that provides the stimulus to breathe.

Although hypoxia has proved to be a stimulus for ventilation when the Pa_{CO_2} level is chronically high, this effort is unpredictable. The mechanism of "hypoxic drive" occurs via the peripheral chemoreceptors and occurs when the PaO_2 is below 60 mm Hg and the SaO_2 is about 80%.[4] Carefully prescribed, controlled oxygen therapy (F_{IO_2} known and controlled, e.g., 24% Venturi mask) need not depress the hypoxic drive.

Referring back to the oxyhemoglobin dissociation curve (see Fig 5–7), at PaO_2 levels below 60 mm Hg, small changes in the PaO_2 result in large changes in SaO_2 and therefore, the oxygen content transport. A patient with a PaO_2 of 40 mm Hg will have an SaO_2 of 75% and experience severe hypoxemia. The administration of supplemental oxygen to such a patient with the goal of achieving a PaO_2 in the range of 50 to 60 mm Hg, will provide "adequate" tissue oxygenation without eliminating the ventilatory response to hypoxia. Table 5–8 provides the criteria for long-term oxygen therapy.

Nocturnal vs. Continuous Oxygen Therapy

In 1980, the results of a study on continuous nocturnal oxygen therapy conducted by the National Heart, Lung, and Blood Institute were reported.[22] During the same period of time, a similar study was being conducted in England by the Medical Research Council.[19] The results of these two studies have set the standard for long-term oxygen therapy.

The Nocturnal Oxygen Therapy Trial (NOTT study) followed 203 patients in six centers throughout the United States and Winnipeg, Canada. The purpose of this study was to determine if 12 hours use of oxygen per day (including the time spent sleeping) was as effective as 24 hours of continuous oxygen therapy. The criteria for patients to be included in this study were: (1) clinically stable COPD, (2) FEV_1/FVC less than 0.6 and stable, (3) resting PaO_2 of 55 mm Hg or less, or (4) PaO_2 of 60 mm Hg with clinical signs of tissue hypoxia (polycythemia, cor pulmonale, etc.). These patients were then randomly placed in two groups. One group received oxygen for 12 hours each day including sleep time (nocturnal oxygen therapy [NOT] group). The other group received supplemental oxygen 24 hours each day (continuous oxygen therapy [COT] group). Figure 5–10 shows the significant difference between

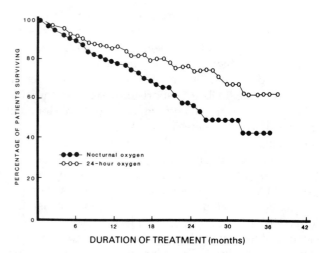

FIG 5–10.
Survival curves of NOTT study. Differences are statistically significant ($P < .01$) at 12, 24, and 36 months. (From Petty TL, Nett LM: History of long-term oxygen therapy. *Respir Care* 1983; 28:859–864. Used with permission.)

the NOT and COT groups based on overall survival rates showing significantly higher survival rates at 12, 24, 36 months for the COT group. The data from this study indicated fewer hospitalizations for the COT group as well.

The British Medical Research Council Study (MRC study) conducted a similar type of project, but in this case, they compared 15 hours of oxygen each day to no supplemental oxygen.[10] The MRC study included nocturnal oxygen in their 15-hour period.

TABLE 5–8.
General Criteria for Long-Term Oxygen Therapy

1. PaO_2 less than 55 mm Hg at rest on room air
2. PaO_2 less than 60 mm Hg when compensatory or secondary polycythemia present
3. Evidence of tissue hypoxia:
   Pulmonary hypertension
   Compensatory polycythemia
   Cor pulmonale
4. Evidence of central cyanosis
5. Severe arterial hypoxemia on exercise
6. Improvement of hypoxemic state with low-flow oxygen therapy (1 to 3 L/min; F_{IO_2}, 0.24 to 0.30)

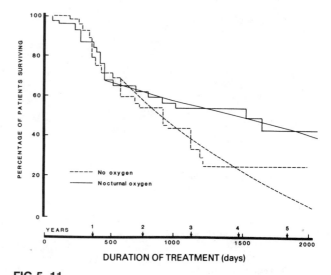

FIG 5–11.
Survival curves of British MRC study. Differences begin after 500 days of oxygen therapy. (From Petty TL, Nett LM: History of long-term oxygen therapy. *Respir Care* 1983; 28:859–864. Used with permission.)

The results of this study are equally significant (Fig 5–11), showing significantly higher survival rates for the nocturnal oxygen group vs. the no oxygen group.

These two studies are not exactly comparable. The results do indicate, however, that continuous oxygen therapy is better than nocturnal oxygen therapy and that nocturnal oxygen therapy is superior to no oxygen therapy.

PHYSIOLOGIC EFFECTS OF OXYGEN THERAPY

As stated previously, the transport and delivery of oxygen to the body tissues is dependent upon a complex interaction of several factors including an adequate: (1) PaO_2; (2) SaO_2; (3) hemoglobin concentration; (4) cardiac output; (5) regional blood blow; and (6) functioning hemoglobin.

The proper clinical use of oxygen therapy requires that one understand and be able to: (1) recognize the symptoms of tissue hypoxia, (2) recognize the indications (parameters) for initiating oxygen therapy, (3) know the impact that supplemental oxygen may have on the pathophysiology of a disease or disorder, and (4) know which pulmonary and nonpulmonary diseases may require oxygen therapy. Given this information, a reasonable prediction can be made as to which patients will benefit from oxygen therapy. Finally, in patients in whom oxygen therapy is warranted, optimal dosage and an evaluation of the ratio between the benefits of oxygen therapy and the risk of oxygen toxicity must be determined.

Acute Hypoxia

In clinical situations in which acute hypoxemia exists, the symptoms are general and nonspecific. They include the hemodynamic compensatory mechanisms (adrenergic mechanisms) that are associated with stress. One should be suspicious of the presence of cellular hypoxia in any acute patient who demonstrates sudden changes in mental status and unexplained hemodynamic parameters such as a change in pulse, change in blood pressure, or cardiac arrhythmia. Table 5–9 lists clinical conditions in the acute setting that indicate the potential for severe tissue hypoxia.

Oxygen therapy should be initiated in these conditions when PaO_2 is less than 60 mm Hg and the

TABLE 5–9.

Clinical Situations in the Acute Care Setting Where There Is a High Incidence of Hypoxia

Myocardial infarction
Congestive heart failure
Acute pulmonary disorders
Hypovolemic shock
Sepsis
Blunt chest trauma
Drug overdose (abuse)
Exacerbation of neuromuscular disease
Liver failure
Acute pancreatitis
Head trauma
Extensive general trauma

SaO_2 is less than 90%. The intended benefits of oxygen therapy at this point are twofold:

1. Oxygen administration may increase the PaO_2 and move the oxygen content to the flattened portion of the oxyhemoglobin dissociation curve. This will allow for nearly maximal oxygen content to be delivered to the tissues at normobaric conditions.
2. Oxygen administration may reduce or eliminate the compensatory hemodynamic changes. This will reduce the oxygen consumption by the heart and, theoretically, should reduce the potential for more serious cardiac arrhythmias. The dosage of oxygen in these cases, as well as the duration of supplemental oxygen, should be minimized to prevent the potential for oxygen-induced pulmonary damage.

Finally, there are acute clinical conditions in which oxygen administration is indicated even in the absence of hypoxemia. These include a fall in the cardiac output, suspected acute myocardial infarction, and abnormalities of oxyhemoglobin saturation (carbon monoxide poisoning, sickle cell crisis). In these situations, arterial blood gases should be drawn as soon as possible and the role of oxygen therapy reevaluated based on the laboratory data and patient status.

Chronic Hypoxemia

Chronic hypoxemia is seen most often in patients with COPD, generally with associated cor pulmonale. In these patients, compensatory mechanisms have developed during the gradual development of the hypoxemic state. These mechanisms include:

1. *Secondary or compensatory polycythemia.* Chronic hypoxia stimulates the production of erythropoietin, which stimulates the bone marrow to produce increased numbers of red blood cells. This polycythemia, in turn, increases the oxygen carrying capacity. At a given PaO_2, the oxygen content will be elevated (see Fig 5–6).

2. *Pulmonary hypertension.* Pulmonary arterial hypertension is a result of hypoxia, with or without acidosis. This causes an increase in the work load of the right ventricle and precipitates cor pulmonale.

The combination of these two mechanisms results in an increased burden on the patient's cardiovascular system and contributes to the general deterioration of the patient's condition with time. Oxygen administration (low-flow oxygen) has been shown to decrease hematocrit, lower pulmonary artery pressures, and reduce those symptoms associated with cor pulmonale. Studies on low-flow oxygen therapy have also shown a marked reduction in mortality for these patients.[20]

PATIENT CONDITIONS REQUIRING OXYGEN THERAPY

Adult Respiratory Distress Syndrome

The adult respiratory distress syndrome (ARDS) represents one of the most difficult clinical problems with respect to oxygenation and oxygen therapy. ARDS is characterized by a rapid onset of dyspnea, tachypnea, hypoxemia, diffuse pulmonary infiltrates, and reduced pulmonary lung volumes. The ARDS patient suffers from generalized atelectasis, pulmonary edema, hyaline membrane formation, and interstitial and alveolar hemorrhage.

ARDS is a nonspecific pulmonary response to a variety of injuries (Table 5–10). The pathophysiology of ARDS is not entirely known. The overall scheme of the progression of ARDS is shown in Figure 5–12. ARDS is a syndrome that centers around the hypoxemic state of a patient. Although the exact etiology and mechanism of the onset and progression of ARDS are not totally understood, hypoxia is a hallmark of this syndrome.

In studying the etiology of ARDS, one readily sees that the primary causes all have the effect of creating either transient or more prolonged hypoxia. Hypoxia, whether the result of fat emboli, trauma, an immune reaction, cardiac failure, drug overdose, or any number of other causes, can set into motion a series of events that perpetuate the hypoxic state

TABLE 5–10.

Causes of Adult Respiratory Distress Syndrome

Pulmonary
  Thoracic trauma
  Prolonged mechanical ventilation
  Pulmonary aspiration
  Pulmonary infection
  Viral pneumonia
  Oxygen toxicity
  Fat embolism
  Prolonged cardiopulmonary bypass
  Near-drowning
  Congestive atelectasis
  Inhalation of toxins and irritants
Nonpulmonary
  Sepsis
  Hemorrhagic shock
  Viral infection (viremia)
  Pancreatitis
  Disseminated intravascular coagulation
  Drug overdose
  CNS disorder
  Congestive heart failure
  Fluid overload
  Immunologic reaction
  Blood transfusions
  Nonthoracic trauma
  Shock (hypovolemia)
  Uremia

and facilitate progression of the clinical manifestations of ARDS (Fig 5–13). The diagnosis of ARDS is generally made on the clinical signs and symptoms presented by the patient:

1. Primary factor or cause present.
2. Sudden marked tachypnea.
3. Dyspnea.
4. Cyanosis.
5. Elevated pulse, blood pressure, and cardiac output.
6. Refractory hypoxemia (PaO_2, <50 mm Hg; FI_{O_2} >0.60).
7. Decrease in lung compliance.
8. Chest radiograph shows diffuse alveolar infiltration.
9. Pulmonary congestion (rales, rhonchi, wheezes).
10. Onset of syndrome generally within 24 to 36 hours following injury or illness.

Blood gas analysis in the early stages of ARDS shows a decreased PaO_2, a normal or low Pa_{CO_2}, and normal pH. As the syndrome progresses and in the

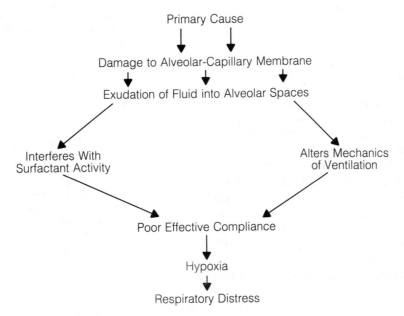

FIG 5–12.
ARDS is considered a severe alveolar-capillary membrane injury that follows this general scheme.

latter stages, the arterial blood gases change: PaO_2 decreased, the Pa_{CO_2} elevated, and the pH decreased.

The goals of oxygen therapy in the managment of ARDS are (1) correction of the hypoxemia, and (2) reduction of the potential further injury secondary to oxygen toxicity.

In the early stages, these goals may be possible through controlled oxygen administration. As the syndrome progresses, shunting becomes more characteristic of the disorder, thus hypoxemia responds very poorly to oxygen administration. If it is not possible to maintain a PaO_2 greater than 60 mm Hg at an FI_{O_2} of 0.8, the patient should be considered a candidate for continuous positive-airway pressure (CPAP).[25] If the patient shows signs of impending ventilatory failure (increasing Pa_{CO_2} and decreasing PaO_2) or is unable to tolerate CPAP, the patient

ADULT RESPIRATORY DISTRESS SYNDROME

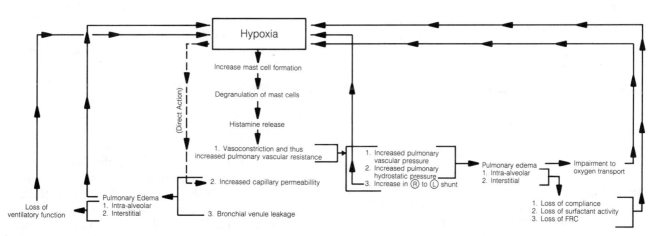

FIG 5–13.
Theoretical model for the role of hypoxia in ARDS.

should be evaluated for mechanical ventilation. Further blood gas evaluation may indicate the need for the application of PEEP.

Acute Respiratory Failure

Acute respiratory failure represents that clinical situation where the rapid progression of a respiratory disease or disorder does not permit the compensatory mechanisms to maintain an adequate ventilatory or respiratory state. Severe tissue hypoxia and hypercarbia will develop as the compensatory mechanisms fail (Fig 5–14). Acute respiratory failure is generally defined as that clinical condition where the blood gas abnormalities meet the following criteria: PaO_2, >50 mm Hg, $PaCO_2$, >50 mm Hg, pH, <7.35 (P_B standard at 760 mm Hg). Acute respiratory failure may result from (1) diseases or disorders of the neuromuscular system; (2) diseases of the thorax; (3) parenchymal lung disease; (4) diseases or disorders of the CNS respiratory center; and (5) airway disease/obstruction.

Acute respiratory failure can also be associated with viral and bacterial infections, drug overdose, inhalation of toxins, aspiration of gastric contents and toxic materials, and cardiovascular failure. Table 5–11 provides a listing of the primary causes of acute respiratory failure.

TABLE 5–11.

Diseases or Disorders That Can Result in Acute Respiratory Failure

Pulmonary disorders
  Airway obstruction
  Chronic bronchitis
  Asthma
  Pulmonary emphysema
  Pneumonia
  Pulmonary edema
  Pulmonary embolism
  Pulmonary fibrosis
  Adult respiratory distress syndrome (ARDS)
Nonpulmonary disorders
  Central nervous system
    Drug overdose
    Cerebrovascular accident
    Head trauma
    Sleep apnea
  Chest wall disease
    Pneumothorax
    Pleural effusion
    Flail chest
  Neuromuscular diseases
    Myasthenia gravis
    Muscular dystrophy
    Multiple sclerosis
    Guillian-Barré syndrome
  Cardiovascular disease
    Cardiac failure
    Shock

Acute hypoxemia in respiratory failure is generally not well tolerated by most patients since the compensatory mechanisms are not present at this stage of failure. The goals of oxygen therapy are threefold:

1. Increase the PaO_2 by increasing the FIO_2.
2. Increase the PaO_2 by improving the distribution of gas in the lungs.
3. Decrease ventilatory work necessary to maintain the PaO_2 at a given level.

Patients with hypoxemia who have an elevated $PaCO_2$, oxygen administration should be utilized with great caution. Patients who are hypoxemic and hypercapneic often have a decreased ventilatory response to PCO_2 and H^+. If this is the case, these patients may be breathing in response to their hypoxic drives. In this case, controlled oxygen therapy should be administered to achieve a PaO_2 between 50 to 60 mm Hg. This will do two things: (1) move the PaO_2 up on the oxyhemoglobin dissociation curve and provide 83% to 90% saturation, and (2) not inhibit the hypoxic drive to breathe.

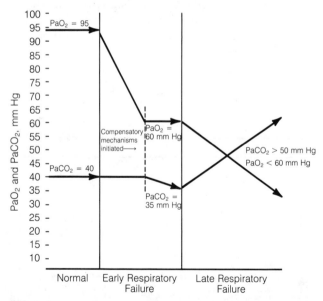

FIG 5–14.

The progression of acute respiratory failure. As the PaO_2 falls, compensatory mechanisms set in to correct/maintain the PaO_2. These mechanisms are an increase in respiratory rate and volume. As these mechanisms are no longer able to maintain the blood gas levels, the patient moves into late respiratory failure which is characterized by increasing $PaCO_2$ and decreasing PaO_2.

In both acute and chronic respiratory failure, the patient should be evaluated for an adequate cardiac output, tissue perfusion, and the hemoglobin level for oxygen carrying capacity. If patients in respiratory failure do not respond to oxygen therapy and, potentially, if the Pa_{CO_2} continues to rise and the acidosis persists, these patients should be evaluated for intubation and mechanical ventilation.

Chronic Obstructive Pulmonary Disease

The term COPD (chronic obstructive pulmonary disease) refers to a group of conditions or disorders associated with the chronic obstruction to the flow of air within the lungs. In general, COPD is the most common form of chronic lung disease. Asthma, cystic fibrosis, and bronchiectasis are sometimes included in the term COPD. However, both chronic bronchitis and emphysema are generally present in the patient with a diagnosis of COPD.

Chronic bronchitis is defined as the excessive production of mucus from bronchi which are free of specific disease. The most important factor in the development of chronic bronchitis is cigarette smoking. Chronic bronchitis is said to exist clinically when the patient complains of cough and increased sputum production for a minimum of 3 consecutive months per year for 2 successive years.[6]

Pulmonary emphysema is defined as the permanent enlargement of the alveoli and alveolar sacs secondary to destruction of the alveolar walls.[6] Cigarette smoking is thought to be the primary etiological factor; as such, this explains why both chronic bronchitis and emphysema are seen in COPD. There are also those who have pulmonary emphysema secondary to a deficiency in alpha[1] antitrypsin.

It is important to approach oxygen therapy from two clinical perspectives: (1) acute oxygen therapy for patients with COPD, and (2) long-term or domiciliary oxygen therapy.

Acute oxygen therapy for the COPD patient must have the goal of providing adequate tissue oxygenation without compromising the patient's "hypoxic drive" to ventilate. Since these patients suffer from chronic hypercarbia, their ventilatory drive or stimulus comes from the stimulation of oxygen chemoreceptors. The administration of controlled oxygen (a defined, known, and controlled FI_{O_2}, e.g., 24% Venturi mask) to elevate other methods can be utilized to correct the precipitating factors for the COPD exacerbation.

Long-term or domiciliary oxygen therapy can be very helpful in the outpatient management of pa-

tients with severe COPD. Long-term oxygen therapy can be used for patients who have been clinically stable for at least 30 days and who have a Pa_{O_2} less than 55 mm Hg at rest or during exercise. Patients with a Pa_{O_2} less than 60 mm Hg who show signs of polycythemia, cor pulmonale, or pulmonary hypertension should also be considered possible candidates for domiciliary oxygen therapy.[13] In these patients, low flow-oxygen (1 to 3 L/min via a nasal cannula) is generally adequate to relieve the severe hypoxemia without compromising the ventilatory status. Low-flow oxygen administration systems do not provide a precise FI_{O_2}. The inspired oxygen concentration will vary with the patient's ventilatory rate and pattern. Low-flow oxygen administration systems are not recommended for patients who are not in a stable condition nor in patients where the diagnosis and baseline arterial blood gas values have not been documented. Table 5–12 provides appropriate FI_{O_2} ranges for controlled and noncontrolled systems.

Pulmonary Edema

Pulmonary edema is defined as the abnormal accumulation of fluid in the interstitial and alveolar spaces in the lung. Pulmonary edema can be divided into two primary categories: cardiogenic pulmonary edema and noncardiogenic pulmonary edema (Table 5–13). Cardiogenic pulmonary edema results from those conditions where the hydrostatic pressure in

TABLE 5–12.

Oxygen Concentrations for Controlled* and Noncontrolled† Oxygen Delivery Systems for Long-Term Oxygen Administration

CONTROLLED SYSTEM	O₂ FLOW RATE, L/MIN	TOTAL FLOW, L/MIN	FI_{O_2}
Venturi masks	4	84	0.24
	6	66	0.28
	8	48	0.35
	8	32	0.40
	15	30	0.60

NONCONTROLLED SYSTEM	O₂ FLOW RATE, L/MIN	FI_{O_2} RANGE
Nasal cannula	1–6	0.24–0.44
Nasal catheter	1–6	0.24–0.50
Simple mask	5–8	0.30–0.60
Partial rebreathing mask	5–10	0.40–1.00

*Controlled systems are those in which an accurate FI_{O_2} is delivered independent of the patient's respiratory rate and ventilatory pattern. High-flow oxygen systems supply oxygen at a total flow rate (oxygen flow plus entrained air) that meets the patient's inspiratory demand. The FI_{O_2} will be accurate and predictable.
†Noncontrolled systems are those in which the FI_{O_2} fluctuates with the respiratory rate and ventilatory pattern. Low-flow oxygen systems supply oxygen at flow rates less than the patient's inspiratory demand. The FI_{O_2} will fluctuate as a result.

TABLE 5-13.

Causes of Pulmonary Edema

Cardiac pulmonary edema
    Cardiac arrhythmias
    Fluid overload
    Systemic and/or pulmonary hypertension
    Myocardial infarction
    Mitral valve disease
    Left ventricular failure
    Pulmonary embolus
Noncardiac pulmonary edema
    Adult respiratory distress syndrome
    Pneumonia
    Renal failure
    Inhalation of toxic gases
    Head trauma
    Anaphylactic shock
    CNS disorders

the pulmonary system is elevated and thus causes the movement of fluid into the lungs as well as abnormal cardiac function.

Oxygen therapy in pulmonary edema is geared to correcting the hypoxemia that is caused by the $\dot{V}/\dot{Q}$ abnormality. The patient should be placed on a controlled (high-flow) oxygen delivery system with an initial $F_{I_{O_2}}$ at 0.40 to 0.60, depending on the severity of the hypoxemia, and blood gases should be measured. In cases where the patient does not initially respond to oxygen administration, IPPB powered by an oxygen source may be an option to consider. The rationale is twofold: (1) in patients with both right and left ventricular cardiac failure, the IPPB may reduce the venous return and lower the cardiac preload; (2) elevated $F_{I_{O_2}}$ via the intermittent positive-pressure breathing (IPPB) may help correct the hypoxemia. In some patients, however, IPPB may prove to be detrimental and should be discontinued if the patient does not benefit. In severe cases of pulmonary edema, particularly if a large shunt is present, the patient may need to be treated via CPAP or mechanical ventilation with PEEP to improve oxygenation.

Asthma

Asthma is characterized by the constriction of the smooth muscles in the small airways. This results in a decrease in the diameter of the airways, increased airway resistance, increased secretion production, bronchospasm, and swelling of the airway mucosa. Airtrapping and hyperinflation of the alveoli follow. The combination of the increased resistance, decreased flow rate, and hyperinflation result in a $\dot{V}/\dot{Q}$ mismatch and hypoxemia. During an asthma attack, arterial blood gases will show mild to moderate hypoxemia and hypocapnea.

Hypoxemia is generally considered to be present during all acute asthma attacks. In patients with status asthmaticus, the hypoxemia can be severe. Arterial blood gases should be drawn in order to determine the degree of arterial hypoxemia present as well as to determine the ventilatory and acid-base status of the patient.

1. *Mild hypoxemia:* Low-flow oxygen via a nasal cannula is appropriate to deliver supplemental oxygen. The oxygen should be humidified and a flow rate of 2 to 4 L/min should be adequate to provide an $F_{I_{O_2}}$ of 0.30 to 0.40.

2. *Moderate hypoxemia:* When the hypoxemia is more pronounced, a higher $F_{I_{O_2}}$ will be required. At this point a controlled oxygen system should be used. A simple mask or a Venturi mask at higher flow rates can provide $F_{I_{O_2}}$ ranges of 0.40 to 0.60.

3. *Severe hypoxemia:* In cases of severe hypoxemia, particularly in status asthmaticus, high $F_{I_{O_2}}$ will be required. In this situation, a tight-fitting partial rebreathing mask or nonrebreathing mask can provide an $F_{I_{O_2}}$ in the range of 0.60 to 1.00.

In monitoring patients in an acute asthma attack, it is important to watch for signs of general worsening of the patient's condition and the possible onset of acute ventilatory failure. The term *status asthmaticus* describes a point in the clinical course of asthma when bronchospasm no longer responds to bronchodilators. Respirations may become shallow and rapid, and there may be so little air moving because of bronchospasm, that rales and wheezes suddenly can no longer be heard. When the patient shows signs of a quiet chest, physical exhaustion, increasing airway obstruction, and an increase in the Pa_{CO_2} with decreasing Pa_{O_2} (despite supplemental oxygen), mechanical ventilation should be considered.

Cor Pulmonale

The major effect of chronic hypoxemia in the COPD patient is an increase in the pulmonary vascular resistance and pulmonary artery pressure secondary to pulmonary vasoconstriction. Hypoxic pulmonary vasoconstriction is thought to be more directly a result of alveolar hypoxia (Pa_{O_2}) rather than a low-oxygen tension in the mixed venous blood (P$\bar{v}O_2$) or the arterial oxygen tension (PaO$_2$).[9]

The physiologic effect of this hypoxic pulmonary vasoconstriction is to direct the blood away from the regions of alveolar hypoxia and thus provide a more effective $\dot{V}/\dot{Q}$ ratio. As the COPD progresses and greater areas of the lung suffer from alveolar hypoxia, this mechanism is no longer effective. At this point there is overall pulmonary hypertension that, along with the polycythemia which is associated with COPD, will lead to: (1) right ventricular hypertrophy secondary to the increased work load on the right ventricle, (2) dilation of the right ventricular wall as a result of the stretching of the muscle fibers, and (3) right ventricular failure (Fig 5–15).

When the right ventricle fails, an adequate cardiac output cannot be sustained. Subsequent to this, the venous return is reduced and stasis or pooling of blood occurs in the systemic system.

The treatment of cor pulmonale ideally should be directed at the primary cause—alveolar hypoxemia (low PaO$_2$). Prior to beginning a long-term oxygen program, it is important to understand the condition of the lung. In patients with cor pulmonale secondary to an increased vascular resistance where there is a destructive process, the circulation pattern in the lung may be somewhat fixed. The use of supplemental oxygen may have little impact on

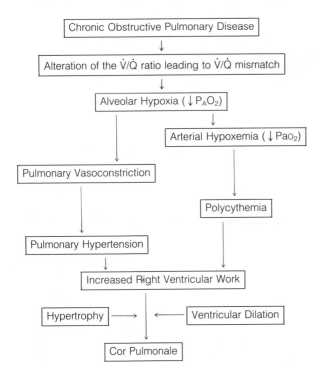

FIG 5–15.
Effect of COPD and associated alveolar hypoxemia on the development of cor pulmonale.

reducing the pulmonary hypertension. However, in those patients with cor pulmonale, where the pulmonary hypertension is primarily the result of alveolar hypoxia, the pulmonary vasoconstriction and subsequent pressure may be reduced or even normalized with supplemental oxygen. For this reason, the patient who is given supplemental oxygen should be monitored carefully to evaluate the benefits in this clinical situation. The general guidelines for prescribing continuous low-flow oxygen at 1 to 3 L/min in COPD are followed.

Carbon Monoxide Poisoning

Carbon monoxide (CO) is an odorless, tasteless, and colorless gas that is a byproduct of incomplete combustion and oxidation. Carbon monoxide is found in cigarette smoke, automobile exhaust, smoke from coal and wood, and sewers and mines. Carbon monoxide has no direct effect on the lung, but does have an affinity for hemoglobin that is nearly 210 times greater than oxygen. Because of this affinity for hemoglobin, carbon monoxide will displace oxygen from the hemoglobin molecule and thus interfere with oxygen transport and delivery to the tissues. When carbon monoxide is bound to hemoglobin, carboxyhemoglobin (COHb) is formed. Normally less than 1% of the available hemoglobin is in the form of carboxyhemoglobin. In normal healthy individuals, no clinical manifestations of carbon monoxide poisoning are observed at COHb levels less than 10%.[11]

The toxic effect of carbon monoxide poisoning are the result of two factors:

1. Since carbon monoxide displaces oxygen on the hemoglobin molecule, the oxygen content of the blood is greatly reduced and tissue hypoxia will result.

2. The presence of COHb will shift the oxyhemoglobin dissociation curve to the left and the shape of the curve will change from S-shaped to a hyperbolic shape. This will reduce the ability of the hemoglobin molecule to release what oxygen is present to the tissues, again resulting in tissue hypoxia.

Contrary to most textbooks, the cherry-red color of the skin mucous membranes are not often observed in patients with carbon monoxide poisoning.[11] The best clue for the clinician is the patient history. The arterial blood gas analysis in these patients will show a normal PaO$_2$ and a normal/low PaCO$_2$. The measured SaO$_2$ will be significantly lower than the estimated or calculated SaO_2 from the oxyhemoglobin dissociation curve. The pH will be low (metabolic acidosis) due to the lactic acid production in the hypoxic tissues. The diagnosis should be made by the measurement of the carboxyhemoglobin level.

The primary treatment once the patient is removed from the toxic environment is the administration of 100% oxygen. This will elevate the PaO_2 and increase the speed at which the carbon monoxide is eliminated. The primary factors for effective elimination are (1) alveolar ventilation and (2) PaO_2.

The half-life for eliminating carbon monoxide from the blood is 5 hours with a normal alveolar ventilation at room air. This means that it will take 5 hours to eliminate one-half of the COHb. This half-life is inversely proportional to the PaO_2; therefore, the half-life can be reduced from 5 hours to 1 hour when the FIO_2 is increased from 0.21 to 1.00. This half-life can be further shortened by placing the patient in a hyperbaric oxygen chamber, although most facilities do not have such capabilities. The patient should be placed on 100% oxygen until the COHb is less than 10%. After the COHb level falls below 10%, administration of supplemental oxygen can be discontinued.

Hyaline Membrane Disease

Hyaline membrane disease is a condition that is characterized by atelectasis and flow of blood to poorly ventilated regions of the lung. Hyaline membrane disease (neonatal respiratory distress syndrome, idiopathic respiratory distress syndrome) results from lung immaturity. The major pathologic changes observed in hyaline membrane disease includes alveolar consolidation, interstitial and intraalveolar pulmonary edema, atelectasis, and pulmonary surfactant deficiency.

The lack of lung maturity in the preterm infant is the overriding causative factor in the respiratory distress syndrome (RDS). RDS occurs in approximately 60% of infants less than 28 weeks' gestational age and is rarely observed in full-term babies.[11] Additional risk factors for the development of RDS are listed in Table 5–14. The surface tension in the preterm is very high due to the lack of surfactant which is normally produced by the alveolar type II cells. Normally, during this time, surfactant is synthesized and stored during the last few weeks of gestation. Premature birth inhibits this process.

The lack of surfactant results in atelectasis, a reduction in pulmonary compliance, an increased work of breathing and hypoxemia. The hypoxia

TABLE 5–14.

Risk Factors for the Development of Respiratory Distress Syndrome (Hyaline Membrane Disease)

Delivery by cesarean birth
Complicated pregnancy
Prolonged labor
Prenatal asphyxia
Diabetic mother
Birth weight below 2.5 kg

causes pulmonary vasoconstriction resulting in pulmonary hypoperfusion. The blood that normally would perfuse ventilated alveoli instead is shunted through the patent ductus arteriosus and the foramen ovale. This shunting is further complicated by the pulmonary hypoperfusion. This results in ischemia of lung tissue, a decrease in lung metabolic functions resulting in a further decline in the production of surfactant. The inadequate ventilation and gas exchange cause hypoxemia, hypercapnea, and severe acidosis. Injury to the alveolar capillary membrane allows the leaking of fluid into the interstitial spaces and alveoli, and the formation of the hyaline membrane (Fig 5–16).

The clinical manifestations of RDS are an increased work of breathing evidenced by an increased respiratory rate, intercostal retractions, substernal retractions, nasal flaring, and respiratory grunting. The respiratory rates often range from 60 to 120 breaths/min. Heart rate, cardiac output, and blood pressure are all elevated secondary to hypoxemia. Chest films show increased opacity with a ground glass appearance.

The severe hypoxemia is the result of shunting, $\dot{V}/\dot{Q}$ mismatch, persistent fetal circulation, and fatigue (see Fig 5–16). If the cycle in the development and progression of RDS is not broken, death will occur.

Respiratory distress syndrome is a self-limited disorder, provided that the severe hypoxemia can be controlled. The overall goal of oxygen therapy is to correct the hypoxemia with the least amount of intervention. The initial course of therapy is oxygen therapy alone. In infants with mild hypoxemia, supplemental oxygen should be provided to bring the PaO_2 into the 50 to 70 mm Hg range at an FIO_2 less than 0.60. In moderate to severe hypoxemia, constant positive airway pressure (CPAP) is the method of choice. The use of CPAP will (1) increase the functional residual capacity (FRC), (2) decrease the work of breathing, and (3) improve arterial oxygenation. The use of CPAP allows for better oxygenation at lower FI_{O_2} levels. CPAP should be initiated when the Pa_{O_2} is less than 50 mm Hg at an FI_{O_2} greater than or equal to 0.60. Because of the poor mortality rate of preterm infants with mechanical ventilation, this form of therapy is avoided if at all possible. Table 5–15 provides general guidelines for the treatment of RDS with supplemental oxygen.

Babies suffering from respiratory distress syndrome are at high risk of developing serious therapeutic complications such as bronchopulmonary dysplasia, retrolental fibroplasia, pulmonary oxygen toxic response, and barotrauma. Since these complications are due to therapeutic intervention, one must be aware of the goals of therapy, the criteria for evaluating the success of therapy, and the risk-benefit ratio of each therapy initiated.

Postoperative Care

Alteration in oxygenation occurs commonly in surgical patients both during and for a period of time following surgery. These changes include a decrease in the functional residual capacity, the ratio

TABLE 5–15.

Guidelines for the Oxygen Treatment of Infants With Respiratory Distress Syndrome*

Indications for increased FI_{O_2} (0.40 to 0.60)
  Normal Pa_{CO_2} range (stable)
  Adequate ventilatory effort
  Ability to maintain Pa_{O_2} ≥50 mm Hg at FI_{O_2} ≤0.60
  No impending complications
Indications for CPAP
  Pa_{CO_2} <60 to 65 mm Hg (and stable)
  Inability to maintain Pa_{O_2} ≥50 mm Hg at FI_{O_2} ≤0.60
  pH >7.25
  No apnea
Indications for mechanical ventilation (PEEP)
  Apnea
  Pa_{CO_2} ≥65 mm Hg (and increasing)
  Pa_{O_2} <50 mm Hg at FI_{O_2} ≥0.80
  pH <7.25

*The guidelines are based primarily on arterial blood gas values and do not represent clinical absolutes. Other clinical factors must also be taken into account such as gestational age, presence of complicating factors, quality of blood gas sample, and size of the baby.

between the functional residual capacity and the closing capacity (FRC/CC ratio), the $\dot{V}/\dot{Q}$ match or ratio, and the saturation of mixed venous blood $S\bar{v}_{O_2}$. Because of these alterations, hypoxemia is frequently observed during the first few hours following surgery. In normal patients, this hypoxemia is transient and not severe enough to create major problems for the patient. Postoperative hypoxemia occurs most frequently in elderly patients, those patients who are significantly obese, those patients with a history of pulmonary or cardiac disease, and, finally, those patients with thoracic or upper abdominal surgery.[10]

Many factors contribute to the changes that occur in a patient's lung function after surgery. Atelectasis, shallow tidal ventilations, and related incomplete alveolar inflation are the normal changes observed. These changes begin during the surgical procedure, are fully present immediately following surgery, and subside generally 1 to 2 days following surgery.

After a surgical procedure, it is very important to breathe deeply to maximum inflation to reexpand areas of atelectasis in the lung. Because of pain, the use of narcotic analgesics, and effects of anesthesia, most patients will have difficulty completing maximal inflation maneuvers. The atelectasis prevalent in patients following surgery is generally due to immobility, sedation, pain, and diaphragmatic splinting. Atelectasis, however, can also be associated with fluid overload, pleural effusion, pneumothorax,

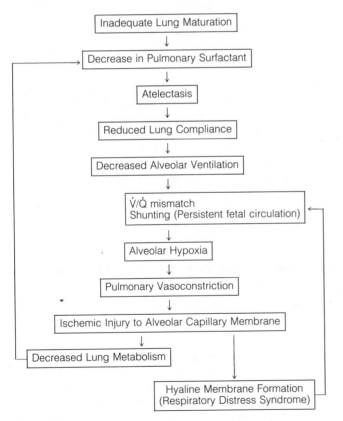

FIG 5–16.
Pathophysiology of the development of respiratory distress syndrome in the preterm infant.

pulmonary embolism, or pulmonary infection. These possible factors should not be overlooked. The pulmonary atelectasis, regardless of the precipitating cause, results in intrapulmonary shunting and hypoxemia.

In postoperative patients, oxygen therapy will not prove highly beneficial to correcting the causes of hypoxemia. In fact, oxygen therapy should initially be utilized to correct moderate to severe hypoxemia and then secondarily to other therapeutic modalities geared toward lung expansion and correction of atelectasis (such as incentive measures that can help reinflate the lung and prevent further atelectasis and hypoxemia). Proper bronchial hygiene, monitoring of the ventilatory status, arterial blood gas analysis, and chest x-ray films are needed to properly manage the hypoxemia in postsurgical patients. Patients who suffer no major complications following surgery and who experience significant hypoxemia will generally respond to low concentrations of oxygen (F_{IO_2} of 0.30 to 0.40) given via a nasal cannula. More significant clinical cases of hypoxemia may require a higher F_{IO_2} via a controlled oxygen system or high concentration noncontrolled system (Venturi mask, partial/nonrebreathing mask). In more severe cases of hypoxemia where CO_2 retention is not present, the use of CPAP will help correct hypoxemia. Patients who suffer acute ventilatory failure (Pa_{CO_2}, >50 mm Hg; pH, <7.30; decreased Pa_{O_2}) should be evaluated for ventilatory support. Patients who are at *high risk* for postsurgical complications, such as those having a history of pulmonary disease, should continue on mechanical ventilation with low F_{IO_2} supplemental oxygen for a few hours postsurgery.

For normal patients and patients with no history of cardiorespiratory disease or disorder, there is no indication for routine oxygen therapy following surgery. In patients with thoracic and cardiac surgery, supplemental oxygen should be given until arterial blood gas analyses indicate the absence of hypoxemia or impending ventilatory failure. Patients with chronic obstructive pulmonary disease who are not on mechanical ventilation and controlled oxygen after surgery should be given low-flow oxygen to maintain the Pa_{O_2} between 50 to 60 mm Hg. In addition, these patients should be monitored closely for signs of ventilatory failure.

HYPERBARIC OXYGEN THERAPY

Hyperbaric oxygen therapy is the administration of oxygen at pressures greater than atmospheric.

The Undersea Medical Society defines hyperbaric oxygenation as "a mode of medical treatment in which the patient is entirely enclosed in a pressure chamber breathing oxygen at a pressure greater than one atmosphere. Treatment may be carried out either in a monoplace chamber with pure oxygen or a larger, multiplace chamber pressurized with compressed air, in which case the patient receives pure oxygen by mask, head tent, or endotracheal tube. Breathing 100% oxygen at one atmosphere pressure or applying oxygen topically to parts of the body without the use of a pressurized chamber which encloses the patient completely is not considered hyperbaric oxygenation."[7]

Figure 5–17 shows an example of a monoplace chamber (single occupant) and a multiplace chamber (more than one occupant) for the therapeutic application of hyperbaric oxygen. As indicated in the definition, monoplace chambers use 100% oxygen in the pressurized chamber; where as in the multiplace chamber, the patient breathes 100% oxygen through a mask or an artificial airway while the chamber is pressurized with compressed air.

Hyperbaric oxygen increases the amount of oxygen in the blood and tissues. This is accomplished by forcing greater amounts of oxygen into solution in the plasma by using high pressure. For example, at one atmosphere (760 mm Hg or 14.7 psi), the Pa_{O_2} is approximately 100 mm Hg at room air. At a Pa_{O_2} of 100 mm Hg, about 0.3 vol% (ml O_2/100 ml blood) oxygen is dissolved in the plasma. At three atmospheres (2,280 mm Hg or 44.1 psi), the Pa_{O_2} is approximately 1,800 mm Hg, at 100% oxygen concentration, and the amount dissolved in plasma is nearly 6.2 vol% (ml O_2/100 ml blood).

The use of hyperbaric oxygen results in several important physiologic changes:

1. A reduction in cardiac output.
2. Generalized vasoconstriction.
3. New capillary bed formation.
4. Reduction in the size of bubbles dissolved in the blood.
5. Altered metabolic function of aerobic and anaerobic organisms in the body.

Because of these physiologic changes, the use of hyperbaric oxygenation has many theoretical applications. The Undersea Medical Society has developed a four-category system for recommending hyperbaric oxygenation (Table 5–16).

Various treatment protocols have been developed for hyperbaric oxygenation (HBO). This generally consists of placing patients in the chamber for

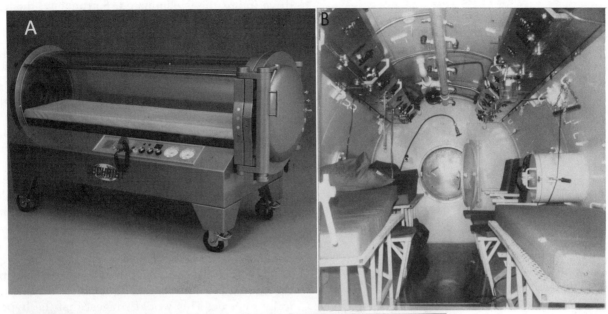

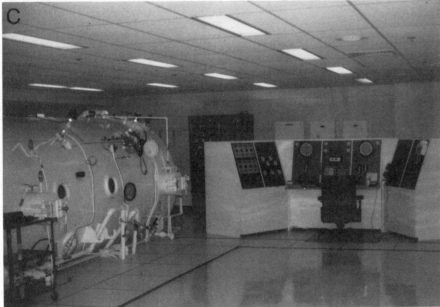

FIG 5–17.

A, monoplace hyperbaric chamber. (Courtesy of Sechrist Industries, Inc.) **B** interior of multiplace hyperbaric chamber. **C,** exterior of multiplace hyperbaric chamber. (Courtesy of Reimers Engineering, Inc.)

prescribed periods of time at 2 to 3 atmospheres. This is called a "dive." A given protocol may require 2 to 4 "dives" each day over several days, weeks, or even months. Table 5–17 shows the relationship between hyperbaric pressures and oxygen carrying capacity.

Hazards of Oxygen Therapy

Oxygen therapy is an important and complex drug used in the treatment of many disorders of the pulmonary system. Prior to the early 1970s, the methods of oxygen delivery were not precise. With the exception of the perinatal care areas, it was not generally possible to administer supplemental oxygen over a prolonged period of time and at a sufficient F_{IO_2} to be alarmed at the potential hazards associated with O_2 therapy.

The predominant use of adult oxygen tents (pediatric croup tents as a mode of oxygen delivery) probably protected many patients. As the field of respiratory care developed and more precise meth-

TABLE 5–16.

Categories for the Use of Hyperbaric Oxygenation*

Category I: Disorders in which hyperbaric oxygen is the primary
mode of therapy
    Acute carbon monoxide poisoning
    Gas gangrene
    Decompression sickness ("bends")
    Acute cyanide poisoning (severe)
    Acute gas embolism
Category II: Disorders in which hyperbaric oxygen may be useful
as an adjunctive therapy to other more traditional modes of
therapy
    Refractory osteomyelitis
    Soft tissue necrosis and refractory anaerobic/aerobic
        infections
    Crush injury with acute traumatic ischemia
    Compromised skin grafts
    Actinomycoses
Category III: Disorder in which there is theoretical indications and
some experimental data for hyperbaric oxygenation
    Traumatic head and spinal cord injury
    Bone grafts
    Lepromatous leprosy
    Sickle-cell crisis
Category IV: Disorders in which there is a theoretical basis;
however, no extensive studies have been done to establish use
    Multiple sclerosis
    Arthritis
    Emphysema

*From Undersea Medical Society, publication no. 30CR (HBO), 1979.

ods of controlled oxygen therapy became common
clinical standards, the dangers and toxicities of oxygen therapy took on greater clinical importance.

Oxygen-Induced Hypoventilation

Oxygen-induced apnea may occur in severely
hypoxic patients where the respiratory center is not
responsive to CO_2 levels. These patients are breathing as a result of the stimulation of the aortic and
carotid chemoreceptors secondarily to the severe hypoxia. When supplemental oxygen is given, the
stimulus for breathing is eliminated. Because the
respiratory centers are not responsive to the CO_2 as
a result of the drug overdose or head trauma, the

drive to breathe is eliminated. Fortunately, this clinical situation does not occur frequently.

The depression of the ventilatory drive as a result of oxygen therapy is more often the case than
oxygen-induced apnea. Oxygen-induced hypoventilation is an extremely important clinical entity in patients with COPD. In these patients where the hypercapnea and hypoxemia develop gradually as the
COPD progresses, the supplemental oxygen should
be given carefully and the patient monitored for a
change in the ventilatory status.

Supplemental oxygen will not cause a significant
depression of the patient's ventilatory status unless
(1) the patient's baseline Pa_{CO_2} is greater than 50 mm
Hg, (2) the baseline Sa_{O_2} is less than 90%, or (3) with
the administration of supplemental oxygen, the patient's Pa_{O_2} exceeds 60 mm Hg.

The first two criteria provide the premise that
the patient is a carbon dioxide retainer and is chronically hypoxic. This would suggest that the hypoxic
drive to breathe is present to some degree. The third
criteria is important once oxygen therapy begins.
The Pa_{O_2} should be elevated to a level greater than
50 mm Hg but should not exceed 60 mm Hg. In this
range, the patient's hemoglobin will be between
84% and 90% saturated. The arterial blood will be at
the flattened portion of the oxyhemoglobin dissociation curve. This position on the curve will provide
an adequate oxygen-carrying capacity without eliminating the hypoxic drive.

In these patients, low-flow oxygen at 1 to 2
L/min should not significantly change the ventilatory
status. However, it is important to follow changes in
the hypoxic drive to breathe by monitoring blood
gases. A small increase in the Pa_{CO_2} may be observed initially, but this will generally stabilize
within acceptable limits. When an increase in the
Pa_{CO_2} is observed, it is important not to withdraw
the oxygen. To do so could cause the Pa_{O_2} to drop
to levels lower than originally observed. That is, a
more severe hypoxemia may result. If necessary,
mechanical ventilation may be initiated to control
the acute ventilatory failure.

TABLE 5–17.

Relationship Between Hyperbaric Pressures and Oxygen-Carrying Capacities (Fi_{O_2} = 1.0)*

ATA	MM HG	PSI	BELOW SEA LEVEL, FT	Pa_{O_2}, MM HG	Sa_{O_2}, %	Hb_{O_2}, VOL %	DISSOLVED O_2, VOL %
1	760	14.7	Sea level	640	100	20.1	2.1
2	1,520	29.4	33	1,313	100	20.1	4.6
3	2,280	44.1	66	2,026	100	20.1	6.2

*Assume Hb = 15 gm%; 1.34 ml of O_2 per gm of Hb; 0.3 ml of O_2 dissolved/Pa_{O_2} = 100; ATA = 1
atmosphere absolute.

Absorption Atelectasis

Atelectasis can occur in regions of the lung as a result of breathing 100% oxygen. This occurs as a result of the elimination of nitrogen or "nitrogen washout" that occurs secondary to the high $F_{I_{O_2}}$. Breathing inspired gas with an $F_{I_{O_2}}$ greater than 0.50 can actually create a shunt effect in the lungs.

Nitrogen is often called a "balance gas" because of the role it plays in Dalton's law. Dalton's law states that the total pressure within a gas is equal to the sum of the partial pressures:

$$P_T = P_A + P_B + P_C + \ldots P_N$$

For practical purposes, the pressure of the gases of alveolar air at sea level would equal:

$$P_B = P_{A_{O_2}} + P_{A_{CO_2}} + P_{A_{N_2}} + P_{A_{H_2O}}$$

If the $F_{I_{O_2}}$ were increased and the $P_{A_{CO_2}}$ and $P_{A_{H_2O}}$ remained unchanged, then the $P_{A_{N_2}}$ would decrease proportionally to the increase in the $P_{A_{O_2}}$ so that the P_B would remain the same. For example, given:

$$P_B = 760 \text{ mm Hg}$$
$$F_{I_{O_2}} = 0.21$$
$$P_{A_{O_2}} = 100 \text{ mm Hg}$$
$$P_{A_{CO_2}} = 40 \text{ mm Hg}$$
$$P_{A_{H_2O}} = 47 \text{ mm Hg}$$

The $P_{A_{N_2}}$ could be calculated:

$$P_B = P_{A_{O_2}} + P_{A_{CO_2}} + P_{A_{H_2O}} + P_{A_{N_2}}$$
$$760 = 100 + 40 + 47 + P_{A_{N_2}}$$
$$573 = P_{A_{N_2}}$$

Now, if the $F_{I_{O_2}}$ were elevated so that the $P_{A_{O_2}}$ equals 300 mm Hg the $P_{A_{N_2}}$ would fall:

$$P_B = 760 \text{ mm Hg}$$
$$P_{A_{O_2}} = 300 \text{ mm Hg}$$
$$P_{A_{CO_2}} = 40 \text{ mm Hg}$$
$$P_{A_{H_2O}} = 47 \text{ mm Hg}$$

the $P_{A_{N_2}}$ would be:

$$P_B = P_{A_{O_2}} + P_{A_{CO_2}} + P_{A_{H_2O}} + P_{A_{N_2}}$$
$$760 = 300 + 40 + 47 + P_{A_{N_2}}$$
$$373 = P_{A_{N_2}}$$

In other words, nitrogen is the "balance gas." Increasing the $F_{I_{O_2}}$ results in an increase $P_{A_{O_2}}$ and the reciprocal decrease in $P_{A_{N_2}}$. Since nitrogen is the most prevalent gas in the aveoli, and since nitrogen is inert and not highly soluble in blood, it helps maintain the gas volume within the alveoli. If a pa-

tient is placed on 100% O_2, as the $P_{A_{O_2}}$ increases, the $P_{A_{N_2}}$ decreases. At the point of "N_2 washout," the alveolar gases are composed of the $P_{A_{O_2}}$, $P_{A_{CO_2}}$, and $P_{A_{H_2O}}$. In areas of the lung where the tidal breathing is reduced secondary to significant airway obstruction, the oxygen will diffuse into the pulmonary blood flow faster than it can be replenished via ventilation. As a result, alveolar volume continually decreases to a point where the surface tension is so great, the alveolus collapses. This results in an increase in the physiologic shunt.

Retrolental Fibroplasia

Retrolental fibroplasia, a vascular proliferation disease of the retina, was first described in 1942.[33] By the early 1950s, researchers had speculated an association between supplemental oxygen administration and the clinical incidence of retrolental fibroplasia. It is believed that the administration of oxygen causes the blood vessels behind the retina to vasoconstrict. This vasoconstriction is severe enough and persistent enough to damage the endothelial cells. The end result of this physiologic response is a fibrotic change in the tissues that results in partial to total blindness. By the late 1940s, retrolental fibroplasia accounted for more than one-third of all blindness in preschool children.[28] For many years, it was not known whether the retrolental fibroplasia was the result of the $F_{I_{O_2}}$ ($P_{I_{O_2}}$) or the $P_{a_{O_2}}$; however, well-controlled clinical studies have indicated that the $P_{a_{O_2}}$ is the cause.[16] Other important factors include the level of immaturity in the preterm infant, the length of oxygen exposure, and the environmental $F_{I_{O_2}}$ (which ultimately affects the $P_{a_{O_2}}$).

Studies indicate that when the $A-a$ gradient is grossly normal, an $F_{I_{O_2}}$ of less than 0.40 minimizes the risk to the preterm infant.[17] At this level of inspired oxygen and depending on the infant's status, the $P_{a_{O_2}}$ should be between the normal newborn limits of 60 and 100 mm Hg.[16, 24] Obviously, since the $P_{a_{O_2}}$ is the causative factor, the $F_{I_{O_2}}$ must be monitored closely and adjusted so that the $P_{a_{O_2}}$ is kept within an acceptable range (60 to 100 mm Hg).[24] Length of exposure to an elevated oxygen level is the significant factor. In long-term oxygen administration, greater than 7 to 10 days, retrolental fibroplasia can occur at a much lower $F_{I_{O_2}}$.[18]

Oxygen Toxicity

Oxygen therapy has been an extremely valuable therapeutic drug in the treatment of a wider variety of diseases and disorders by controlling or eliminating the hypoxemia and subsequent tissue hypoxia. Elevated oxygen levels in body tissues, however, can have a negative effect and ultimately injure these cells.

The pathology of oxygen was first described in 1897.[31] Since early studies, many researchers have demonstrated the toxicity of oxygen in animal models. Clinical interest in oxygen toxicity as a significant problem has occurred in recent years due primarily to our increased sophistication in oxygen administration. With the widespread use of controlled oxygen systems, artificial airways, and PEEP/CPAP, pulmonary abnormalities associated with oxygen administration have received greater attention. Several factors appear to affect the toxic response to oxygen including previous exposure to oxygen, length of exposure, nutritional status, and age.[8] The pathology of oxygen toxicity is nonspecific and consists of atelectasis, edema, alveolar hemorrhage, inflammation, fibrin deposition, and thickening and hyalinization of the alveolar membranes.[8]

Once distributed throughout the body, oxygen is utilized in three ways: (1) the formation of oxygen-bound substances in metabolizing cells, which aids in normal cell function (this accounts for 9% of the body's oxygen consumption); (2) the biosynthesis of important molecules such as steroids, pigments, and fatty acids (this accounts for only 1% oxygen consumption); and (3) the electron-transfer system within the mitochondria for the production of energy (Fig 5–18). This is also called the mitochondrial respiratory chain and accounts for nearly 90% of oxygen consumption.[5]

Both hypoxia and oxygen toxic responses are biochemical, subcellular phenomena with striking similarities. In hypoxia, when the delivery of oxygen to the mitochondrial respiratory chain is impaired due to the lack of oxygen molecules, the electron transfer system slows and ceases, and energy is no longer produced. This ultimately results in the clinical manifestations of hypoxia that can be observed. In oxygen toxic response, the excess oxygen molecules made available to the electron-transfer system in the mitochondria interfere with the normal electron transfer system and energy is no longer produced.[34]

Oxygen toxic response can be divided into two phases based on pathologic findings:

1. *Exudative phase.* This is the early phase (24 to 72 hours) of oxygen toxicity. In this phase, there are

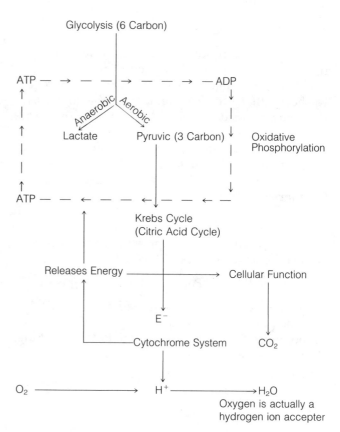

FIG 5–18.
The role of oxygen in cell metabolism. Within the mitochondria of the cell, the electron-transfer system (cytochrome system) utilizes oxygen to produce energy (ATP). The specific function of molecular oxygen is to bind with the H^+ to form cellular water (H^+ is a by-product of energy production).

changes in the alveolar type II cells, destruction of the pulmonary capillary endothelial cells, and necrosis of alveolar type I cells. This results in interstitial and intra-alveolar pulmonary edema, hemorrhage, and hyaline membrane formation.[8, 33]

2. *Proliferation phase.* This later phase occurs after 72 hours. Hyperplasia of alveolar type II cells is observed. In addition, there is a thickening of the alveolar septa, hyperplasia of pulmonary capillaries, and fibroblastic proliferation.[8, 33]

Recovery from oxygen toxicity when the patient has entered the proliferation phase is not without some degree of permanent lung damage. The lungs demonstrate scarring, fibrosis, alveolar septal thickening, capillary dilation, and an increased number of capillaries. In the newborn who is highly susceptible to oxygen toxicity, this change in the lung is referred to as bronchopulmonary dysplasia.

Table 5–18 lists the clinical signs and symptoms

TABLE 5–18.

Clinical Signs and Symptoms of Oxygen Toxicity

Symptoms
   Substernal stress/pain
   Cough
   Dyspnea
   Anxiety
   Paresthesia
   Fatigue
Signs
   Pulmonary infiltrates on chest film
   Decreased Pao_2
   Decreased compliance
   Pulmonary edema
   Atelectasis
   Increased right-to-left shunt
   Decreased vital capacity

TABLE 5–19.

Factors Affecting the Onset of Oxygen Toxic Response

Factors that hasten onset or increase severity
   of oxygen toxic response
      Adrenocortical hormones
      CO_2 inhalation-retention
      Amphetamines
      Epinephrine
      Insulin
      Norepinephrine
      Thyroid hormones
      Vitamin E deficiency
Factors that delay onset or decrease severity
   of oxygen toxic response
      Acclimatization to hypoxia
      Adrenergic-blocking drugs
      Anesthesia
      Ganglionic-blocking drugs
      Hypothermia
      Intermittent exposure
      Hypothyroidism
      Vitamin E

observed in oxygen toxicity. Oxygen toxic response not only affects the lungs but other body systems as well, including the central nervous system, the endocrine system, and the blood-producing or hematopoietic system.

The toxic effect of oxygen is thought to relate to the length of exposure and the partial pressure of oxygen. Individuals exposed to high F_{IO_2} (100% O_2) will develop substernal distress or pain, a nonproductive cough, and a change in the breathing pattern. Pulmonary function evaluation will show a decrease in the vital capacity, a decrease in the diffusion capacity, and a decrease in the compliance.[33] These changes, however, do not occur early in the development of oxygen toxicity. They occur secondary to the increase in lung water, which would not be clinically evident for many hours (18 to 24 hours) after exposure to the high F_{IO_2}. The interstitial pulmonary edema results in the shunting of blood, atelectasis, and signals the early stages of adult respiratory distress syndrome (ARDS).

The response and susceptibility to oxygen toxic effects varies greatly and makes it difficult to establish specific guidelines to prevent the onset of oxygen toxicity. Table 5–19 provides a list of factors that seem either to hasten or delay the onset of oxygen toxicity. Overall, there appears to be a general relationship between the duration of exposure and the F_{IO_2}. At normal barometric pressure, an F_{IO_2} less than or equal to 0.50 will not result in a significant incidence in oxygen toxic response.[23] The clinical management principles should be to improve oxygenation at the lowest possible F_{IO_2} using an F_{IO_2} of 0.50 as the critical level at which oxygen toxic effects

should be considered a major risk in adults. This would further suggest the CPAP and mechanical ventilation with PEEP should be considered as mechanisms to reduce the F_{IO_2} needed for clinically acceptable blood gases.

MIXED GAS THERAPY

Helium-Oxygen Therapy

Helium is a chemically inert gas that is nearly seven times lighter than air. Helium is not used in body metabolism and normally exists as a trace element in the atmosphere. Helium has a density of 0.1758 gm/L as compared to oxygen, which has a density of 1.43 gm/L or air, which has a density of 1.293 gm/L. Because of the low density and inert characteristics of helium, it can be used as a substitute for nitrogen in oxygen mixtures. When helium is used in combination with oxygen as a medical gas, the force required to move the gas through airways is greatly reduced.

Helium is a relatively rare gas. The major source of most commercial helium is the natural gas fields. The helium recovered from such fields is the result of the liquefaction and purification of natural gas. The production of helium for medical as well as commercial and industrial use is under the control of the federal government.

The most common use of helium in the medical

setting is found in the pulmonary function laboratory where helium is used in the "helium dilution test for functional residual capacity." Although helium-oxygen therapy has been written about in medical texts for many years,[23] it has never received wide use in respiratory care. Table 5–20 provides comparative information on helium-oxygen mixtures. From this table, one can see that the density of an 80/20 helium-oxygen mixture is nearly one-third that of air. As a result, it should take about one-third less effort to move a volume of the helium-oxygen mixture than the same volume of air. For this reason, helium-oxygen mixtures can be helpful in upper airway obstructions, bronchospasms, status asthmaticus, and refractory viral croup.[21] Helium-oxygen mixtures greater than 70%/30% are not commercially available because as the percentage of oxygen increases in the mixture, the low-density property is lost.

When administering helium-oxygen mixtures, several factors must be kept in mind:[31]

1. Helium-oxygen therapy must be administered via a tight-fitting closed system (a non-rebreathing mask). Small leaks will allow helium to escape due to the low density. Helium-oxygen mixtures can also be administered via a cuffed artificial airway.

2. A compensated flowmeter calibrated to the helium-oxygen mixture should be used if available. Because of the difference in densities, an air or oxygen flowmeter will not provide an accurate reading. This problem can be corrected using the following conversion factor. For each L/min reading on a compensated *oxygen* flowmeter, 1.8 L/min of the helium-oxygen mixture is being delivered.

3. Helium-oxygen gas mixtures are poor vehicles for the deposition of aerosol due to the low density of the gas mixture.

A benign side effect of helium is the distortion (high pitch) of the patient's voice. This distortion goes away as soon as the gas mixture is removed and the higher density air or oxygen replaces the mixture in the lungs. Helium-oxygen actually has no curative or permanent corrective properties. Any interruption in the helium-oxygen therapy and a return to air or an oxygen mixture will cause a return in the original symptoms unless the primary problem is corrected. As a result, helium-oxygen should be considered a temporary adjunct therapy.

Carbon Dioxide–Oxygen Therapy

Like helium-oxygen therapy, carbon dioxide-oxygen therapy has never gained widespread clinical use in the United States. Carbon dioxide is a colorless, odorless gas with a density about 1.5 times that of air. Carbon dioxide is a byproduct of combustion, fermentation, and organic decay. Carbon dioxide will not support life. While carbon dioxide itself is nontoxic, without adequate oxygen present, carbon dioxide will cause asphyxiation.

Carbon dioxide is a strong central nervous system stimulant for respiration. In normal individuals, the Pa_{CO_2} is the primary regulator of ventilation. Elevated amounts of CO_2 in the blood will increase the ventilatory drive. The therapeutic mixtures of carbon dioxide and oxygen are commonly called "carbogen" mixtures. The physiologic effects of carbogen therapy are:[32]

1. Stimulation of the respiratory center. Maximum response is observed with the 10%/90% CO_2/O_2 carbogen mixture. Stimulation results in an increase in both rate and depth of ventilation.

2. Cardiovascular stimulation. Increased levels of carbon dioxide in the blood will cause an increase in both the systolic and diastolic blood pressure, an increase in force of myocardial contraction, vasoconstriction, and an increase in heart rate.

3. Local vasodilation. The vascular bed in skeletal muscle will dilate in response to an increase in the carbon dioxide level in exercising muscles.

The clinical indications for carbogen therapy are based on the physiologic response:

1. Improvement of cerebral blood flow. The general cardiovascular responses have the net effect of decreasing the peripheral blood vasculature and shunting or forcing more blood to the brain. Clinically, the cerebral blood flow changes as a result of carbogen therapy have been disappointing. This is likely due to the atherosclerosis seen in stroke patients where this therapy has been attempted.

TABLE 5–20.

Densities of Selected Medical Gases

GAS	MIXTURE, %	DENSITY, GM/L
Air	100	1.293
Oxygen	100	1.429
Helium	100	0.179
Helium-oxygen	80/20	0.429
Helium-oxygen	70/30	0.554

2. Stimulation of deep breathing. Carbogen therapy has been used to increase both the rate and depth of ventilation. The increase in the ventilatory drive overcomes the tendency for hypoventilation that is seen in physically weak patients. Carbogen therapy can also be used during the postoperative period to prevent or reduce atelectasis.

3. Treatment of singulation (hiccups). Hiccups are a result of spasms occurring in the diaphragm secondary to irritation of the phrenic nerve. The increased carbon dioxide stimulates the medullary respiratory center which sends out impulses to the diaphragm that override the activity of the phrenic nerve.

Carbogen therapy is considered dangerous by some physicians and therapists. It should be administered only when ordered by a physician and only the 5/95 (5% carbon dioxide, 95% oxygen) mixture should be given. Potential side effects of carbogen therapy include headache, nausea, dyspnea, tachycardia, unconsciousness, and convulsions. Carbogen mixtures should be administered via a tight closed system such as a nonrebreathing mask. The mask should be hand-held and not strapped to the patient to allow for rapid removal if necessary.

Therapy should not be given with the 5/95 mixture for more than 4 to 6 minutes. If the pulse rate increases more than 20 beats/min or if there is a 40 mm Hg increase in the systolic blood pressure, therapy should be discontinued. Finally, carbogen should never be given to patients with acute or chronic pulmonary problems, especially where carbon dioxide retention is a problem. Patients with COPD will not be responsive to carbogen therapy and the increased carbon dioxide level will complicate their acid-base status. Patients with upper airway obstruction should not be given carbogen therapy in an attempt to stimulate ventilation. This will tend to increase their work of breathing and can precipitate acute ventilatory failure as a result of fatigue.

OXYGEN AND MIXED GAS THERAPY ORDERS

The evaluation of the physician order for both completeness and appropriateness represents one of the more delicate areas in the relationship between the physician and the respiratory care practitioner. Ambiguity in the physician order can create potential problems for the respiratory care practitioner in trying to "figure out" what the order is trying to accomplish. On the other hand, orders that are too specific (when not necessary) can restrict the practitioner's latitude in providing the most appropriate therapy.

All respiratory care departments should have standard protocols for all of the services provided through the respiratory care service. In the areas of medical gas therapy, the protocol should delineate the following:

1. The goals of the specific therapy.
2. The indications, contraindications, and hazards of the therapy.
3. The criteria to be utilized in evaluating the therapy.
4. The information that should be included in the physician order, i.e., an oxygen therapy order should include:

- Date and time therapy is to begin.
- The specific oxygen concentrations desired at the liter flow desired.
- The type of equipment desired (e.g., nasal cannula, catheter, mask, etc.).
- Frequency of therapy (e.g., continuous, during ambulation, sleep, or other specific times).
- Duration of therapy.

5. The procedure that will be followed when the order is incomplete or inappropriate.
6. What latitude the respiratory care services will exercise in carrying out the physician's order. For example, if the physician orders "supplemental oxygen via a mask, to achieve 40% oxygen concentrations," the department may select an aerosol mask with a 40% setting via the nebulizer, or the department may select a simple mask with the needed liter flow to achieve an estimated 40% concentration.
7. The criteria and/or conditions under which the therapy will be interrupted or discontinued. For example, if the physician orders "a 5/95 carbon dioxide-oxygen therapy for 5 minutes, b.i.d.," the respiratory care service may have standard protocols to stop treatment if the pulse rate increases more than 20 beats/min regardless of the time factor requested by the physician.
8. What "standard orders" the respiratory care service will use when the orders are incomplete.

The medical staff should understand that their orders will be evaluated against the appropriate protocols in order to allow for quality assurance and standard care. It is important to provide the respiratory care services area with the needed flexibility to carry out physician orders. The field of respiratory therapy and the provision for quality care necessitates the use of a variety of complex and everchanging medical equipment. It is not realistic that the entire medical staff can or will stay up-to-date on all the technological advances. For this reason, a respiratory care advisory committee established by the hospital and consisting of the respiratory care service medical director, technical director, physicians, respiratory therapist, and other appropriate health practitioners is vital. Such a committee can revise and modify department policies and procedures as needed. Furthermore, the committee can serve a continuing education function for the medical and nursing staff. Most importantly, however, the members of the committee can serve a valuable communication function which will result in better care for the patient and the most efficient utilization of the respiratory care practitioner. Each hospital must determine its own standard of practice based on its physical and personnel resources, the quality of practitioners available, and other overall expectations of the medical staff in respiratory care.

REFERENCES

1. Albritton EC (ed): *Standard Value in Blood.* Philadelphia, WB Saunders Co, 1952.
2. Anthonisen NR: Hypoxemia and O_2 therapy. *Am Rev Respir Dis* 1982; 126:729–732.
3. Barach AL: The therapeutic use of oxygen. *JAMA* 1922; 79:693–699.
4. Block AJ: Low flow oxygen therapy. *Am Rev Respir Dis* 1974; 110 (suppl):71–80.
5. Cohen PG: The metabolic function of oxygen and biochemical lesions of hypoxemia. *Anesthesiology* 1972; 37:2.
6. Burton GG: Differential diagnosis of various obstructive pulmonary diseases and implications for therapy, in Burton GG, Hodgkins JE (eds): *Respiratory Care: A Guide to Clinical Practice,* ed 2. Philadelphia, JB Lippincott Co, 1984.
7. Davis JC: *Hyperbaric Oxygen Therapy: A Committee Report.* Bethesda, Md, Undersea Medical Society Inc, 1983.
8. Deneke SM, Fanburg BL: Normobaric oxygen toxicity of the lung. *N Engl J Med* 1980; 303:2.
9. Des Jardins TR: *Clinical Manifestations of Respiratory Disease.* Chicago, Year Book Medical Publishers, 1984.
10. Fairley HB: Oxygen therapy for surgical patients. *Am Rev Respir Dis* 1980; 122 (pt 2):37–42.
11. Farzan SA: *A Concise Handbook of Respiratory Diseases,* ed 2. Reston, Va, Reston Publishing Co, 1985.
12. Flasterstein F, Klocke R: Outpatient oxygen therapy. *Primary Care* 1982; 9:127–133.
13. Fulmer JD, Snider GL: ACCP-NHLBI National Conference on Oxygen Therapy. *Chest* 1982; 86:2.
14. Hodgkin JE, Collier CA: Blood gas analysis and acid-base physiology. *Respiratory Care: A Guide to Clinical Practice,* ed 2. Philadelphia, JB Lippincott, Co, 1984.
15. Hodgkin JE, Zorn EG, Gee G: *Respiratory Rehabilitation: A Comprehensive Approach.* Detroit, Parke-Davis, 1979.
16. James LS, Lanman JT: History of oxygen therapy and retrolental fibroplasia. *Pediatrics* 1976; 57:592–628.
17. Kensey V, et al: Retrolental fibroplasia and the use of oxygen. *Arch Ophthalmol* 1956; 56:481.
18. Klaus MH, Fanaroff AA (ed): *Care of the High Risk Neonate,* ed 2. Philadelphia, WB Saunders Co, 1979.
19. Medical Research Council Working Party: Long term domiciliary oxygen therapy in chronic cor pulmonale complicating chronic bronchitis and emphysema. *Lancet* 1981; 1:681–686.
20. Neff TA, Petty TL: Long-term continuous oxygen therapy in chronic airway obstruction. *Ann Intern Med* 1970; 72:621–625.
21. Nelson DS, McClellan L: Helium-oxygen mixtures as adjunctive support to refractory viral croup. *Ohio Med J* 1982; 78:729–730.
22. Nocturnal Oxygen Therapy Trial Group: Continuous or nocturnal oxygen therapy in hypoxemic chronic obstructive lung disease. A Clinical Trial. *Ann Intern Med* 1980; 93:391–398.
23. Petty TL, Nett LM: The history of long-term oxygen therapy. *Respir Care* 1983; 28:859–864.
24. Phibbs RH: Oxygen therapy: A continuous hazard to the premature infant. *Anesthesiology* 1977; 47:486–487.
25. Pilbean SP: *Mechanical Ventilation: Physiological and Clinical Applications.* St Louis, CV Mosby Co, 1986.
26. Powner DJ: Assessment of oxygen transport and availability. *Postgrad Med* 1981; 70:211–218.
27. Rarey KP, Youtsey JW: *Respiratory Patient Care.* Englewood Cliffs, NJ, Prentice-Hall, Inc, 1981.
28. Reese E: Persistence and hyperplasia of primary vitreous, retrolental fibroplasia. *Arch Ophthalmol* 1949; 41:527–552.
29. Ryerson GG, Block AJ: Oxygen as a drug: Chemical properties, benefits, and hazards of administration, in Burton GG, Hodgkin JE: *Respiratory Care: A Guide to Clinical Practice.* Philadelphia, JB Lippincott Co, 1984.
30. Shapiro BA, Harrison RA, Walton JR: *Clinical Application of Blood Gases,* ed 3. Chicago, Year Book Medical Publishers, 1982.
31. Smith JL: The influence of pathological conditions on active absorption of oxygen toxicity of the lung. *N Engl J Med* 1897; 22:307–318.
32. Spearman CB, Sheldon RL, Egan DF: *Egan's Fundamentals of Respiratory Therapy,* ed 4. St Louis, CV Mosby Co, 1982.

33. Terry TL: Extreme prematurity and fibroblastic overgrowth of persistent vascular sheath behind each crystalline lens. Preliminary report. *Am J Ophthalmol* 1942; 25:203–204.

34. Winter PM, Smith G: The toxicity of oxygen. *Anesthesiology* 1972; 37:210–241..

35. Wintrobe MM: *Clinical Hematology*, ed 6. Philadelphia, Lea & Febiger, 1967.

SUGGESTED READING

Abraham AS, et al: Reversal of pulmonary hypertension by prolonged oxygen administration to patients with chronic bronchitis. *Circ Res* 1963; 23:147.

Adamson JW, Finch CA: Hemoglobin function, oxygen affinity, and erythropoietin. *Ann Rev Physiol* 1975; 37:351.

Anderson PB, et al: Long-term oxygen therapy in cor pulmonale. *Q J Med* 1973; 42:563.

Bartlett RH: Respiratory therapy to prevent pulmonary complications of surgery. *Respir Care* 1984; 29:667–676.

Bland RD: Special considerations in oxygen therapy for infants and children. *Am Rev Respir Dis* 1980; 122 (pt 1).

Bradley BL, Garner AE, Billiu D, et al: Oxygen-assisted exercise in chronic obstructive lung disease. *Am Rev Respir Dis* 1978; 118:239.

Braun HA, Cheney FW, Lochman CP: *Introduction to Respiratory Physiology*, ed 2. Boston, Little, Brown & Co, 1980.

Brodsky JB: Oxygen: A drug. *Int Anesthesiol Clin* 1981; 19:1–8.

Burton GG, Hodgkin JE: *Respiratory Care: A Guide to Clinical Practice*, ed 2. Philadelphia, JB Lippincott, Co, 1984.

Comroe JH: *Physiology of Respiration*. Chicago, Year Book Medical Publishers, 1965.

Cullen JH, Kaemmerlen JT: Effect of oxygen administration at low rates of flow in hypercapnic patients. *Am Rev Respir Dis* 1967; 95:

Des Jardins TR: *Clinical Manifestations of Respiratory Disease*. Chicago, Year Book Medical Publishers, 1984.

Embury SH, Garcia JF, et al: Effects of oxygen inhalation on endogenous erythropoietin kinetics, erythropoiesis, and properties of blood cells in sickle-cell anemia. *N Engl J Med* 1984; 311:291–295.

Fishman AP: Chronic cor pulmonale. *Am Rev Respir Dis* 1976; 114:775–790.

Fishman AP: Hypoxia on the pulmonary circulation—how and where it acts. *Circ Res* 1976; 38:221–231.

Grambau GR, Dirks JW: in Belland JC (ed): *Data Gathering in Respiratory Disease*. Arlington, American Academy of Physician Assistants, 1982.

Guyton AC: *Basic Human Physiology*, ed 2. Philadelphia, WB Saunders Co, 1977.

Katz JA: PEEP and CPAP in perioperative respiratory care. *Respir Care* 1984; 29:614–622.

Kettel LJ, Bigelow DB, Levine BE: Recommendations for continuous oxygen therapy in chronic obstructive lung disease: Committee report of ACCP. *Chest* 1973; 64:505.

Leggett RJ, et al: Long-term domiciliary oxygen in cor pulmonale complicating chronic bronchitis and emphysema. *Thorax* 1976; 31:414.

Luce JM: Clinical risk factors for postoperative pulmonary complications. *Respir Care* 1984; 29:484–490.

Luce JM: Long-term oxygen therapy: Physiologic and economic considerations. *Respir Care* 1983; 28:866–875.

Marini JJ: Postoperative atelectasis: Pathophysiology, clinical importance, and principles of management. *Respir Care* 1984; 29:516–521.

Marshall BE, Wyche MQ: Hypoxemia during and after anesthesia. *Anesthesiology* 1972; 37:178–201.

Mithoefer J: Indications for oxygen therapy in chronic obstructive pulmonary disease. *Am Rev Respir Dis* 1974; 110(pt 2):35–39.

Neff TA, Petty TL: Long-term oxygen therapy in chronic airway obstruction. *Ann Intern Med* 1970; 72:621–626.

Petty TL: *Intensive and Rehabilitative Respiratory Care*, ed 3. Philadelphia, Lea & Febiger, 1982.

Shankar PS: Oxygen therapy. *Q Med Rev* 1980; 31:1–18.

Shapiro BA, Harrison RA, Trout CA: *Clinical Application of Respiratory Care*, ed 2. Chicago, Year Book Medical Publishers, 1979.

Shapiro BA, et al: Changes in intrapulmonary shunting with administration of 100% oxygen. *Chest* 1980; 77:138–140.

Snider GL, Renaldo JE: Oxygen therapy in medical patients hospitalized outside of the intensive care unit. *Am Rev Respir Dis* 1980; 122(pt 2):29–35.

Slonim NB, Hamilton LH: *Respiratory Physiology*, ed 2. St Louis, CV Mosby Co, 1971.

Thibeault DW, Gregory GA (eds): *Neonatal Pulmonary Care*. Reading, Massachusetts. Addison-Wesley Publishing Co, 1979.

Tinitis P: Oxygen therapy and oxygen toxicity. *Ann Emerg Med* 1972; 12:321–328.

6

Humidity and Aerosol Therapy

Joseph L. Rau, Jr., Ph.D., R.R.T.

The topics of humidity and aerosol therapy will be treated separately, although the relationship between the two will be discussed. With each topic, a presentation of relevant physical principles and physiological considerations is intended to form the foundation for a discussion of specific indications, hazards, contraindications (if any), and assessment of the therapy. The emphasis with humidity and aerosol therapies will be on the clinical application. Equipment used for humidity or aerosol production is treated in Chapter 13, and only the clinical implications of such equipment will be mentioned.

HUMIDITY THERAPY

Physical Principles

Matter exists in three states: solid, liquid, and gas. In the case of water, or the compound H_2O, we refer to the solid phase as *ice*, to the liquid phase as *water*, and to the gaseous phase as *water vapor*. The existence of a substance in a particular state is a function of temperature and pressure, and depends on the nature of the particular substance. At an atmospheric pressure of 760 torr, water freezes/melts at 0°C, and vaporizes/liquifies at 100°C. The change of state of pure water, at 760 torr, defines these points on the Celsius scale.

A certain amount of thermal energy, or heat, measured in calories per gram is required to raise the temperature of a substance. With 1 gm of pure water at 1 atmosphere of pressure, a single calorie will raise the temperature of water approximately 1°C. However, at the freezing and boiling points, ex-

tra thermal energy is required for the change of state (Fig 6–1).

For 1 gm of water to change from ice at 0°C to liquid water at 0°C, a total of 80 cal of heat must be supplied. This is referred to as the *latent heat of fusion* (Δh_f). It is for this reason that an ice-water mixture remains at 0°C until all of the ice has melted. All of the heat goes to melt the ice, before the heat can cause a rise in temperature. To change from liquid to gas, a similar phenomenon occurs, and the amount of thermal energy is referred to as the *latent heat of vaporization* (Δh_v).

In addition to the conversion from liquid to gas at the boiling point of water, evaporation also occurs with water at temperatures below 100°C. During its liquid phase, the temperature of water represents the average kinetic activity of all the molecules. If a container of water has a surface area exposed to the ambient air, some individual molecules with *higher* kinetic energies can escape from the liquid phase to the gas phase. This process is called *evaporation*, and the temperature of the liquid water is slightly lower since the average kinetic energy of the remaining molecules is now lower with the removal of the higher-energy molecules. This is referred to as *evaporative cooling*, and can significantly lower the temperature. Transfer of heat from the environment may then raise the temperature of the liquid to ambient, and the process of evaporation continues until all of the liquid water is gone, or until the air cannot contain any more water as a gas. The water molecules that transfer from the liquid to the gas phase and enter the surrounding air are generally referred to as *humidity*.

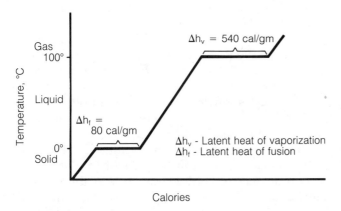

FIG 6–1.
Conceptual illustration of the latent heats of fusion and vaporization for water.

Humidity is water in the gas phase, can be one of the constituent gases in a gas mixture, and is also referred to as water vapor or molecular water. As a gas, humidity is not visible, is not steam, a vapor trail or a mist. As a gas, humidity exerts a pressure, symbolized by P_{H_2O}, and in a mixture of gases, contributes to the total pressure, according to Dalton's law. For example, if room air has a total pressure of 760 torr, and a P_{H_2O} of 47 torr due to humidity, then the *dry* gas mixture has a total pressure of 760 − 47 or 713 torr.

The process of evaporation is dependent on surface area, and temperature.

1. Increased surface area increases evaporation.
2. Applying heat energy and warming liquid water increases evaporation.

The maximum amount of water vapor that a gas mixture can hold is also temperature dependent. Warmer gas mixtures can hold more water as a gas than cool gas mixtures. When a gas mixture contains all of the water in gas form that is possible at a given temperature, the gas mixture is *saturated*. If the temperature of a saturated gas mixture drops, there will be an excess of water in the gas phase, which will condense from the gaseous state back to the liquid state. The *dew point* of a gas mixture is the temperature at which the gas mixture becomes saturated, given the actual amount of water held as a gas in the mixture. Humidity is more specifically quantified as *relative* and *absolute*.

Absolute humidity is the actual mass or weight of water existing as a gas, in a gas mixture, and which is measured in grams per cubic meter or milligrams per liter. Relative humidity is the actual ab-

solute humidity as a percentage of the maximum absolute humidity at a given temperature. As a formula, relative humidity is as follows:

$$\text{Relative humidity (\%)} = \frac{\text{content}}{\text{capacity}}(100)$$

The content may be in absolute humidity which is the weight of water as a gas, or we may use the partial pressure, with the actual partial pressure as a percentage of the maximum partial pressure at capacity. Table 6–1 gives the capacity for absolute humidity and the corresponding partial pressure for the specified temperatures. The capacity is the absolute humidity at saturation. Table 6–2 illustrates a calculation of absolute humidity, for the conditions of typical room air: 21°C, 40% relative humidity. There are 7.34 mg/L of water as a gas in the sur-

TABLE 6–1.

Water Content (Absolute Humidity) and Partial Pressures of a Saturated Gas at Varying Temperatures

TEMPERATURE, °C	WATER CONTENT, MG/L	WATER VAPOR PRESSURE (P_{H_2O}), MM HG
0	4.85	4.58
5	6.80	6.54
10	9.40	9.20
15	12.83	12.79
16	13.64	13.62
17	14.47	14.51
18	15.36	15.46
19	16.31	16.45
20	17.30	17.51
21	18.35	18.62
22	19.42	19.79
23	20.58	21.02
24	21.78	22.32
25	23.04	23.69
26	24.36	25.13
27	25.75	26.65
28	27.22	28.25
29	28.75	29.94
30	30.35	31.71
31	32.01	33.58
32	33.76	35.53
33	35.61	37.59
34	37.57	39.75
35	39.60	42.02
36	41.70	44.40
37	43.90	46.90
38	46.19	49.51
39	48.59	52.26
40	51.10	55.13
41	53.70	58.14
42	56.50	61.30
43	59.50	64.59
44	62.50	68.05
100	598.00	760.00

TABLE 6–2.

Sample Calculation of Absolute Humidity, Given Temperature, and Relative Humidity

Conditions
  21°C
  40% relative humidity
Formula

  Relative humidity $= \dfrac{content}{capacity} \times (100)$

Calculation
  From Table 1, capacity at 21°C is 18.35 mg/L

  $40\% = \dfrac{content}{18.35} \times (100)$

  (40%/100) 18.35 = content
  Content = 7.34 mg/L

rounding air at these conditions. Since the formula for relative humidity involves a relationship of three terms, one of the three may be solved for using algebraic rearrangement given values for the other two. In the example used, if we knew that the absolute humidity (actual) was 7.34 mg/L, and capacity at 21°C is 18.35 mg/L, then we can solve for relative humidity:

$$\text{Relative humidity (\%)} = \frac{7.34}{18.34} \times 100 = 40\%$$

Likewise, we could solve for capacity, knowing the relative humidity and actual absolute humidity:

$$40\% = \frac{7.34}{\text{capacity}} \times 100$$

$$\text{Capacity} = \frac{7.34}{40\%} \times 100 = 18.35 \text{ mg/L}$$

Table 6–1 illustrates the direct relationship of capacity for water in the gaseous state to temperature. As temperature increases, the capacity for water as a gas in a gas mixture increases. Identical relative humidities at different temperatures can mean different absolute humidities. Fifty percent relative humidity at 0°C is much less water than 50% relative humidity at 20°C. At 0°C, we would have 2.43 mg/L of actual water content as a gas, and at 20°C, 8.65 mg/L. With the same relative humidity, the air is much dryer at 0°C than at 20°C.

Physiological Considerations

When air or any gas mixture is inspired in a normally functioning airway, the inspired gas is filtered, warmed, and humidified. The condition of gas in the lungs is generally designated by the reference point of BTPS, for body temperature and pressure, saturated. Values at this reference point are as follows: body temperature, 37°C; body pressure, ambient barometric pressure; saturated, 100% relative humidity (P_{H_2O}, 47 torr; absolute humidity, 43.9 mg/L).

With a normally functioning upper airway (mouth, nose, larynx), inspired air is warmed to 37°C and saturated by the time it reaches the area of the major tracheal bifurcation or carina.[12, 15] Even inspired air at −100°C can be brought to within one or two degrees of body temperature at the tracheal bifurcation.[44, 76] A more recent study states that full saturation of inspired gas occurs approximately 5 cm beyond the major carina.[12, 15] The point at which full saturation at body temperature occurs is referred to as the *isothermic saturation boundary*. The movement of this point in the airway under differing inspired air conditions may be of theoretical interest for influencing airway reactions to cold air. It has been reported that there is a difference in mouth vs. nose breathing for conditioning inspired gas[66]: nose breathing (in oropharynx): 34°C, 80% to 90% relative humidity; mouth breathing (in oropharynx): 21°C, 60% relative humidity. With mouth or nose breathing, inspired gas is still saturated at body temperature by the region at the carina. Even with a bypassed airway using an endotracheal tube, warming and humidification are complete by the second or third tracheal bifurcation.[37]

The warming of inspired gas is accomplished by *convection*, at a rate of 0.340 cal/L/°C.[12, 67] The humidification of inspired gas is by means of *evaporation* of water from the respiratory tract, which has a significant cooling effect on respiratory mucosa due to the latent heat of vaporization, which is 540 cal/gm (see Fig 6–1). The actual amount of water in milliliters contributed by the lung to saturate inspired gas is estimated as 250 ml/day,[66] for average room air ranges of temperature and relative humidity (21°C, 50% relative humidity). The amount of water the respiratory tract actually contributes to reach saturation at body temperature is determined by the actual *humidity deficit*, which is the difference between the humidity of inspired gas and absolute humidity at saturation, body temperature.

If we assume a body temperature of 37°C, absolute humidity in the lungs is approximately 44 mg/L, with a partial pressure, P_{H_2O}, of 47 torr. With an ambient temperature of 21°C, at 50% relative humidity, the humidity deficit is seen to be the difference between body content (44 mg/L) and ambient content, which can also be calculated. Table 6–3 gives

TABLE 6–3.

Calculation of Humidity Deficit
_____

Body Conditions
  37°C
  100% relative humidity
  44 mg/L absolute humidity
Ambient conditions
  21°C
  50% relative humidity
Absolute humidity at 21°C, 50% relative humidity

$$50\% = \frac{content}{18.35} \times (100)$$

  Content = 9.175 mg/L
Humidity deficit
  Deficit = content (body) − content (ambient)
  Deficit = 44 mg/L − 9.175 mg/L
  Deficit = 34.825 mg/L

the details of calculation. Adequate systemic hydration provides the water necessary for humidification of inspired gases, under a variety of ambient conditions.

Humidity Therapy

Humidity therapy is the supplying of increased levels of humidity in inspired gas, as a direct therapeutic procedure or as an adjunct to other therapies. The use of aerosol therapy to achieve humidification of inspired gases will be discussed separately.

Purposes and Indications

1. Humidification of dry inspired therapeutic medical gases, such as oxygen or helium-oxygen mixtures, except at flow rates of 1 to 4 L/min.
2. Humidification of inspired gas to approximately BTPS conditions, with a bypassed upper airway, or with infant head enclosures, with the application of therapeutic gas mixtures.
3. The possible reduction of airway resistance in exercise-induced asthma,[67] nocturnal asthma[8] or other asthmatic episodes,[34] and in laryngotracheobronchitis (croup).[31]

Indication 1.—Medical gases such as O_2, CO_2, or helium, from tanks or central piping systems, are completely free of humidity. Even if such gases are mixed with ambient air of normal humidity levels and the upper airway is intact, a completely dry therapeutic gas can lower inspired humidity levels, increase the humidity deficit, and irritate the nasal and oropharyngeal surfaces.

The first indication for supplemental humidity combines the use of unheated bubble devices with low-flow oxygen delivery systems. The use of aerosols, either heated or unheated, with high-flow gas delivery systems, will be discussed as part of aerosol therapy.

With low oxygen percentages during oxygen therapy, using a low-flow delivery system or a Venturi mask (a high-flow system), large amounts of ambient air are mixed with the dry oxygen, and thus inspired humidity is not significantly lower than room air. For this reason, the National Conference on Oxygen Therapy of the American College of Chest Physicians (1984) stated that there was no evidence to indicate the need for routine humidification of oxygen at flow rates of 1 to 4 L/min, when environmental humidity is adequate. "Adequate" environmental humidity is not further defined. Widely accepted rational criteria for an inadequate water content in inspired gas are not currently available.[12] Although the normal respiratory tract *can* saturate a dry inspired gas, this may not be desirable, especially in persons with preexisting pulmonary disease. It is generally accepted that a dry gas acts as an antiexpectorant and has a dessicating effect on the upper airway. The airway is not usually exposed to perfectly dry gas.

Scuba divers are well aware of the drying effect of breathing dry air from a tank for 45 to 60 minutes through the mouth, and of the accompanying acute thirst. Recently it has been suggested that an inspired absolute humidity of at least 12 mg/L be maintained when delivering dry gas.[12] With masks and suitable low flow rates, no *supplemental* humidification may be needed to achieve this, but with cannulae or catheters in *direct contact* with the mucosal epithelium of the nose or nasopharynx, at least 12 mg/L should be added to the dry gas to prevent topical irritation. This suggestion is based on evidence that ciliary activity decreases when exposed to less than 13 mg/L of absolute humidity, and that pseudostratified ciliated epithelial cells undergo deteriorative (loss of cilia, abnormal morphology) changes if exposed to gas with less than 12 mg/L of absolute humidity.[6] The flow of dry oxygen from a cannula or nasal catheter is in direct contact with the nasal or nasopharyngeal mucosa. However, guidelines of the National Conference on Oxygen Therapy would exclude supplemental humidity with cannulae and catheters, if flows are below 4 L/min. An absolute humidity of 12 mg/L gives 65% relative humidity at 21°C, and 27% relative humidity at 37°C. Tests on unheated bubbler devices have shown that most can deliver relative humidities of 35% to 45% at 37°C, in the normal ranges of oxygen flow rates for low-flow devices.[13, 16, 37] Until a universal guideline is established and accepted for minimal inspired absolute humidity, the first indication for humidity therapy suggests that dry therapeutic gases used with non-bypassed upper airways and delivered by low-flow systems should be humidified with unheated bubbler devices. The exception is a Venturi mask or low-flow system delivering 4 L/min or less of dry gas to the mouth and/or nose.

Indication 2.—The second indication for humidity is based on evidence that dry inspired gas with a bypassed upper airway can cause mucosal drying, crusting, and mucus plugs with endotracheal tubes.[6, 66] To prevent this, inspired gas should be at a temperature of 32° to 37°C, and fully saturated, with intubated patients. To achieve this, a heated humidfying device will have to be warmer than 32° to 37°C, since cooling of the inspired gas will occur in the delivery tubing. The amount of cooling, and hence the temperature needed at the humidifier, is dependent on the length of tubing, ambient room temperature, and flow and temperature of the source gas to be humidified. The practical approach is to monitor the gas temperature close to a patient's airway and adjust the humidifier temperature accordingly. Such humidity is prophylactic, to prevent drying of the airway and secretions, and does not directly add water to the respiratory mucosa. However, the airway normally contributes approximately 250 ml/day of water to humidify air on inspiration, and full humidification of inspired gases will prevent this water loss, which in turn can contribute to a positive fluid balance in an intubated mechanically ventilated patient. In order to match BTPS conditions with a bypassed upper airway, *only humidity* and not the addition of liquid or particulate humidity will be discussed (aerosols will be discussed separately). Patients with permanent tracheostomies do adapt to ambient conditions of temperature and humidity without requiring supplemental warming and humidifying of inspired gas. Such patients are not receiving dry therapeutic gases, as is the case with intubated patients on ventilators.

The delivery of medical gas mixtures to neonates and infants, using an oxyhood (a clear Plexiglas device fitting over the head) requires warmed and humidified gas to prevent cooling of the head and loss of body heat. Both warming and humidity are important with the premature infant (an infant who at birth is not fully developed because of shortened gestation, low birth weight, or both) or when there is failure to thrive, and calories are needed for body metabolism rather than heat production and temperature regulation. Cool gas mixtures flowing over the face and head can provide undesirable cold stress in such applications.

Indication 3.—The third indication for humidity therapy has not been traditionally cited in the literature. However, there is growing evidence that warm, humidified air can reduce airway resistance[5, 34] and may prevent or lessen bronchoconstriction of exercise-induced asthma (EIA).[9, 14, 67] Such evidence offers a new, rational basis for the old practice of holding asthmatic children in steam-filled bathrooms to ameliorate asthmatic episodes.

Cold air seems to increase airway resistance even in normal persons. A recent study found decreased peak flows and flows at 50% of forced vital capacity in marathon runners participating in $-2°$ to $-4°C$ conditions.[40] Normal subjects performing hyperventilation maneuvers in subfreezing air demonstrate significant falls in $FEV_{1.0}$ and maximum mid-expiratory flow, but are much less sensitive to airway cooling than asthmatics.[53] Other investigators studied airway cooling and concluded that in normal subjects increased airway resistance is via neural, specifically cholinergic mechanisms, whereas in asthma additional mechanisms seemed to operate.[30] The anticholinergic agent, ipratropium, blocked the fall in $FEV_{1.0}$ for normals, but in asthmatics both ipratropium and cromolyn sodium, a mast cell stabilizer, were required to abolish the response. It has been suggested that the bronchospastic response of exercise-induced asthma is stimulated by *cooling* of the airway mucosa.[14, 65, 76] Furthermore, this effect is produced primarily by *evaporative* cooling, not convective, which is more pronounced the greater the humidity deficit. Cold inspired air has less absolute humidity than warm air, and thus requires more vaporization at the airway surface to saturate the inspired gas. Heat loss with vaporization of water is much greater than with convection as previously seen. The shifting of the isothermic saturation boundary, previously defined, deeper within the lung may cause additional mechanisms of bronchoconstriction, such as mast cell degranulation, with asthmatics. The fact that swimming does not effectively produce exercise-induced asthma confirms the role of a humidity deficit and evaporative cooling as a stimulus to airway reactivity.[75] The worsening of asthma at night, or nocturnal asthma, may be caused by airway cooling secondary to body cooling which normally occurs at night.[8] Administering air at 37°C and 100% relative humidity during the night, compared to ambient air at 23°C, 20% relative humidity, may reduce bronchoconstriction measured by pulmonary function tests.[8] Also, asthma attacks induced by exposing the body to cold showers at 15°C or wind may be substantially prevented by breathing warm humidified air.[34]

A recent study reported a significant decrease in the frequency of cough, sputum, and abnormal physical signs in the chest in patients receiving warm, humidified air following upper abdominal surgery.[22] In addition, the arterial oxygen tension of this group was greater than that of the control group on the first and third day postoperatively. These studies suggest that mucosal cooling by evaporation seems to be a common factor in increasing airway resistance in normal subjects and to an even greater degree in asthmatics. Preliminary evidence suggests that warmed and humidified air may improve the postoperative course of surgical patients. While additional research questions are raised by these results, the implication is that humidity therapy, with other forms of treatment, may be effective in treating the bronchoconstriction of certain types of asthma.

Evaluation and Assessment

Humidity is a relatively safe form of supportive or preventive therapy, but depending on the patient situation and the configuration of equipment used to supply humidity, the following means are suggested to assess effectiveness and prevent accidents.

1. Check the subjective response of the patient.
2. Monitor the temperature with heated gases delivered by mask or to an endotracheal tube.
3. Remove and drain condensate in delivery tubing, especially with heated delivery systems.
   - Heating wires inside delivery tubing can prevent condensation as gas cools beyond the dew point.
   - Water traps can drain condensation in delivery tubing.
4. Assess the nature and amount of respiratory tract secretions produced with cough or obtained by aspiration.
5. Assess breath sounds to detect adequate and bilateral ventilation or sounds indicative of secretions.
6. Utilize appropriate pulmonary function mea-

sures or arterial blood gas analyses with asthmatic patients receiving humidity, depending on the acuteness and severity of bronchoconstriction.

In addition, the usual clinical information on a patient should be monitored, such as vital signs, and especially respiratory rate and pattern. The equipment should also be checked for any problems unique to the particular delivery method used.

AEROSOL THERAPY

Aerosol therapy is the delivery and deposition of aerosol particles to the pulmonary system for a variety of therapeutic reasons. The use of aerosol for treatment of the lung has been documented since the beginning of the field of respiratory therapy in the mid-1940s.[1] Although there are widespread standard clinical practices such as cool aerosols, the efficacy of certain practices such as cool mists for upper airway disorders or inflammation, bland aerosols of water for retained secretions, and water aerosols for humidification purposes, has yet to be established.[31, 74] The following discussion of aerosol therapy will provide the terminology needed to describe therapeutic aerosols, and summarize available data concerning lung deposition. With this background, the established uses of aerosols will be listed, and then critically discussed in the light of available research findings.[39, 48] Hazards of aerosol therapy and assessment of such therapy will complete this section of the chapter.

Physical Characteristics of Aerosols

A discussion of the clinical applications of aerosols is complicated by the fact that the physical characteristics of aerosols represent a complex topic. Terms used to describe the clinically relevant aspects of aerosols are described first and followed by information on how aerosols are deposited in the human lung.

An aerosol is a suspension of particulate matter, either solid or liquid, in a carrier gas. The size range of particles in an aerosol is between 10^{-3} μ and 100 μ, although the size range of interest for pulmonary applications is between 1 and 10 μ.[39, 45] The two general techniques for producing aerosols are *condensation* of gas molecules into the liquid or solid state and *comminution* of solid or liquid substances. Comminution involves shattering or pulverizing a solid or liquid into minute particles, requires energy, and is the general method by which therapeutic aerosols are produced in respiratory care. Specific methods of comminution are provided by jet nebulizers using a jet mixing and shearing action; by the Babington principle (a device in which a gas flows at a high velocity from an orifice in a small glass sphere over which a liquid film is deposited, to produce aerosol particles), and by ultrasonic nebulization using acoustic energy. Dry (solid) particles of bronchoactive agents are also produced using pressurized canisters in the fluorocarbon propellants or a turbo inhaler which pierces a capsule of dry powder. When an aerosol consists of water, the greatly increased surface area provided by the numerous minute particles leads to increased ambient humidity through enhanced evaporation. Although a water aerosol is *not itself* humidity, it supplies increased relative humidity, and therefore aerosols of water have been used for humidification. The use of such aerosols will be discussed under clinical application. Since the heat of evaporation is large, significant cooling of unheated nebulizers can occur, lowering a nebulizer as much as 10°C below ambient.[68]

Although it is possible to produce aerosol particles of fairly precise sizes, methods of aerosol generation do result in a *distribution* of sizes. This is especially true of *therapeutic* as opposed to diagnostic or research use of aerosols. When the distribution of sizes is very restricted and has a narrow range, an aerosol is termed *monodispersed*, while a broader size range is referred to as *heterodispersed* or alternately *polydispersed*. Therapeutic aerosols currently used in respiratory care are considered heterodispersed.

Since aerosols are produced as a *range* of sizes, and not all one size, it is important to understand the relation between *particle size* and *mass*. Most particles are spheroidal in shape. At a fixed density (mass per unit volume), the volume of a particle varies with (or is proportional to) the amount of mass, and the relation between volume and size of a sphere is:

$$\text{Volume} = 4/3 \ \pi \ r^3$$

Eliminating the constants 4/3 and π, the volume of a particle is directly proportional to the cube of the radius, so that a small decrease in particle size dramatically lowers the available mass, while an increase in size increases mass by the third power of the radius. The relationship of size to mass is illustrated in Table 6–4.

A single 10-μ particle has the same mass as 1,000 particles of 1-μ size, and 1,000,000 particles of 0.1-μ

TABLE 6–4.

Relation of Particle Size to Its Volume and Mass*†

PARTICLE SIZE (RADIUS), μ	MASS OF SINGLE PARTICLE, $v \doteq r^3$	EQUIVALENT MASS
10	$V \doteq 10^3 = 1,000$	1 particle
1	$V \doteq 1^3 = 1$	1,000 particles
0.1	$V \doteq .1^3 = .001$	1,000,000 particles

*Volume = $4/3\pi r^3$, where π = 3.1416 and r = particle radius.
†Assume equal density for all particles, so that volume indicates mass.

size. Therapeutic applications of aerosols require certain amounts of the aerosolized substance to be deposited in the lung if an adequate effect is to be obtained. Below 1 μ, the mass of a particle is considered inadequate to provide sufficient quantities for therapeutic purposes, although aerosols of 0.1 to 0.01 μ are entirely feasible.

Since mass is so important in therapeutic use of aerosols, the mass median diameter (MMD) is a descriptive measure used to characterize the distribution (range) of particle sizes. A distribution is usually well-described by a measure of its center and a measure of its spread. Measures of central tendency with an aerosol are given by the count median diameter and the mass median diameter.

Count median diameter (CMD) is the particle size above and below which 50% of the *number* of particles is found. Mass median diameter (MMD) is the particle size above and below which 50% of the *mass* of particles is found.

The two values, CMD and MMD, in a given distribution of particle sizes, will be different, since most of the mass occurs in a few of the larger particles, as seen previously. The MMD indicates where the *mass* of the aerosol is centering, which is the particle size of interest when we are concerned with obtaining a certain *amount* of an aerosolized substance for clinical applications. Figure 6–2 illustrates that the CMD is lower than the MMD, even with a positively skewed distribution of sizes. A skewed distribution (most particles occur at the low end of the range) is more typical of actual heterodisperse aerosols than a symmetrical normal distributional shape.

Because of the difficulty in measuring particle sizes with aerosols, a simplified approach has been used which results in an aerodynamic mass diameter (AD) is a measure of a particle's terminal settling velocity under gravity, where the particle is assigned the diameter of a unit density sphere that has that identical settling velocity.

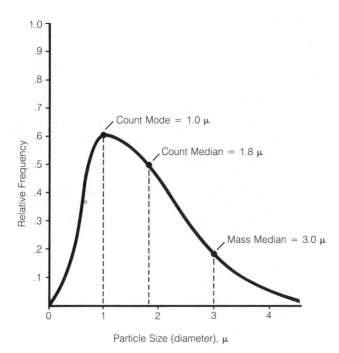

FIG 6–2.
A hypothetical skewed distribution of aerosol particle sizes, illustrating the differences among the mode, the count, and mass median diameters.

In other words, regardless of the particle's size, shape, or density, if it settles at the same point as a reference sphere with a given diameter, the particle is said to have that diameter (AD). For example, if a particle settles at the same point as a 10-μ reference sphere when projected horizontally, the particle is said to have an aerodynamic mass diameter of 10 μ. At times, the AD will be used to characterize an aerosol in the literature or by the manufacturer. Other characteristics of an aerosol that are useful when comparing aerosol-producing devices are the number and mass concentration. Number concentration is the number of particles per liter of gas. Mass concentration is the mass of the particles per liter of gas, in grams per liter.

Two physical properties of aerosol particles are hygroscopicity and electric charge. Hygroscopic growth refers to the increase in size of a particle due to condensation of humidity. Whether a particle grows or further evaporates and becomes smaller is a function of the particle's substance (water, drug, etc.), ambient humidity, and temperature. Generally, particle size will remain stable as long as temperature and humidity remain relatively unchanging. Once in the lung, conditions are stabilized at approximately 37°C and 100% relative humidity. With pure water, a 1-μ droplet should evaporate completely in approximately 0.5 seconds at 20°C, saturated, whereas a 10-μ particle requires around 1 minute.[45]

Most aerosol particles produced by comminution have electric charges but the clinical relevance of this to pulmonary deposition has not been established.[45] *Coalescence* of particles can also occur leading to fewer but larger particles; however, extremely dense aerosols of 10[10] number per liter are needed, with prolonged residence times (>1 minute), which does not occur in therapeutic applications.[68]

It would be useful for clinical practitioners in respiratory care to have aerosol-producing devices described in terms of the following physical characteristics:

1. Mass median diameter or alternatively aerodynamic mass diameter.
2. Geometric standard deviation.
3. Range of particle size produced.
4. The number and/or the mass concentration.

Unfortunately, there is no standardized protocol followed by manufacturers in characterizing their aerosol devices. There is also lack of descriptive research on the output of aerosol devices in the published literature, particularly for large reservoir disposable jet nebulizers and small gas-powered handheld nebulizers. Table 6–5 summarizes avail-

TABLE 6–5.
Particle Sizes for Various Methods of Aerosol Production*

	MMD (REFERENCE)	CMD	GSD
Babington and Ultrasonics			
Babington	1.2[47]		
Monaghan 650	5.2[9, 24]		1.6–2.0
Monaghan 670	6.5[9, 24]		1.5
DeVilbiss 900	2.8[54]		2.1
DeVilbiss 35	6.9[24, 27]	3.8	1.6
DeVilbiss Pulmosonic	5.0[20]	3.5	1.5
Mist-O$_2$-Gen En 140	6.5[24]	3.7	1.4
Gas-powered jet nebulizers			
Air Shields Jet	6.0[54]		2.5
Heyer	7.4[9]		2.0
DeVilbiss 40	2.8–4.2[27]		1.8–1.9
Raindrop	7.9[20]	2.5	2.3
Acorn	4.8[20]	2.4	2.0
Metered-dose inhalers (MDIs)			
Alupent (Boehringer Ingelheim)	3.5[19]	0.65	1.7
Metaprel (Dorsey)	3.5[19]	0.67	1.5
Beclomethasone	2.0[20]	0.6	2.1
Isuprel Mistometer	4.3[19]	0.82	2.1
Bronkometer (isoetharine)	3.5[19]	0.74	1.7

*MMD = mass median diameter; CMD = count median diameter; and GSD = geometric standard deviation.

able information on certain aerosol devices, using the physical characteristics previously defined.

The physical characteristics of aerosols that are important for their clinical application and that have been discussed can be summarized as follows:

1. The *large surface area* of aerosolized water particles allows more evaporation and increased humidity of a gas.
2. Therapeutic aerosols are heterodispersed and form a distribution of particle sizes.
3. Therapeutic aerosols are in the 1- to 10-μ range.
4. The volume of an aerosol particle is proportional to the cube of its radius, so that the mass median diameter is an important descriptive feature when we are concerned with *amounts* of an agent.
5. Below the 1-μ size, the mass carried by an aerosol becomes negligible in relation to amounts desired for pulmonary deposition.

Pulmonary Deposition of Aerosols

Deposition of aerosol particles in the lungs is difficult to specify precisely, since such deposition is a function of a number of variables, whose net interaction is difficult to determine. For example, there is a low probability of particles greater than 10 μ penetrating beyond the nose or mouth into the lung.[68] Particles of 0.01 to 1 μ have such stability to remain in suspension that they are considered as an inhaled and exhaled gas, rather than as particles to be deposited. In addition, the mass carried by particles less than 1 μ is considered negligible for therapeutic pulmonary applications. In the 1- to 10-μ size range, two physical factors affect deposition: *inertial impaction* and *gravitational settling* (sedimentation).

Inertial impaction is a mechanism of deposition for dense, fast-moving particles which are unable to negotiate changes in airway direction, and consequently impact on airway surfaces. Inertial impaction increases with high particle velocity and small airway size. This mechanism applies primarily to particles of 5 to 10 μ that deposit in the nose, mouth, pharynx, larynx, and the first 6 to 10 generations of the tracheobronchial tree, down to airways of 2 mm diameter. In this region of the pulmonary system, carrier gas velocity is highest and *total* cross-sectional area is lowest, conditions which maximize inertial impaction.

Gravitational settling (sedimentation) is a mech-

anism of deposition which applies to particles larger than 1 μ, and is time-dependent. Longer residence times increase the probability that a particle will deposit on an airway. This mechanism is operative in small airways of less than 2 mm diameter, in the last 5 to 6 airway generations. Here the carrier gas velocity is lowest and total cross-sectional area of the airways is the highest, which allows sedimentation to be maximized. Slow inspiratory flows and breathholding should minimize inertial impaction in the upper airway (nasopharyngeal region, above the larynx) and maximize sedimentation in the lower airways, down to the alveolar level.[49]

Brownian motion is a mechanism of deposition which affects small particles of less than 1 μ size, when airflow velocity is low. It is based on bombardment of small particles by carrier gas molecules, and the resulting random movement of the particles leads to airway deposition. Since the particle size affected (<1 μ) is not in the current therapeutic range, this mechanism is not considered applicable to clinical practice.

Given the mechanisms of inertial impaction operative in the upper airway and larger bronchi, and sedimentation in the periphery of the lung, penetration and deposition of particles in the pulmonary system is largely a function of particle size. The literature is varied on how particle size affects penetration in the lung.[38, 45, 71] Table 6–6 lists the percentage of lung deposition for given particle size and locations, based on actual measurements, and calculations.[38, 71] A graphic representation of pulmonary deposition versus particle size is shown in Figure 6–3. There is general consensus in the literature on the following points.

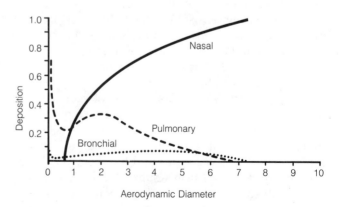

FIG 6–3.
Aerosol deposition in the respiratory tract as a function of particle size. Rate = 15/min, V_T = 1,450 cc. (From the Task Group on Lung Dynamics: *Health Physics*, vol 12. New York, Pergamon Press, 1966. Used with permission.)

TABLE 6–6.

Percentage of Deposition in Specified Portions of the Airway for Given Aerosol Particle Sizes

PARTICLE SIZE, μ	MEAN % DEPOSITION			
	MOUTH*	N-P†‡	T-B†‡	P†‡
1.0	0	3.6	2.7	25
2.0	0	40.6	5.1	34.6
3.0	5	55.2	7.1	30.8
4.0	10	65.4	8.4	23.8
6.0	30	79.9	9.1	10.3
10.0	65	99.2	0.7	0.2
12.0	75	—	—	—
14.0	85	—	—	—
>16.0	100	—	—	—

*Data from Lippman, 1977.[38] Using mouthpiece, flow = 30 L/min.

†Data from Task Group on Lung Dynamics, 1966.[71] Data obtained by calculation, assuming V_T = 750 cc, rate = 15/min.

‡N-P = nasopharynx, nares to larynx; T-B = tracheobronchial, trachea to terminal bronchioles; and P = pulmonary, respiratory bronchioles to alveolar sacs.

1. With mouth breathing, particles greater than 15 μ are removed above the larynx.
2. With nose breathing, particles greater than 10 μ are completely removed above the larynx.
3. With mouth breathing, particles in the 5- to 10-μ range may impact within the first six airway generations.[45, 68]
4. Particles of 1 to 5 μ tend to deposit toward the lung periphery, in the last few airway generations, with maximal deposition in the 2- to 4-μ range.[45, 68]

Table 6–6 and Figure 6–3 also show that little deposition occurs between the larger bronchi and the lung periphery; this is the region of the small airways, which is of major clinical importance.

The method of inhalation is an important variable for the deposition of particles in the lung. When inhaling an aerosol, the variables include inspiratory flow rate, nose vs. mouth breathing, and lung volume at which inspiration begins. Low flows of less than 30 L/min give greater peripheral deposition than high flows.[26, 47] Nasal breathing results in impaction of most particles greater than 5 μ in the nasopharynx.[45] Mouth breathing increases the impaction of 5 to 10 μ particles in the oropharynx, and the first six tracheobronchial generations.[45]

Some investigators have found a better response to bronchodilator when the drug was inhaled at 80% of vital capacity (that is, during the last part of inspiration).[62, 72] By contrast, another study found that actuating an aerosol at 20% of vital capacity gave greater whole lung (conducting airways and alveolar) deposition than actuation at 50% or 80% vital capacity.[52] However, regardless of the lung volume, it has been noted that the greatest whole lung deposition occurred with a 30-L/min flow and a 10-second breath-hold.[52] Part of the difference between these results relates to what is being measured. One study considered changes in airway resistance as an effect of the drug,[62] whereas another measured actual lung deposition.[52] Because of absorption into the bloodstream, a clinical effect of a drug on the lung can be achieved with oropharyngeal impaction and deposition as well as by direct lung deposition. Both studies agree that a slow inhalation with a long breath-hold maximizes deposition and response.

It has also been shown that less than 10% of the total dose delivered with an aerosol goes to the lungs.[50, 78] One of the studies reported the following mean distribution of an inhaled aerosol with eight patients:[50] mouth, 80.4%; lung, 8.8%; actuator (pressurized canister), 9.8%; and exhalation, 1.0%.

Some of the particles deposited in the mouth are ultimately swallowed and go to the stomach. The amount of aerosol impacting in the oropharynx has been shown to be significantly reduced when using pressurized canisters (metered-dose inhalers [MDIs]) if the mouthpiece is held 4 cm from the open mouth and actuated after inhalation begins. An alternative to holding the MDI 4 cm from the mouth is to introduce a spacer device, such as an extension tube, between the canister and the mouth.[19, 28, 56] Then the initial burst of aerosol loses velocity and gathers in the tube spacer instead of impacting in the throat. An extension tube also requires less coordination than holding the canister 4 cm away, aiming for the mouth and actuating the canister at the appropriate moment of inhalation.[17, 24, 27]

Coupled with the difficulty of coordinating breathing and canister actuation is the lack of proper instruction and physician ignorance of proper nebulizer use.[36, 61] Two devices have been marketed which simplify correct use of MDI devices: the InhalAid and the InspirEase both by Key Pharmaceutical.[35, 64, 73] The first device incorporates an incentive indicator for a deep breath with a pause, and both have a reservoir for the aerosol to minimize oropharyngeal impaction and eliminate the need to coordinate the breath and actuation.

Based on current results concerning pulmonary deposition of aerosols, general guidelines could be offered for the clinical application of aerosols.

1. For peripheral pulmonary deposition, such as with a bronchodilator, corticosteroid, or cromolyn sodium, particle sizes with an MMD of 2 to 4 μ, slow inspiratory flow rates, and an inspiratory hold are recommended. There is not complete agreement on optimal lung volume for aerosol actuation, but one investigator suggests that lung volume at which actuation occurs is less important than flow rate and an adequate breath-hold.[52] A breath-hold of 10 seconds was found to give superior deposition compared to 4 seconds.[52, 62] Extension tubes and reservoir devices reduce oral impaction and patient coordination needs.[51]

2. For treatment of the nasopharynx, as in nasal congestion, rhinitis, or for passage of nasal tubes (endotracheal, bronchoscopes), coarse particles of 5 to 15 μ, nose breathing, and normal inspiratory flows below 30 L/min could be suitable.[45, 71]

3. Treatment of the *oropharynx, larynx,* and *first few airway generations* would require particle sizes of 5 to 10 μ and mouth breathing. This would be desirable for bronchoscopy preparation and in general for topical anesthesia of the upper airway or for decongestant effect with upper airway edema, following extubation or due to other inflammation such as laryngotracheitis. Higher inspiratory flow rates (30 L/min or above) with this particle size would tend to shift greater deposition toward the oropharynx while normal flow rates peaking at 30 L/min would shift deposition to the trachea and bronchi for particles of 6 to 8 μ.[68]

4. There is little control over deposition of particles between the larger airways and the peripheral airways less than 2 mm diameter (see Fig 6–3).[45] Particles of 5 to 10 μ preferentially deposit in the upper airway and trachea due to higher velocities and inertial impaction, whereas particles of 1 to 5 μ tend to preferentially deposit in the periphery, where lower velocities and sedimentation occur.

Indications and Uses for Aerosol Therapy

1. Deposition of bronchoactive aerosols.
2. Enhancement of secretion clearance.
3. Sputum induction.
4. Humidification of inspired gases.
5. Treatment of upper airway inflammation with unheated bland aerosols.

Indication 1.—The term *bronchoactive aerosol* refers to all drugs currently given in respiratory care by aerosol for topical treatment of the pulmonary system. This excludes distilled water and saline solutions, which are referred to as bland aerosols and will be discussed separately. The rationale for the aerosol delivery of bronchoactive agents is to treat the lung locally to minimize systemic exposure and increased side effects. Drug groups that have been given by aerosol are listed in Table 6–7 and include bronchodilators for relaxing bronchial smooth muscle, mucolytics to reduce mucus gel to a more liquid state, corticosteroids as anti-inflammatory agents in asthma, and cromolyn sodium as a prophylactic agent in asthma. Racemic epinephrine and phenylephrine, 1/4%, have been used as a topical vasoconstrictor and decongestant, and lidocaine 2% as a topical anesthesia. Both phenylephrine and lidocaine can be useful with elective nasal intubations or as agents to prepare the upper airway for bronchoscopy. In addition, antimicrobial therapy has been attempted by the aerosol route, and is more commonly used in pediatric applications, especially cystic fibrosis, but in conjunction with systemic antimicrobial therapy. Table 6–7 lists the dosage amounts for antimicrobial drugs that have been reported.[60] The use of aerosolized antimicrobials remains controversial despite their use by this route.[74]

The pharmacology of bronchoactive agents has been detailed elsewhere.[60, 79] The difference in dosage strength between a gas-powered nebulizer delivery vehicle and an MDI can be seen in Table 6–7, with a more controlled delivery from the MDI requiring much smaller amounts of a given drug. Dosages for nebulizer delivery are given in milligrams of the active ingredient, based on the available percentage strength and the standard amount in cubic centimeters. Optimal use of MDIs is achieved with the reservoir devices, such as the InspirEase (Key Pharmaceutical) or less optimally with extension devices such as the Aerochamber (Monaghan), and has been previously discussed. Decongestant therapy and topical anesthesia of the nasal passages, oropharyngeal area, and the larynx can be achieved with larger particle sizes from an atomizer, from a gas-powered nebulizer, or even with an ultrasonic nebulizer using slightly higher inspiratory flow rates to maximize oropharyngeal impaction.

Indication 2.—Nebulization of bland aerosols (water, saline) has traditionally been used, usually in short-term intermittent treatments of 10 to 15 minutes on a 3- to 4-day schedule, to aid with secretion clearance. The original view was that secretions could be liquefied with such aerosol therapy. This view has been superseded by the more realistic concept that bland aerosols stimulate irritant subepithe-

TABLE 6–7.

Categories of Aerosolized Bronchoactive Drugs, With Dosage Amounts* Indicated for
Gas-Powered Nebulizers and MDI, Where Applicable

	NEBULIZER SOLUTION	MDI	USE
Bronchodilators			
Isoproterenol	1.25–2.5 mg	0.125–0.250 mg	Short-term bronchodilation
Isoetharine	2.5–5.0 mg	0.34–0.68 mg	Short-term bronchodilation
Metaproterenol	15 mg	1.3–1.95 mg	Maintenance bronchodilator therapy
Terbutaline	—	0.40 mg	Maintenance bronchodilator therapy
Albuterol	2.5 mg	0.18 mg	Maintenance bronchodilator therapy
Atropine	0.05 mg/kg	—	Bronchodilator (anticholinergic)
Ipratropium	—	0.036 mg	Bronchodilator (anticholinergic)
Mucolytics			
Acetylcysteine	200–300 mg	—	Reduce viscosity and elasticity of mucus gel
Corticosteroids			
Dexamethasone	—	0.3 mg	Anti-inflammatory, with asthma
Beclomethasone	—	0.1 mg	Anti-inflammatory; treatment of nasal rhinitis
Triamcinolone	—	0.4 mg	Anti-inflammatory
Flunisolide	—	0.5 mg	Anti-inflammatory
Antiasthmatic			
Cromolyn sodium	20 mg	—	Asthma prophylaxis
Decongestants			
Racemic epinephrine	5.6–11.25 mg	—	Vasoconstriction and reduction of mucosal edema
Phenylephrine	2.5–5.0 mg	—	Vasoconstriction and reduction of mucosal edema
Lidocaine	40–60 mg	—	Anesthesia of the upper airway
Antimicrobial			
Kanamycin	250 mg		Pulmonary infections, especially gram-negative
Gentamicin	80 mg		
Polymixin B	5–10 mg		
Amphotericin B	5 mg/day		Fungal pulmonary infections
Nystatin	100,000 units		Fungal pulmonary infections

*Dosages are per administration. For example, flunisolide is 0.5 mg per 2 puffs, the usual amount prescribed for each dosing.

lial receptors (cough receptors) in the trachea and bronchi, thereby initiating a vagally mediated reflex mucus production, cough, and, to some extent, increased airway resistance.[55] It is thought that stimulation of the cough receptors initiates a vagal afferent impulse to the spinal cord, with reflex arc via efferent vagal fibers to the lung. This mechanism has been termed vagally mediated reflex bronchoconstriction, and can be triggered by cold air or high flow rates in hyperreactive airways, as well as by aerosol particles.[25] A concomitant increase in mucus production by the submucosal glands, which are under vagal control, results in increased expectoration, productive cough, and enhanced secretion clearance. This view is supported by the fact that a 10-minute aerosol treatment delivers less than 1 cc of solution to the airway surface, and the mucus gel is relatively impervious to absorption of water.[3, 18, 55] A study has demonstrated a greater mean weight of sputum production with hypertonic saline (1.21 M) breathed from an ultrasonic nebulizer for 11 minutes, compared to a control. They attributed the accelerated clearance to an increase in productive coughing.[55]

Aerosols in general are irritants to the lung, and this results in an expectorant action, giving a productive cough and increased clearance of secretions. Bland aerosols are basically expectorants, an effect caused by topical irritation. This is the same property of aerosols utilized for sputum induction. It may be that the general irritant effect of aerosols was the cause of *insignificant* differences in sputum production when four medications (neosynephrine, isoproterenol, normal saline, and sterile water) were aerosolized (one at a time) preceding postural drainage in cystic fibrosis patients.[54] Whether bland aerosol therapy is a desirable method of clearing secretions or should be discarded in favor of alternative methods less irritating to the airway such as systemic hydration and bronchial hygiene techniques (percussion, postural drainage) remains to be established.[60, 74] Certainly the advent of superior *mucus-controlling* agents, as opposed to mucolytics, which simply liquefy, may provide better aerosol therapy for states of hypersecretion, both acute and chronic. Such agents are not currently available, but are being investigated, and would be capable of selectively altering the rheologic properties (viscosity, elasticity) of mucus gel to optimize transport by the ciliary system.[59]

Indication 3.—The mechanism of sputum induction using aerosols is probably the same as that described for the enhancement of secretion clearance. Irritation of the large airways with a bland aerosol of sterile water or hypertonic saline provokes an expectorant effect via a vagally mediated reflex. The result is increased production of mucus from the vagally innervated submucosal glands and a productive cough. Ultrasonic nebulizers have usually been employed to produce the aerosol because of the density of its output and the small particle size obtained.

Indication 4.—Water aerosols have generally been used for humidification in two applications: as an unheated aerosol to humidify dry therapeutic gases in high-flow oxygen delivery systems such as aerosol masks or face shields and as a heated aerosol to achieve BTPS conditions with a bypassed upper airway receiving therapeutic gas mixtures. Because of the tremendous surface area available for evaporation with an aerosol of sterile water, it is possible to increase relative humidity of an oxygen-air mixture by nebulizing water. If the carrier gas is raised to body temperature, 100% relative humidity at 37°C is possible.

Although the use of cold aerosols for humidity with high flow oxygen delivery is relatively safe, it can cause increased airway resistance, especially in hyperreactive airways.[25, 66] However, the more hazardous use is the heated aerosol to achieve BTPS conditions with an intubated patient. Increased airway resistance, deposition of large amounts of fluid in the lung over prolonged times, and chance of infection become possible risks.[11, 70] The essential problem with heated aerosols of water is that in addition to the humidity delivered, particles of liquid

water are also deposited, which are not required by the lung. Heated pass-over, bubble-through or saturated wick devices can all match BTPS *without* the addition of liquid particles. In view of the hazards associated with aerosols, such devices should be used wherever possible with intubated patients, in place of heated nebulizers. Although a short-term aerosol treatment with a mouth-breathing patient deposits little actual volume of liquid in the lung, a continuous heated aerosol with an intubated patient, over prolonged periods of time, deposits considerably more liquid volume. The longer the time period of administration and the smaller the person, the greater the chance of excess liquid in the airways, causing pooling of secretions, impaired mucociliary clearance, and possible growth of organisms. It is estimated that approximately 50 ml of water from an ultrasonic could be deposited in the lung over a 24-hour period with a nose-breathing adult; and 20 ml for a 4-year-old child.[77] Investigators have demonstrated a 37% reduction in viscosity for sputum exposed to a water aerosol for 3 hours, and since decreased viscosity may actually impair mucus transport, the addition of liquid water to the lung in the form of an aerosol should be minimized, if not eliminated when *only humidity* is required.[18]

Indication 5.—Use of unheated bland aerosols with upper airway inflammation has been traditionally applied in two clinical situations: pediatric croup and following extubation. The use of "mist tents" with cystic fibrosis patients, to deliver water to peripheral airways, has been shown to be at best ineffective, and actually to cause deterioration of pulmonary function.[7, 46] This has contradicted the previous findings, which were influenced by the method of measuring functional residual capacity (FRC) and by the use of the vital capacity (VC) and maximal ventilatory volume (MVV).[42] In general, mist tents have been considered ineffective in treating *lower* respiratory tract disorders, such as cystic fibrosis, bronchiolitis, or pneumonia.[23, 46] Little water is actually deposited in the lower airway, and bacterial contamination or bronchospasm can be caused. This conclusion was reiterated in the 1979 Conference on the Scientific Basis of In-Hospital Respiratory Therapy.[74]

In the upper airway, the beneficial effect of unheated bland aerosol remains to be demonstrated.[74] There are three variables involved in applying cool aerosols to the upper airway: temperature, humidity, and the particles of water. The effect of warm or cool humidified gas with or without aerosol particles on transglottic airflow resistance remains to be systematically investigated. It may be that the high humidity achieved with water aerosols has a beneficial effect on the airway, and there is no need for additional particulate water. In the case of croup (acute viral laryngotracheitis), investigators recently suggested that holding a child in a warm, humid atmosphere, e.g., a bathroom with a hot shower running, is harmless at least, and probably comforting and anxiety reducing; they questioned the placement of children in cold, damp tents.[31] In the case of postextubation edema, would cool, high-humidity gas be as good or better than an unheated bland aerosol? The use of topical vasoconstricting agents (phenylephrine, racemic epinephrine) or of corticosteroids in managing upper airway inflammation has *not* been questioned.[4, 58]

Hazards

Hazards associated with aerosol therapy relate to the agent used, the delivery device, the gas temperature, and the patient's age, size, history, and current status.

1. Drug reaction. One of the most common applications of aerosol therapy is deposition of bronchoactive drugs. Common side effects that can be hazardous if not corrected can be given for each major category used.

• Sympathomimetics: tachycardia, palpitations, nervousness, and muscle tremor
• Corticosteroids: oral candidiasis, laryngitis
• Cromolyn sodium: bronchospasm
• Antimicrobials: bronchospasm, sensitivity reactions

2. Bronchospasm is a hazard whenever particulate matter is introduced into the airway. This effect of increased airway resistance is especially likely with 20% acetylcysteine, aerosol antibiotics, dry powdered cromolyn sodium, and water or hypertonic aerosols. Bronchospasm has also been documented as a significant hazard with ultrasonic nebulizers, especially in the presence of hyperreactive airways.[21, 41, 57, 69] A separate pretreatment bronchodilator with a rapid, short-acting agent such as isoetharine may be necessary.

3. Bacterial contamination can occur with aerosols, either through introduction of bacteria-laden particles in the respiratory tract or through autoinfection from tubing condensate. A recent study demonstrated that aerosols containing *Pseudomonas aeruginosa* could be recovered up to 15 ft away from the exhalation of infected animals receiving continuous heated aerosol therapy, leading to potential cross infection.[11] Although the nebulizers were sterile, tubing condensate was also heavily contaminated. Since humidifiers with no aerosol do not transmit particles, direct infection is not possible as with a contaminated nebulizer. Tubing condensate should be drained away from the patient, and ventilator circuits should be changed daily to minimize autoinfection.

4. Upper airway burns may become possible with overheated aerosol therapy. Measurement of gas temperature close to the airway should insure that overheating, above 37°C, should not occur.

5. Fluid overload can occur with continuous heated and/or high-output aerosol generators (ultrasonic, solosphere, heated jet nebulizers) used for humidity with intubated patients. Although a small amount of water volume is deposited in the lungs with a 10-minute, short-term aerosol treatment, over a prolonged period of time under the above conditions, substantial liquid can accumulate in the airways. In addition to the particulate liquid deposited, the usual pulmonary water loss of approximately 250 ml/day no longer occurs. The extra liquid can produce a positive fluid balance systemically, as well as a topical pooling of secretions. The risk of fluid overload increases with decreases in the size of the patient. Two cases have been reported concerning pediatric applications, with a heated Puritan all-purpose nebulizer used with nasal CPAP, and with an ultrasonic nebulizer, as a humidifier for a ventilator.[63, 70] Heated aerosols cannot be recommended for humidity with bypassed upper airways, although the practice continues. If aerosols are used in such applications, then patients should be monitored for fever, runny, watery secretions, edema, polyuria, and hyponatremia as clinical indicators of fluid overload.

6. Aspiration of foreign body with an MDI. A case in which a 51-year-old asthmatic carpenter aspirated a penny using an MDI has been reported.[29] It was found that all inhalers except that for Intal could accommodate and eject dimes and pennies during inspiration. Since an MDI device may be carried in pockets with small-sized objects, patients should be alerted to this hazard.

7. Specific hazards with mist tents. Whatever the final conclusion regarding the *efficacy* of mist tents for croup or upper airway inflammation and the use of aerosols in tents in general, there are def-

inite hazards to such therapy. Assuming a pediatric application, the following can occur:[31]

- Chilling due to evaporation, and dampness.
- Bacterial contamination.
- Increased airway resistance secondary to airway irritation with aerosols.
- Anxiety and separation from family causing hyperventilation and increased Vo_2.
- Less accessibility for patient care.

Assessment

The primary assessment of aerosol therapy relates to the goal of the therapy. With bronchoactive drugs, expiratory flow rates and secretion clearance should be monitored. Specific techniques to do this include bedside spirometry or peak expiratory flows, inspection of respiratory pattern and rate, sputum collection and chest auscultation, as well as questioning the patient concerning breathing and sputum production. Sputum cultures and the chest radiograph should be reviewed as these are available.

In using water aerosols for humidity, gas temperature should be monitored to avoid overheating or underheating. The use of bland aerosols for upper airway inflammation can be assessed through physical examination, especially inspection of respiratory rate, pattern (use of accessory muscles, retraction), skin color and tone, and breath sounds.

In general, assessment of vital signs, especially pulse rate, and respiratory status will alert the clinician to potential adverse effects of aerosol therapy.

REFERENCES

1. Abramson HA: Principles and practice of aerosol of the lungs and bronchi. *Ann Allergy* 1946; 4:440.
2. American College of Chest Physicians—National Heart, Lung, and Blood Institute: National Conference on Oxygen Therapy. *Respir Care* 1984; 29:922–935.
3. Asmundsson T: Efficiency of nebulizers for depositing saline in human lung. *Am Rev Respir Dis* 1973; 108:506.
4. Barker GA: Current management of croup and epiglottitis. *Pediatr Clin North Am* 1979; 26:565.
5. Bar-Or O, Neuman I, Dotan R: Effects of dry and humid climates on exercise-induced asthma in children and preadolescents. *J Allergy Clin Immunol* 1977; 60:163–168.
6. Chamney AR: Humidification requirements and techniques. *Anesthesia* 1969; 24:602–617.
7. Chang N, et al: An evaluation of nightly mist tent therapy for patients with cystic fibrosis. *Am Rev Respir Dis* 1973; 107:672–675.
8. Chen WY, Chai H: Airway cooling and nocturnal asthma. *Chest* 1982; 81:675–680.
9. Chen WY, Horton DJ: Heat and water loss from the airways and exercise-induced asthma. *Respiration* 1977; 34:305–313.
10. Chen WY, Horton DJ: Airways obstruction in asthmatics induced by body cooling. *Scand J Respir Dis* 1978; 59:13–20.
11. Christopher KL, et al: The potential role of respiratory therapy equipment in cross infection: A study using a canine model for pneumonia. *Am Rev Respir Dis* 1983; 128:271–275.
12. Darin J: The need for rational criteria for the use of unheated bubble humidifiers (editorial). *Respir Care* 1982; 27:945–947.
13. Darin JD, Broadwell J, MacDonell R: An evaluation of water-vapor output from four brands of unheated, prefilled bubble humidifiers. *Respir Care* 1982; 27:41–50.
14. Deal EC, Jr, et al: Role of respiratory heat exchange in production of exercise-induced asthma. *J Appl Physiol* 1979; 46:467–475.
15. Dery R: The evolution of heat and moisture in the respiratory tract during anesthesia with a non-rebreathing system. *Can Anaesth Soc J* 1973; 20:296–309.
16. Dolan GK, Zawadski JJ: Performance characteristics of low-flow humidifiers. *Respir Care* 1976; 21:393–403.
17. Dolovich M, et al: Optimal delivery of aerosols from metered dose inhalers. *Chest* 1981; 80(suppl):911–915.
18. Dulfano JJ, Adler KB: Physical properties of sputum: VII. Rheologic properties and mucociliary transport. *Am Rev Respir Dis* 1973; 107:130.
19. Eriksson NE, Haglind K, Hidinger KG: A new inhalation technique for freon aerosols: Terbutaline aerosol with a tube extension in a 2-day cross-over comparison with salbutamol aerosol. *Allergy* 1980; 35:617–622.
20. Ferron GA, Kerrebijn KF, Weber J: Properties of aerosols produced with three nebulizers. *Am Rev Respir Dis* 1976; 114:899–908.
21. Flick MR, Moody LE, Block AJ: Effect of ultrasonic nebulization on arterial oxygen saturation in chronic obstructive pulmonary disease. *Chest* 1977; 71:366–370.
22. Gawley TH, Dundee JW: Attempts to reduce respiratory complications following upper abdominal operations. *Br J Anaesth* 1981; 53:1073–1078.
23. Gibson LE: Use of water vapor in the treatment of lower respiratory disease. *Am Rev Respir Dis (Suppl)* 1974; 110:100–103.
24. Godden DJ, Crompton GK: An objective assessment of the tube spacer in patients unable to use a conventional pressurized aerosol efficiently. *Br J Dis Chest* 1981; 75:165–168.
25. Gold WM: Vagally-mediated reflex bronchoconstriction in allergic asthma. *Chest* 1973; 63(suppl):11.

26. Goldberg IS, Lourenco RV: Deposition of aerosols in pulmonary disease. *Arch Intern Med* 1973; 131:88–91.

27. Gomm SA, et al: Effect of an extension tube on the bronchodilator efficacy of terbutaline delivered from a metered dose inhaler. *Thorax* 1980; 35:552–556.

28. Gurwitz D, et al: Assessment of a new device (aerochamber) for use with aerosol drugs in asthmatic children. *Ann Allergy* 1983; 50:166–170.

29. Hannan SE, et al: Foreign body aspiration associated with the use of an aerosol inhaler. *Am Rev Respir Dis* 1984; 129:1025–1027.

30. Heaton RW, et al: The bronchial response to cold air challenge: evidence for different mechanisms in normal and asthmatic subjects. *Thorax* 1983; 38:506–511.

31. Henry R: Moist air in the treatment of laryngotracheitis. *Arch Dis Child* 1983; 58:577.

32. Hiller C, et al: Aerodynamic size distribution of metered-dose bronchodilator aerosols. *Am Rev Respir Dis* 1978; 118:311–317.

33. Hiller FC, et al: Physical properties of therapeutic aerosols. *Chest* 1981; 80(suppl):901–903.

34. Horton DJ, Chen WY: Effects of breathing warm humidified air on bronchoconstriction induced by body cooling and by inhalation of methacholine. *Chest* 1979; 75:24–28.

35. Huntley W, Weinberger M: Evaluation of bronchodilation from aerosol beta-2 agonists delivered by the Inhal-Aid device to young children. *J Asthma* 1984; 21:965–970.

36. Kelling JS, et al: Physician knowledge in the use of canister nebulizers. *Chest* 1983; 83:612–614.

37. Klein EF, Jr, et al: Performance characteristics of conventional and prototype humidifiers and nebulizers. *Chest* 1973; 64:690–696.

38. Lippman M: Regional deposition of particles in the human respiratory tract, in Lee DHK, Falk HL, Murphy SD (eds): *Handbook of Physiology*, section 9. Bethesda, American Physiological Society, 1977.

39. Lourenco RV, Cotromanes E: Clinical aerosols. I. Characterization of aerosols and their diagnostic uses. *Arch Intern Med* 1982; 142:2163–2172.

40. Mahler DA, Loke J: Lung function after marathon running at warm and cold ambient temperatures. *Am Rev Respir Dis* 1981; 124:154–157.

41. Malik SK, Jenkins DE: Alterations in airway dynamics following inhalation of ultrasonic mist. *Chest* 1972; 62:660.

42. Matthews LW, Doershuk CF, Spector S: Mist tent therapy of the obstructive pulmonary lesion of cystic fibrosis. *Pediatrics* 1967; 39:176–185.

43. Mercer TT: Production and characterization of aerosols. *Arch Intern Med* 1973; 131:39–50.

44. Moritz AR, Weisiger JR: Effects of cold air on air passages and lungs: experimental investigation. *Arch Intern Med* 1945; 75:233–240.

45. Morrow PE: Aerosol characterization and deposition. *Am Rev Respir Dis* 1974; 110:88–99.

46. Motoyama EK, Gibson LE, Zigas CJ: Evaluation of mist tent therapy in cystic fibrosis using maximum expiratory flow volume curve. *Pediatrics* 1972; 50:299–306.

47. Newhouse MT, Ruffin RE: Deposition and fate of aerosolized drugs. *Chest* 1978; 73(suppl):936–943.

48. Newman SP, Clarke SW: Therapeutic aerosols 1—Physical and practical considerations (editorial). *Thorax* 1983; 38:881–886.

49. Newman SP, Pavia D, Clarke SW: Improving the bronchial deposition of pressurized aerosols. *Chest* 1981; 80(suppl):909–911.

50. Newman SP, et al: Deposition of pressurized aerosols in the human respiratory tract. *Thorax* 1981; 36:52–55.

51. Newman SP, et al: Deposition of pressurized suspension aerosols inhaled through extension devices. *Am Rev Respir Dis* 1981; 124:317–320.

52. Newman SP, et al: Effects of various inhalation modes on the deposition of radioactive pressurized aerosols. *Eur J Respir Dis* 1982; 119(suppl):57–65.

53. O'Cain CF, et al: Airway effects of respiratory heat loss in normal subjects. *J Appl Physiol* 1980; 49:875–880.

54. Olson DL, et al: Effectiveness of aerosol therapy preceding postural drainage in cystic fibrosis. *Respir Care* 1976; 21:333–334.

55. Pavia D, Thomson ML, Clarke SW: Enhanced clearance of secretions from the human lung after the administration of hypertonic saline aerosol. *Am Rev Respir Dis* 1978; 117:199.

56. Pedersen S: Aerosol treatment of bronchoconstriction in children with or without a tube spacer. *N Engl J Med* 1983; 308:1328–1330.

57. Pflug AE, Cheney FW, Jr, Butler J: The effects of an ultrasonic aerosol on pulmonary mechanics and arterial blood gases in patients with chronic bronchitis. *Am Rev Respir Dis* 1970; 101:710–714.

58. Postma DS, Jones RO, Pillsbury HC, III: Severe hospitalized croup: Treatment trends and prognosis. *Laryngoscope* 1984; 94:1170–1175.

59. Puchelle E, et al: Drug effects on viscoelasticity of mucus. *Eur J Respir Dis* 1980; 61(suppl 110):195.

60. Rau JL, Jr: *Respiratory Therapy Pharmacology*, ed 2. Chicago, Year Book Medical Publishers, 1984.

61. Riley DJ: The proper use of canister nebulizers, plain and fancy (editorial). *Chest* 1983; 83:590–591.

62. Riley DJ, Liu RT, Edelman NH: Enhanced responses to aerosolized bronchodilator therapy in asthma using respiratory maneuvers. *Chest* 1979; 76:501–507.

63. Rosenfeld WP, Linshaw M, Fox HA: Water intoxication: A complication of nebulization with nasal CPAP. *J Pediatr* 1976; 89:113–114.

64. Sackner MA, Brown LK, Kin LS: Basis of an improved metered aerosol delivery system. *Chest* 1981; 80(suppl):915–918.

65. Schachter EN, Witek TJ, Kolak B: Airway response to cold air and exercise in healthy subjects. *Respir Therapy* 1985; 15:36–43.

66. Shapiro BA, Harrison RA, Trout CA: *Clinical Applica-*

tion of Respiratory Care. Chicago, Year Book Medical Publishers, 1975.

67. Strauss RH, et al: Influence of heat and humidity on the airway obstruction induced by exercise in asthma. *J Clin Invest* 1978; 61:433–440.

68. Swift DL: Aerosols and humidity therapy: Generation and respiratory deposition of therapeutic aerosols. *Am Rev Respir Therapy* 1980; 122(suppl):71–77.

69. Taguchi JT: Effect of ultrasonic nebulization on blood gas tensions in chronic obstructive lung disease. *Chest* 1971; 60:356–361.

70. Tamer MA, Modell JH, Rieffel CN: Hyponatremia secondary to ultrasonic aerosol therapy in the newborn infant. *J Pediatr* 1970; 77:1051–1054.

71. Task Group on Lung Dynamics: Deposition and retention models for internal dosimetry of the human respiratory tract. *Health Physics,* vol 12. New York, Pergamon Press, 1966, pp 173–207.

72. Thomas P, et al: Modifying delivery technique of fenoterol from a metered dose inhaler. *Ann Allergy* 1984; 52:279–281.

73. Tobin MJ, et al: Response to bronchodilator drug administration by a new reservoir aerosol delivery system and a review of other auxiliary delivery systems. *Am Rev Respir Dis* 1982; 126:670–675.

74. Wanner A, Rao A: Clinical indications for and effects of bland, mucolytic, and antimicrobial aerosols. *Am Rev Respir Dis* 1980; 122(suppl):79–87.

75. Weinstein RE, et al: Effects of humidification on exercise-induced asthma (EIA) (abstract). *J Allergy Clin Immunol* 1976; 57:250–251.

76. Wells RE, Walker JEC, Hickler RB: Effects of cold air on respiratory airflow resistance in patients with respiratory-tract disease. *N Engl J Med* 1960; 263:268–273.

77. Wolfsdorf J, Swift DL, Avery ME: Mist therapy reconsidered; an evaluation of the respiratory deposition of labelled water aerosols produced by jet and ultrasonic nebulizers. *Pediatrics* 1969; 43:799–808.

78. Ziment I: Why are they saying bad things about IPPB? *Respir Care* 1973; 18:673.

79. Ziment I: *Respiratory Pharmacology and Therapeutics.* Philadelphia, WB Saunders Co, 1978.

Chest Physical Therapy and Airway Care

Donna L. Frownfelter, P.T., R.R.T.

The basic techniques of chest physical therapy have been utilized since the early 1900s.[15] The efficacy of therapy has been expanded to treat various forms of respiratory dysfunction of both an acute and chronic nature resulting from medical or surgical origins. In general usage, "chest PT" is often synonymous with the techniques of postural drainage, percussion, and vibration. This is a very limited and incomplete definition. The cardiopulmonary section of the American Physical Therapy Association has adopted a more inclusive and appropriate definition of chest physical therapy (see below). Airway clearance techniques are very important in the respiratory therapist's armamentarium for the patient who needs bronchial hygiene. Accordingly, this chapter emphasizes airway clearance and breathing exercise techniques.

A DEFINITION OF CHEST PHYSICAL THERAPY[4]

Chest physical therapy is an area of practice concerned with evaluation and treatment of patients of all ages with acute and chronic chest disorders. These disorders may be primary diseases or may be secondary to other medical and surgical conditions. The term *chest physical therapy* has come to mean gravity-assisted bronchial drainage with chest percussion. This unfortunately narrow definition, which is found in contemporary scientific literature, fails to recognize the many other modalities that may be employed to evaluate and treat the patient with cardiopulmonary dysfunction.

The physical therapy evaluation of the spontaneously breathing and mechanically ventilated patient may include, but not be limited to:

- Analysis of medical information from the patient's record.
- Chest assessment (auscultation, palpitation, chest wall mobility, posture analysis, breathing pattern, identification, mediate percussion).
- Assessment of degree of stress and tension patient exhibits.
- Muscle strength testing.
- Joint range-of-motion (ROM) testing.
- Noninvasive oxygen monitoring (ear oximetry, transcutaneous oximetry).
- Exercise stress and tolerance testing.
- Identification of respiratory therapy appliances which might enhance chest PT.
- Functional evaluation of mechanically ventilated patient.

Treatment is based on the results of initial and subsequent continuous evaluation. Most of the techniques used fall into the categories of airway clearance (secretion removal) or therapeutic exercise. Airway clearance techniques facilitate loosening and removal of secretions from the tracheobronchial tree. These techniques may include, but are not limited to:

- Positioning for gravity drainage.
- Chest percussion.
- Chest vibration.
- Chest shaking.
- Rib springing.
- Cough training, stimulation, and assistance.

- Airway suctioning.
- Oxygen, bronchodilator, and humidity therapy utilization in conjunction with chest PT treatments.

Therapeutic exercise programs with appropriate oxygen support may include but are not limited to:

- Posture correction.
- Relaxation training.
- Manual stretching of the thorax.
- Chest mobilization.
- Exercise techniques to improve and maintain ROM, i.e., postthoracotomy, strength and coordination of the trunk and extremities (i.e., passive and active ROM exercises, proprioceptive neuromuscular facilitation (PNF) techniques, progressive resistive exercise). Respiratory muscle strengthening and endurance exercises and breathing exercises (diaphragmatic, costal, pursed-lip, incentive spirometry, sustained maximal inspiration, paced breathing).
- Glossopharyngeal breathing.
- General conditioning exercises.
- Energy conservation and life-pacing.
- Instruction in home care programs.
- Patient and family education.

Goals of treatment include improvement of airway clearance, ventilation, and exercise tolerance; reduction in the work of breathing and ultimately restoration of the patient to his full potential (pulmonary rehabilitation) in the inpatient, outpatient, and home care settings. Optimal pulmonary rehabilitation includes home program planning which helps the patient and family understand and participate in self-care. A follow-up program should include restructuring of the treatment plan and identification of interdisciplinary resources for information and assistance.

PATIENT ASSESSMENT

Prior to the formulation of an appropriate respiratory care plan for the patient with ineffective airway clearance, a thorough assessment of the patient's condition must be made. The patient's chart should be read daily or prior to treating each patient. All of the information listed below should be evaluated when planning for chest physical therapy treatments. The evaluation is essential as it will enable the therapist to:

1. Understand the underlying medical or surgical condition as it affects the patient's respiratory dysfunction.
2. Plan appropriate intervention techniques.
3. Evaluate the effectiveness of the chosen techniques administered.
4. Change and progress therapy as indicated.
5. Suggest that therapy be discontinued when it is no longer needed.
6. Formulate an appropriate home care plan for patients with chronic respiratory dysfunction who need to continue therapy at home.

SPECIFIC INFORMATION TO BE OBTAINED FROM THE PATIENT'S RECORD

- Is the respiratory dysfunction acute or chronic?
- Is the patient in acute respiratory distress? How long has the acute distress been present?
- What is the current cardiovascular status (i.e., blood pressure, heart rate, arrhythmias)?
- Is the cardiovascular status being supported by vasopressors (i.e., dopamine drip)?
- Is an intra-aortic balloon pump in use?
- Is the patient producing mucus? If not, is there a reason (i.e., dehydrated, unable to cough due to decreased strength)?
- What surgery has the patient experienced? Where is the incision, chest tubes, etc.?
- How long was the anesthetic course during the surgery?
- How well is the patient deep breathing and coughing postoperatively?
- How much pain medication is the patient requiring?
- Is the patient ambulating? Is he able to sit in a chair?
- What is the nutritional status of the patient?
- Has the patient been sleeping well, able to rest, or sleep deprived?
- Are the laboratory values stable (i.e., platelets, hemoglobin, hematocrit)?
- What is the chest x-ray report? Is it current (i.e., within 24 hours)?

When an assessment has been performed (see chapters 1 through 4), this should be used to formulate the goals for the chest physical therapy treatment. The therapist needs to determine what he is attempting to do for the patient in order to select the appropriate techniques (Table 7–1). This process separates a "routine technician treatment" (sometimes referred as "bang, breathe and cough") from a well-designed, effective, individually tailored therapist-designed treatment program. In addition to the routine chest assessment procedures, the patient's posture, muscle tone, and general physical fitness level, ability to cough, breathing pattern, and relaxation state should be evaluated. There are other indicators of success as related to chest physical therapy treatments. Things to consider in patient evaluation are also motor ability—patient coordination, ability to follow directions in the proper sequence such as, "take a deep breath, hold it and cough," or the simple maneuver of an incentive spirometer are extremely difficult for many patients. In these individuals, chest physical therapy may be indicated for a longer period of time than one would expect in a more coordinated individual. The patient's desire to cooperate and independently continue therapy to improve his pulmonary status is also extremely important. These other criteria may at times be the key to success in a chest physical therapy program. Goals may be both short- and long-term. The patient may initially receive postural drainage with percussion and vibration for bronchiectasis. However, the long-term goal will be to teach the patient how to do his therapy independently at home.

INDICATIONS FOR CHEST PHYSICAL THERAPY

The indications for chest physical therapy may be either prophylactic or therapeutic. Prophylactic treatment seems more rational; however, with cost containment issues being strongly raised, this is often not the case. Examples of prophylactic chest physical therapy would be the high-risk abdominal or thoracic surgery patient that has a long smoking history and abnormal pulmonary functions preoperatively.[12, 22, 24, 52] This patient would benefit from preoperative bronchial hygiene and breathing and cough facilitation. The same patient would be aggressively treated postoperatively to prevent respiratory complications rather than wait until an atelectasis due to secretions has occurred. Other examples of prophylactic care are noted in Table 7–2.

PRECAUTIONS TO CHEST PHYSICAL THERAPY

Chest physical therapy treatment is not without potential hazard to some patients.[12, 22, 39, 48] Caution must be used with many patients that are medically unstable. Examples of precautions are listed below.

1. Untreated tension pneumothorax (an absolute contraindication, however, when treated, i.e., chest tube placement, chest PT should be initiated to assist in more rapid reinforcement of the lung.

2. Abnormal coagulation profile, in particular severely decreased platelets, i.e., below 30,000/cu mm, may choose to do postural drainage and breathing exercise rather than use percussion techniques. Platelet counts may be monitored and treatment given when the infusion has increased the platelets.

3. In status epilepticus or status asthmaticus, the increased stimulation may worsen the patient's unstable condition.

4. Immediately following intracranial surgery, head-down positions should be modified until the neurosurgeon believes it is appropriate. This may be

TABLE 7–1.

Goals of Chest Physical Therapy

Prevent the accumulation of secretions
Improve the mobilization and drainage of secretions
Promote relaxation to improve breathing patterns
Promote improved respiratory function developing respiratory strength *and* endurance
Improve cardiopulmonary exercise tolerance
Teach bronchial hygiene programs to patients with chronic respiratory dysfunction in airway clearance

TABLE 7–2.

Indications for Chest Physical Therapy

Prophylactic indications
   The preoperative high-risk surgical patient
   The postoperative patient who is unable to mobilize secretions
   The neurologic patient who is unable to cough effectively
   The ventilator patient who has a tendency to retain secretions
   The patient with a primary pulmonary disease, i.e., cystic fibrosis or bronchiectasis, that needs to improve bronchial hygiene
Therapeutic indications
   The patient with atelectasis due to secretions
   The patient with retained secretions
   The patient with an abnormal breathing pattern due to primary or secondary pulmonary dysfunction
   The patient with COPD and resultant decreased exercise tolerance
   The patient with a musculoskeletal deformity that makes his breathing pattern and cough ineffective

a one-time treatment if a patient develops a profound atelectasis.

5. "Brittle" bones may tend to fracture with aggressive percussion. Caution should be used with patients with osteoporosis, long-term steroids, and metastasis to the ribs.

6. Following esophageal anastomosis, head-down positions should be modified to prevent gastric reflux from the suture line.

7. Patients who have recently suffered an acute MI or cerebrovascular accident (CVA) should be relatively stable (i.e., blood enzymes, blood pressure, ECG) before any extreme positioning is undertaken.

8. Recent rib fractures should be avoided, however; postural drainage combined with a gentle vibration may be utilized, as well as breathing exercises.

9. Tube feedings should be allowed to infuse (approximately 1 to 1½ hours) and be ingested on spontaneously breathing patients prior to Trendelenburg positions. However, patients with artificial airways can usually tolerate Trendelenburg with the cuff inflated.

Modification of treatment may mean not tipping the bed in Trendelenburg but using the proper postural drainage position on a flat bed. It may mean more gentle percussion or withholding percussion from a fragile patient with decreased platelets. These are only two modifications. This is the area where appropriate therapeutic judgment must be applied.

A physician's order for chest physical therapy may be very general or very specific. There are *chest physical therapy orders* or *postural drainage to right lower lobe in Trendelenburg position* orders. Either way, the order has certain drawbacks and benefits. The general order leaves the responsibility on the therapist to do an appropriate patient and chart evaluation to determine what is the specific respiratory dysfunction. A well-educated therapist is capable of this judgment. However, someone very new to performing chest physical therapy may flounder and need more guidance. The very specific order limits the therapist legally to doing *only* what is requested, i.e., the right lower lobe. In actuality, if there is a right lower lobe problem, the left side should also be treated to prevent complication as the patient will be lying more frequently on the left side to drain the right lower lobe and may have dependent secretions. If the therapist feels a need for more information or clarificatioin of the order, the physician should be contacted.

PHYSIOLOGIC EFFECTS OF CHEST PHYSICAL THERAPY

Many articles published in the last 10 years attempt to document the physiologic effects of chest physical therapy (see bibliography). The emphasis in this chapter is on the effects of postural drainage, percussion, vibration, and breathing exercises.

Postural Drainage and Positioning

Positioning for bronchial drainage is stated to facilitate the mucus flow by the effect of gravity.[6, 7, 37, 45, 47, 54, 55] Positioning also effects diaphragmatic movement.[11, 17, 21, 30] Diaphragmatic excursion improves when the patient is turned from supine to sidewise (Fig 7–1). The airflow to the dependent lung is improved initially. Later the pressure of the

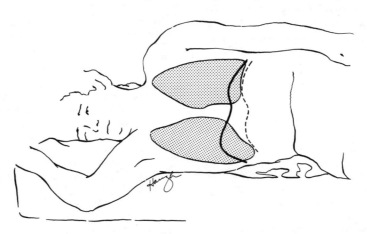

FIG 7–1.
When the patient is lying on his side, the dome of the diaphragm on the lower side rises further in the thorax than the dome on the upper side. (From Frownfelter DL: *Chest Physical Therapy and Pulmonary Rehabilitation: An Interdisciplinary Approach*, ed 2. Chicago, Year Book Medical Publishers, 1987, p 9. Used with permission.)

bed on the chest wall restricts movement of the dependent thorax. There are less frequent ventilatory pattern changes in bedridden patients. This, combined with the effects of anesthesia on mucociliary clearance, may cause atelectasis in the dependent lung.[18]

Studies have shown changes in PaO_2 with positioning. In patients with unilateral lung disease, when the patient is placed with the *good* lung down, PaO_2 improves; when the diseased lung is down, PaO_2 decreases.[39] When patients in respiratory failure were positioned prone, the PO_2 improved.[13, 35, 50]

Percussion and Vibration, Shaking

Percussion seems to loosen mucus from the tracheobronchial tree.[6, 7, 44] Vibration is thought to assist in the movement of secretions toward the trachea. Shaking is a more vigorous form of vibration with more chest compression. Shaking is used when secretions are thick and more force is needed to mobilize them.[44, 47] There is not agreement on the force or speed of percussion and vibration.[42, 44, 47]

Studies have shown that the combination of techniques of postural drainage, percussion, and vibration are effective in secretion removal.[7, 10, 34, 37, 42] Observation by fiberoptic bronchoscopy of dogs after instillation of propyliodone demonstrated that percussion resulted in "spattering of plugs" and that vibration appeared to cause a "more directional flow of propyliodone."[23]

Chest physical therapy has also been seen to reverse lobar atelectasis in postoperative, traumatic injury, and nonsurgical patients.[18, 22] The effects of chest physical therapy were seen to be equal to fiberoptic bronchoscopy.[34]

The postoperative and total lung/thorax compliance is often seen to improve following a chest physical therapy treatment.[32] It seems there is less shunting as a result of increased ventilation.[33]

Breathing Exercise

Breathing exercise has been shown to decrease respiratory rate and increase tidal volume.[1, 14, 19] Specific breathing exercises will increase lateral costal expansion and have been shown to prevent atelectasis in many patients postoperatively.[3, 16, 17, 24, 38, 53]

Cough

Coughing effectiveness can be impaired by surgery (decreased inspiratory volume secondary to

diaphragmatic embarrassment; position, neuromuscular weakness and pain).[20] Increased airway resistance and submaximal airflow can also contribute to poor cough.[6, 26, 28, 29, 31]

Postural Drainage

Postural drainage is a method of facilitating the removal of secretions from the tracheobronchial tree by proper positioning of the patient and utilization of gravity (Fig 7–2). The segmental bronchus to be drained is placed in a vertical position so that gravity can assist drainage of mucus from that segment.[3]

Postural drainage is appropriate in patients with increased, retained secretions, lung abscess, atelectasis, and when there are neurologic or neuromuscular weakening diseases that decrease the patient's ability to cough.[4, 56] It is also used prophylactically in high-risk patients to prevent respiratory complications. These may be medical patients (i.e., ventilated patients) or postoperative surgical patients (i.e., thoracic or abdominal surgery).

It is important to know the specific segments involved so the proper postural drainage position may be utilized (Fig 7–3). Positions should be modified when the patient's condition is unstable (i.e., high blood pressure, arrhythmias, severe shortness of breath, pain). An attempt should be made to place the patient in as close to the proper position as possible within the necessary modifications.

Before positioning patients, the procedure should be explained to the patient. Loosen clothing for comfort, especially around the neck and waist. Determine where all wires and tubes are positioned (i.e., ECG, IVs, catheters) and what will happen to them when the patient is positioned. Make adjustments prior to moving patient.

When the patient is in the appropriate position, assess that the joints are well-supported and the patient is reasonably comfortable and able to remain in position for 5 to 10 minutes. Assess the patient's tolerance to the treatment and whether modifications are necessary (i.e., pain medication prior to treatment).

Following the treatment, assess and chart the results—productivity, ease of breathing, breath sound improvement, or more effective cough.

Percussion

Percussion is applied over the surface landmarks of the bronchial segment being drained (Fig 7–4). The hand is cupped and wrists are loose. The hands rhythmically and alternately strike the chest wall.

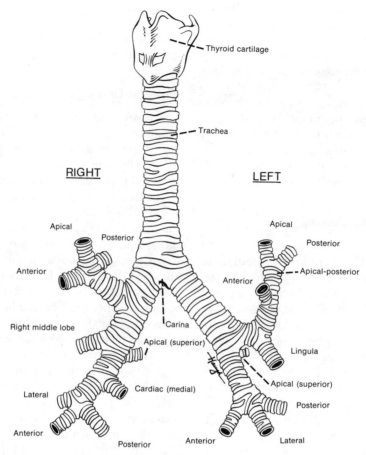

FIG 7–2.
Tracheobronchial tree (a three-quarters view, rotated towards the right side). (From Frownfelter DL: *Chest Physical Therapy and Pulmonary Rehabilitation: An Interdisciplinary Approach,* ed 2. Chicago, Year Book Medical Publishers, 1987, p 23. Used with permission.)

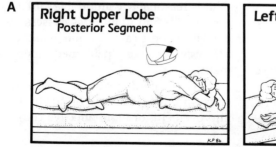

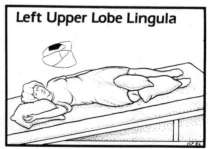

FIG 7–3.
A and **B,** postural drainage positions. (From Frownfelter DL: *Chest Physical Therapy and Pulmonary Rehabilitation: An Interdisciplinary Approach,* ed 2. Chicago, Year Book Medical Publishers, 1987, pp 276–277. Used with permission.) *(Continued.)*

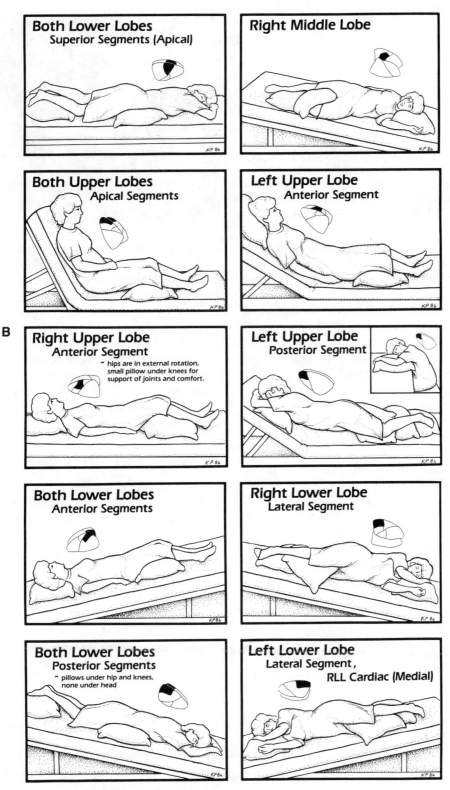

FIG 7–3. (Cont.)

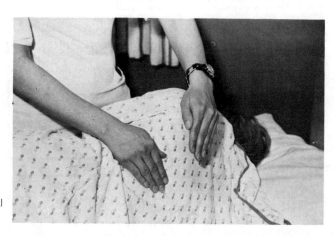

FIG 7–4.
Chest percussion. (From Frownfelter DL: *Chest Physical Therapy and Pulmonary Rehabilitation: An Interdisciplinary Approach*, ed 2. Year Book Medical Publishers, 1987, p 289. Used with permission.)

The patient's skin condition should be evaluated prior to and following treatment. Incisions, bony prominences, and inflamed areas should be avoided during percussion.

Percussion is usually done over a thin layer of cloth, i.e., hospital gown or sheet. A terry cloth towel or blanket may detract from the effectiveness of the technique. Usually percussion is done for approximately 5 minutes. If the patient is very productive or secretions very thick, treatment may be lengthened if the patient is tolerating it well.

Vibration

Vibration is a shaking movement used to move loosened mucus plugs to larger airways so they can be coughed or suctioned out. The technique is usually administered with postural drainage following percussion. Vibration may be used alone when percussion may be contraindicated. Vibration is applied only during the exhalation phase. The patient is asked to take a deep breath or given a deep ventilation by bag or ventilator.

Hand position is important in vibration (Fig 7–5). The therapist's hands may be placed side by side or one on top of the other. The fingers and palm should be flat on the chest to avoid *digging in* with the fingertips. Even pressure should be exerted with the whole hand.

Vibration is usually done for 5 to 10 deep breaths. The chest wall should be compressed during exhalation and vibration done in the normal mechanical manner (ribs down and in during exhalation).

Shaking

Shaking is a vigorous form of vibration. It is usually used with thick secretions that might be difficult to mobilize through usual methods. As with vibration, the patient takes a deep breath, then during exhalation the chest wall is vigorously *pumped* to forcefully expel the breath. Shaking is vibration and is usually performed in the proper postural drainage position.

Care needs to be observed to use "shaking" only with patients that have a compliant chest wall. Patients with osteoporosis, history of rib fractures, long-term steroids, metastatic carcinoma of the ribs, or large barrel chests would not be appropriate for this technique.

Special Considerations for the Neonate and Child

In applying chest physical therapy to infants and children, a special understanding of the differences from the adult must be appreciated. Structural differences are seen that have strong functional implications. For example, the infant's narrower airways create more resistance to airflow and are obstructed more easily. In addition the ribs are more circular and horizontal. The angle of insertion of the diaphragm on the ribs is more horizontal and the ribs are more cartilaginous. Consequently the chest wall mechanics are less efficient, more distortion of the chest wall occurs, and the result can be increased work of breathing.[27]

The neonate has a higher laryngeal position. It has been assumed that this results in obligatory mouth breathing for the first few months of life. This theory is now being questioned.[40] There are also notable physiological differences. The newborn's diaphragm has fewer type I high oxidative muscle fibers (25% compared to 50% in an adult).[15] This may predispose an infant to earlier diaphragmatic fatigue when stressed. There are also fewer collateral ventilatory channels than in the adult. Because the number of channels in the right middle and upper lobes

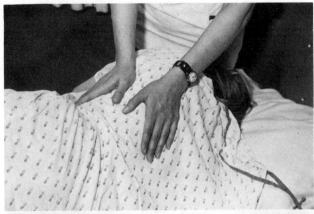
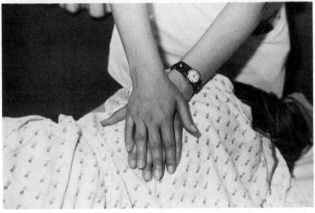

FIG 7–5.
Chest vibration, hands separated *(top)*, hand placement one on top of the other *(bottom)*. (From Frownfelter DL: *Chest Physical Therapy and Pulmonary Rehabilitation: An Interdisciplinary Approach*, ed 2. Year Book Medical Publishers, 1987, p 293. Used with permission.)

of neonates are especially reduced, there seems to be a relatively higher incidence of atelectasis in those lobes.[15]

These factors lead to neonates and infants having less functional reserve and being more prone to respiratory compromise.[15] These factors must be considered when providing chest physical therapy and during suctioning. One must use extreme care and caution not to overly stress these patients.

The more common disease states encountered in the neonatal and pediatric population are: meconium aspiration syndrome, pneumonia, bronchopulmonary dysplasia, transient tachypnea of the newborn, cystic fibrosis, respiratory problems secondary to CNS depression, immobile cilia syndrome, asthma, and neuromuscular disease.

The basic techniques for chest physical therapy need a little alteration but are basically the same for bronchial hygiene. The same postural drainage positions are utilized. Generally, instead of just concentrating on one specific drainage position a full range of drainage positions will be used. The infants airways are so small that it is easy for mucus plugging. If one position is used frequently the opposite lung segment will be seen to have mucus plugging or atelectasis. Consequently, it is recommended that

a full range of positions be utilized. This may be modified according to the infant's tolerance level. If the child cannot tolerate all positions in one treatment, it can be divided into two treatments. Aggressive positioning should be done between treatments.

In tiny infants below 800 gm, modifications of the Trendelenburg position can be used. This is due to the high incidence of intraventricular hemorrhage in premature infants. Chest percussion and vibration are modified in the infants. "Tenting" of the index, middle, and ring finger forms a natural cup (Fig 7–6). Percussion may be done with a small anesthesia mask or one of the small palm cups commercially available (although this author's preference is to do percussion manually). Tented fingers have the advantage of allowing one to feel the amount of pressure and contact with the infant's body. Vibration can be done with the fingers in a much gentler form than for adults. If the respiratory rate is high, vibration may be done at every other breath.

Suctioning should be done with great care while watching monitors carefully. Bagging should be done attached to a pressure manometer to monitor appropriate pressure. Shorter time periods for suc-

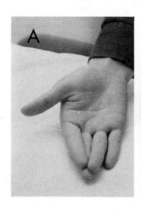
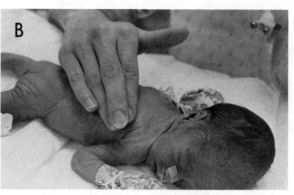

FIG 7–6.
Chest percussion for infants—"tenting." **A,** position. **B,** use in chest percussion. (From Frownfelter DL: *Chest Physical Therapy and Pulmonary Rehabilitation: An Interdisciplinary Approach*, ed 2. Chicago, Year Book Medical Publishers, 1987, p 689. Used with permission.)

tioning are recommended (5 seconds). The primary point to remember when treating infants and children is that they are not just little adults and must be treated with consideration for their unique structure and physiology.

BREATHING EXERCISE

Breathing exercise is an important part of the chest physical therapy regimen for medical and surgical chest conditions.[4, 38, 49, 55] They are indicated in all patients receiving chest physical therapy. Breathing exercises may be the primary technique used or may accompany postural drainage, vibration, and coughing.

Diaphragmatic Breathing

As a basic principle, diaphragmatic breathing needs to be taught and reinforced in various positions and during activities (Figs 7–7 through 7–12).

The initial teaching is usually best done in a supine semifowler's position with knees bent. The patient should be comfortable and fully supported so all his attention is on breathing. Rather than a great deal of explanation, it is more helpful to have the patient experience the proper breathing, to become aware of the appropriate movement of breathing.

The patient should be as relaxed as possible prior to starting the breathing exercise. Jacobsen's relaxation exercise may be modified to relax the patient's neck and shoulders.[52] Jacobsen believed that a maximal muscle contraction leads to maximal muscle relaxation. Ask the patient to shrug his shoulders, hold them up, and let them drop. He can make a fist and tighten his arms and chest, hold it, and then let it go. This has been an effective, relatively quick system to relax neck and shoulders.

The therapist places his hand on the patient's upper abdomen and asks the patient to breath normally (see Fig 7–7,A and B). The therapist feels the breathing pattern and depth. Then at the end of an exhalation, a stretch is given downward and inward

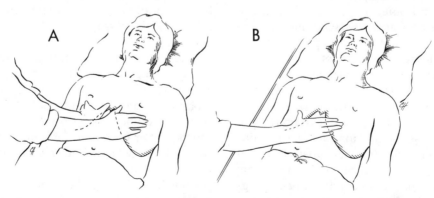

FIG 7–7.
(A), placement of hands for diaphragmatic breathing (especially for a large patient where one hand is inadequate. **(B),** therapist's hand placement for diaphragmatic breathing. (From Frownfelter DL: *Chest Physical Therapy and Rehabilitation: An Interdisciplinary Approach*, ed 2. Chicago, Year Book Medical Publishers, 1987, p 237. Used with permission.)

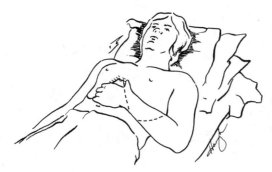

FIG 7–8.
The patient is encouraged to continue practicing diaphragmatic breathing to become aware of his breathing pattern. This is usually the first position of the diaphragmatic breathing teaching sequence. (From Frownfelter DL: *Chest Physical Therapy and Rehabilitation: An Interdisciplinary Approach,* ed 2. Chicago, Year Book Medical Publishers, 1987, p 238. Used with permission.)

and the patient is told, "Now push my hand up." The therapist continues to use end expiratory stretch to facilitate diaphragmatic breathing.

In order to make the patient aware of his breathing pattern, the patient is asked, "Do you feel the breathing is from your abdomen?" Then the patient's hand is placed on the upper abdomen, and he is taught to feel the breathing independently (see Fig 7–8). He would then be instructed to reinforce this hourly and do self-checks that he is breathing properly.

If the patient has difficulty with diaphragmatic breathing a change of position may help. Some patients with distended or obese abdomens may feel relief when lying on their sides. Another position for ease of breathing may be a hands-knees position where the diaphragm is able to move in a gravity eliminated position.

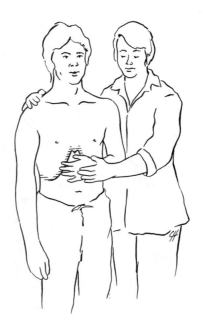

FIG 7–10.
The third position in the sequence is standing. Full-length mirrors are helpful at this point. (From Frownfelter DL: *Chest Physical Therapy and Rehabilitation: An Interdisciplinary Approach,* ed 2. Chicago, Year Book Medical Publishers, 1987, p 239. Used with permission.)

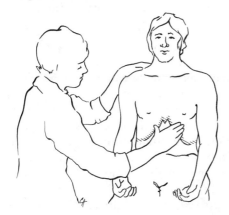

FIG 7–9.
The patient advances to the sitting position for breathing retraining. Note the relaxed position of the patient's shoulders and hands. (From Frownfelter DL: *Chest Physical Therapy and Rehabilitation: An Interdisciplinary Approach,* ed 2. Chicago, Year Book Medical Publishers, 1987, p 238. Used with permission.)

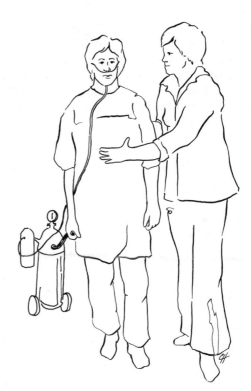

FIG 7–11.
Walking is the fourth stage of retraining. The patient is encouraged to relax, control his breathing, take long steps and slow down. (From Frownfelter DL: *Chest Physical Therapy and Rehabilitation: An Interdisciplinary Approach,* ed 2. Chicago, Year Book Medical Publishers, 1987, p 239. Used with permission.)

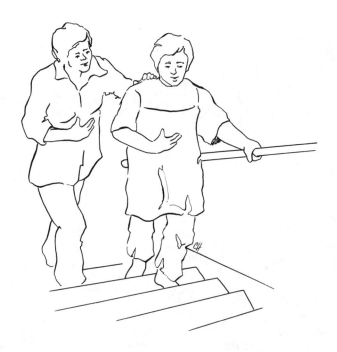

FIG 7–12.
Stairs are important, especially if the patient has them at home. He is instructed to pause slightly as he breathes in and to exhale as he climbs one to two stairs. (From Frownfelter DL: *Chest Physical* *Therapy and Rehabilitation: An Interdisciplinary Approach,* ed 2. Chicago, Year Book Medical Publishers, 1987, p 240. Used with permission.)

The next progression of diaphragmatic breathing instruction is in a sitting position, then standing and walking. It is task-specific, and one cannot assume that because a patient is able to perform diaphragmatic breathing supine in bed that he will also be able to perform it sitting, standing, and walking. It needs to be reinforced in all positions and activities (see Figs 7–9 through 7–12).

Segmental Breathing (Localized Breathing)

In segmental or localized breathing exercises, the patient is asked to attempt to ventilate specific areas of the lungs. The therapist's or patient's hand is placed over the surface landmark of the lung segments to be ventilated. For example, if the inferior segment of the lingular area needs to be emphasized, the therapist's hand is placed over the left anterior chest over the fourth, fifth, and six intercostal spaces (Figs 7–13 through 7–15). Slight stretch pressure is given and the patient is asked to try to push the therapist's hand (or his own hand) up as he inspires. The tactile input and stretch will facilitate a deeper inspiration.

Lateral Costal Breathing Exercise

Unilateral or bilateral costal breathing exercise will increase ventilation to the lower lobes and will also facilitate diaphragmatic breathing. The diaphragm is responsible for lower chest lateral costal expansion so these exercises are very effective in increasing ventilation. These exercises are especially helpful following abdominal surgery, when patients prefer to have the therapist's hands on the lateral thorax rather than their abdomen (Fig 7–16). They are also helpful with patients with large distended abdomens (i.e., pregnant, ascites).

Pursed Lip Breathing/Dyspnea Training

Patients in respiratory distress will often be seen to utilize pursed lip breathing. However, they often appear very stressed and try to force the air out. This force may actually cause an increase in cardiovascular pressure as noted by increased jugular vein distention. Increased airway collapse may also be seen with the stressed forceful pursed lip breathing. The patients are attempting to expel air from their lungs. In order to do this effectively, a relaxed form of pursed lip breathing should be taught and reinforced.[19, 46, 51]

The pursed lip breathing exerts a positive back pressure on the airways which allows the patient to exhale without the airways collapsing and trapping air in the lungs.[14, 19, 46] Patients should be reminded to do pursed lip breathing when they become dyspneic in order to regain control of their breathing.

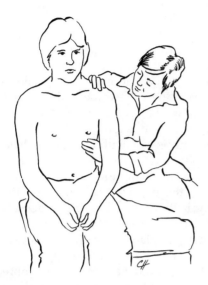

FIG 7–13.
Unilateral (segmental) breathing emphasizing the left lower lobe. Note that the patient's shoulder must remain down, with hands placed on ulnar border or palm up in his lap. (From Frownfelter DL: *Chest Physical Therapy and Rehabilitation: An Interdisciplinary Approach*, ed 2. Chicago, Year Book Medical Publishers, 1987, p 247. Used with permission.)

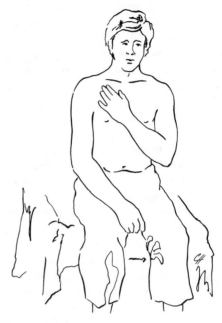

FIG 7–15.
Segmental right upper lobe expansion exercise. (From Frownfelter DL: *Chest Physical Therapy and Rehabilitation: An Interdisciplinary Approach*, ed 2. Chicago, Year Book Medical Publishers, 1987, p 248. Used with permission.)

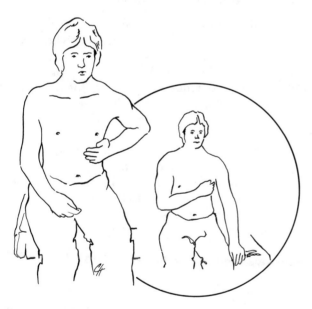

FIG 7–14.
The patient can perform unilateral (segmental) breathing by placing either hand on the side of the chest to be emphasized. The patient can also perform midchest expansion by moving his hand up. (From Frownfelter DL: *Chest Physical Therapy and Pulmonary Rehabilitation: An Interdisciplinary Approach*, ed 2. Chicago, Year Book Medical Publishers, 1987, p 247. Used with permission.)

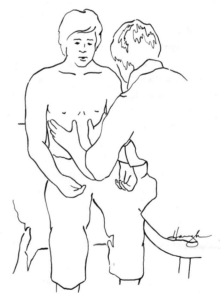

FIG 7–16.
Bilateral lower lobe expansion (this also facilitates diaphragmatic movement). (From Frownfelter DL: *Chest Physical Therapy and Pulmonary Rehabilitation: An Interdisciplinary Approach*, ed 2. Chicago, Year Book Medical Publishers, 1987, p 244. Used with permission.)

They can then go a step further and utilize proper breathing patterns to attempt to prevent dyspnea during activities.

Patients can be encouraged to exhale during activities that require increased exertion. Even getting out of a chair can be stressful for a compromised patient. The patient is encouraged to use energy-conserving techniques with proper breathing 'to maintain control of their breathing. For example, the patient having difficulty rising from the chair is encouraged to move forward in the chair, bend forward, take a breath in, and exhale as he rises from the chair.[52, 53] Generally, the patient is asked to exhale during exertional activities. Patients can learn to anticipate their activities and how to prepare for and breathe during them in order not be dyspneic. Planning for different activities is important. A patient should pause and take several deep relaxing breaths prior to each activity. A sequence for getting out of bed and walking would be: (1) take a few deep breaths; (2) breath in, exhale, and sit up on the side of the bed; (3) take a few more deep breaths while sitting at the side of the bed; (4) breathe in, exhale, and stand; (5) take a few deep breaths while standing at bedside; (6) take a deep breath, exhale, and start to walk.

The therapist needs to discuss with the patient what type of activity makes him dyspneic. A plan for dealing with the exertional dyspnea in a way that allows some motor activity should be prepared. Although the relaxation and breathing strategies suggested need to be individualized, a tremendous improvement in the patient's quality of life can occur.

Energy conservation techniques should also be taught in dyspnea training. Patients should be encouraged to sit for as many activities as possible, i.e., shaving, washing, preparing food, dressing, combing hair, and so on. Practical advice such as putting on a terry cloth bathrobe instead of drying off with towels is helpful.

Patients should pace their activities. Adequate time should be planned so patients do not need to rush for appointments or activities. If walking, patients should note areas where they can rest—benches, coffee shops, malls, and so on. Life-pacing also involves spacing activities so everything is not scheduled too close together.

Patients need to know they can usually continue with activities they enjoy; however, they need to do more planning, organize, and pace their activities. The goal is to accomplish what they chose to and not to get it done quickly without consideration of their abilities and limitations.

AIRWAY CARE

Normal bronchial hygiene is usually accomplished by the mucociliary escalator. Coughing may be affected when additional effort is needed to clear the airways. When these methods are not effective in maintaining effective bronchial hygiene, tracheobronchial aspiration is indicated.[2, 25, 36, 51]

Suctioning is not without potential hazards.[9, 41] The therapist must always be cognizant of potential complications of suctioning. Some complications are: irritation to the nasotracheal mucosa with bleeding (especially if there are abnormally decreased platelets or abnormalities in clotting), abrupt drops in the PaO_2, vagal stimulation, bradycardia, patient irritability, and fear. All therapists should experience suctioning. They would be much more appreciative of the maneuver following the experience. Preoxygenation and limiting time suctioning has been shown to decrease or eliminate the fall in PO_2.[9, 36]

General Suctioning Guidelines

1. All equipment should be checked for working order prior to attempting to suction. If a chest physical therapy treatment is being given, the suction equipment should be checked and set up prior to the treatment in order not to waste time if the patient needs suctioning.

2. If the patient is being monitored, the ECG pattern should be noted as well as the patient's heart rate. In neonates, the transcutaneous oxygen ($TcPO_2$) should be monitored if available.

3. Suctioning should only be used when the normal bronchial hygiene mechanisms are dysfunctional. The therapist should not assume that because a patient needed suctioning at one point, he continues to need it. The patient should be asked to cough regularly, and assessment should be ongoing whether or not suctioning is necessary.

4. If the patient has swallowing dysfunction and increased oral secretions, he can be instructed to independently aspirate his oral secretions. Swallowing exercises should also be considered to strengthen the muscles and teach the patient the necessary swallowing procedures.

5. The external diameter of the suction catheter may be estimated by dividing the size by 3 (i.e., 12 French catheter = 12 + 3 − 4 mm). The catheter should be no larger than half the cross-sectional diameter of the tube.

Nasotracheal Suction Procedure

1. Check equipment.
2. Check monitors.
3. Inform patient of the procedure.
4. Preoxygenate patient.
5. Place patient's neck in mild extension (Fig 7–17).
6. Lubricate catheter with water-soluble gel.
7. Pass catheter (without suction) upward and backward with short increments, continue until an obstruction (the carina is reached).
8. Pull back catheter slightly, then apply suction while withdrawing catheter.
9. Limit aspiration time to 10 to 15 seconds total. A good guideline is for the therapist to hold his breath during suctioning as the patient is also not breathing; it gives the therapist a better sensitivity for what the patient experiences.
10. Allow the patient to rest for several seconds and reoxygenate.
11. Repeat procedure if necessary to remove more secretions.

Endotracheal or Tracheostomy Suctioning

The procedures are the same except sterile technique is followed and no lubrication is usually necessary although it may be used if there is difficulty passing the catheter. Following the suctioning of the artificial airway, the oral and nasal passages should be evaluated to see if suction is needed. Once the catheter is used for nasal and oral suction, it is contaminated. If the artificial airway needs additional aspiration, a new glove and catheter should be used.

ARTIFICIAL AIRWAYS

An artificial airway consists of a tube that is inserted in the trachea, either through the mouth or nose (oral or nasal endotracheal tube) or by a surgical incision (tracheotomy). The appropriate artificial airway is chosen based on the goal that is to be achieved. The indications for an artificial airway are listed in Table 7–3.

Nasopharyngeal Airway

The simplest airway to facilitate suctioning is the nasopharyngeal airway.[51] This airway is usually soft latex and provides ready access to the trachea for suctioning or the insertion of a fiberoptic bronchoscope. The airway helps guide the catheter directly to the trachea instead of a blind nasotracheal attempt. In patients that need frequent suctioning, this airway will help to protect the nasal and pharyngeal mucosa. Often the immediate use of this airway will avert a later intubation or tracheotomy by the facilitation of good respiratory care (Fig 7–18). The tube should be well-anchored with tape so it has little movement. The tube should be alternated in the nares for skin protection. The area around the nares should be kept clean and dry.

Oral and Nasal Endotracheal Tubes

Endotracheal tubes may be indicated when, in addition to suctioning, the patient is in need of mechanical ventilation or CPAP. They provide the necessary mechanical adaptions with a cuff around the portion of the tube in the trachea to allow all the

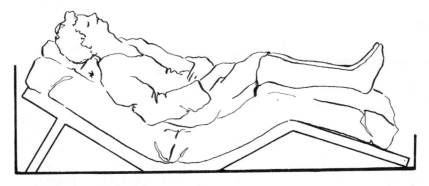

Semi-Fowler 10-12"

FIG 7–17.
Position for nasotracheal suctioning (semi-Fowlers's 10 to 12 in.). (From Frownfelter DL: *Chest Physical Therapy and Pulmonary Re-* *habilitation: An Interdisciplinary Approach*, ed 2. Chicago, Year Book Medical Publishers, 1987, p 738. Used with permission.)

TABLE 7–3.

The Indications for an Artificial Airway

Establish and maintain a patient's airway
Bypass upper airway obstruction
Facilitate suctioning
Provide access for mechanical ventilation or CPAP
Prevent aspiration of stomach contents (protection
   of the airway)

volume of gas to be delivered through the tube to the lungs.

Oral endotracheal tubes are usually chosen during crisis situations such as cardiac arrests. It is generally an easier access to the lungs, and a larger tube can be used. This tube has the disadvantage that the patient can bite down; the patient also feels more irritation if conscious (Fig 7–19).

Nasotracheal Airways

Nasotracheal airways are usually chosen for more long-term ventilation. They are often better tolerated for comfort. They have some drawbacks since a smaller size tube must be used, and it may be more difficult to suction due to the increased curvature of the tube.

Early Complications of Tracheal Intubation

Complications may occur (1) during intubation, (2) while the tube is in place, and (3) during extubation (Table 7–4).[5, 8, 43] A prospective study of 150 critically ill adult patients reported the following complications and consequences of endotracheal intubation and tracheotomy[43]:

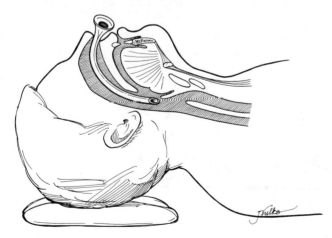

FIG 7–18.
Schematic of the position of the nasopharyngeal airway in situ.

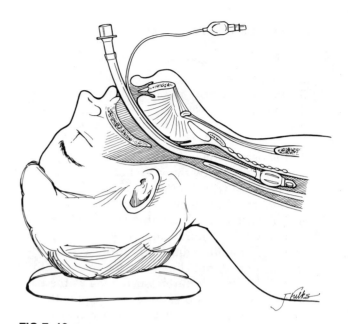

FIG 7–19.
The orotracheal tube in proper position in the trachea.

1. Tooth avulsion (1% to 2% oral intubations).
2. Nasal bleeding (54% in nasal intubations).
3. Retropharyngeal or hypopharyngeal perforation leading to abscess formation, subcutaneous emphysema, and mediastinitis.
4. Vocal fold hematomas, dislocation of arytenoids.
5. Pulmonary aspiration (8%).
6. Right mainstem intubated (9%).
7. Cardiac arrhythmias (32%).
8. Tracheal edema, ulceration, and stenosis (most tracheal injury at the site of the cuff or the tip of the endotracheal tube).
9. Nutrition may be inadequate if a feeding tube is not used.
10. Communication is altered as patients get discouraged about their condition and lack of ability to communicate.

After extubation, patients may experience hoarseness, which will usually resolve spontaneously. Damage to the vocal cords and glottis may occur if the cuff is not deflated prior to removing the tube.[5] Laryngeal edema may be the result of intubation trauma, hypersensitivity to local anesthetics, lubricants, or by ethylene oxide released from polyvinylchloride tubes.[5] Tracheal stenosis (or tracheomalacia) may occur at the cuff site several weeks or months after extubation. Several other late complications of tracheal intubation have been reported (Table 7–5).[5, 8, 43]

TABLE 7–4.

Early Complications of Tracheal Intubation*

	DURING INTUBATION	WITH TUBE IN PLACE	DURING EXTUBATION
Traumatic-mechanical	Fracture-luxation cervical spinal column (spinal cord injury)	Fracture—luxation of cervical spinal cord	Trauma to glottis by inflated cuff
	Eye trauma	Ventilatory obstruction	Difficult or impossible extubation
	Epistaxis	Rupture of trachea	Ventilatory obstruction
	Tooth trauma	Emphysema, pneumothorax	
	Retropharyngeal dissection	Ruptured cuff	
	Subcutaneous, mediastinal emphysema	Tracheal bleeding	
	Perforation of esophagus or pharynx	Aspiration	
	Laceration of pharynx or larynx		
	Arytenoid dislocation		
	Aspiration (blood, tooth, laryngoscope bulb, gastric contents, tumor tissue, adenoid)		
	Pneumothorax		
	Esophageal intubation (gastric distention)		
	Bronchial intubation (hypoxemia)		
Reflex	Laryngeal spasm		Laryngeal spasm
	Bronchospasm		
	Cardiac arrhythmias		
	Arterial hypotension		

*From Applebaum EL, Bruce DL: *Tracheal Intubation*. Philadelphia, WB Saunders Co, 1976. Used by permission.

Tracheotomy

Tracheotomy is indicated when intubation may need to be more permanent or long-term. Aspiration of secretions is usually easier. It may be indicated when there is a need to bypass the upper airways (i.e., tumor obstruction, facial injuries). Tracheot-

TABLE 7–5.

Late Complications of Tracheal Intubation*

Sore jaw
Sore throat, dysphagia
Sore skeletal muscles
Paresis or paralysis of tongue
Paresis or paralysis of vocal cords
Lingual nerve injury
Ulceration of lips, mouth, pharynx
Laryngitis, sinusitis, respiratory tract infection
Stricture of nostril
Laryngeal edema
Laryngeal ulceration
Laryngeal granulomas or polyps
Synechiae of vocal cords
Laryngotracheal membranes and webs
Perichondritis or chondritis of larynx
Tracheal stenosis

*From Applebaum EL, Bruce DL: *Tracheal Intubation*. Philadelphia, WB Saunders Co, 1976. Used by permission.

omy has surgical risks such as bleeding, infection, subcutaneous emphysema, pneumothorax, recurrent laryngeal nerve injury, air embolism, and tracheoesophageal fistula (Table 7–6). The tracheostomy tube can cause swallowing dysfunction.[5]

Tracheostomy Care

The important components of tracheostomy care are to maintain patency of the tube, keep the wound site clean, assess for proper ventilation and humidity, and observe any changes that may be pertinent. Supplemental humidity is used after the tracheostomy is performed. Secretions should be monitored and aerosol therapy recommended if secretions are very thick and tenacious. The patient will be unable to cough properly since the tube is below the vocal folds. Postural drainage may be recommended in tracheostomy patients with retained secretions.

The tracheostomy tube should be well anchored (Fig 7–20). A square knot should be used to tie the flange in place. It should be placed on one side of the patient's neck. The dressing under the tracheostomy tube should be changed whenever it is soiled to prevent bacterial contamination. The skin around the incision should be cleansed regularly and kept dry.

TABLE 7–6.

Complications of Tracheotomy*

I. Immediate
   A. Hemorrhage
   B. Apnea; cardiac arrest
   C. Hypotension
   D. Obstruction; displaced tube
   E. Subcutaneous emphysema
   F. Pneumothorax; pneumomediastinum
   G. Aspiration and atelectasis
   H. Recurrent laryngeal nerve injury
   I. Tracheoesophageal fistula
   J. Aerophagia
II. Delayed
   A. Hemorrhage
   B. Obstruction
   C. Tracheitis
   D. Pneumonia
   E. Wound infection
   F. Subglottic edema
   G. Tracheal stenosis
   H. Tracheoesophageal fistula
   I. Dysphagia
   J. Persistent tracheocutaneous fistula
   K. Difficult decannulation
   L. Unsightly scar

*From Applebaum EL, Bruce DL: *Tracheal Intubation.* Philadelphia, WB Saunders Co, 1976. Used by permission.

An additional tracheostomy tube of the same size should be taped near the patient's bedside to be used for emergency situations. During the first few days after a tracheostomy, it may be disastrous if the tube is dislodged, so extreme care is given to caring for the patient (tube should only be changed within first 3 days by surgeon who put it in). Tubing should be positioned without pulling on the tube. Extreme care should be taken with postural drainage and suction procedures especially with ventilated patients.

Tracheal Instillations

Many authorities feel that when the patient is well-hydrated or given aerosol and humidity therapy, tracheal instillation is unnecessary.[10] Often only the instilled fluid is suctioned and bronchoconstriction may occur. In a small group of patients, in particular neonates who have very small endotracheal or tracheostomy tubes and a few adult patients with abnormally thick tenacious secretions that do not respond well to aerosol and humidity therapy, instillation of saline may prove beneficial.

The volume of saline should be gauged to the patient. Usually in neonates, 0.5 to 1.0 cc of sterile normal saline would be used prior to suction. This is accompanied by hyperventilation and preoxygenation. In adults, 1 to 2 cc may be instilled. Aggressive suction should follow immediately after instillation of saline.

Instillation of saline should not be routine (other than in neonates) and should be based on rationale and proper clinical judgment related to each individual patient. When assessing response to instillation, it is important to decide whether to attempt the procedure again.

In summary, techniques of chest physical therapy and airway care are utilized to prevent and treat ineffective airway clearance and alteration in breathing patterns. Sound clinical judgment must be utilized to select and properly execute appropriate therapeutic techniques based on goals set for each individual patient. The goals should be evaluated daily and changes in therapy made when necessary.

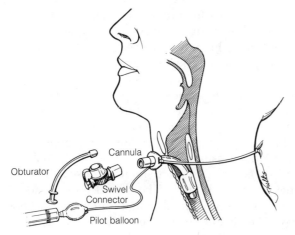

FIG 7–20.
Tracheostomy tube with low-pressure cuff and pilot balloon to monitor cuff pressure and inflation, inserted and tied in place.

REFERENCES

1. Acee S: Helping patients breathe more easily. *Geriatric Nurse* 1984; 230:233.
2. Albanese AJ, Toplitz AD: A hassle-free guide to suctioning a tracheostomy. *RN* 1982; 24:29.
3. Alvarez SE, et al: Respiratory treatment of the adult patient with spinal cord injury. *Phys Ther* 1981; 61:1737.
4. American Physical Therapy Association—Cardiopulmonary Section; Definition of Chest Physical Therapy. Adopted 1982.
5. Applebaum EL, Bruce DL: *Tracheal Intubation.* Philadelphia, WB Saunders Co, 1976.

6. Bateman JR, Newman SP, et al: Is cough as effective as chest physical therapy in the removal of excessive tracheal bronchial secretions? *Thorax* 1981; 36:683–687.

7. Bateman JRM, Newman SP, Caunt KM, et al: Regional lung clearance of excessive bronchial secretions during chest physiotherapy in patients with stable chronic airways obstruction. *Lancet* 1979; 1:294–297.

8. Blanc VF, Tremblay NA: The complications of tracheal intubation. *Anesth Analg* 1974; 53:203.

9. Brandstater B, Maullem M: Atelectasis following tracheal suctioning in infants. *Anesthesiology* 1979; 31:294–297.

10. Chopra SK, Taplin GV, Simmons DH, et al: Effects of hydration and physical therapy on tracheal transport velocity. *Am Rev Respir Dis* 1974; 115:1009–1014.

11. Clauss RH, Scalabrini BY, Ray JF, et al: Effects of changing body position upon improved ventilation-perfusion relationships. *Circulation* 1968; 37(suppl 2):214–217.

12. Craig DB: Postoperative recovery of pulmonary function. *Anesth Analg* 1981; 60(1):25–40.

13. Douglas WW, Rehder K, Beynen FM, et al: Improved oxygenation in patients with acute respiratory failure: The prone position. *Am Rev Respir Dis* 1977; 115:559–566.

14. Evans TW, Howard P: Whistle for your wind. *Br Med J* 1984; 289:449–450.

15. Frownfelter D: *Chest Physical Therapy and Pulmonary Rehabilitation.* Chicago, Year Book Medical Publishers, 1987.

16. Goyeche JR, Abo Y, Ikemi Y: Asthma: The yoga perspective: II. Yoga therapy in the treatment of asthma. *J Asthma* 1982; 19:189–201.

17. Grassino A, Bellemare F, Laporta D: Diaphragm fatigue and the strategy of breathing in COPD. *Chest* 1984; 85(suppl 6):515–545.

18. Hammond WE, Martin FJ: Chest physical therapy for acute atelectasis. *Phys Ther* 1981; 61:217–220.

19. Ingram RH, Schilder DP: Effect of pursed lips expiration on the pulmonary pressure-flow relationship in obstructive lung disease. *Am Rev Respir Dis* 1967; 95:381–388.

20. Irwin RS, et al: Cough: A comprehensive review. *Arch Intern Med* 1977; 137:1189.

21. Kaneko K, Mille-Emili J, Dolowich MB: Regional distribution of ventilation and perfusion as a function of body position. *J Appl Physiol* 1966; 21:767–777.

22. Kigin CM: Chest physical therapy for the postoperative or traumatic injury patient. *Phys Ther* 1981; 61:1724.

23. Kigin CM: Personal communication, 1986.

24. Krastins IRB, Corey ML, McLead A, et al: An evaluation of incentive spirometry in the management of pulmonary complications after cardiac surgery in a pediatric population. *Crit Care Med* 1982; 10:525–528.

25. Landa JF, et al: Effects of suctioning on mucociliary transport. *Chest* 1980; 77:202–207.

26. Langerson J: The cough—its effectiveness depends on you. *Respir Care* 1979; 24:142–149.

27. Laitman JT, Crelin ES: Developmental change in the upper respiratory system of human infants. *Perinatol Neonatol* 1980; 4:15.

28. Leith DL: Cough, in Brain JD, Proctor DF, Reid LM (eds): *Respiratory Defense Mechanisms.* New York, Marcel Dekker, 1977.

29. Leith DL: Cough. *Phys Ther* 1968; 48:439–447.

30. Livingston JL: Variations in the volume of the chest with changes of posture. *Lancet* 1928; 1:754–755.

31. Loudon RG: Cough, a symptom and a sign. *Basics Respir Dis* 1981; 9:4.

32. Mackenzie CF, Shin B, McAslan TC: Total lung/thorax compliance changes following chest physiotherapy. *Anesth Analg* 1980; 59:207–210.

33. MacKenzie CF, Shin B, McAslan TC: Chest physiotherapy: The effect on arterial oxygenation. *Anesth Analg* 1978; 57:28–30.

34. Marini JJ, Person DJ, Hudson LD: A prosective comparison of fiberoptic bronchoscopy and respiratory therapy. *Am Rev Dis* 1979; 119:971–978.

35. Martin RJ, Herrell N, Rubin D, et al: Effect of supine and prone positions on arterial oxygen tension in the preterm infant. *Pediatrics* 1979; 63:528–531.

36. McFadden R: Decreasing respiratory compromise during infant suctioning. *Am J Nurs* 1981; 12:2158–2161.

37. Oldenburg FA, Dolovich MB, Montgomery JM, et al: Effects of postural drainage, exercise and cough on mucus clearance in chronic bronchitis. *Am Rev Respir Dis* 1979; 12:730–745.

38. Ratnam KV, Sim MK: Treatment of disease without the use of drugs. Self-treatment of asthma by thought control and breathing exercises. *Singapore Med J* 1980; 21:604–608.

39. Remolina C, et al: Positional hypoxemia in unilateral lung disease. *N Engl J Med* 1981; 304:523–525.

40. Rodenstein DO, Perlmutter N, Stanesw DC: Infants are not obligatory nasal breathers. *Am Rev Respir Dis* 1985; 131:343–347.

41. Roper PC, Vonwiller JB, Fisk GC, et al: Lobar atelectasis after nasotracheal intubation in newborn infants. *Aust Paediat J* 1982; 12:272–275.

42. Rossman CM, et al: Effect of chest physiotherapy on the removal of mucus in patients with cystic fibrosis. *Am Rev Respir Dis* 1982; 126:131.

43. Stauffer JL, Olsen DE, Petty TL: Complications and consequences of endotracheal intubation and tracheotomy, a prospective study of 150 critically ill adult patients. *Am J Med* 1981; 70:65–75.

44. Sutton P, Lopez-Vidriero MT, Pavia D, et al: Assessment of percussion, vibratory shaking and breathing exercises in chest physiotherapy. *Eur J Respir Dis* 1985; 66:147–152.

45. Tecklin JS: Positioning, percussing, and vibrating patients for effective bronchial drainage. *Nursing* 1979; 9:64–71.

46. Thoman RL, Stoker GL, Ross JC: The efficacy of pursed lips breathing in patients with chronic obstructive pulmonary disease. *Am Rev Respir Dis* 1966; 3:100–106.

47. Torrington KG, Sorenson DE, Sherwood LM: Postoperative chest percussion with postural drainage in obese patients following gastric stapling. *Chest* 1984; 86:891–895.

48. Tyler ML: Complications of positioning and chest physiotherapy. *Respir Care* 1982; 27:458.

49. Vraciu J, Vraciu R: Effectiveness of breathing exercises in preventing pulmonary complications following open heart surgery. *Phys Ther* 1977; 57:1367–1370.

50. Wagoman MJ, Shutack JG, Moomjian AS: Improved oxygenation and lung compliance with prone positioning of neonates. *J Pediatr* 1979; 99:787–791.

51. Wanner A: Nasopharyngeal airway: A facilitated access to the trachea. *Ann Intern Med* 1971; 75:593–595.

52. Watson CA, Ross JE, Ramsey M: Identification of neurosurgical patients susceptible to pulmonary infection. *J Neurosurg Nurs* 1984; 16:123–127.

53. Williams IP, Smith CM, McGavin CR: Diaphragmatic breathing training and walking performance in chronic airways obstruction. *Br J Dis Chest* 1982; 76:164–166.

54. Wong JW, Keens TG, Wannamaker EM, et al: Effects of gravity in tracheal transport rates in normal subjects and in patients with cystic fibrosis. *Pediatrics* 1977; 60:146–152.

55. Zadai C: Physical therapy for the acutely ill medical patient. *Phys Ther* 1981; 61:1746.

56. Zausmer E: Bronchial drainage, evidence supporting the procedures. *Phys Ther* 1968; 48:586–591.

SUGGESTED READING

Abraham AS, et al: Reversal of pulmonary hypertension by prolonged oxygen administration to patients with chronic bronchitis. *Circ Res* 1963, vol 23.

Adamson JW, Finch CA: Hemoglobin function, oxygen affinity, and erythropoietin. *Ann Rev Physiol* 1975; 37:351.

Anderson PB, et al: Long-term oxygen therapy in cor pulmonale. *Q J Med* 1973; 42:563–573.

Bartlett RH: Respiratory therapy to prevent pulmonary complications of surgery. *Respir Care* 1984; 29:667–679.

Bland RD: Special considerations in oxygen therapy for infants and children. *Am Rev Respir Dis* 1980; 122:45–54.

Bradley BL, Garner AE, Billiu D, et al: Oxygen-assisted exercise in chronic obstructive lung disease. *Am Rev Respir Dis* 1978; 118:239–243.

Braun HA, Cheney FW, Lochman CP: *Introduction to Respiratory Physiology*, ed 2. Boston, Little, Brown, & Co, 1980.

Brodsky JB: Oxygen: A drug. *Int Anesthesiol Clin* 1981; 19:1–8.

Burton GG, Hodgkin JE: *Respiratory Care: A Guide to Clinical Practice*, ed 2. Philadelphia, JB Lippincott, Co, 1984.

Comroe JH: *Physiology of Respiration*, ed 2. Chicago, Year Book Medical Publishers, 1974.

Cullen JH, Kaemmerlen JT: Effect of oxygen administration at low rates of flow in hypercapnic patients. *Am Rev Respir Dis* 1967; 95:116–120.

Des Jardins TR: *Clinical Manifestations of Respiratory Disease*. Chicago, Year Book Medical Publishers, 1984.

Embury SH, Garcia JF, et al: Effects of oxygen inhalation on endogenous erythropoietin kinetics, erythropoiesis, and properties of blood cells in sickle-cell anemia. *N Engl J Med* 1984; 311:291–295.

Fishman AP: Chronic cor pulmonale. *Am Rev Respir Dis* 1976; 114:775–794.

Grambau GR, Dirks JW: in Belland JC (ed): *Data Gathering in Respiratory Disease*. Arlington, Va, American Academy of Physician Assistants, 1982.

Guyton AC: *Basic Human Physiology*, ed 2. Philadelphia, WB Saunders Co, 1977.

Katz JA: PEEP and CPAP in perioperative espiratory care. *Respir Care* 1984; 29:614–629.

Leggett RJ, et al: Long-term domiciliary oxygen in cor pulmonale complicating chronic bronchitis and emphysema. *Thorax* 1976; 31:414–418.

Marini JJ: Postoperative atelectasis: Pathophysiology, clinical importance, and principles of management. *Respir Care* 1984; 29:515–522.

Marshall BE, Wyche MQ: Hypoxemia during and after anesthesia. *Anesthesiology* 1976; 172:37.

Petty TL: *Intensive and Rehabilitative Respiratory Care*, ed 3. Philadelphia, Lea & Febiger, 1982.

Shankar PS: Oxygen therapy. *Q Med Rev* 1980; 31:1–20.

Shapiro BA, Harrison RA, Kacmarek R; et al: *Clinical Application of Respiratory Care*, ed 3. Chicago, Year Book Medical Publishers, 1985.

Shapiro BA, et al: Changes in intrapulmonary shunting with administration of 100% oxygen. *Chest* 1980; 77:138–141.

Snider GL, Renaldo JE: Oxygen therapy in medical patients hospitalized outside of the intensive care unit. *Am Rev Respir Dis* 1980; 122:29–36.

Slonim NB, Hamilton LH: *Respiratory Physiology*, ed 5. St Louis, CV Mosby Co, 1987.

Thibeault DW, Gregory GA (eds): *Neonatal Pulmonary Care* Reading, Addison-Wesley Publishing Co, 1979.

Tinitis P: Oxygen therapy and oxygen toxicity. *Ann Emerg Med* 1983; 12:321–328.

8

Intermittent Positive-Pressure Breathing

Carl P. Wiezalis, M.S., R.R.T.

Intermittent positive-pressure breathing (IPPB) is a form of short-duration hyperinflation therapy that subjects the lungs and chest of the patient to respiratory volumes at higher than atmospheric pressure. IPPB treatment is administered to the spontaneously breathing patient by specifically engineered pressure-cycled ventilators collectively referred to as "IPPB machines" (the mechanical characteristics of these devices are described in Chapter 14). The pneumatically driven devices delivering the driving gas, oxygen, compressed air, or some mixture of oxygen and entrained air when set on "air dilution." The F_{IO_2} in the air dilution mode is not accurately controlled by the machine and can range from 40% to 100%. Electrically driven IPPB machines deliver room air only.

THE PRESCRIPTION

As with most therapeutic modalities, IPPB is ordered by the physician by prescription. The established hospital protocols and respiratory care department's procedure manual should guide decisions about the form and propriety of the prescription. The prescription for IPPB should include:

1. Therapeutic modality (IPPB).
2. Adjunctive equipment (in-line ultrasonic nebulizer).
3. Duration and frequency of the procedure.
4. Preset pressure and/or tidal volume.
5. F_{IO_2} (air, oxygen, or air dilution).
6. Therapeutic objective(s) (if the department follows this protocol).

7. Pharmacologic agents—dilution and volume.
8. Physician's signature.

PHYSIOLOGIC EFFECTS OF IPPB

Much of the dogma of the 1940s, 1950s, and 1960s turned out to be the hypotheses of the 1970s.[4] Many claims have been made about the physiologic effects of IPPB since the renaissance of its use after World War II.[12] Not until the mid-1970s did IPPB come under rigorous scrutiny; this was exacerbated by fiscal constraint as well as physiologic concerns. Even then, the majority of clinical studies were performed in the outpatient setting.[9, 14, 18] Shapiro et al. state the four following physiologic effects of IPPB:[21] (1) increase in mean airway pressure; (2) decrease in work of breathing; (3) manipulation of I:E ratio; and (4) increase in tidal volume.

By form and function, IPPB applies supra-atmospheric pressure to the airways during the inspiratory phase. This pressure is reflected down the tracheobronchial tree to the alveolar space. The transpulmonary pressure, which is the absolute pressure difference between the alveolar space and the pleural space, dictates lung volume. Transpulmonary pressure gradients as seen in IPPB tend to increase intrapleural pressure, decrease right atrial filling, and decrease venous return from the superior and inferior vena cavae. This in turn may decrease pulmonary perfusion, left ventricular filling, and cardiac output. In addition, inhibition of venous return may cause increased intracranial pressure, which is particularly dangerous to patients with brain injury or disease. Minimizing the period of positive pressure, interrupting therapy and coaching an extended inhalation phase was thought to reduce risk.[21]

Decreased work of breathing is frequently listed as a physiologic justification for I.P.P.B. The machine pressure and flowing gases are visualized as replacing the muscles of ventilation, allowing them to rest as long as the patient is cooperative physiologically and psychologically. Any patient with a disease that results in increased work of breathing, thus, at least theoretically, may benefit from I.P.P.B. However, when the treatment ends, so does the reduction in work of breathing.

The effectiveness of IPPB therapy is highly dependent upon the practitioner's ability to help the patient understand the objectives of the care plan, the operation of the equipment, and how he should functionally interact with the machine.[15] The effectiveness of the therapy is measured by patient performance against the standard as instructed and coached. Words of wisdom must be accurately understood by a functionally capable patient before directed actions are performed. Therefore, full patient participation in therapy requires: (1) a conscious patient capable of understanding oral and/or written direction; (2) a psychologically stable patient under reasonable emotional control; and (3) a patient capable of coordinated interaction with the respiratory equipment by instruction and/or coaching.

Periodic evaluation visits after the training period are essential to measure compliance and correct lapses in memory or the development of bad habits. Some institutions *never* allow patient administration of IPPB equipment in the hospital setting.

The coachable patient, with the assistance of IPPB, may be capable of altering his inspiratory-expiratory ratio to achieve physiologic benefit. The benefit of such "normalized" I:E ratios in diseased patients frequently ends with the IPPB treatment, but may be helpful in reprogramming the patient on an extended or permanent basis.

In the absence of voluntary splinting of the chest wall with the associated decrease in compliance, IPPB may increase tidal volumes over those in spontaneously breathing patients.[5] This, when seen, is due to a greater change in transpulmonary pressure with IPPB as opposed to spontaneous breathing. The increase in tidal volume lasts only as long as the therapy is applied. Voluntary splinting of the chest wall decreases compliance, decreases the transpulmonary pressure gradient, and limits the volume increase with increasing pressure. It has been shown that while IPPB increases the transpulmonary pres-

sure gradient 109% over spontaneous breathing, incentive spirometry resulted in a 183% increase in the transpulmonary pressure gradient and proportional increase in tidal volume.[11]

These responses to instruction and coaching with incentive spirometry depend on the neuromuscular health of the patient, freedom from restrictive pulmonary disease, and the ability of the patient to understand, coordinate, and cooperate in coached deep breathing. One cannot expect a partially sedated patient to perform either IPPB or incentive spirometry to the levels quantified above.

QUESTIONABLE THERAPEUTIC OBJECTIVES

The following is a list of therapeutic objectives frequently mentioned in the literature for IPPB:[7]

1. Improve cough.
2. Mobilize secretions.
3. Decrease the work.
4. Improve the distribution and deposition of aerosols.
5. Prevent atelectasis.
6. Treat atelectasis.
7. Improve ventilatory pattern.
8. Treat acute pulmonary edema.
9. Decrease Pa_{CO_2}.

Support for achievement of these objectives in the research literature is mixed and at times contradictory. One should review this literature with a critical eye, being prepared to carefully evaluate the methods, results, and conclusions of past, current, and forthcoming research attempting to determine the scientific basis for IPPB. Controls such as equipment, patient education, and performance must be held constant. Variables must be limited. One must not confuse the responses of chronically ill pulmonary patients in the home-outpatient setting with those of the acutely ill. Volume-oriented IPPB should not be confused with maximum volume IPPB. Clinicians must sort out collateral pathophysiology for serial pathophysiology. IPPB is all but dead in many hospitals across America. Perhaps it deserves extinction. Equally compelling is the possibility that the machine is good but its application has been faulty.

IPPB is a costly alternative to coached deep breathing and cough, incentive spirometry, postural drainage, and chest physical therapy. Where the favorable results can be achieved by these less costly modes of care, we are obligated to do so.[8]

The cardinal indication for IPPB is inability to inspire adequately. The "pneumatic power" of the ventilator, theoretically at least, compensates for a variety of human failures. This inability must be measured by both (1) vital capacity (VC) below 15 ml/kg, and (2) IPPB tidal volume delivered must exceed 75% of the deficient VC.[21]

METHODS OF ATTACHMENT

The IPPB machine is connected to the patient by way of a breathing circuit (permanent or disposable) and attached by transparent mask, straight mouthpiece, or mouthpiece with a broad lip flange called a mouth seal. Mouthpieces are frequently used with nose clips if the patient cannot control volume loss during inspiration through closure of the posterior nares. Occasionally IPPB is administered to a patient via tracheostomy tube, and suitable adapters must be used. Clear plastic masks are specified so that the practitioner can visualize the mouth and nose and quickly terminate the treatment if the patient should vomit or expectorate.

A good seal is essential for full inflation. If the patient wears dentures, the seal is more easily accomplished if they are in place. The use of gauze pads under the mask over facial depressions can help attain a seal. Head straps were used in the past to attach the mask to the patient's head. These frequently were very uncomfortable, difficult to use, and dangerous if vomiting occurred. Straps also allowed the practitioner to move physically away from the fragile patient, and this resulted, at times, in decreased coaching and evaluation.

TREATMENT PROTOCOL

The following steps should be followed in performing IPPB therapy:

1. Appropriately sterilized IPPB machine, breathing circuit, and adjunctive equipment should be assembled and tested *outside* of the patient's room. Masks and mouthpieces should be kept in sealed containers until the therapy begins.

2. The patient should be identified, and his chart, x-rays, and orders reviewed.

3. The objectives of the therapy, procedures, and the need for cooperation should be explained to the patient in simple terms.

4. The following parameters must be measured and/or evaluated prior to therapy:

- Tidal volume.
- Vital capacity: below 15 ml/kg.
- Physical examination of the chest.
- Vital signs (pulse rate, blood pressure, respiratory rate).

5. The patient should be positioned either sitting upright in an armchair or lying in a semi-Fowler's position. Children may be held on the practitioner's lap with the child's back against the practitioner's chest.

6. Equipment should be set to maximum sensitivity without self-cycling (negative 1 to 2 cm H_2O pressure), the peak pressure set, initially, between 10 and 15 cm H_2O and peak flow at as low settings as patient can comfortably tolerate.

7. In-line ultrasonic machines should be articulated with the IPPB circuitry.

8. Pharmacologic agents or normal saline should be placed in the medication nebulizer or in the ultrasonic cup according to protocol.

9. Before connecting the mask or mouthpiece to the IPPB tubing circuit, the first-time patient should be allowed to apply the appliance to his mouth so that he may get accustomed to the contact.

10. The mask/mouthpiece is then attached to the circuit. With the machine in the passive (expiratory) mode, the patient is asked to breathe normally. The machine should switch to the positive pressure inspiratory mode with the next patient inhalation. The machine automatically changes to the expiratory mode when the preset peak pressure is reached. If inspiratory flow continues after the patient spontaneously exhales, the following should be looked for:

- Air leak through nose, around mouthpiece, or mask.
- Disconnected or perforated expiratory valve tubing.
- Defective expiratory mushroom valve or valve housing.
- Holes in large bore circuit tubing.

11. Peak pressure settings—techniques and outcomes.

- The IPPB tidal volume must exceed 75% of the limited vital capacity. Otherwise, consult with

the patient's physician relative to alternatives.
- Volume-oriented IPPB:
  Prescribed volume = 3–4 ml × ideal body
  $$\text{weight (lb)}$$
  $$= 10 \text{ ml} \times \text{weight (kg)}[19]$$
- Maximum volume IPPB (Table 8–1)
  —Measure inspiratory capacity (IC).
  —Inspiratory pressure is slowly increased until inspiratory capacity is reached (usually 35–45 cm H_2O).
  —10 deep, high-pressure breaths repeated 3 to 4 times per treatment (rest 1 to 2 minutes between sets)—every 2 hours during day; less at night.
- Old method: peak pressure slowly elevated to between 15 to 20 cm H_2O or to prescribed peak pressure limit (tidal volume varies with compliance).[17]

12. Therapy is continued for duration specified on the prescription.

13. The patient is directed to avoid premature termination of the inspiratory cycle by voluntary splinting of the chest wall or closure of the epiglottis or placing the tongue over mouthpiece orifice.

14. The patient is coached to pause at the end inspiration for a 1- to 2-second inspiratory hold or plateau. (This provides for better distribution of gases.)

15. Vital signs are monitored at least once during the treatment period.

16. The mask/mouthpiece or tracheal tube adapter is removed for coughing, expectoration, or suctioning. Splinting with hands or towel may be necessary to control pain over fractures, wounds, and surgical incisions.

17. If the patient experiences anxiety or pain, the therapy is terminated and the physician is consulted.

18. When the treatment period is over, the equipment is removed, vital signs are again monitored, and the chest is auscultated. Deep breathing and coughing instruction is repeated.

19. The circuit and mask/mouthpiece are placed in appropriate plastic bags, labeled, and stored in appropriate cabinets.

20. The patient is encouraged to deep breathe and cough as much as possible between treatments.

21. Inquiry is made about any pain or discomfort experienced during the treatment. The record of therapy and patient response is charted. This report should include:

- Duration of therapy.
- Peak pressure used.
- Volume achieved/maintained if significant to protocol.
- Medication, dilution, and volume delivered.
- Sputum production volume, color, texture, smell.
- Patient's response to therapy, including vital signs.
- Additional information, special needs, equipment problems.

HAZARDS ASSOCIATED WITH IPPB THERAPY[20, 21, 22]

The Impact of Increased Intrathoracic Pressure

The return of blood from the body to the vena cavae and right ventricle is facilitated by blood under positive venous pressure flowing into a box-like structure with subatmospheric pressure. The increased transmural pressure gradient in the thorax

TABLE 8–1.

Volume Measurements and Arterial Blood Gases in Patients Receiving Maximum Volume IPPB

CATEGORY	PATIENT 1	PATIENT 2	PATIENT 3	PATIENT 4
Tidal volume, ml	515	425	490	330
Respiratory rate, breaths/min	18	22	20	35
Inspiratory capacity, ml	1,075	765	1,160	545
IPPB inspiratory volume, ml	1,635	1,370	1,850	1,155
Pa_{O_2} before IPPB, mm Hg	56 (4 L/min)†	61 (FI_{O_2} 0.40)‡	54 (2 L/min)†	49 (FI_{O_2} 0.60)
Pa_{CO_2} before IPPB, mm Hg	31	34	41	28
Pa_{O_2} after IPPB, mm Hg	85 (3 L/min)†	76 (FI_{O_2} 0.35)‡	81 (2 L/min)†	96 (4 L/min)†
Pa_{CO_2} after IPPB, mm Hg	35	32	39	34

*From O'Donahue WJ, Jr: Maximum IPPB for the management of pulmonary atelectasis. *Chest* 1979; 76:6.
†Oxygen by nasal cannula.
‡Oxygen by mask.

tends to dilate the vessels and chambers, thereby increasing the flow to and through the chest. Cyclical elevation of the intrapleural and intrathoracic pressure above atmospheric pressure during IPPB-assisted inspiration is pneumatically the opposite of normal spontaneous inspiration. The so-called thoracic pump, functional in the spontaneously breathing person, is subverted by excessively high intrapleural pressures caused by reversed transpulmonary pressure gradients.

Blood flows into the thorax and heart according to the venous gradient (VG). The larger the VG, the greater the flow. The following calculations will clearly illustrate the opposite effect IPPB has on the venous gradient and venous return.[11]

EXPIRATION

Central venous pressure	$+15$ cm H_2O
Intrapleural pressure	$-\ \ 4$ cm H_2O
Venous gradient	19 cm H_2O

NORMAL INSPIRATION

Central venous pressure	$+15$ cm H_2O
Intrapleural pressure	-10 cm H_2O
Venous gradient	25 cm H_2O

IPPB INSPIRATION (20 cm H_2O)

Central venous pressure	$+15$ cm H_2O
Intrapleural pressure	$+10$ cm H_2O
Venous gradient	5 cm H_2O

Therefore, the higher the IPPB peak pressure, the higher the transpulmonary pressure gradient and the higher the intrapleural pressure. When the intrapleural pressure meets or exceeds the venous pressure, the great veins will collapse and halt venous return until the intrapleural pressure falls and a positive gradient is once again established. Given the fact that Central Venous Pressure (CVP) has a normal range of 5 to 15 cm H_2O pressure, the thoracic pump mechanism may be interfered with at pressures less than the example (IPPB inspiration, 20 cm H_2O), given above.

Any time the CVP is lowered, the patient receiving IPPB comes under greater risk. Since we rarely have the luxury of a CVP catheter in place, the adequacy of venous return must be indirectly measured by looking for tachycardia as a response to decreased left ventricular filling and decreased blood pressure due to decreased cardiac output.[22]

Dizziness and headache during IPPB may be related to profound hemodynamic alteration and are not necessarily psychosomatic. Decreased venous return may result in increased intracranial pressure and cause these and other neurologic signs and symptoms.

Measuring vital signs *before*, *during*, and *after* IPPB therapy will help the therapist understand the full physiologic impact of his therapy. Termination of therapy and resting the patient should allow vital signs to return to normal, if caused by pneumatic effects on hemodynamics. Persistent tachycardia, however, may be the result of aerosolized drugs administered. Any increase in heart rate of 20 or more over pretherapy levels should prompt termination of therapy and discussion with the patient's physician.

Hyperventilation and Respiratory Alkalosis[23]

The effects of acute alveolar hyperventilation are the same whether mitigated by spontaneous inspiration or IPPB inspiration. Breathing is generally easier with IPPB equipment and tidal volumes are generally larger. Add an anxiety factor to this and one can readily see the potential for increasing minute ventilation leading to decreased arterial P_{CO_2}. This, in time, may cause dizziness and/or fainting, tetany, and paresthesias. The careful therapist should be looking for these side effects and be prepared to rest the patient until symptoms disappear. Coaching, monitoring, or education should prevent hyperventilation from occurring in the first place.

Effects on Hypoxic Drive[10]

Patients with chronic lung disease who have inadequate minute ventilation may eventually retain so much carbon dioxide that the stimulation for ventilation shifts from elevated Pa_{CO_2} to decreased Pa_{O_2}. This "hypoxic drive" condition may be subverted and apnea induced by supplemental oxygen administered by pneumatic IPPB supported inspiration. Even on air dilution, these devices deliver mixtures containing over 40% oxygen. Blood gases should always be reviewed prior to commencing therapy on a chronically diseased patient. Values like the following should forewarn hypoxic drive potential:

$Pa_{CO_2} > 50$ mm Hg
$Pa_{O_2} < 60$ mm Hg
Compensated pH $(7.35 - 7.40)$

Gastric Insufflation

IPPB can cause a sometimes serious gastric problem when part of the volume delivered by the machine finds its way into the stomach. This is possible because IPPB therapy is usually delivered to the oropharynx and both the larynx and the esophagus receive equal pressure exposures. If the peak pressure is greater than the opening pressure of the esophagus, variable volumes may enter the stomach, causing discomfort, pain, belching, and vomiting. Of these, vomiting is chronically the most hazardous, for if the vomitus with its low pH is aspirated into the lungs, serious pneumonitis may result.

Air in the stomach may also interfere with downward excursion of the hemi-diaphragms, thereby decreasing inspiratory volumes. The patient with gastric insufflation should be removed from the therapy and the condition resolved before going on at a lower peak pressure, if possible.

Pneumothorax

Pneumothorax is a potentially life-threatening condition that may occur secondary to IPPB therapy. Weakened areas of the lung, blebs, and bullae, may become hyperinflated and rupture from high machine pressure or trapped air and coughing. Sharp chest pain is the primary symptom of pneumothorax. Therefore, chest pain should always be carefully evaluated by the physician and practitioner. Application of IPPB to a pneumothorax can lead to higher than atmospheric pressures in the pleural space and tension pneumothorax. This, in time, can lead to mediastinal shift, cardiac tamponade, and compression of the healthy lung.

Hemoptysis

The expectoration of blood during or after an IPPB (or any other) treatment is always dramatic and upsetting for all involved. The blood may be related to a variety of conditions, minor or serious, and should be discussed immediately with the physician. Continuing IPPB with hemoptysis may force air into the bloodstream and cause an air embolism.

Dehydrated Sputum

Pneumatically driven IPPB mechanisms in the 100% O_2 mode are driven by perfectly dry gas. Unless steps are taken to humidify the gas, the patient's secretions will become dehydrated and thick. This should never happen with an informed patient and family. Even on the air dilution setting, dry air/oxygen is mixing with ambient air that may not contain adequate water to prevent inspissation of secre-

tions. The patient must be reminded about the relationship between fluid intake and secretion viscosity.

Drug Reactions

Agents administered to the lungs by way of aerosolization and IPPB may cause a variety of side effects both troublesome and dangerous. The most serious is anaphylaxis. Other difficulties include cough, tachycardia, bronchospasm, hypotension, and dermatitis. Even sterile distilled water may prompt strong asthma-like reactions in some patients. Negative side effects must be recognized early and therapy discontinued until discussed with the physician.

Cross-Infection

IPPB equipment has long been implicated as a source of nosocomial infection. Contaminated equipment and circuits can blow aerosolized microorganisms into the patient's lungs and cause infection. Breathing circuits should be changed every 24 hours and should *never* be shared with other patients. Appropriate filters should be used to prevent machinery contamination and gas source contamination from getting into the patient's breathing circuit.

SUMMARY OF CONTRAINDICATIONS[8]

Absolute Contraindications

1. Tension pneumothorax *without* chest tube.
2. Massive pulmonary hemorrhage.

Relative Contraindications

1. Active tuberculosis.
2. Needle biopsy within 24 hours.
3. Hyperventilation.
4. COPD with air-trapping.
5. Decreased cardiac output.
6. Hypovolemia.
7. Intracranial injury with elevated pressure.
8. Angina exacerbated by IPPB-tamponade effect.
9. Uncooperative or combative patient.

IPPB is a costly potentially hazardous form of respiratory therapy.[2, 6] The patient capable of adequate spontaneous ventilation is not a candidate for this mode of therapy.[1, 13] The future of IPPB hopefully lies in the truth found in quality scientific research and not in the most current opinion expressed in a letter to the editor. Many physicians and respiratory care practitioners continue to feel that IPPB is at times important in the successful resolution of a challenging case.[16] This empirical base is reason enough to continue to question, appropriately use, and monitor this form of therapy in the clinical setting.

REFERENCES

1. Ali J, Serrette C, Wood LD, et al: Effects of postoperative intermittent positive-pressure breathing on lung function. *Chest* 1984; 85:192–196.
2. Baker JP: Magnitude of usage of intermittent positive pressure breathing. *Ann Intern Med* 1983; 99:170–177.
3. Barach AL, Segal MS: The indiscriminate use of IPPB. *JAMA* 1975; 231:11.
4. Brewer LA: A historical account of the "wet lung trauma" and the introduction of intermittent positive pressure oxygen therapy in World War II. *Ann Thorac Surg* 1981; 4:386–389.
5. Cheney FW, Nelson EJ, Horton W: Function of intermittent positive pressure breathing related to breathing patterns. *Am Rev Respir Dis* 1974; 110:183–187.
6. Emory WB: Intermittent positive-pressure breathing: Good medicine or gadgetry? *J MSMA* 1976; 17:295–297.
7. Eubanks DH, Bone RC: *Comprehensive Respiratory Care.* St Louis, CV Mosby Co, 1985.
8. Fouts JB, Brashear RE: Intermittent positive-pressure breathing—a critical appraisal. *Postgrad Med* 1976; 59:5.
9. Intermittent Positive Pressure Breathing Trial Group: Intermittent positive pressure breathing therapy of chronic obstructive pulmonary diseases: A clinical trial. *Ann Intern Med* 1983; 99:612.
10. Israel RH, Poe RH: Insidious onset of acute alveolar hypoventilation following intermittent positive-pressure breathing. *Respiration* 1981; 41:199–201.
11. McConnell DH, Maloney JV, Buckberg GD: Postoperative intermittent positive-pressure breathing treatments: Physiologic considerations. *J Thorac Cardiovasc Surg* 1974; 68:944–952.
12. Motley HL, Werko L, Cournand A, et al: Observations on the clinical use of intermittent positive pressure. *J Aviation Med* 1947; 18:417.
13. Murray JF: Review of the state of the art in intermittent positive-pressure breathing therapy. *Am Rev Respir Dis* 1974; 110:6.
14. Murray JF: Indications for mechanical aids to assist lung inflation in medical patients. *Am Rev Respir Dis* 1980; 122:121.
15. Noehren TH: Indications for I.P.P.B. *Respir Care* 1976; 21:717–723.
16. Noehren TH, Klauber MR: Controversy over intermittent positive-pressure breathing. *Chest* 1978; 73:282–283.
17. O'Donohue WJ Jr: Maximum volume IPPB for the management of pulmonary atelectasis. *Chest* 1979; 76:6.
18. Pierce AK (ed): Conference on the scientific basis of respiratory therapy. Temple University Conference at Sugarloaf, Pennsylvania. *Am Rev Respir Dis* 1974; 110.
19. Rarey KP, Youtsey JW: *Respiratory Patient Care.* Englewood Cliffs, NJ, Prentice-Hall Inc, 1981.
20. Rau J, Rau M: To breathe or be breathed: Understanding IPPB. *Am J Nursing* 1977; 77:4.
21. Shapiro B, Harrison R, Trout C: *Clinical Applications of Respiratory Care.* Chicago, Year Book Medical Publishers, 1983.
22. West JB: *Pulmonary Pathophysiology—The Essentials.* Baltimore, Williams & Wilkins Co, 1978.
23. West JB: *Respiratory Physiology—The Essentials.* Baltimore, Williams & Wilkins Co, 1974.

Incentive Spirometry and Other Aids to Lung Inflation

F. Herbert Douce, M.S., R.R.T.

Expiratory resistance breathing and "blow-bottles" were once routinely used to prevent and reverse atelectasis, but these expiratory techniques may decrease transpulmonary pressure and functional residual capacity, and commonly have been replaced by inspiratory techniques.[6, 13, 17] In addition to intermittently applying positive pressure to the airway, there are other lung inflation techniques that share the primary therapeutic goal of preventing and reversing atelectasis. These techniques include incentive spirometry, which is also known as incentive breathing or sustained maximal inspiration (SMI), the periodic use of continuous positive-airway pressure (CPAP), and periodically inspiring increased concentration of carbon dioxide.[43] The purpose of each of these techniques is to reinflate collapsed alveoli by increasing the transpulmonary pressure and functional residual capacity (FRC). This chapter addresses the etiology of atelectasis and the physiologic rationale of spontaneous deep breathing for the correction of atelectasis. In addition, recommendations for determining therapeutic appropriateness, procedural steps, and effectiveness of incentive breathing therapy are discussed.

ETIOLOGY AND PATHOPHYSIOLOGY OF ATELECTASIS

Incentive spirometry and other techniques that aid lung inflation are primarily performed to prevent and reverse alveolar collapse or atelectasis. Many factors have been implicated in the etiology of at-

electasis, especially for surgical patients (Fig 9–1). Preoperatively, patients with advanced age,[45] a smoking history,[11, 31 36] obesity,[31, 40] general debilitation or malnutrition,[26] concurrent infection,[26] and underlying cardiovascular and pulmonary diseases[49] have been identified as being at risk for developing postoperative pulmonary complications, including atelectasis. Patients with these characteristics may be at further risk for developing atelectasis if they receive general anesthesia,[42] if the surgical procedure involves the thoracic cage or upper abdominal musculature,[2, 24, 35, 45] or if their respiratory tract is dehydrated.[54]

Patients with some of these characteristics may objectively demonstrate their predisposition to develop postoperative atelectasis and pneumonitis if their lung mechanics are measured preoperatively by spirometry. Patients may be classified as "at risk" or "at high risk" for developing postoperative pulmonary complications as a result of their preoperative spirometry (Table 9–1).[26, 49]

There are two primary pathological factors implicated in the etiology of atelectasis: airway obstruction and an altered sigh mechanism. When retained secretions, mucosal edema, bronchospasm, or a mechanical obstruction occlude an airway, the pulmonary perfusion to the affected alveoli does not immediately cease. Alveolar collapse occurs when the gases trapped distally to the occluded airway transfer to the pulmonary blood. The rate of alveolar collapse is related to the partial pressures of the trapped gases with increased rates of reabsorption and collapse for higher oxygen tensions.[15] This

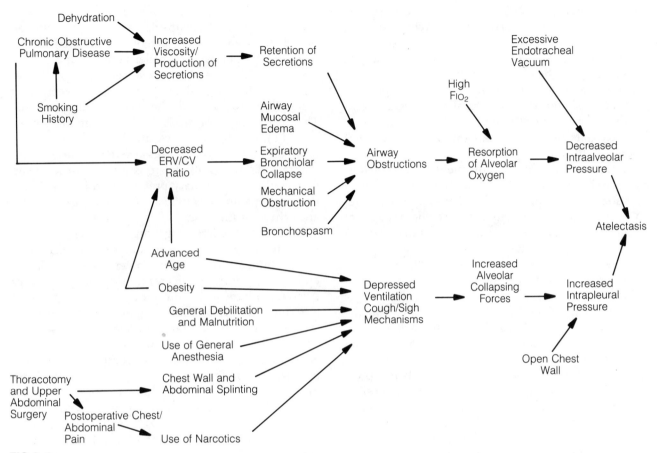

FIG 9–1.
Conditions and mechanisms contributing to the development of atelectasis.

mechanism is commonly known as absorption atelectasis, and may occur more frequently when supplemental oxygen is administered to patients who have retained secretions and airway obstruction.

A postoperative decrease in expiratory reserve volume (ERV) in relation to the closing volume (CV) may predispose patients to bronchiolar collapse and atelectasis.[4, 10] When the CV exceeds the ERV, airways close during normal tidal breathing, and atelectasis can occur, probably through the absorption mechanism. Obese patients have a decrease in ERV

related to their weight.[37] An increased CV has been associated with advanced age and with a smoking history.[4, 33] Patients with chronic obstructive airway disease may have a decreased ERV and an increased CV.[10] The ERV/CV ratio may explain why patients who are obese, advanced in age, smoke, and who have chronic airway obstruction are at risk for developing atelectasis postoperatively.

A sigh is an involuntary, slow, deep breath with an end-inspiratory pause which opens collapsed alveoli by increasing the transpulmonary pressure.[14] Beginning at the functional residual capacity (FRC), the volume of a sigh breath approximates the inspiratory capacity (IC), and the lung volume during the postinspiratory pause approximates the total lung capacity (TLC). Normally, we sigh approximately 10 times each hour.[8] An altered sigh mechanism produces a breathing pattern that can be observed as shallow, rapid tidal volumes with fewer periodic deep breaths than normal.[22, 34, 38] The monotonous breathing pattern may begin intraoperatively if periodic sigh breaths are not provided for the patient

TABLE 9–1.

Spirometric Indicators of Risk and High Risk for Postoperative Pulmonary Complications

MEASUREMENT	AT RISK	AT HIGH RISK
FVC	<50% predicted	<1.5 L
FEV$_1$	<50% predicted	<1.0 L
FEV$_1$	<2.0 L	
FEV$_1$/FVC	<50%	<35%
FEF$_{25\%-75\%}$	<50% predicted	
MVV		<50% predicted

under general anesthesia or neuromuscular paralysis. In addition to the preoperative factors, postoperative pain and restrictive bandages may contribute to the development of the monotonous breathing pattern due to chest wall splinting and immobility. Narcotics used for the treatment of postoperative pain may also depress the natural sigh mechanism.[20]

In the absence of the sigh breath, the number of adjacent collapsed alveoli can increase to the point where air flow to an entire ancinus is reduced or even eliminated.[3] Ciliary movement, which is normally assisted by expiratory air flow, by itself may be inadequate to propel lower respiratory tract secretions, and these secretions may become a stagnant bacteriologic media. These mechanisms help explain the development of atelectasis and pneumonitis and the interrelationship of these two conditions which are often termed postoperative pulmonary complications.

Other clinical factors that can contribute to the development of atelectasis include thoracic trauma, excessive endotracheal suctioning, and breathing high concentrations of oxygen.[14, 15, 17] When an opening in the chest wall occurs, the pleural pressure becomes atmospheric and the transpulmonary pressure is decreased because the force of thoracic expansion no longer opposes the force of lung collapse. Depending on the size of the opening, massive atelectasis or whole lung collapse can occur. When endotracheal suctioning is performed with an excessive amount of vacuum or for an excessive amount of time, or with a catheter that is too large, the intrapulmonary pressure may be reduced as the FRC is aspirated, and atelectasis will develop. Strict adherence to proper technique and hyperinflation after each suctioning procedure should minimize this etiology of atelectasis.[18]

The law of Laplace ($P = ST/r$) may also help explain the development of atelectasis. The periodic expansion of an alveolus may stimulate the alveolar type II cell to secrete surfactant by moving the lamellar bodies to the cell membrane for exocytosis of surfactant.[39] Therefore, in the absence of periodic expansion, surfactant production may be decreased, and surface tension slowly increases as the existing surfactant becomes deactivated. When the volume and the radius of an alveolus are not periodically increased by inhalation and as the force of surface tension slowly increases, the recoil pressure of the alveolus increases to the point when the air is expelled and the alveolus collapses. Periodically inflating an alveolus, by inhaling a tidal volume or a sigh, increases the volume and radius of the alveolus and stimulates surfactant secretion; as a result, the surface tension and collapsing pressure remain reduced. Of course, more alveoli are affected by the sigh breath than by the smaller tidal volume.[14]

The pathophysiology of atelectasis can be described in terms of the relationship between lung distending pressure and the resultant lung volume. The distending pressure is the transpulmonary pressure (PL), which is the pressure difference across the lung, or intrapulmonary pressure (Palv) minus intrapleural pressure (Ppl). There is a direct relationship between transpulmonary pressure and lung volume; the relationship is nonlinear, following the compliance curve of the lung.[17]

In general, decreasing transpulmonary pressure promotes lung and alveolar collapse and increasing transpulmonary pressure promotes alveolar inflation and expansion.[17] A decrease in transpulmonary pressure occurs when the intrapulmonary pressure is reduced or when the intrapleural pressure is increased. An increase in transpulmonary pressure occurs when intrapulmonary pressure is increased or when intrapleural pressure is reduced. When the opposing recoil forces of the lung and chest wall are in equilibrium, the intrapulmonary pressure is atmospheric (0 cm H_2O) and the mean intrapleural pressure is normally 5 cm H_2O below atmospheric (-5 cm H_2O). The resultant transpulmonary pressure is 5 cm H_2O, and the lung volume is the FRC. At the end of a spontaneous, maximal inspiration as the contracted inspiratory muscles counteract the recoil forces of the lung and chest wall, the intrapulmonary pressure remains atmospheric, and the mean intrapleural pressure can vary from 32 cm H_2O to 40 cm H_2O below atmospheric. The variations in intrapleural pressures are due to the vertical pressure gradient of the lung; the more subatmospheric pressures occur at the lung apex. After a full spontaneous inspiration, the resultant mean transpulmonary pressure can exceed the alveolar critical opening pressure of 7 to 20 cm H_2O when surfactant is present, and collapsed alveoli become reinflated (Fig 9–2).[41]

MANIFESTATIONS OF ATELECTASIS: INDICATIONS FOR INCENTIVE SPIROMETRY

There are several manifestations of atelectasis. The characteristics of atelectasis on chest x-ray include diminished lung volume with displaced interlobar fissures, increased radiopacity, vascular or

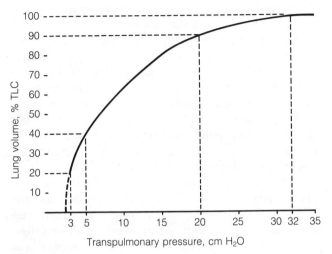

FIG 9–2.
The relationship of transpulmonary pressure and lung volume.
(Adapted from Comroe JH: *Physiology of Respiration.* Chicago,
Year Book Medical Publishers, 1974.)

bronchial crowding, and hilar displacement.[21] A low-grade fever is sometimes associated with the pneumonitis that may accompany atelectasis.[30] Patients with massive atelectasis may occasionally complain of chest pain as the parietal and visceral pleura separate. If atelectasis is unilateral, there may be a shift of the mediastinum toward the atelectatic lung, the chest overlying the affected lung may be less distensible, and chest movement may be diminished. Percussion sounds may be dull and tactile fremitus and breath sounds may be diminished or absent (Table 9–2).[52]

The physiological manifestations of atelectasis include a reduced lung compliance with a resultant increase in the work of breathing, a decreased FRC with resultant ventilation-perfusion mismatch, an increased physiologic shunt, and a decrease in arterial oxygen tension.[12] Periodic sigh breaths are presumed to reinflate collapsed alveoli and keep pul-

monary compliance, work of breathing and the physiologic shunt within their normal ranges (see Table 9–2).[3]

The factors implicated in the etiology of atelectasis and the characteristics of patients who are predisposed to develop atelectasis serve as indications for incentive breathing therapy when preventing atelectasis is the primary goal. The continuing absence of the clinical and physiological manifestations of atelectasis indicates that prevention was successful. The clinical and physiological manifestations of atelectasis serve as indications for incentive breathing therapy when treating and reversing atelectasis are the primary goals. The therapeutic goals for incentive breathing therapy are to increase FRC, lung compliance, and arterial oxygen tension, and to decrease the work of breathing, physiologic shunt, and fever associated with accompanying pneumonitis.[30] Increasing lung volume as seen on chest x-ray, reducing radiopacity, and increasing breath sounds in the affected lung segment are also important therapeutic goals.

CLINICAL APPLICATIONS

The ideal maneuver to reinflate collapsed alveoli would achieve and maintain the greatest transpulmonary pressure; clinically, the inspired volume is the critical measurement.[6, 17] A maximal inspiration produces the greatest transpulmonary pressure, and the postinspiratory pause that maintains the pressure has been associated with increases in arterial oxygen tensions presumably by recruiting alveoli and reducing the percent physiologic shunt.[51] Once inflated, normal alveoli remain inflated for approximately 1 hour.[3, 22] Consequently, the therapeutic objective of each treatment is to achieve and maintain the greatest transpulmonary pressure by inspiring the IC, and patients should perform sustained maximal inspirations (SMI) at least hourly for maximum benefits. During the incentive breathing session, the therapist should motivate and encourage the patient to mimic sigh breaths. From the resting position of the FRC, the patient should inspire slowly, as deeply as possible, with a postinspiratory pause of 3 to 5 seconds. The general procedural steps for incentive breathing therapy are listed in Table 9–3.

Incentive breathing therapy incorporates a device called an incentive spirometer or incentive breathing exerciser. These devices provide visual feedback and evidence that a volume is being inspired and held. These devices are designed to mo-

TABLE 9–2.
The Clinical and Physiological Signs Associated With
Atelectasis

CLINICAL SIGNS	PHYSIOLOGICAL SIGNS
Positive chest x-ray	Reduced lung compliance
Fever, with pneumonitis	Increased work of breathing
Chest pain, if massive	Decreased FRC
Mediastinal shift, if unilateral	$\dot{V}/\dot{Q}$ mismatch
Decreased chest expansion	Increased Q_S/Q_T
Dull percussion note	Decreased Pa_{O_2}
Diminished breath sounds and tactile fremitus	

TABLE 9–3.

Procedural Steps for Incentive Breathing Therapy

Preparation
1. Verify and interpret the medical prescription
2. Review the medical record to confirm/formulate therapeutic goals
3. Wash your hands
4. Select, gather, assemble, and test the incentive breathing device
5. Identify the patient; introduce yourself
6. Explain the purpose and methodology of the procedure; confirm the patient's understanding and cooperation

Implementation
1. Place the patient in a semi-Fowler's position; assure patient comfort/safety
2. Place the incentive breathing device in position for proper functioning
3. Set the volume level of the device above the previous level of patient achievement or at maximal level if preoperative
4. Compare the maximal inspired volume to the preoperative or predicted IC or to the positive pressure breath; formulate a therapeutic objective
5. Readjust the volume level of the device to match the current patient achievement
6. Observe the patient performance/condition; verbally coach the patient to inspire a set volume level and breath-hold; reinforce the achievement
7. Readjust the volume level according to patient achievement and assessment of strength/effort
8. Repeat the SMI at least 10 times; provide rest periods between SMI
9. Terminate the treatment if adverse reaction occurs

Completion
1. Provide the patient instruction for unsupervised use of incentive device
2. Evaluate patient progress; document pertinent data in medical and departmental records
3. Notify appropriate health team members of adverse reaction, if any

tivate patients to inspire as deeply as possible and to hold their breath. The operation and mechanisms of these devices are discussed in Chapter 15. Candidates for incentive breathing therapy must be alert and conscious with the ability and desire to follow instructions; they should have eyesight which is adequate to see the device and watch it function. Children under the age of 4 years are generally not able to perform incentive breathing therapy. The ability of the therapist to motivate the patient and actively coach each SMI cannot be overemphasized. The effectiveness of incentive breathing therapy may be as dependent on the therapist as the frequency of SMI and the incentive device.

It is common and preferable to teach patients how to perform SMI preoperatively, so that therapy can begin as early as possible following recovery from anesthesia. When performed preoperatively, the initial session provides the therapist with an opportunity to measure the inspiratory capacity which is used as the therapeutic objective to be reached postoperatively. In the absence of a preoperative measurement of the IC, predicting the normal IC is a suitable substitute. No specific regression equations have been developed to predict the normal inspiratory capacity, but several equations have been developed to predict normal TLC and FRC.[25, 34] The predicted normal IC would be the difference between the predicted normal TLC and FRC.

The efficacy of incentive breathing therapy has been studied by several investigators, but the frequency of performing SMI during a treatment session has not been well documented by all investigators. In a randomized study of 150 patients who underwent laparotomy, Bartlett reported that patients who used an incentive spirometer ten times hourly while awake had 9% postoperative pulmonary complications and 32% had chest x-rays that were positive for atelectasis.[7] Craven instructed his post-upper-abdominal surgery patients to perform SMI ten times each hour for 5 days; he reported that 37% had positive chest x-rays for atelectasis and 46% had complications; compliance with his instructions was not confirmed.[16] In a sample of 15 patients, Van de Water reported 20% postoperative pulmonary complications following bilateral adrenalectomy and hourly incentive breathing therapy; the number of sustained maximal inspirations was not reported.[50] Dohi reported 29% pulmonary complications and 26% positive chest x-rays following abdominal surgery and hourly incentive breathing; the number of SMI performed each hour and the volumes inspired were not reported and apparently not controlled.[19] The incidence of postoperative complications has been reported by Lyager as low as 4.7% when incentive breathing and chest physical therapy, which included modified postural drainage, percussion and coughing, are combined and performed hourly following laparotomy.[32] Inverson studied the effects of 3 to 5 SMI every 3 hours following thoracotomy and open heart surgery; 15% developed significant pulmonary atelectasis.[28] Gale also studied postoperative cardiac patients and reported 84% abnormal chest radiographs when incentive breathing was used four times daily; his frequency of SMI was not specified.[23] Indihar reported 20% postoperative pulmonary complications after 3 days of performing SMI 15 times in 15-minute periods every 4 hours.[27] Jung reported that 48% of his post-upper-laparotomy patients developed postoperative pulmonary complications after being treated with incentive breathing therapy, but his patients performed an unspecified number of SMI only four times a day.[29]

It is difficult to compare these studies because of differences in the surgical sites, patient groups, definitions of postop complications, and the intensity of the therapy; most reports omit the number of SMI performed and the volume inspired relevant to the preoperative or predicted inspiratory capacity. In virtually every study, incentive breathing reduced postoperative complications in relation to either control or comparison groups if performed at least ten times each hour while awake. Bakow adds "that a minimum of 10 breaths per hour seems to be therapeutic."[5]

Since the introduction of incentive breathing therapy, no documented complications have appeared in the literature, although two potential complications have been suggested.[7, 44, 51] Hyperventilation may occur if the sustained maximal inhalations are performed too rapidly, without rest periods between deep breaths. Patients who experience hyperventilation may develop dizziness, lightheadedness, a tingling sensation in the extremities, and possible muscle tremors. If hyperventilation is suspected, the treatment session should be temporarily terminated to provide a period for carbon dioxide levels to return to normal, and the patient should be reinstructed on proper technique, including emphasis on rest periods between maximal inspirations. A second potential complication is barotrauma resulting in alveolar hyperinflation and rupture. Patients who experience barotrauma may complain of acute chest pain, and depending upon the degree of barotrauma, appropriate health team members should be immediately informed of the patient's adverse response, the treatment session should be terminated, and patient safety should be assured.

Incentive breathing therapy is a normal physiologic maneuver with no documented complications or hazards. It costs less than other procedures with similar therapeutic goals and is the procedure of choice when the inspired volume exceeds the volumes produced by other methods. The recommended hourly frequency and the relative simplicity of incentive breathing therapy make this technique ideally suited for some patients to perform without direct supervision. The following should be monitored at least daily (more frequently for 48 hours postoperatively): preoperative inspiratory capacity; patient understanding and compliance with instructions; setting new volume objectives; and assessment of development of symptoms associated with atelectasis. When a patient demonstrates the ability to inspire 80% of the preoperative inspiratory capacity, there is no longer a need for daily assessments by the therapist. Using a disposable device, unsupervised incentive breathing therapy may continue through convalescence.

At least three types of postoperative respiratory care protocols have evolved for nonintubated patients. In the first type, the inspired volume is compared to the preoperative volume or to the predicted normal inspiratory capacity (IC) when preoperative measurements are lacking. When the postoperative IC is less than 50% of the preoperative or predicted volume, aggressive therapy *may* include IPPB (see Chapter 8), chest physical therapy (see Chapter 7), and endotracheal suctioning. When the postoperative IC is between 50% and 80% of the preoperative or predicted volume, incentive breathing therapy using SMI is utilized. When the postoperative IC is 80% of the preoperative or predicted volume, no postoperative respiratory care is indicated unless manifestations of atelectasis and pulmonary complications are present.

In the second type of protocol, the volume inspired with incentive spirometry is compared to the volume inspired with IPPB at various inflation pressures. When the IPPB volume exceeds the spontaneous volume by 10% or more, IPPB is utilized postoperatively.

The third type of protocol is a combination of the first two types. Comparisons are made between preoperative or predicted IC, postoperative IC, and positive pressure volumes to determine if lung expansion therapy is indicated and which technique would produce the larger inspired volume and transpulmonary pressure (see Fig 9–2).

In a university teaching hospital, Zibrak has shown that when therapists use established protocols to postoperatively evaluate patient progress toward individualized inspiratory volume goals, unnecessary incentive spirometry treatments can be reduced.[53] According to Zibrak, the elimination of unnecessary procedures reduced their hospital costs, length of stay, and the incidence of postoperative pneumonia in high-risk groups. He suggests that therapists concentrate on providing respiratory care to patients at risk for postoperative complications who are unable to achieve inspiratory volume goals.

For nonintubated patients who are unable or unwilling to perform SMI or IPPB, breathing increased concentrations of carbon dioxide has been proposed as a substitute. By adding mechanical-type dead space to the airway, Schwartz and Adler reported that volumes larger than resting tidal volumes are inhaled by *normal* spontaneously breathing subjects.[1, 43] Neither investigator compared the volumes inspired through their rebreathing devices with the IC of their subjects; and it is doubtful that the two volumes would be comparable. Schwartz also demonstrated a decrease in arterial oxygen tension with rebreathing which was reversed with the addition of low-flow oxygen. In patients who are already hypoventilating, rebreathing devices are fraught with danger. Accordingly, rebreathing devices are not commonly used to increase the tidal volumes of patients, since rebreathing could induce a severe respiratory acidosis in patients with CO_2 retention. Carbon dioxide therapy is further discussed in Chapter 5.

Mask CPAP therapy will also increase transpulmonary pressure and lung volumes by increasing the intra-alveolar pressure. The use of mask CPAP seems to reinflate collapsed alveoli and increase arterial oxygen tensions, at least temporarily.[46-48] Mask CPAP also does not require active patient participation and cooperation and has been reported as a successful alternative to incentive breathing. The efficacy of the periodic use of mask CPAP has not been well documented; the continuous use of CPAP is discussed in Chapter 5.[9]

REFERENCES

1. Adler RH: A rebreather for prophylaxis and treatment of postoperative respiratory complications. *Chest* 1967; 52:640–648.
2. Anscombe AR, Buxton R: Effect of abdominal operations on total lung capacity and its subdivisions. *Br Med J* 1958; 2:84.
3. Anthonisen NR: Effect of volume and volume history of the lung on pulmonary shunt flow. *Am J Physiol* 1964; 207:235–238.
4. Anthonisen NR, Danson J, Robertson PC, et al: Airway closure as a function of age. *Respir Physiol* 1969; 8:58.
5. Bakow ED: Sustained maximal inspiration—a rationale for its use. *Respir Care* 1977; 22:379.
6. Bartlett RH, Gazzaniga AB, Geraghty TR: Respiratory maneuvers to prevent postoperative pulmonary complications. *JAMA* 1973; 224:1017.
7. Bartlett R, Krop R, Hanson EL, et al: The physiology of yawning and its application to postoperative care. *Surg Forum* 1970; 21:222–224.
8. Bendixen HH, Smith GM, Mead J: Pattern of ventilation in young adults. *J Appl Physiol* 1964; 19:195–198.
9. Branson RD, Hurst JM, DeHaven CB: Mask CPAP: State of the art. *Respir Care* 1985; 30:846–857.
10. Buist S, Ross B: Predicted values for closing volumes using a modified single breath nitrogen test. *Am Rev Respir Dis* 1973; 107:744.
11. Chalon J, Tayyab JA, Ramanathan S: Cytology of respiratory epithelium as a predictor of respiratory complications after operation. *Chest* 1975; 67:32–35.
12. Cherniack RM, Cherniack L: *Respiration in Health and Disease*. Philadelphia, WB Saunders Co, 1983, p 223.
13. Colgan FJ, Mahoney PD, Fanning GL: Resistance breathing (blow bottles) and sustained hyperinflations in the treatment of atelectasis. *Anesthesiology* 1970; 32:11–18.
14. Comroe JH: *Physiology of Respiration*, ed 2. Chicago, Year Book Medical Publishers, 1974, p 232.
15. Coryloss PN, Birnbaum GL: Studies in pulmonary gas absorption in bronchial obstruction: Behavior and absorption times of oxygen, carbon dioxide, nitrogen, hydrogen, helium, ethylene, nitrous oxide, ethylene chloride and ether in the lung. *Am J Med Sci* 1932; 183:347.
16. Craven JL, Evans GA, Davenport JL, et al: Prevention of postoperative pulmonary complications. *Br J Surg* 1972; 61:793.
17. Demers RR, Saklad M: The etiology, pathology, and treatment of atelectasis. *Respir Care* 1976; 21:234–239.
18. Demers RR, Saklad M: Mechanical aspiration: A reappraisal of its hazards. *Respir Care* 1975; 20:661.
19. Dohi S, Gold MI: Comparison of two methods of postoperative respiratory care. *Chest* 1973; 73:592–595.
20. Egbert LD, Bendixen HH: Effect of morphine on breathing pattern. *JAMA* 1964; 188:485–488.
21. Felson B, Weinstein A, Spitz H: *Principles of Chest Radiology*. Philadelphia, WB Saunders Co, 1965, p 129.
22. Ferris BG, Pollard DS: Effect of deep and quiet breathing on pulmonary compliance in man. *J Clin Invest* 1960; 39:143–151.
23. Gale GD, Saunders DE: The Bartlett-Edwards incentive spirometer: A preliminary assessment of its use in the prevention of atelectasis after cardiopulmonary bypass. *Can Anaesth Soc J* 1977; 24:408.
24. George J, Hornum I, Mellemgard K: The mechanism of hypoxemia after laparotomy. *Thorax* 1966; 22:382.
25. Goldman HI, Becklake MR: Respiratory Function tests: Normal values at median altitudes and the prediction of normal results. *Am Rev Tuberc* 1959; 79:457–467.
26. Hodgkin JE: Preoperative assessment of respiratory function. *Respir Care* 1984; 29:496–503.
27. Indihar FJ, Forsberg DP, Adams AB: A prospective comparison of three procedures used in attempts to prevent postoperative pulmonary complications. *Respir Care* 1982; 27:564.
28. Iverson L, Ecker R, Fox H, et al: A comparative study of IPPB, the incentive spirometer, and blow bottles: The prevention of atelectasis following cardiac surgery. *Ann Thorac Surg* 1978; 25:197–200.
29. Jung R, Wight J, Nusser R, et al: Comparison of three methods of respiratory care following upper abdominal surgery. *Chest* 1980; 78:31–35.

30. Lansing AM, Jamilson WG: Mechanisms of fever in atelectasis. *Arch Surg* 1963; 87:168–171.
31. Lattimer RG, Dickman M, Day WC, et al: Ventilatory patterns and pulmonary complications after upper abdominal surgery determined by preoperative and postoperative computerized spirometry and blood gas analysis. *Am J Surg* 1971; 122:622–628.
32. Lyager S, Wernberg M, Rajani N: Can postoperative pulmonary conditions be improved by treatment with the Bartlett-Edwards incentive spirometer after upper abdominal surgery? *Acta Anaesthesiol Scand* 1979; 23:312.
33. McCarthy DS, Spencer R, Green R, et al: Measurement of "closing volume" as a single and sensitive test for early detection of small airways disease. *Am J Med* 1972; 52:747.
34. Mead J, Collier C: Relation of volume history of lungs to respiratory mechanics in dogs. *J Appl Physiol* 1959; 14:669.
35. Mittman C: Assessment of operative risk in thoracic surgery. *Am Rev Respir Dis* 1961; 84:197.
36. Morton HJV, Camb DA: Tobacco smoking and pulmonary complications after operation. *Lancet* 1944; 1:368–372.
37. Needham CD, Rogan MC, McDonald I: Normal standards for lung volumes, intrapulmonary gas mixing and maximum breathing capacity. *Thorax* 1954; 9:313–325.
38. Okinaka AJ: Postoperative pattern of breathing and compliance. *Arch Surg* 1966; 92:887–891.
39. Oyarzun ML, Clements JA: Ventilatory and cholinergic control of pulmonary surfactant in the rabbit. *J Appl Physiol* 1977; 43:39–45.
40. Putnam H, Jenicek JA, Cellan CA, et al: Anesthesia in the morbidly obese. *South Med J* 1974; 67:1411.
41. Radford EP: Static mechanical properties of mammalian lungs, in *Handbook of Physiology*, sec 3, Respiration, vol 1. Washington DC, American Physiological Society, 1964; pp 429–449.
42. Rehder K, Sessler AD, Marsch HJ: General anesthesia and the lung. *Am Rev Respir Dis* 1975; 112:541.
43. Schwartz SI, Dale WA, Rahn H: Dead-space rebreathing tube for prevention of atelectasis. *JAMA* 1957; 163:1248–1251.
44. Shapiro B, Peterson J, Cane R: Complications of mechanical aids to intermittent lung inflation. *Respir Care* 1982; 27:467.
45. Stein M, Kotta GM, Simon M, et al: Pulmonary evaluation of surgical patients. *JAMA* 1962; 181:765–770.
46. Stock MC, Downs JB, Gauer PK, et al: Prevention of atelectasis after upper abdominal operations. *Crit Care Med* 1983; 11:220–224.
47. Stock MC, Downs JB, et al: Comparison of CPAP, incentive spirometry, and conservative therapy after cardiac operations. *Crit Care Med* 1984; 12:969–972.
48. Stock MC, Downs JB, Corkran ML: Pulmonary function before and after prolonged CPAP by mask. *Crit Care Med* 1984; 12:973–974.
49. Tisi GM: Preoperative evaluation of pulmonary function. *Am Rev Respir Dis* 1979; 119:293–308.
50. Van de Water JM, Watring WG, Linton LA, et al: Prevention of postoperative pulmonary complications. *Surg Gynecol Obstet* 1972; 135:1–5.
51. Ward RJ, Danziger F, Bonica JJ, et al: An evaluation of postoperative respiratory maneuvers. *Surg Gynecol Obstet* 1966; 123:51–54.
52. Wilkins R, Sheldon R, Krider S: *Clinical Assessment in Respiratory Care*. St Louis, CV Mosby Co, 1985, p 174–177.
53. Zibrak JD, Rossetti P, Wood E: Effect of reductions in respiratory therapy on patient outcome. *N Engl J Med* 1986; 315:292–295.
54. Ziment I: Mucokinesis—the methodology of moving mucus. *Respir Ther* 1974; 4:15–19.

Mechanical Ventilation

Thomas A. Barnes, Ed.D., R.R.T.

INDICATIONS

The indications for mechanically ventilating a patient can be divided into three categories related to functions of the lungs: (1) ventilation, (2) oxygenation, and (3) mechanics. Numerical guidelines for each of these areas have been described by Pontoppidan et al. based on their experience in the respiratory care unit at Massachusetts General Hospital, and can be found in Table 10–1. Computer and space-age technology has contributed to improvements in the capabilities of ventilators since these guidelines were published in 1973. However, the physiologic indications for mechanical ventilation remain virtually unchanged from the past. The criteria are only guidelines, and each patient should be evaluated carefully using vital signs and other important physical data. The pattern that the data forms is more relevant than any single criteria for instituting mechanical ventilation.

The prophylactic use of mechanical ventilation is appropriate when paralysis of the respiratory muscles is imminent, such as with myasthenia gravis, Guillain-Barré syndrome, and barbiturate poisoning.[17, 26, 30, 45] Severe respiratory insufficiency resulting from infant or adult respiratory distress syndromes will cause severe hypoxemia and hypercarbia that may require mechanical ventilation until pulmonary function improves.[1, 23, 43, 56] Mechanical ventilation or continuous positive-airway pressure (CPAP) is frequently used to provide internal stabilization of the chest wall following blunt or penetrating trauma to the chest.[25, 61, 65] The use of a ventilator prevents paradoxical breathing where the injured area of the chest moves in instead of out during inspiration.

Cardiac, upper abdominal, thoracic, or neurosurgical operations may lead to postoperative respiratory failure caused by anesthesia and drugs given for pain which depress the respiratory centers. Many aspects of major surgery may lead to deteriorating pulmonary function and decreased lung volume (FRC).[33] If postoperative pain is not adequately treated or the patient is exposed to long periods of hypoxemia during or after surgery, the pulmonary capillaries may leak making the lungs stiff and difficult to ventilate.[27]

GOALS

Adequate Ventilation

A primary goal of mechanical ventilation is to provide the right volume of oxygen-enriched and CO_2-free gas to the alveoli. The best indicator of adequate alveolar ventilation is a normal arterial carbon dioxide tension. A normal arterial CO_2 tension is usually 40 mm Hg unless the patient has chronic obstructive pulmonary disease, in which case the baseline value may be much higher. Carbon dioxide is 20 times more soluble in body fluids than oxygen and moves rapidly from pulmonary capillaries to alveoli. The amount of CO_2 removed from the patient's blood is dependent only on the amount of fresh gas moving in and out of the alveolar spaces. Gases move between pulmonary capillary blood and alveoli because of a difference in their partial pressures. A direct relationship between arterial CO_2 tension and alveolar ventilation exists because: (1) the partial pressure of CO_2 in alveoli is a function of the volume of gas being moved in and out of the alveoli, and (2) there is an equilibrium for CO_2 found

TABLE 10–1.

Guidelines for Ventilatory Support in Adults With Acute Respiratory Failure*‖

DATUM	NORMAL RANGE	TRACHEAL INTUBATION AND VENTILATION INDICATED
Mechanics		
Respiratory rate, breaths/min	12–20	>35
Vital capacity, ml/kg of body weight†	65–75	<15
FEV_1, ml/kg of body weight†	50–60	<10
Inspiratory force, cm H_2O	75–100	<25
Oxygenation		
Pao_2, mm Hg	100–75 (air)	<70 (on mask O_2)
$P(A-aDO_2)^{1.0}$, mm Hg‡	25–65	>450
Ventilation		
Pa_{CO_2}, mm Hg	35–45	>55§
V_D/V_T	0.25–0.40	>0.60

*From Pontoppidan H, Geffin G, Lowenstein E: *Acute Respiratory Failure in the Adult.* Boston, Little, Brown & Co, 1973. Used with permission.
†"Ideal" weight is used if weight appears grossly abnormal.
‡After 20 minutes of 100% oxygen.
§Except in patients with chronic hypercapnia.
‖The trend of values is of utmost importance. The numerical guidelines should obviously not be adopted to the exclusion of clinical judgment. For example, a vital capacity below 15 ml/kg may prove sufficient provided the patient can still cough "effectively," if hypoxemia is prevented and if hypercapnia is not progressive. However, such a patient needs frequent blood gas analyses and must be closely observed in a well-equipped, adequately staffed recovery room or intensive care unit.

between alveolar gas and oxygenated blood leaving the pulmonary capillaries (Fig 10–1).

Oxygen is less soluble in body fluids than carbon dioxide, and although the arterial oxygen tension will fall when alveolar ventilation is inadequate, there are several other variables which may also cause PaO_2 to decrease. The oxygen saturation of hemoglobin may still be high in some cases when a patient is in ventilatory failure and may not begin to decrease sharply until the arterial CO_2 tension has risen to over 70 mm Hg (Fig 10–2). A high CO_2 tension can be dangerous since it causes high blood pressure, cerebral congestion, increased cerebrospinal fluid pressure, and ultimately coma. The clinical signs of hypercarbia include skin that is hot, flushed, and moist from capillary engorgement. Moderately high CO_2 tensions cause tachycardia and if unchecked will lead to heart block and ventricular bradycardia.[54]

Adequate Oxygenation

The term *respiratory failure* is more appropriate than *ventilatory failure* to describe a patient who needs mechanical ventilation. The term *respiratory failure* has the advantage of covering both potential problems: (1) lack of ability to mechanically move "oxygen in" and "CO_2 out" of the lungs and (2) insufficient ability to rapidly diffuse the appropriate amounts of oxygen into the pulmonary capillary blood. Acute respiratory failure should be rapidly reversible in most cases if aggressive measures such as mechanical ventilation, optimal PEEP, cardiovascular support, and monitoring are employed early in the course of the disease with the intent of reversing functional impairment

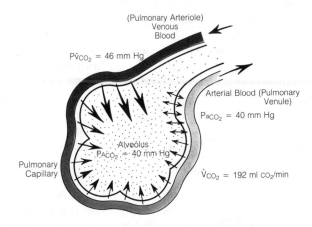

FIG 10–1.

A schematic representation of the CO_2 equilibrium established between alveolar gas and blood leaving pulmonary capillaries.

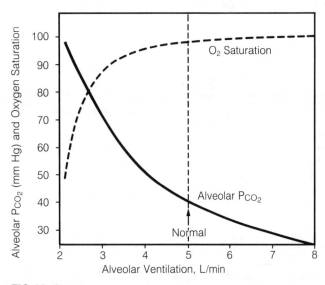

FIG 10–2.
The relationship between alveolar ventilation, arterial carbon dioxide tension, and oxygen saturation. (Modified from Mushin WW, Rendell-Baker L, Thompson PW: *Automatic Ventilation of the Lungs*, ed 3. Oxford, Blackwell Scientific Publications, 1980.)

rather than only employing such measures to improve oxygenation to satisfactory levels.[10, 11]

Reduced Work of Breathing

The third primary goal of mechanical ventilation is to lower the metabolic cost of breathing. The work of breathing normally is approximately 0.5 kg·M/min and requires only 2% to 3% of total oxygen consumption. In severe acute respiratory failure, decreased pulmonary compliance and increased resistance to gas flow in the airways may cause a 200% to 300% increase in the work of breathing. Tolerance to an increased ventilatory work load will vary according to several factors that limit the mechanical capacity of the muscles of respiration. Respiratory muscles will eventually become fatigued in response to large ventilatory requirements, and mechanical ventilation must be provided until elastic and resistive forces are restored to normal.

COMPLICATIONS AND HAZARDS

Effects on the Systemic Circulation

The manner in which a ventilator delivers gas to the lungs may have adverse effects on the systemic circulation.[41, 44, 48, 57, 62, 70] The parameters that need to be controlled to minimize the increase in mean intrathoracic pressure, which adversely effects circulation, include respiratory frequency, tidal volume, I:E ratio, sigh volume and frequency, peak inspiratory flow rate and pattern, airway pressure, and inspiratory pause time. The effect of the ventilatory pattern on cardiac output has been well-documented by studies on animals and humans.[3, 16, 38, 49, 53]

Steps can be taken to lower mean intrathoracic pressure.[66, 67, 71–73] For example, the use of intermittent mandatory ventilation (IMV) will decrease the number of positive pressure tidal volumes delivered to the lungs. Also, smaller tidal volumes (i.e., 10 ml/kg) should be used when the patient is first placed on a ventilator to allow time for a compensatory rise in peripheral venous tone. A key factor that determines whether cardiac output will increase or decrease is fluid balance. Hypovolemic patients (negative fluid balance) will be likely to have a decrease in cardiac output when the mean intrathoracic pressure is high. However, patients that have a normal fluid balance or those that are hypervolemic (i.e., positive fluid balance) will usually not have a drop in cardiac output even with a high mean intrathoracic pressure.[52] Accordingly, the infusion of the correct amount of blood, electrolyte solutions, or plasma expanders to maintain blood volume slightly above normal should help to minimize the decrease in cardiac output due to high intrathoracic pressure. The use of higher levels of positive end-expiratory pressure (PEEP) (>5 cm H_2O) and larger tidal volumes (>10 ml/kg) should be attempted only after the cardiovascular system has been stabilized.

Several factors determine the degree to which airway pressure will be communicated to blood vessels in the thorax. The lung is normally a relatively dry organ (the estimated pulmonary capillary blood volume is 90 ml) with alveolar epithelial membranes separated from pulmonary capillaries by a small distance equivalent to one ply of tissue paper. However, there are several pathologic states in which fluid may leak from capillaries that surround alveoli.[2, 5] The result is a heavy, noncompliant lung called the adult respiratory distress syndrome (ARDS). The distance for diffusion of oxygen between gas and blood increases when fluid leaks from the pulmonary capillaries. Fortunately, most of the high airway pressure needed to ventilate ARDS patients is absorbed by the noncompliant lung before it can be transmitted to the pulmonary capillaries and large vessels within the thorax.

Barotrauma

The possibility of a pneumothorax developing as a result of high alveolar pressure is unlikely in patients with ARDS since their lungs are noncompliant and filled with fluid. The high airway pressure needed to provide ventilation is counterbalanced by all the forces that are trying to collapse alveoli and small airways. Once the patient's pulmonary function improves, the danger of alveolar rupture and air leaks into the pleural space increases. Studies have shown that the incidence of pneumothorax even with high levels of PEEP and peak airway pressure was only 10% when patients were supported with IMV.[10, 11] The increased use of synchronized intermittent mandatory ventilation (SIMV) may decrease the incidence of tension pneumothorax related to mechanical ventilation even further.[51] Caution is required when using IMV instead of SIMV since the patient may have a mandatory tidal volume delivered on top of his spontaneous inspiration. The pressure limit control on all modern ventilators is designed to prevent high pressures from developing in the lungs and to sound an alarm if the limit is reached. Since a tension pneumothorax may occasionally develop without high airway pressures, the clinical signs of air in the pleural space should be well-understood and the patient carefully monitored for this complication (Table 10–2).

Hyperventilation

Hyperventilation can be defined as excessive ventilation of the alveoli which causes increased carbon dioxide excretion above and beyond that needed to maintain a patient's normal arterial CO_2 tension. A blood gas study should be done whenever there is any question regarding the adequacy of ventilation because of the physiologic and acid-base conse-

quences of allowing hyperventilation to occur for too long.[68] For a patient without chronic lung disease, a CO_2 tension below 35 mm Hg could indicate too much alveolar ventilation unless the goal was to lower intracranial pressure by decreasing the cerebral blood flow.[24, 34] The excess removal of CO_2 will result in respiratory alkalosis, since for every molecule of CO_2 excreted by the lungs, a hydrogen ion is converted to water ($H^+ + HCO_3^- \rightarrow H_2CO_3 \rightarrow CO_2 + H_2O$). Overbreathing accelerates and underbreathing slows this process. The problems caused by hyperventilation are severe and represent an important hazard of mechanical ventilation, especially when the patient is not allowed or is unable to breathe spontaneously while connected to the ventilator. The respiratory alkalosis that develops with sustained hyperventilation leads to metabolic compensation such as increased renal excretion of bicarbonate, retention of chloride, decreased production of ammonia, and excretion of acid salts, all tending to reduce the rise in pH. However, the decrease in hydrogen ions results in a subsequent decrease in the concentration of serum potassium (hypokalemia) which may cause life-threatening cardiac arrhythmias. Another complication of the alkalosis caused by hyperventilation is a shift of the oxyhemoglobin dissociation curve to left which results in less oxygen being released to the tissues (Fig 10–3).

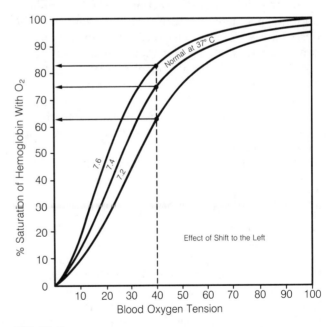

FIG 10–3.
Oxyhemoglobin dissociation curve at 37°C. A shift to the left increases oxygen affinity for hemoglobin, which results in less oxygen being released to the tissues at any given oxygen tension.

TABLE 10–2.

Common Physical Findings of a Tension Pneumothorax

Absent or distant bilateral breath sounds
Hyperresonant percussion note over affected area
Shift of trachea away from affected side
Presence of subcutaneous emphysema
Decrease in arterial blood pressure, venous return, and cardiac output
Decrease in ventilation
Sharp pain over affected side
Changes in heart rate

Patients who are hyperventilated often complain of tingling or numbness of their extremities (paresthesia), feel lightheaded, and may have hyperactive reflexes. If the arterial CO_2 is low enough, tetanic muscular contractions and seizures may develop. The cerebral arterioles respond to the decreased CO_2 tension by contracting and limiting cerebral blood flow to levels that may cause brain damage. The greatest danger is to patients with chronic pulmonary disease who live in a constant state of compensated respiratory acidosis, with consistently elevated arterial CO_2 tensions. The chronic hypercarbia, hypoxemia, and low pH found with these patients results in cerebral vascular dilation and an above normal cerebral blood flow. Consequently, when a hypercarbic patient is hyperventilated, the arterial P_{CO_2} may decrease too quickly causing a sudden drop in cerebral blood flow, thereby depriving the brain of adequate amounts of oxygen.

VENTILATOR SELECTION

Functional Characteristics and Capability

Classification Systems

Respiratory care practitioners must have a good understanding of the functional characteristics of different types of mechanical ventilators. This knowledge is critical to selecting the right ventilator for a given situation. Mushin classifies ventilators by describing functional characteristics under varying conditions (pulmonary compliance and airway resistance) found in normal and abnormal lungs.[54] Although most modern mechanical ventilators provide a high level of functional capability, a decision still needs to be made regarding which combination of ventilation parameters are best for a specific respiratory problem.

For example, several ventilators allow the clinician to select from among two or more inspiratory flow waveforms, modes of ventilation, and other functional characteristics. Therefore, a knowledge of classification systems facilitates selection of the best ventilator and provides the information needed to select the most appropriate ventilation parameters.

The use of negative pressure applied to the outside of the chest to facilitate chest excursion and the flow of gas at atmospheric pressure into the lungs was used before the development of positive pressure ventilators. Since so few of these negative pressure "chest cuirass" or "iron lung" type ventilators are in use today, only positive pressure ventilators will be covered in this chapter. High-frequency ventilation (HFV) and high-frequency oscillation (HFO) may not be advisable as the initial respiratory support method, and thus are not presented here.[8, 64]

Termination of Inspiration

The various ways a ventilator can be set to terminate the inspiratory phase is an important classification category. The practitioner's goal when using a ventilator should be to provide adequate ventilation and oxygenation with the least adverse effect on other physiologic parameters. The patient needs to receive an adequate tidal volume and minute ventilation regardless of changes in airway resistance and pulmonary compliance. Therefore, several components of the classification system must define the delivery of a tidal volume during the inspiratory phase. The focus naturally falls on a ventilator's capability to deliver all of the required tidal volume before the inspiratory phase terminates. Accordingly, the terms *pressure-cycled* and *volume-cycled* form a major classification category since they relate directly to a ventilator's capability to deliver a preset tidal volume. A pressure-cycled ventilator can be defined as one that will terminate the inspiratory phase at the preset *pressure limit* even though the needed tidal volume may not have been delivered (see Fig 10–6, panel C).

Conversely, a volume-cycled ventilator will terminate the inspiratory phase after delivering the *preset tidal volume* regardless of the peak airway pressure (Fig 10–4, panel C). Since many ventilators are *time cycled* and most have pressure limiting capabilities, some clinicians prefer to use the term *volume preset* to identify ventilators in which the tidal volume can be adjusted and guaranteed to be delivered within certain airway pressure and time limits. If the pressure limit is set correctly, at 10 cm H_2O above peak airway pressure, then small changes in airway resistance and pulmonary compliance will not affect delivery of the tidal volume. In summary, a ventilator may be cycled from the inspiratory to expiratory phase when a preset tidal volume has been delivered, a preset pressure reached, or when a minimum flow limit occurs, and/or when a preset time period has elapsed.

Inspiratory Waveforms

Ventilators are commonly classified according to the type of flow, pressure, and volume waveforms produced during the inspiratory phase. Waveforms are usually discussed in terms of whether the ventilator generates a constant gas flow or pressure during inspiration.

Ventilators that are flow generators can be clas-

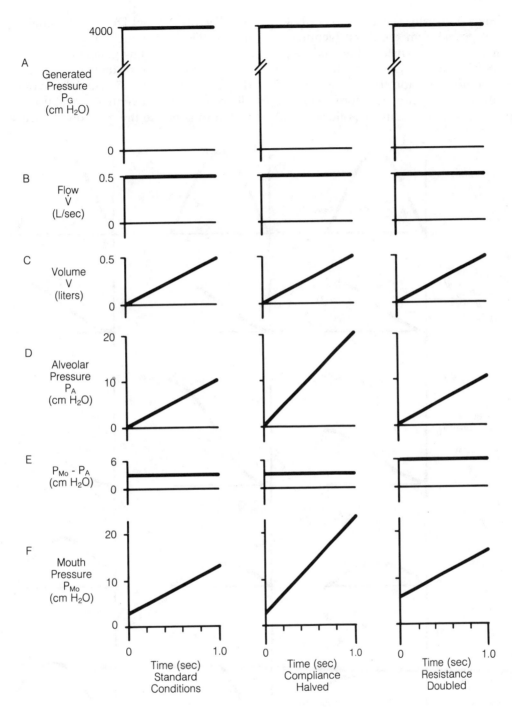

FIG 10–4.
Theoretical inspiratory waveforms by a ventilator generating a very high constant pressure and having a very high internal resistance. This type of ventilator is classified as a constant-flow generator.

(Modified from Mushin WW, Rendell-Baker L, Thompson PW: *Automatic Ventilation of the Lungs*, ed 3. Oxford, Blackwell Scientific Publications, 1980.)

sified further according to whether they produce constant or nonconstant flow waveforms. Those that produce a constant flow waveform (square wave) during inspiration often develop high-driving pressure (100 to 4,000 cm H_2O) across an internal, high-

resistance orifice (Fig 10–4, panel A). Constant-flow generators deliver gas at a constant rate into the lungs regardless of changes in pulmonary compliance and airway resistance (Fig 10–4, panel B). Since the change in pressure needed to move the tidal volume into the lungs is usually less than 50 cm H_2O, the high internal pressure on the distal (ventilator) side of the orifice assures a constant flow and delivery of a preset tidal volume. Inspiratory time will be determined by the flow rate and the size of the tidal volume. The alveolar pressure waveform will rise from the expiratory phase baseline in a linear man-

ner (Fig 10–4, panel D) until the tidal volume is delivered (Fig 10–4, panel C).

Nonconstant flow generators usually are categorized by the shape of their inspiratory flow pattern (Fig 10–5, panel A). Sinusoidal waveforms are usually produced by a ventilator that uses a rotary-drive piston to generate the gas flow. However, there are

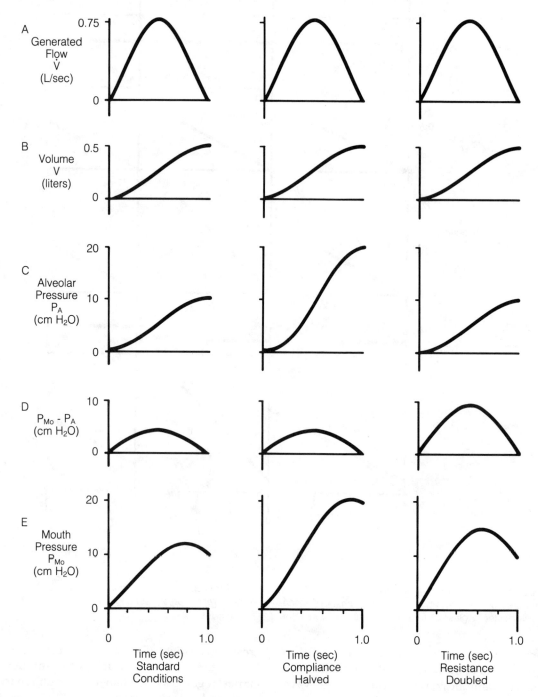

FIG 10–5.
Theoretical inspiratory waveforms by a ventilator with a sine wave (half cycle) flow pattern. (Modified from Mushin WW, Rendell-Baker L, Thompson PW: *Automatic Ventilation of the Lungs,* ed 3. Oxford, Blackwell Scientific Publications, 1980.)

several ventilators without pistons that are also able to create *sine wave* flow patterns under certain conditions by using high-technology valves that can rapidly change diameter to control flow rate (see Chapter 16). Since the pressure waveform is integrally related to changes in flow, it also forms a nonlinear shape.

Ventilators that develop low pressure, such as pressure-cycled IPPB machines, will have flow curve that rise rapidly at first and then gradually taper and slow down as airway back pressure reduces the inspiratory flow rate (Fig 10–6, panel B). Therefore, pressure-cycled ventilators set at a low cycling pressure are likely to prematurely end the inspiratory

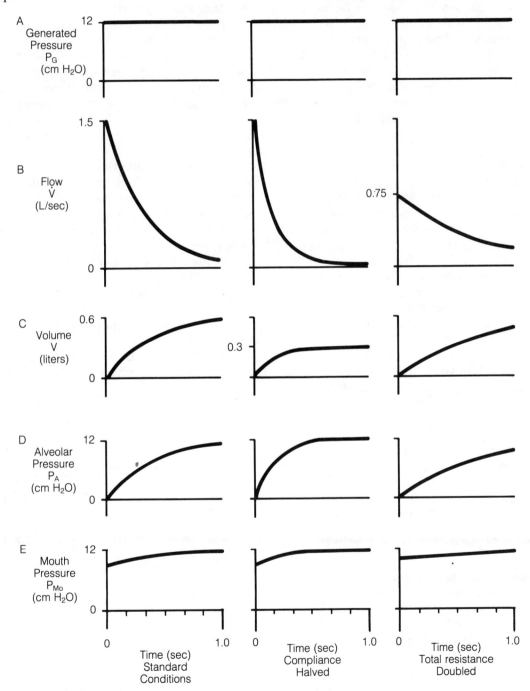

FIG 10–6.

Theoretical inspiratory waveforms by a ventilator generating a low-constant pressure. This type of ventilator is classified as a constant-pressure generator and used for short-term ventilation such as IPPB treatments. (Modified from Mushin WW, Rendell-Baker L, Thompson PW: *Automatic Ventilation of the Lungs*, ed 3. Oxford, Blackwell Scientific Publications, 1980.)

phase without delivering an adequate tidal volume when the pulmonary compliance decreases and/or the airway resistance increases (Fig 10–6, panel C). Ventilators with low driving pressures are usually used only for short periods of time when the patient's pulmonary mechanics are almost normal and not expected to change. Some ventilators such as the Puritan-Bennett 7200 ventilator have the capability to provide a choice of decelerating, square wave, or sine wave inspiratory flow patterns and also allow the clinician to preset other ventilation parameters, i.e., tidal volume, SIMV rate. Therefore, in some instances, classification of the inspiratory phase waveforms that are available only serves the purpose of describing the functional capability of a ventilator rather than separating it into a specific category.

Power and Control Sources

The way that a ventilator receives the power needed to mechanically ventilate a patient is an important category in all classification systems. A clinician needs only to have lived through a major power failure to appreciate this category. The source of power for ventilators is either electricity or compressed gases, and some ventilators are pneumatically powered and electrically controlled. Ventilators that are pneumatically powered and controlled are good standby units if the hospital is in an area subject to frequent electrical power failures.

The Siemens Servo 900B and 900C ventilators are examples of ventilators that are pneumatically powered but also need electricity to control the inspiratory and expiratory valves. Other ventilators such as the Monaghan 225/SIMV are pneumatically powered and controlled through the use of the *Coanda Effect* (phenomenon that causes a jet stream to attach to a nearby wall). Some ventilators, such as the Emerson IMV ventilator, are powered and controlled by electricity. They rely on a pneumatic mixing valve as their source of oxygen-enriched gas and will continue to provide mechanical ventilation with room air when there is a malfunction in the source of compressed gases.

In summary, ventilators should be classified into categories related to how they are powered and controlled. The category for power is described as electrical or pneumatic, and control mechanisms are categorized as either electronic or fluidic logic.

Flow Generation and Circuits

A pressure gradient between the ventilator and the alveolar spaces must be developed for gas to flow into the lungs. The way that ventilators generate the necessary flow of gases into the lungs is an important part of classification systems. The major divisions of this "flow generation" category are (1) pistons, (2) bellows, and (3) pneumatic devices. The ventilators are further divided into those with single versus double circuits. A ventilator using a "single circuit" has gas flow directly from the drive mechanism to the breathing circuit and then into the lungs, i.e., from the cylinder of a piston directly to the lungs. "Double circuit" ventilators have gas from the driving mechanism compress a bellows or bag, which causes the gas inside the bellows to flow into the patient's breathing circuit and onward to the lungs, i.e., the gas that compresses the bellows or bag is not delivered to the patient (Fig 10–7). Gas from a high-pressure source such as a compressor or external piping system is allowed to flow into the "box" until the bag or bellows is compressed. Since the pressure generated in the box is usually 100 cm H_2O or higher, the flow rate out of the bag or bellows is held constant throughout the inspiratory phase.

Ventilators that use a piston to generate flow usually produce an inspiratory waveform with the shape of one-half of a sine wave. Examples are the Emerson 3PV postoperative and 3MV IMV ventilators, which have their pistons connected to a rotating cam (Fig 10–8). The rotation of the cam causes the piston to force gas out of the cylinder, at a "nonconstant" flow rate. The sinusoidal shape of the flow waveform produced by rotary driven piston ventilators has important physiologic advantages which

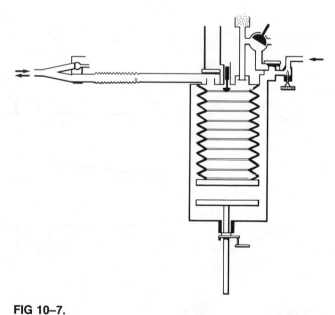

FIG 10–7.
Double-circuit, "bellows in a box," constant mechanism-flow generator.

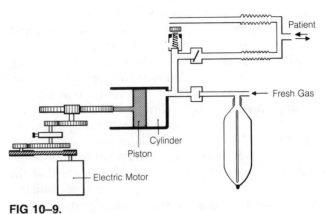

FIG 10–9.
Single-circuit, square wave, constant-flow generator.

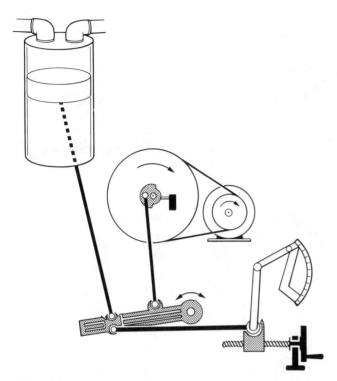

FIG 10–8.
Single-circuit, sine wave, non–constant-flow generator.

are discussed later in this chapter. There are a few ventilators whose pistons are connected to a "linear drive" mechanism, e.g., Bourns LS104–150 infant ventilator (Fig 10–9). A linear-driven piston moves gas out of the cylinder at a "constant flow rate."

The third classification category for flow generation is "pneumatic devices." Ventilators in this category electronically control the inspiratory flow rate by using high precision valves, some of which were originally designed for the space program. The more sophisticated ventilators of this type, such as the Siemens Servo 900B and 900C and the Puritan-Bennett 7200, use proportional solenoids which are either electronically servo-controlled (Servo 900B and 900C) or regulated by a microprocessor (Puritan-Bennett 7200). The pneumatic generation of flow using high internal pressures and electronically controlled inspiratory valves allows several waveforms to be available on a single ventilator, e.g., square, sinusoidal, and tapered (Fig 10–10). Other ventilators are pneumatically powered but fall into the pressure-cycled category, e.g., Bird Mark 7 and Puritan-Bennett PR-2. The flow waveforms generated by pressure-cycled ventilators are controlled by special valves that begin to close when pressure increases or flow decreases.

Modes of Ventilation

The mechanisms that a ventilator has available for ending the expiratory phase and allowing inspiration to begin are called *modes of ventilation* and should be included when a ventilator is classified. Some basic ventilation devices (such as pressure-cycled machines that are used for short-term postoperative or emergency ventilation) provide only the

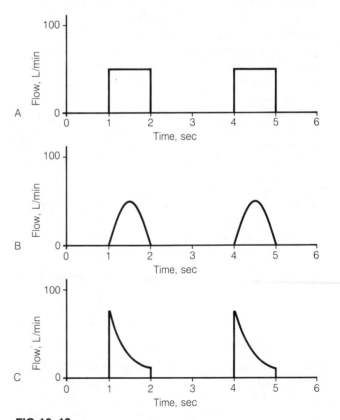

FIG 10–10.
Inspiratory flow waveforms generated by electronically controlled pneumatic valves. **A,** square wave. **B,** sine wave. **C,** decelerating flow.

assist-mode (patient-triggered), *control mode* (machine-triggered), or *assist-control mode* (patient-triggered with machine triggering, if necessary). All three triggering categories—assist mode of ventilation (AMV), control mode of ventilation (CMV), and assist-control mode (AMV/CMV)—bring about the delivery of positive-pressure tidal volumes. The distinguishing feature is whether the patient triggers inspiration by starting to inhale or the ventilator automatically triggers the inspiratory phase after a preset time interval. The assist-control mode simply means that the patient can cycle the ventilator at his own initiative only if the CMV rate is exceeded. The advantage of the assist-control mode is that it protects the patient from periods of apnea and guarantees a life-sustaining baseline rate of ventilation. A ventilator operating in the assist-control mode may provide only CMV capability if the control for patient triggering is not adjusted properly, i.e., the sensitivity may be set too low and require a large drop in baseline pressure or a substantial flow of gases toward the lungs to trigger the ventilator. Conversely, when the patient trigger control is too sensitive to inspiratory efforts, the ventilator may begin to cycle automatically at a very high CMV rate. Both the control and assist modes of ventilation result in every breath creating positive pressure in the thorax, which may significantly decrease venous return to the heart, reduce cardiac output, and increase intracranial pressure.

In the early 1970s, a different way to regulate mechanical breaths was introduced; it was termed *intermittent mandatory ventilation* (IMV). IMV allows the patient to breathe spontaneously from the ventilator circuit in addition to receiving mandatory tidal volumes. The more the patient can do on his own, the fewer mandatory machine-delivered breaths will be needed. The intrathoracic pressure is lower with IMV than with controlled or assisted ventilation because of fewer positive pressure waveforms (Fig 10–11). The use of IMV allows the patient to be weaned from the ventilator without trials off the ventilator. The number of IMV breaths delivered by the ventilator can be decreased as the patient's pulmonary function returns to normal (Fig 10–12).[14, 22, 40, 50]

Synchronized intermittent mandatory ventilation (SIMV) is similar to IMV except that mandated breaths are synchronized with the patient's own spontaneous breathing rate. The use of the SIMV mode prevents delivery of a mandatory tidal volume from the ventilator on top of a spontaneous inspiration. Such "stacking" of breaths has in some instances led to overdistention of the lungs and incisional pain in postoperative patients. The use of

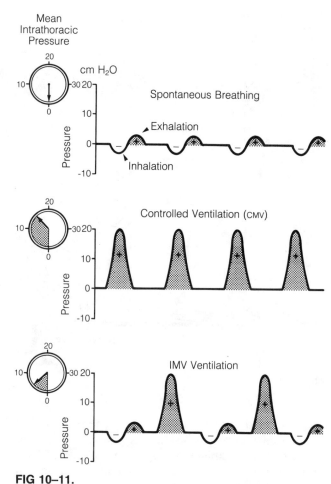

FIG 10–11.
Intrathoracic pressure is lower with IMV than with controlled or assisted ventilations since fewer positive-pressure waveforms are delivered.

PEEP, which increases the functional residual volume, combined with the use of large ventilator delivered tidal volumes, make the stacking of IMV and spontaneous breaths a serious problem that can be resolved by using SIMV.

In summary, the modes of ventilation that are used to trigger the start of the inspiratory phase should be well understood by clinicians and included when the ventilator is classified. The modes that should be considered are: assist mode (AMV), control mode (CMV), assist-control (AMV/CMV), intermittent mandatory ventilation (IMV), and synchronized intermittent mandatory ventilation (SIMV).

Modes of Minute Volume and Pressure Support

One of the goals of mechanical ventilation is to ensure an adequate alveolar minute volume. By using the CMV mode of ventilation, this goal can be accomplished, but the inherent risks related to in-

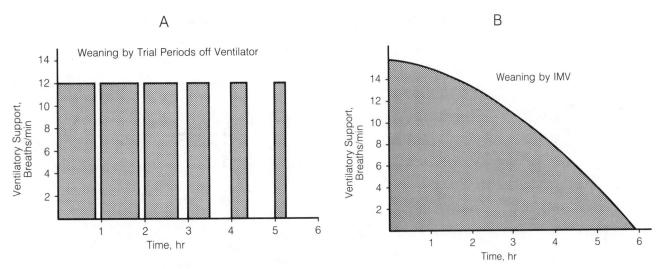

FIG 10–12.

Comparison of weaning by trial **(A)** to the use of IMV **(B)** to gradually lower the number of mandatory breaths per minute delivered by the ventilator.

creased intrathoracic pressure, barotrauma, and hyperventilation discussed earlier in this chapter are serious complications. There are many advantages to using IMV and SIMV (instead of CMV) in terms of providing ventilatory support with fewer complications and hazards since patients are allowed to contribute some of their ventilatory requirement, thereby reducing the number of positive pressure breaths needed.[18, 37, 59] However, the IMV or SIMV rate has to be changed as the patient's spontaneous respiratory rate and tidal volume increase or decrease over time.[9]

The use of *extended mandatory minute ventilation* (EMMV) available on the Engstrom Erica Ventilator guarantees that the patient will receive a preset minute volume over an extended period of time. This is accomplished by the ventilator delivering a mandatory tidal volume whenever the spontaneous ventilation is not adequate to reach the preset minute volume. A constant flow of gases equal to the preset minute volume is fed into a constant pressure reservoir or bellows that the patient breathes from spontaneously. If the patient's spontaneous breathing is not enough to meet the mandatory baseline minute volume, the reservoir or bellows will fill and trigger the ventilator to deliver a mandatory breath, thereby ensuring a minimum minute volume. The mandatory breath is prevented from being delivered during or immediately after a spontaneous effort by the patient. Accordingly, there is no danger of stacking spontaneous and mandatory tidal volumes, since these are not IMV breaths delivered at preset intervals.[38]

The *pressure support* mode allows a spontaneous breath to be assisted by a preset amount of constant pressure which is added to the baseline pressure level and applied throughout the inspiratory phase. The inspiratory flow rate will be high at first and taper in order to maintain the constant pressure as air flows into the lungs. An example of a ventilator with this capability is the Siemens Servo 900C. It measures the peak inspiratory flow and triggers the ventilator into the expiratory phase when the flow tapers to 25% of the peak flow generated. The inspiration will also be terminated if the pressure rises to 3 cm H_2O above the inspiratory pressure support level or if the inspiratory time exceeds 80% of the total cycle time of the rate control setting. Also, the Siemens Servo 900C allows pressure support to be used with SIMV. Other ventilators such as the Engstrom Erica allow pressure support to be used with SIMV, EMMV, and other spontaneous breathing modes. The Servo 900C ventilator also allows what has been called a *pressure control* mode where the pressure support is applied throughout inspiration but the breaths/minute, inspiratory time percentage, and pause time percentage controls all function to provide an assist-control mode of ventilation. However, the preset minute volume control on the Servo 900C is not operative with the pressure control mode in use (Fig 10–13).

Positive End-Expiratory Pressure

The capability of the ventilator to apply greater than ambient pressure to the airways during both inspiratory and expiratory phases in all modes of ventilation is a critical performance characteristic of ventilators. The term *continuous positive-airway pres-*

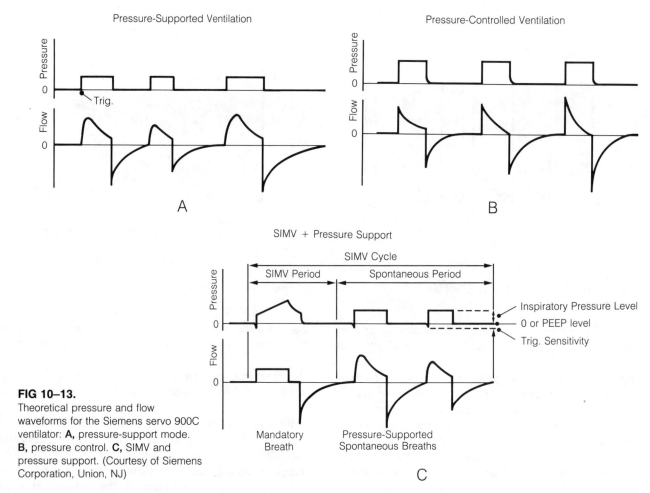

FIG 10–13.
Theoretical pressure and flow waveforms for the Siemens servo 900C ventilator: **A,** pressure-support mode. **B,** pressure control. **C,** SIMV and pressure support. (Courtesy of Siemens Corporation, Union, NJ)

sure (CPAP) is used when above-ambient pressure is applied to a breathing circuit when there are no ventilator-delivered tidal volumes being provided, i.e., during spontaneous breathing (Fig 10–14). When CPAP and mechanical ventilation are applied together, the increased baseline pressure is called PEEP *(positive end-expiratory pressure).* The result of CPAP or PEEP is continuous positive-pressure breathing (CPPB), which helps to reverse underlying pathophysiologic changes (such as small airway and alveolar collapse) by increasing the functional residual capacity and splinting the lung in a position of function (Fig 10–15).[32, 41, 63]

Expiratory Flow Waveforms

The capability of a ventilator to retard expiratory flow should be described when classifying a ventilator. Expiratory resistance can be selectively used to limit or retard the expiratory flow rate of some patients who have chronic obstructive pulmonary disease. These patients normally "purse lip" breathe when not being mechanically ventilated. The col-

lapse of their small airways does not allow them to exhale completely unless a small back pressure is created in their airways. The expiratory flow rate control on a ventilator retards the flow of gas by decreasing the aperture of the exhalation valve. The back pressure created allows small airways to stay open long enough for the patient to exhale their tidal volume. The slower expiratory flow rate requires an I:E ratio, which provides substantially more time for exhalation (Fig 10–16).[12]

THE EFFECT OF CHANGES IN PULMONARY COMPLIANCE AND RESISTANCE

Low-Pressure Generators

The functional characteristics of low-pressure generators were only of academic interest until *pressure support* became available to assist spontaneous breathing of ventilator patients. In the past this type

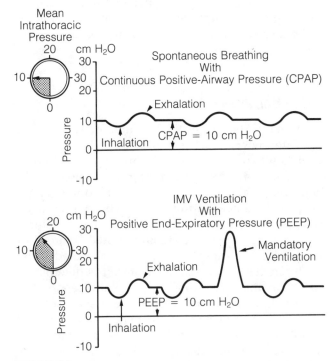

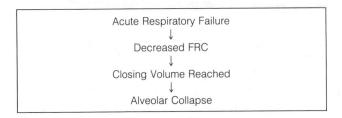

FIG 10–14.
Continuous positive-pressure breathing (CPPB).

of pressure generator was used almost exclusively to administer intermittent positive-pressure breathing (IPPB) over short periods of time using machines such as the Bennett PR-2. With low generated pressure, flow and volume waveforms are affected by changes in pulmonary compliance and airway resistance. The most significant aspect is a 50% decrease in tidal volume seen when the compliance is halved (see Fig 10–6). Doubling the airway resistance also reduces the tidal volume but to a lesser degree. Obviously, a ventilator with a low-driving pressure is not well-suited to long-term mechanical ventilation where frequent changes in compliance and resistance can occur.

Acute Respiratory Failure
↓
Decreased FRC
↓
Closing Volume Reached
↓
Alveolar Collapse

Splint the Lung in a Position of Function

FIG 10–15.
Continuous positive-pressure breathing increases the functional residual capacity and splints the lung in position of function.

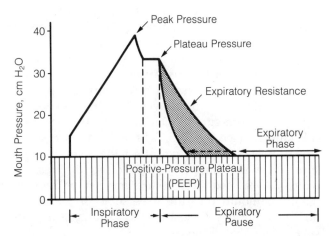

FIG 10–16.
Pressure waveforms seen with and without apparatus resistance during expiration. Mouth pressure rises to a peak from the PEEP level followed by a drop to the plateau pressure after the tidal volume has been delivered. Pressure falls to the positive-pressure plateau (PEEP level) at a rate determined by the amount of expiratory resistance.

Constant Flow Generators

Ventilators that generate high pressure across an internal resistance commonly are classified and referred to as *constant flow generators*. A major advantage of constant flow generators is their capability of delivering a preset tidal volume using an square wave inspiratory flow waveform.[20] Ventilators that generate a very high pressure across an internal resistance (i.e., 100 to 4,000 cm H_2O) will have flow and volume waveforms that are not affected by changes in pulmonary compliance or airway resistance (see Fig 10–4). However, proportional step valves that have the capability of varying the internal resistance against which these high pressures are applied allow the inspiratory flow rate to be held constant or to change several times during the inspiratory phase. Therefore, several commonly used ventilators have the functional capability of providing four different inspiratory flow waveforms: (1) square wave (constant flow), (2) decelerating wave (peak flow initially that declines throughout inspiration), (3) accelerating wave and (4) sine wave (see Fig 10–10). When the *pressure support* mode is used, a decelerating inspiratory flow waveform occurs during spontaneous breathing that varies according to the amount of constant pressure generated and the pneumatic characteristics of the lung (see Fig 10–13).

Sine Wave Flow Generators

Some ventilators generate flow by using a rotary-driven piston that creates a sine wave pattern or waveform with each inspiration regardless of the compliance and airway resistance. The flow rate will change throughout the inspiratory phase and the peak flow will be determined by the tidal volume (stroke volume of the piston) and the preset inspiratory time. A decrease in pulmonary compliance will not affect the flow waveform, but the alveolar and mouth pressure waveforms will be increased substantially (see Fig 10–5,C–E). Also, an increase in airway resistance does not affect the alveolar pressure but will result in a higher mouth pressure which may exceed the pressure limit set on the ventilator. If mouth pressure rises some of the preset tidal volume may be lost by the venting of a pressure relief valve in the circuit.

Pressure-Cycled Ventilators

One of the goals of mechanical ventilation is to provide adequate ventilation. This can only be done if the ventilator used has the capability of delivering a preset tidal volume in the face of a decrease in pulmonary compliance and/or increase in airway resistance. Pressure-cycled ventilators are poor choices for long-term mechanical ventilation since small increases in peak airway pressure (caused by changes in compliance and/or resistance) will prematurely cycle the ventilator into expiration.

For long-term ventilation, *volume-cycled* (or volume preset) ventilators, capable of generating high pressure, are best. Volume preset ventilators have pressure-limiting devices that will either vent some of the tidal volume or terminate inspiration when a preset pressure limit is reached. Therefore, the pressure limit on a volume preset ventilator, should be set 10 cm H_2O above the observed peak inspiratory pressure to assure that preset tidal volume is delivered.

VENTILATOR BREATHING CIRCUITS

A ventilator breathing circuit represents a classic example of a machine-to-man interface. The circuit must act as a conduit for gas to flow during inspiration from ventilator to lungs and provide a route during expiration for removing gas. It must be flexible, yet strong enough not to tear, develop leaks, or kink; and must have ports for monitoring several important parameters such as (1) proximal airway pressure, (2) proximal gas temperature, and (3) inspired oxygen concentration. The circuit is comprised of several critical components that direct the flow of gases, control the temperature and humidity of the inspired gases, and establish a baseline pressure (PEEP or CPAP) during the expiratory phase.

Circuit Compliance

Some of the preset tidal volume delivered by a ventilator never reaches the airways because it is used to fill and distend the breathing circuit, which stretches to a larger size during inspiration. If circuits were made of rigid metal pipes, additional gas would still be needed to fill the circuit during inspiration, since gas is compressed to a smaller volume at higher pressures. The amount of tidal volume lost in the circuit during inspiration is calculated using the *tubing compliance factor*. This factor is determined for all circuits before they are used and reported in ml of volume lost per cm H_2O of pressure (see Appendix B). The average permanent (nondisposable) circuit has a compliance factor of approximately 3 ml/cm H_2O, which means a pressure increase of 40 cm H_2O (peak airway pressure − PEEP or baseline pressure) would result in 120 ml of tidal volume being lost in the circuit and not delivered to the lungs. Some ventilators such as the Puritan-Bennett 7200 automatically correct for volume lost in the circuit and actually deliver all of the preset tidal volume to the lungs. The volume lost in the circuit becomes a critical consideration when small tidal volumes are used to ventilate a pediatric or neonatal patient.

IMV Circuits

Occasionally it becomes necessary to modify a ventilator that does not have IMV capability so that a patient can breathe spontaneously from the circuit and also periodically receive mandatory ventilation. The prime considerations in making this modification are (1) to provide a source of humidified gas for spontaneous breathing that has the same fractional oxygen concentration as that provided by mandatory breaths from the ventilator; (2) provide gas for spontaneous breaths at flow rates that exceed the patient's peak inspiratory flow rate (with low trigger effort and fast response time); (3) the use of a low-resistance one-way valve between the spontaneous gas source (demand valve or reservoir bags) and the breathing circuit; and (4) a device for lowering the IMV rate to 2 per minute (Figs 10–17 and 10–18).

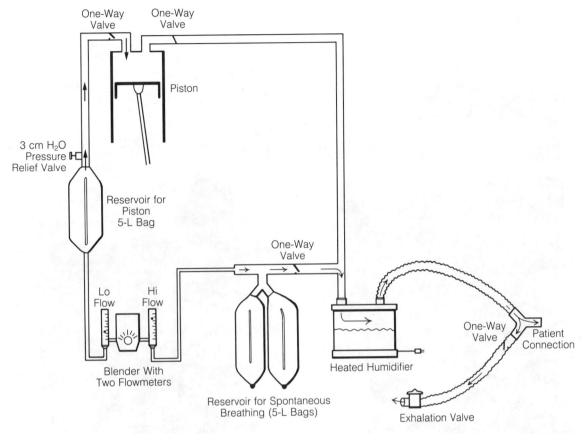

FIG 10–17.
Intermittent mandatory ventilation (IMV) circuit for Emerson 3PV postoperative ventilator. A continuous flow into the spontaneous reservoir bags set higher than patient's peak inspiratory flow rate decreases the work of breathing spontaneously from the circuit.

Positive End-Expiratory Pressure Devices

The use of PEEP during mechanical ventilation allows the clinician to "splint the lung" in a position of function by increasing the functional residual capacity (FRC).[69] An increase in the FRC opens collapsed alveoli and small bronchioles, thereby improving ventilation-to-perfusion ratios. The amount of PEEP needed (ideal or best PEEP) will vary according to the amount of pulmonary and cardiovascular dysfunction. The capability of a ventilator to provide a wide range of accurate PEEP pressures is an important functional characteristic that should be mentioned when a ventilator is classified. Second only in importance to the amount available is the ease with which changes in PEEP level can be made. It can be as simple as entering the PEEP level on a computer keyboard or as complicated as changing the level of a column of water. Since the optimal PEEP level needed may change on an hour-to-hour basis, it is critical that the ventilator have the capa-bility (1) to accurately maintain a preset amount of PEEP, (2) for quick and accurate changes of the level of PEEP, and (3) to monitor the proximal PEEP level.

PEEP devices are best described according to the degree that they are flow dependent. If the entry and exit channels are small in diameter, resistance will be high and peak inspiratory pressure may take longer to return to the baseline (PEEP level). A few ventilators have *threshold* PEEP devices that are not flow dependent. Threshold PEEP devices do not retard exhalation, and consequently mean airway pressure is lower. Examples of devices that are used to create PEEP are illustrated in Figure 10–19.

FLUIDIC CONTROL DEVICES

Coanda Effect

The *Coanda effect* is named after Henri Coanda, who studied wall attraction effects in 1930. Twenty

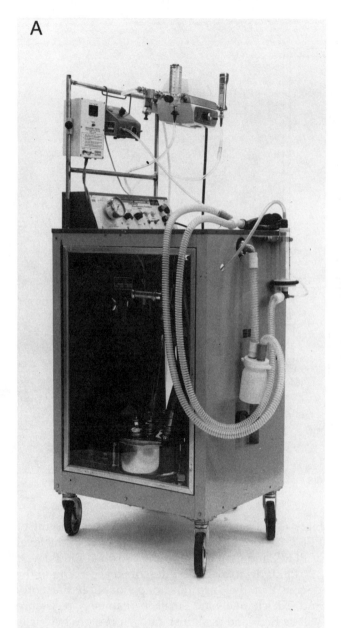

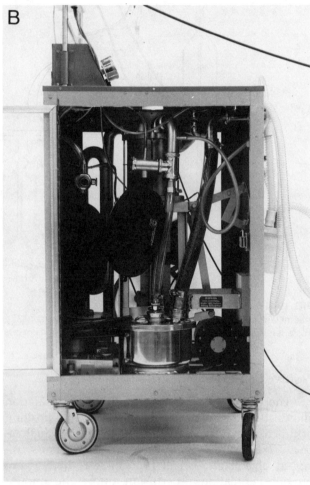

FIG 10–18.
A and **B,** Emerson 3PV postoperative ventilator modified for intermittent mandatory ventilation.

years earlier he was taught firsthand about wall attachment when an experimental jet plane he built and piloted crashed after the jet exhaust flames became attached to the fuselage.[54] Wall attachment occurs because gases leaving a jet have a lower pressure surrounding the high velocity stream (Bernoulli principle). The surrounding air will be entrained into the jet stream and if a wall is placed adjacent to the jet stream, the pressure next to the wall will drop quickly since air cannot easily enter from that side. The lower pressure causes the jet stream to be pulled over against the wall and a small separation bubble helps to keep the stream attached to the wall (Fig 10–20). A simple application of the Coanda effect is used with a fundamental fluidic device called a *flip-flop* element where a jet stream enters from a power source and attaches to one of two adjacent walls and subsequently exits either through the right or left outlet. If the pressure of the two control ports is equal the gas will attach without preference to the wall of one of the outlet channels (Fig 10–21,A). A small momentary increase or decrease in pressure in

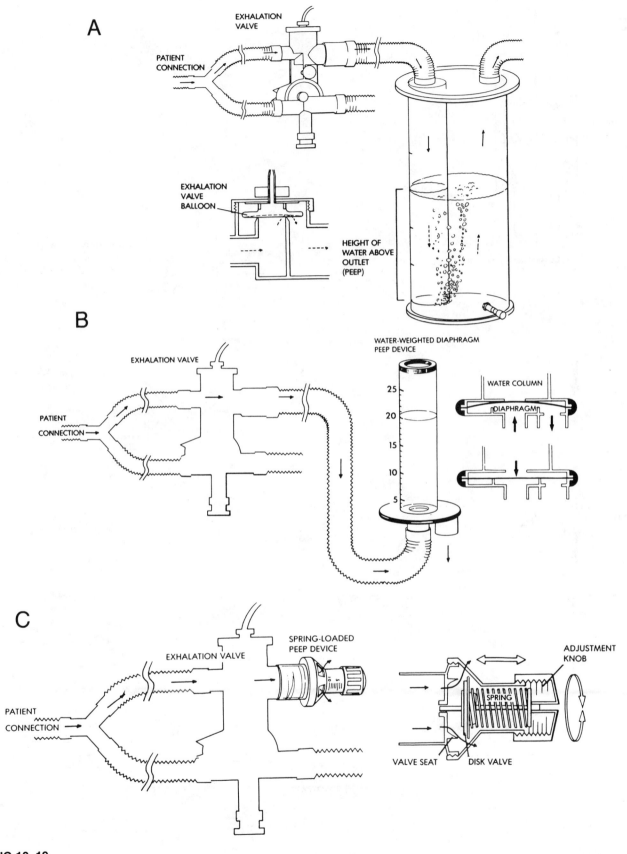

FIG 10–19.
Devices used to create positive end expiratory pressure (PEEP):
A, water column. **B,** water-weighted diaphragm. **C,** spring-loaded disk valve. **D,** weighted ball valve. **E,** Venturi system. **F,** pressur-ized balloon valve. **G,** magnet attraction valve. (From Kirby RR, Smith RA, Desautels DA: *Mechanical Ventilation.* New York, Churchill Livingstone, 1985. Used with permission.) *(Continued.)*

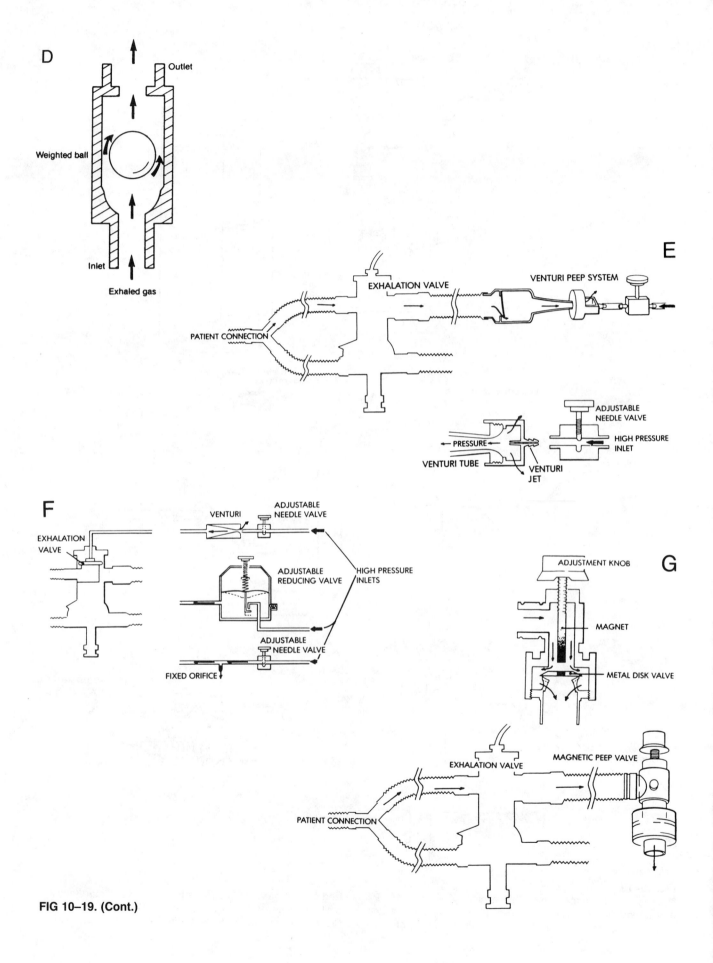

D

Outlet

Weighted ball

Inlet

Exhaled gas

E

EXHALATION VALVE

VENTURI PEEP SYSTEM

PATIENT CONNECTION

ADJUSTABLE
NEEDLE VALVE

PRESSURE

HIGH PRESSURE
INLET

VENTURI TUBE

VENTURI
JET

F

EXHALATION
VALVE

VENTURI

ADJUSTABLE
NEEDLE VALVE

ADJUSTABLE
REDUCING VALVE

HIGH PRESSURE
INLETS

ADJUSTABLE
NEEDLE VALVE

FIXED ORIFICE

G

ADJUSTMENT KNOB

MAGNET

METAL DISK VALVE

EXHALATION VALVE

MAGNETIC PEEP VALVE

PATIENT CONNECTION

FIG 10–19. (Cont.)

A

Jet Stream of Gas

B

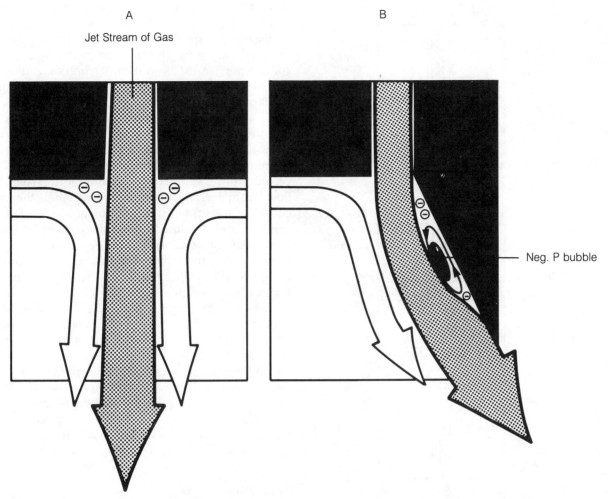

Neg. P bubble

FIG 10–20.
Wall attachment or Coanda effect. **A,** gas leaving from a high-velocity jet causes a fall in lateral pressure which entrains air from both sides. **B,** if a wall is placed on one side, air entrainment is blocked and the fall in pressure attaches the jet stream to the wall.

one of the control ports will attach the jet stream to the opposite outlet channel (Fig 10–21,B).

Fluidic Elements

Six basic fluidic elements that use the Coanda effect form a foundation for more sophisticated fluidic circuits which in many ways are similar to electronic circuits. The *flip-flop* element (Fig 10–22,A) uses one or more control ports to direct the jet stream to the wall of an outlet channel. The jet stream will stay attached to the wall of that outlet channel until another signal from the opposite side moves the jet stream to the other outlet channel. The control port signal only needs to be received for a split second since the jet stream once moved will stay attached to the new outlet channel. This tendency to stay attached to a wall when the control port pressure is equalized is called "memory," i.e., the stream remembers the direction of the last signal (Fig 10–21,C).

The *or/nor gate* allows gas to flow from the left outlet until one of the control ports provides a constant increase in pressure which diverts the jet stream to the wall of the outlet channel on the right (Fig 10–22,B). The jet stream will return to the outlet on the left in the absence of any increase in pressure (signal) at the control ports.

The *back pressure switch* (Fig 10–22,C) allows the jet stream to be switched from the left-hand outlet channel when the signal at the sensor port reaches a certain strength. The strength of the signal is regulated by diverting some of the flow from the power source into the control port channel. The more gas that is allowed to exit through the control port, the stronger the signal will need to be to switch the jet

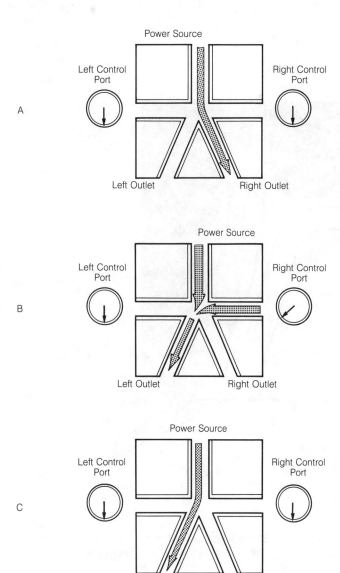

FIG 10–21.
Flip-flop fluidic element. **A,** if the control port pressures are equal, the jet stream randomly attaches to either the right or left outlet when the power source is turned on. **B,** a small momentary increase in pressure by the right control port reattaches the jet stream to the left outlet channel. **C,** the jet stream remains attached to the left outside channel when the control port pressures become equal. This characteristic of flip-flop elements is called "memory," e.g., it remembers the last control port signal.

stream flow from one outlet channel to another.

The *"and/nand gate"* (Fig 10–22,D) allows gas to flow from the outlet on the right when a signal is received at both control ports C1 and C2 simultaneously. The jet stream will continue to flow from the outlet on the right as long as both control port signals continue to be present. If the signal from one of the control ports is turned off, the gas flow from

the active control port will exit through the other control port and the jet stream will attach itself to outlet channel on the left. Both the or/nor gate and the and/nand gate do not have memory, e.g., the control ports must be constantly pressurized in order for the jet stream to be diverted to the right-hand outlet.

The *proportional amplifier* (Fig 10–22,E) allows the jet stream to flow from both outlet ports simultaneously. The amount of flow from each outlet will be proportional to the strength of the signals received from the opposite control port. When the flows from each outlet are added together, they will equal the total flow from the power source. For example, if the pressure at C2 is three times as strong as that found at C1 and the flow from the power source is 40 L/min then the flow from the outlets channels will be 30 L/min from the left side and 10 L/min from the right.

The *Schmitt trigger* (Fig 10–22,F) is used by some ventilators to sense positive or negative pressure. The jet stream will flow from the right-hand outlet until the pressure at C2 is higher than that C1 at which time the jet stream will attach to the left-hand outlet channel. The Schmitt trigger in practice is actually a series of proportional amplifiers and flip-flop elements that connect to each other to compare a varying pressure with an adjustable reference pressure and to provide an on/off signal for outlet ports.

Basic Applications

A simple IPPB machine can be designed using some basic fluidic elements (Fig 10–23). A simple back pressure switch can be used to switch the jet stream and Venturi flow from an outlet connected to the inspiratory line to another outlet for exhalation. The amount of negative pressure the patient has to create to switch the jet stream to the inspiratory channel can be adjusted by varying the amount of pressure at the control port for sensitivity adjustment. The IPPB machine can be pressure-cycled into exhalation by varying the amount of pressure at the control port for pressure limit adjustment. An entrainment port could be designed to be a variable orifice, thereby allowing adjustment of the inspiratory flow rate.

A more complex use of fluidic elements can be found in the design of a prototype ventilator built by the U.S. Army's Harry Dimond Laboratories, Washington, D.C. The U.S. Army volume-cycled ventilator (Fig 10–24) uses two large bi-stable fluid amplifiers and several fluidic elements to provide power

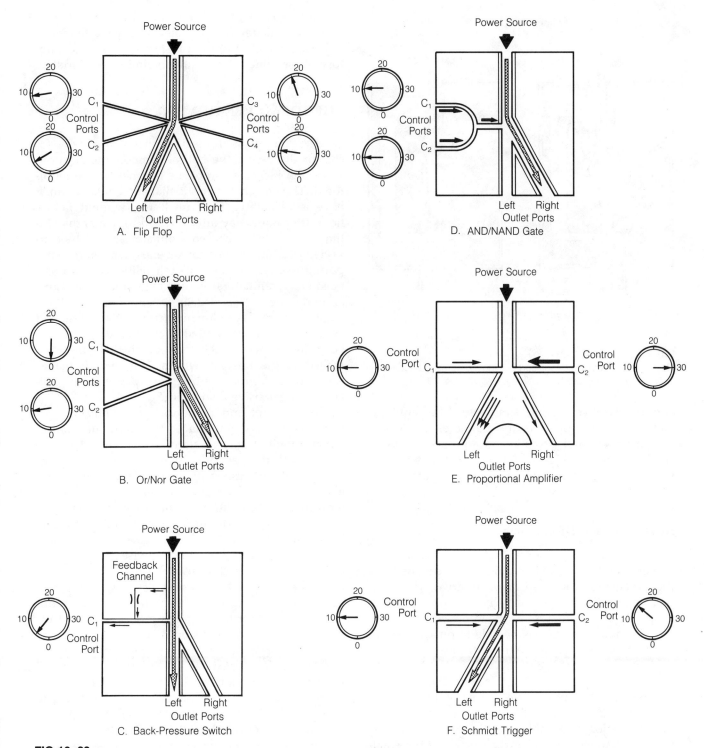

FIG 10–22.
Basic fluidic control elements. **A,** flip flop. **B,** or/nor gate. **C,** back-pressure switch. **D,** AND/NAND gate. **E,** proportional amplifier. **F,** Schmidt trigger.

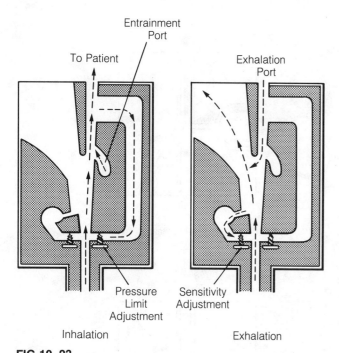

FIG 10–23.
Fluidic IPPB machine. (Modified from McPherson SP: *Respiratory Therapy Equipment*, ed 3. St Louis, CV Mosby Co, 1985.)

and to control ventilation parameters. The ventilator makes good use of all of the fluidic elements discussed above, and practitioners are encouraged to study its simple design as a step toward understanding more complex uses of fluid devices in other ventilators.

Advantages and Disadvantages

The use of ventilators that are pneumatically powered and controlled by fluidic logic circuits have the advantage of safe operation in areas where explosive anesthetic gases may be a problem. Also, hospitals located in areas prone to power failures or electrical interference may be able to put ventilators of this type to good use, either for primary ventilation purposes or as a back-up when electrical problems occur. Since there are a substantially smaller number of mechanical or moving parts, this ventilator should have a longer life than other types.

The major disadvantage is the problem caused by small particles of dirt or dust blocking the small channels that are inherent in fluidic elements. Another problem is the high usage of compressed air as a power source that can run up to 2 cubic ft/min (56 L/min). The high demand for compressed air becomes a problem if several pneumatically driven and fluidically controlled ventilators are connected to the same compressed air system, since they may exceed

the output capacity of the compressor. Finally, this type of ventilator can be noisy and has a tendency to cycle abruptly from the inspiratory to the expiratory phase which some patients find uncomfortable.

THE IDEAL VENTILATOR

The concept of an ideal ventilator provides a focus for discussing the critical components of ventilators and identifies problems that need to be monitored. The one characteristic that all ventilators must have is reliability. They must run without failure hour after hour, day after day, and for months at a time. A newly purchased ventilator should be connected to a lung analog for several days before being put into service to check its reliability. The cost and need for ventilators is so high that the turnaround time for service or repair of malfunctions must be short. Several manufacturers have designed ventilators that use printed circuit boards which can be easily replaced with a new board that can be air mailed to the hospital within 24 hours. It makes sense to use ventilators that have proven to be reliable after extensive field testing.

The control and monitoring of ventilation parameters is very important, therefore the control panel, monitoring, and alarm systems must be designed with the patient's safety in mind. For example, an alarm system that sounds frequent false alarms will soon be ignored or silenced. Alarm systems that can be deliberately or inadvertently turned off can be very dangerous if someone forgets to reactivate them. Simple things, such as all controls turning only one revolution in a clockwise direction with a latch to lock the control in place so that it is not accidentally moved to another setting, are sometimes missing from even the more expensive ventilators. The proper labeling and grouping of controls is necessary so no confusion occurs when changing ventilation or alarm parameters. Important monitoring data such as proximal airway pressure, inspired oxygen concentration, and delivered tidal volumes must be prominently displayed, connected to alarm systems, and easily read from a distance.

The gas delivered to the patient both for mechanical and spontaneous breaths must be adequately humidified (100% relative humidity at body temperature). An inline temperature probe should be placed in the breathing circuit close to where it connects to the patient since there is a danger of burning the patient's airways if the mainstream humidifier becomes empty and overheats. An ideal ventilator would monitor and display the tempera-

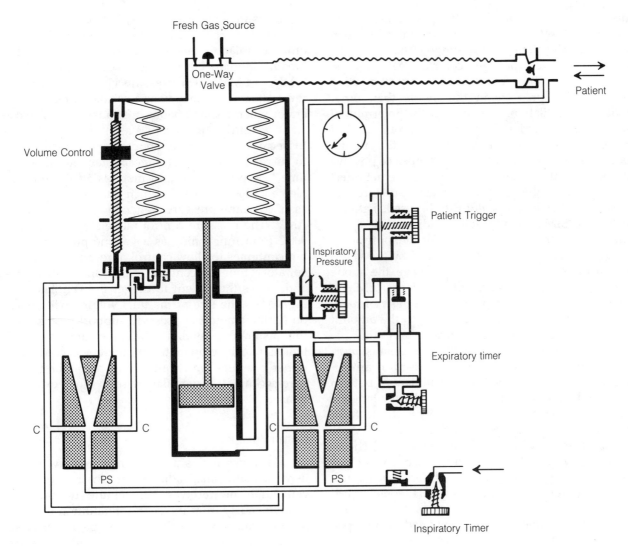

FIG 10–24.
The U.S. Army volume-cycled ventilator. (Modified from Mushin WW, Rendell-Baker L, Thompson PW: *Automatic Ventilation of the Lungs,* ed 3. Oxford, Blackwell Scientific Publications, 1980.)

ture, sound an alarm, and shut off the humidifier if a high temperature occurs. The challenge to engineers is to deliver the humidified gas from a mainstream humidifier to upper airways at the right temperature without large amounts of water condensing and obstructing the inspiratory or expiratory side of the breathing circuit.

ADMINISTERING MECHANICAL VENTILATION

Initial Ventilation Parameters

Modes of Ventilation

The ventilation pattern will be affected by the way a ventilator is cycled from the expiratory to inspiratory phase. If a patient can trigger the ventilator

to deliver a mandatory tidal volume, the mode is called *assisted mechanical ventilation* (AMV). When the tidal volume is delivered by the ventilator at specific time intervals regardless of the patient's inspiratory efforts, the mode is called *controlled mechanical ventilation* (CMV). The assist-control mode is operative when the AMV and CMV modes are combined to deliver a tidal volume every time the patient makes a strong enough inspiratory effort and guarantees that the ventilator will automatically revert to a preset respiratory rate should the patient become apneic or begin to breathe slowly.

The assist mode has the advantage of allowing a patient to determine the minute volume needed. However, a lesion of the respiratory centers, pain, anxiety, or medication may cause the patient to hyperventilate or hypoventilate to dangerous levels.[31]

The control mode will allow the practitioner to inadvertently provide the wrong amount of ventilation, especially if there is a sudden change in the patient's condition. Both the control (CMV) and assist modes (AMV) have the disadvantage of creating more positive pressure in the thorax than other modes of ventilation. The use of the intermittent mandatory ventilation (IMV) or synchronized IMV (SIMV) mode will allow a patient to breathe spontaneously and therefore lower the number of positive pressure breaths required per minute. The net effect will be to lower the mean intrathoracic pressure and to allow higher levels of PEEP to be used. Patients on IMV or SIMV may be able to adjust their spontaneous breathing to correct for inappropriate amounts of ventilation being provided by the ventilator. Conversely, ventilators that have the mode called *extended mandatory minute ventilation* (EMMV) have the advantage of allowing the number of mandatory breaths to fluctuate according to the amount of spontaneous ventilation provided by the patient.[29] The use of EMMV without *pressure support* (inspiratory assist) could potentially lead to an unfavorable and very inefficient ventilation pattern comprised of a large number of small spontaneous tidal volumes that move gas primarily back and forth across anatomical and physiological deadspace.[28, 55] In most cases, EMMV would not be a good choice for the *initial* mode of ventilation since it would be difficult to estimate the amount of deadspace ventilation that would occur during spontaneous breathing.[42]

When first mechanically ventilated, many patients have unstable cardiovascular systems that might be adversely affected by a high mean intrathoracic pressure resulting from the control (CMV) or assist (AMV) mode of ventilation.[60] Accordingly, SIMV without pressure support for spontaneous breaths appears to be the best way to initially provide adequate ventilation. The lowest number of mechanical breaths per minute should be used since a high SIMV rate differs very little from CMV in terms of the ventilation pattern. In cases such as flail chest where spontaneous breathing may work against internal splinting of the chest wall, CMV may be the mode of choice. However, the use of CMV concurrent with the depression of spontaneous ventilation by muscle paralysis or heavy sedation may place the patient in a life-threatening circumstance if the ventilator malfunctions or the patient becomes accidentally disconnected from the ventilator. Therefore, whenever possible, the patient should be allowed and encouraged to breathe spontaneously when being mechanically ventilated.

Pressure support of a spontaneous breathing pattern may be used alone or in conjunction with other ventilation modes that allow the patient to breathe spontaneously from the circuit such as IMV, SIMV, or EMMV. The pressure support mode allows the ventilator to function as a constant pressure generator when a spontaneous breath is taken. The constant pressure applied serves as an inspiratory assist to decrease the work of spontaneous breathing and to increase the size of the spontaneous tidal volume.[36] A pressure control mode is available on the Siemen 900C ventilator which allows it to function as a constant pressure generator during CMV or AMV. The pressure control mode stops the Siemen 900C from functioning as a volume preset machine but continues to allow control of respiratory rate, inspiratory time percentage, pause time percentage, and allows the patient to trigger the ventilator during AMV. The size of the tidal volume will depend on (1) the amount of pressure support provided, (2) the inspiratory time, (3) whether the patient attempts to exhale prematurely, thereby exceeding the upper pressure limit control and prematurely pressure-cycling the ventilation into the expiratory phase.

Respiratory Rate

Many ventilators are designed to allow the patient to make small adjustments in the volume of ventilation he receives per minute by breathing spontaneously from the circuit in addition to receiving mandatory tidal volumes. The patient may still be given too many mandatory IMV breaths (hyperventilated) or too few (hypoventilated). However, small adjustments made by the patient increasing or decreasing his spontaneous respiratory rate will allow small corrections to be made. The mechanical respiratory rate of the ventilator becomes more critical when a patient is completely unable to breathe due to paralysis or a severe decrease in pulmonary function. Many patients in acute respiratory failure will have most of their own breathing efforts wasted on moving small tidal volumes rapidly back and forth to areas of the lung where there is anatomical and physiological deadspace. Accordingly, very little of the gas moved spontaneously by these patients contributes to the ventilation of functional alveoli.

The initial respiratory rate for adults is usually set at 10 per minute until an arterial blood gas study can be done to evaluate the adequacy of ventilation. Then the rate is adjusted up or down based on the arterial CO_2 tension. Since there are advantages to setting the ventilator to deliver a large tidal volume, the respiratory rate becomes the main parameter used to regulate alveolar ventilation. A blood gas study should be done after the patient has been on the ventilator for approximately 10 to 20 minutes and the respiratory rate adjusted accordingly. Changes in respiratory rate usually should not be made unless the CO_2 tension is outside of the clinically acceptable range of 30 to 50 mm Hg, or the patient's spontaneous breathing rate is greater than 30 per minute. Head injuries may require a lower than normal CO_2 tension to be maintained.

The respiratory rates of children, infants, and newborns all need to be set substantially higher than adults. Table 10–3 provides some guidelines for setting the initial respiratory rate and tidal volume.

Tidal Volume

The use of small tidal volumes ($<$10 ml/kg) to mechanically ventilate adult patients seriously affects the efficiency of oxygenation by promoting progressive alveolar and small airway closure. This may result in right-to-left shunting of blood and a large alveolar-arterial oxygen gradient. For adults, the accepted norm for ventilator-delivered tidal volumes is 10 to 15 ml/kg of ideal body weight. Large tidal volumes have been associated with a reduction in the alveolar-arterial oxygen gradient and help to internally stabilize the chest wall when paradoxical breathing is a problem.

The initial tidal volume setting should usually be 10 ml/kg to minimize the increase in pressure. Many patients, when placed on a ventilator, have unstable cardiovascular parameters, and increased intrathoracic pressure may restrict the venous return of blood to the heart.[49, 53, 54, 62] Since the left ventricle can only pump what is sent to it by the right ventricle via the pulmonary circulation, the cardiac output and subsequently the blood pressure may be adversely affected by the use of large tidal volumes. Once the cardiovascular system is stabilized by adequate oxygenation, cardiotonic drugs, and adequate circulating blood volume,[52] the tidal volume should be increased to 13 ml/kg and eventually to 15 ml/kg. The tidal volume should not be adjusted to increase or decrease the arterial CO_2 tension. The alveolar ventilation can be controlled more effectively by changing the respiratory rate and using optimal levels of PEEP.[10, 11]

Positive End-Expiratory Pressure

The use of PEEP is an important way to prevent terminal airway and alveolar collapse. Usually a minimum of 5 cm H_2O of PEEP will be indicated for use during mechanical ventilation since tracheal intubation holds the larynx constantly open which leads to alveolar collapse and a reduction in functional residual capacity.[1, 15] The application of PEEP opens collapsed alveoli and terminal bronchioles, increases the functional residual capacity, and "splints" the lung in a position of function. The ventilator needs to be adjusted to deliver the optimal or best level of PEEP to improve ventilation-perfusion ratios and to allow a lower inspired oxygen concentration to be used. The safe way to arrive at the optimal level is to start with a baseline of zero and add PEEP in 5 cm H_2O increments while monitoring the criteria used to determine the greatest improvement in oxygen transport.

Optimal PEEP is the level of end expiratory pressure that results in the lowering of intrapulmonary shunting, significant improvement in arterial oxygenation, and only a small change in cardiac output, arteriovenous oxygen content difference, or mixed venous oxygen tension (Fig 10–25).[11] The SIMV mode of ventilation, the use of precise cardiovascular monitoring, and interventions to improve cardiovascular function allow the concept of optimal PEEP to be used safely.

Inspiratory Flow Waveforms

Modern ventilators allow practitioners to select both the peak inspiratory flow rate and a specific type of flow waveform. The three most commonly

TABLE 10–3.

Estimated Basal Tidal Volume and Frequency by Age, Weight, and Sex*

AGE, YR	NORMAL FREQUENCY	AVERAGE WEIGHT, LB	TIDAL VOLUME, ML	
			MALE	FEMALE
Newborn	30–40	8	18–22	18–22
1	25–35	22	55–70	55–70
2	±28	27	80	80
3	±25	32	100	100
4–6	20–25	36–44	125–150	125–145
7–9	20–25	50–65	160–180	155–175
10–14	20–25	65–100	200–265	185–245
15–16	16–18	100–115	300–330	280–300
Adult	12–18	120	350	320
		130	370	340
		150	400	360
		175	450	400
		200	500	440
		225	540	460

*From Spearman CE, Sheldon RL, Egan DF: *Egan's Fundamentals of Respiratory Therapy*, ed 4. St Louis, CV Mosby Co, 1982. Used with permission.

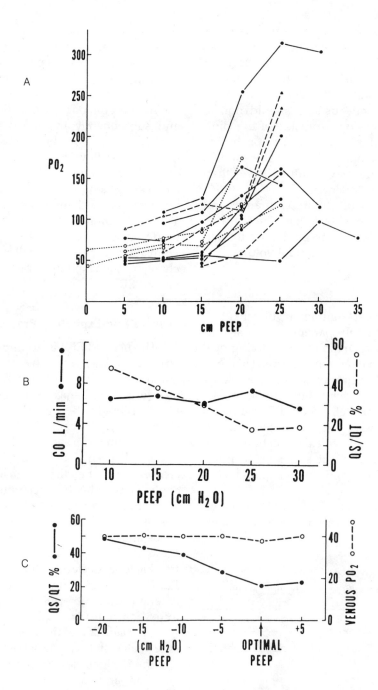

FIG 10–25.
A, arterial Po_2 as a function of the level of PEEP in patients who did not respond to lower levels. Note that little or no improvement occurred until 15 cm H_2O was exceeded. **B,** cardiac output determinations performed at varying levels of end-expiratory pressure. Note lack of change despite use of high levels of end-expiratory pressure, whereas shunt fraction decreased significantly. **C,** venous oxygen tension measurements at different levels of end-ex- piratory pressure. Decreased values were not observed in these patients when PEEP levels were raised. In conjunction with cardiac output data, this supports the thesis that no detrimental cardiovascular effects were produced. (From Civetta JM, Barnes TA, Smith LO: "Optimal PEEP" and intermittent mandatory ventilation in the treatment of acute respiratory failure. *Respir Care* 1975; 20:551– 557. Used with permission.)

used waveforms are shown in Figure 10–10. The inspiratory waveform provided depends on whether the ventilator is functioning as a constant flow, nonconstant flow, or constant pressure generator. Some flow patterns allow the pressure or flow to be held constant while the other parameter increases or decreases in response to the patient's pulmonary compliance and airway resistance. The flow pattern found with some flow generators is a sine wave which retains the same shape despite changes in compliance and resistance.

The constant flow generator is perhaps the easiest to understand since the waveform produced is square and the flow rate does not increase or decrease during the entire inspiratory phase. This type of flow generator requires high driving pressures so that changes in compliance or airway resistance will not cause the inspiratory flow rate to change. Another type of flow generator that uses a rotary-driven piston as a drive mechanism produces a nonconstant flow waveform that has the shape of a sine wave. One of the advantages of ventilators that produce a sine wave is that they come closest to duplicating the inspiratory flow patterns seen with normal spontaneous breathing. The sine wave pattern has slow flow rates at first as the inertia of the lung is overcome and airways stretch to a larger diameter, followed by a sharp increase in flow that delivers almost all the tidal volume, and finishes with a sudden decrease in flow toward the end of the inspiratory phase (Fig 10–26). The result is little or no gas flow during the last part of the inspiratory phase, which has the beneficial effect of allowing time for the gas to move into less compliant areas of the lungs.[35]

Constant flow generators that allow the inspiratory flow rate, tidal volume, and respiratory rate to be set provide a means for controlling inspiratory time and the I:E ratio. A peak inspiratory flow of 30 to 40 L/min usually provides a laminar flow that comes close to matching that seen during quiet spontaneous breathing. A higher peak inspiratory flow may be required for patients that are short of breath, tachypneic, and/or anxious because of moderate hypoxemia, pain, severe chronic airway obstruction, or other sequelae.[12] Some ventilators regulate inspiratory flow by adjusting inspiratory time. The calculations required to determine the mean flow rate are straightforward, and examples can be found in Appendix B.

The choice of which inspiratory flow waveform to use may be influenced by the amount of airway resistance encountered. A sine wave or decelerating

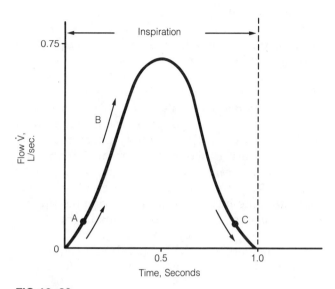

FIG 10–26.
Advantages of a sine wave inspiratory flow pattern. *A*, low flow initially allows the inertia of the lung to be overcome. *B*, a rapid increase in flow allows the tidal volume to be delivered early, which allows *C*, time for distribution of the tidal volume into less compliant areas of the lung.

waveform will allow early delivery of the tidal volume and low flow toward the end of inspiration. A sine wave may be better than a square or decelerating taper waveform if pulmonary edema creates high inertia that must be overcome at the beginning of inspiration. The constant flow (square wave) waveform has the advantage of delivering the tidal volume quickly, thereby allowing a longer expiratory time which helps to reduce the effect of increased mean intrathoracic pressure. The mode of ventilation operative influences the inspiratory flow waveform selected since SIMV and other modes that combine spontaneous breathing with fewer mandatory breaths allow longer inspiratory times and the use of an inspiratory hold.

Inspiratory Hold

One of the advantages of using SIMV is the ability to reduce the number of positive pressure breaths delivered per minute, thereby reducing the mean intrathoracic pressure. A lower mean intrathoracic pressure allows the amount of time spent in the inspiratory phase during SIMV breaths to be extended by setting the ventilator to "hold" the tidal volume in the lungs after being delivered. A control for creating an inspiratory hold is available on most flow generators. A plateau is created in the inspiratory pressure waveform during the hold time which is usually designated as a proportion of the entire ventilatory cycle or in seconds. The inspiratory hold allows the tidal volume to be distributed more evenly into areas of lung with low compliance and high airway resistance.[46] However, this is done at the price of increased intrathoracic pressure, and the degree to which arterial oxygenation is improved has been questioned by some investigators.[21] Inspiratory hold is not often used when a patient is first mechanically ventilated since it may increase mean intrathoracic pressure. The cardiovascular system must first be stabilized and a ventilation pattern established that minimizes the increase in intrathoracic pressure before the inspiratory phase is extended. The use of positive end expiratory pressure (PEEP) to constantly keep areas of the lung with low compliance open has significantly reduced the need for an inspiratory hold.

Inspiratory-Expiratory Ratio

The time allowed for the inspiratory and expiratory phases of mechanical ventilation is commonly referred to as the inspiratory-expiratory (I:E) ratio. The inspiratory part of the ratio includes the time to deliver the tidal volume *plus* the hold time before the exhalation valve opens and exhalation begins. The expiratory part of the ratio includes the time necessary for the tidal volume to exit through the exhalation valve *plus* the pause time before the next inspiration starts. It is important to remember to include the inspiratory hold and expiratory pause times when calculating the I:E ratio (see Fig 10–16). Usually the I:E ratio is determined by calculating the inspiratory time from a knowledge of the size of the tidal volume, the inspiratory flow rate, and inspiratory pause time. The expiratory time is determined by knowing the total cycle time and subtracting the inspiratory time. See Appendix B for examples of how to calculate I:E ratios. The inspiratory time should be long enough to deliver the tidal volume at flow rates that will not result in turbulence and high peak airway pressures. Normally ventilators will be set to deliver tidal volumes at a flow rate of 30 to 40 L/min which usually results in safe I:E ratios of 1:1.5 or 1:2.[6] Inspiratory to expiratory ratios that allow positive pressure to be applied to the lungs for a longer time during inspiration are more likely to raise mean intrathoracic pressure, thereby decreasing cardiac output. For example, a 1:2 I:E ratio is better than 1:1 since above baseline pressure is held in the chest for a shorter period of time.[47] Most ventilators allow several ventilation parameters to be set which may indirectly affect the inspiratory time and I:E ratio. However, many ventilators sound an alarm if the inspiratory phase exceeds the expiratory phase, e.g., I:E ratio of 2:1.

Diverse I:E ratios may have to be used when inspiration cannot be completed in one-third of the respiratory cycle due to low compliance and/or increased airway resistance. This situation occurs in clinical practice with assisted ventilation when the inspiratory time needs to be lengthened and the patient will not tolerate a reduction in the number of mandatory breaths/min.

Inspired Oxygen Concentration

Until the level of hypoxemia is determined, a patient placed on a ventilator should usually receive a F_{IO_2} of 1.00.[4] The oxygen concentration should be systematically lowered as soon as possible; however, this should be done in relatively small increments followed by a blood gas study to ensure that the arterial oxygen tension does not drop below 80 mm Hg. Patients with adult respiratory distress syndrome (ARDS) who are difficult to oxygenate will usually benefit from receiving optimal PEEP, which should allow significantly lower inspired oxygen concentrations to be used. The risk of oxygen toxicity (see Chapter 5) should be avoided if possible but not at the expense of providing adequate tissue oxygenation.[19] Appropriate and sometimes aggressive use of early intubation, optimal CPAP/PEEP, mechanical ventilation, and interventions to improve cardiovascular function usually will allow adequate oxygen transport to occur at F_{IO_2} levels that have not proved to be toxic.

Pressure Limit

A volume-cycled or volume preset ventilator should be adjusted to limit peak inspiratory pressure (PIP) to a safe level. Also, it is useful on a volume preset ventilator to know when the peak inspiratory pressure is rising. A rise in PIP usually means that the airway resistance is rising and/or the pulmonary compliance is falling. Therefore, many practitioners believe the peak inspiratory pressure alarm should be set 10 cm H_2O higher than the observed peak inspiratory pressure so that a change will cause the alarm to sound, alerting someone of a change in the patient's pulmonary mechanics. It may in some cases simply mean that the patient has accumulated secretions in his airways or tracheal tube and needs to be suctioned.

Patient Trigger

The patient trigger control may be set to allow a patient to initiate an assisted or spontaneous breath. Usually the trigger control is set to begin inspiration when the inspiratory effort causes pressure in the breathing circuit to drop 2 cm H_2O below the end expiratory level. If 20 cm H_2O of PEEP were in use and the trigger level were set at 2 cm H_2O below the baseline pressure, the ventilator would cycle into the inspiratory phase whenever the pressure in the circuit dropped to 18 cm H_2O. Most ventilators have a trigger control that is operative over a wide range of pressures to accommodate different PEEP levels and to provide for a larger inspiratory effort in preparation for weaning a patient from mechanical ventilation. Failure to take the PEEP level into consideration when adjusting the patient trigger control may result in the patient having to make a much larger inspiratory effort in order to trigger a breath which would result in an increased work of breathing, increased oxygen consumption, and fatigue. A weak patient may not be able to receive assisted or spontaneous breath from the circuit in this circumstance.[7]

Sigh Volume and Frequency

Intermittent sighing may be necessary to maintain airway patency and to prevent atelectasis. The use of large tidal volumes and PEEP help to prevent atelectasis and reduce the need to periodically sigh a patient being mechanically ventilated. However, when small tidal volumes (10 ml/kg), zero end-expiratory pressure (ZEEP), and nonspontaneous modes of mechanical ventilation (e.g., CMV, AMV) are used, periodic ventilator-delivered sighs may be needed. The sigh volume is usually set at twice the size of the tidal volume and delivered at certain time or frequency intervals of once or twice every 100 breaths or approximately 6 to 12 times per hour.

Alarm Parameters

A ventilator is a complex life support system that interfaces a patient to a machine that by its very mechanical and electrical nature is potentially subject to failure. The elements of support provided by the ventilator such as oxygen, ventilation, and PEEP all must function flawlessly for long periods of time.

The function of alarm systems is to alert the practitioner that a change in ventilation parameters has occurred. The change may be the result of a change in the patient's condition, such as a pressure limit alarm sounding because the patient needs to be suctioned or may indicate a mechanical or electrical failure. The fundamental concept to remember is that *inoperative or inadequately adjusted alarms are dangerous.* It is important that all alarms on a ventilator be properly tested prior to patient use and then again every time a ventilator is checked while in use. The best way to check an alarm is to simulate a life-threatening change in the parameter being monitored while the ventilator is connected to a test lung. For example, if a PEEP pressure alarm is supposed to sound within 10 seconds when the end-expiratory level drops by more than 2 cm H_2O, you should create a small leak in the patient's breathing circuit to drop the PEEP level by 3 cm H_2O and test the alarm's sensitivity and the response time. It is absolutely incorrect and dangerous to change alarm parameters without testing for their proper operation. The alarm systems available vary according to the ventilator being used, but the following parameters are critical: (1) peak inspiratory pressure, (2) I:E ratio, (3) PEEP pressure, (4) inspired oxygen concentration, and (5) exhaled tidal volume.

Control Interaction

Several ventilators are designed in a way that allow control parameters to interact with each other. For example, a change made to the peak inspiratory flow control on many ventilators will affect both the inspiratory time and the I:E ratio. Other examples of controls that interact with each other are inspiratory time, pressure limit, minute volume, respiratory rate, I:E ratio, tidal volume, and mode of ventilation. Practitioners must be able to predict what effect a change in one or more parameter settings will have on the ventilation pattern. A good working knowledge of the functional capability and classification categories of ventilators should allow control interaction to be anticipated. Initial ventilation parameters and the integrity of the breathing circuit should be checked with a test lung prior to connecting the ventilator to a patient. The pressure, flow, and volume waveforms that will occur during the inspiratory and expiratory phases must be determined. Also, the effect of increased airway resistance and/or decreased pulmonary compliance on ventilation waveforms should be considered when selecting the initial set of ventilator parameters.

REFERENCES

1. Annest SJ, et al: Detrimental effects of removing end-respiratory pressure prior to endotracheal extubation. *Ann Surg* 1980; 191:539–545.
2. Ayers SM: Mechanisms and consequences of pulmonary edema: Cardiac lung, shock lung, and principles of ventilatory therapy in adult respiratory distress syndrome. *Am Heart J* 1982; 103:97–112.
3. Baeza OR, Wagner RB, Lowery BD: Pulmonary hyperinflation. A form of barotrauma during mechanical ventilation. *Thorac Cardiovasc Surg* 1975; 70:790–805.
4. Baigelman W, et al: Relation of inspired oxygen fraction to hypoxemia in mechanically ventilated adults. *Crit Care Med* 1984; 12:486–488.
5. Bergquist RE, et al: Comparison of ventilatory patterns in the treatment of freshwater near-drowning in dogs. *Anesthesiology* 1980; 52:142–148.
6. Berman LS, Downs JB, Van Eeden A: Inspiration: expiration ratio: Is mean airway pressure the difference? *Crit Care Med* 1981; 9:775–777.
7. Brach BB, Yin F, Timms R: Reduced inspiratory effort during intermittent mandatory ventilation with PEEP. *Crit Care Med* 1976; 4:142–143.
8. Carlon GC, et al: Early prediction of outcome of respiratory failure. Comparison of high-frequency jet ventilation and volume-cycled ventilation. *Chest* 1984; 86:194–197.
9. Carnevale F, et al: Induced paralysis: When your patient is on Pavulon. *Nurse* 1983; 79:45–48.
10. Civetta JM, Flor RJ, Smith LO: Aggressive treatment of acute respiratory insufficiency. *South Med J* 1976; 69:749–751.
11. Civetta JM, Barnes TA, Smith LO: "Optimal PEEP" and intermittent mandatory ventilation in the treatment of acute respiratory failure. *Respir Care* 1975; 20:551–557.
12. Connors AF Jr, McCaffree DR, Gray BA: Effect of inspiratory flow rate on gas exchange during mechanical ventilation. *Am Rev Respir Dis* 1981; 124:537–543.
13. Cournand A, et al: Physiologic studies of the effects of intermittent positive pressure breathing on cardiac output in man. *Am J Physiol* 1948; 152:162.
14. Cullen P, et al: Treatment of flail chest. Use of intermittent mandatory ventilation and positive end-expiratory pressure. *Arch Surg* 1975; 110:1099–1103.
15. Dechert R, Bandy K, Lanzara R: Use of PEEP in acute respiratory distress syndrome in dogs. *Crit Care Med* 1981; 9:10–3.
16. Delooz HH: Factors influencing successful discontinuance of mechanical ventilation after open heart surgery: A clinical study of 41 patients. *Crit Care Med* 1976; 4:265–270.
17. Douglas JG, Ferguson RJ, Crompton GK, et al: Artificial ventilation for neurological disease: Retrospective analysis. *Br Med J* 1983; 286:1943–1946.
18. Downs JB, Douglass ME, Sanfelippo PM: Ventilatory pattern, intrapleural pressure, and cardiac output. *Anesth Analg* 1977; 56:88–96.
19. Drummond GB, Zhong NS: Inspired oxygen and oxygen transfer during artificial ventilation for respiratory failure. *Br J Anaesth* 1983; 55:3–13.
20. Epstein RA, Epstein MA: Flow to lung compartments with different time constants: Effect of choice of model. *Acta Anaesthesiol Scand* 1981; 25:39–45.
21. Fuleihan SF, Wilson RS, Pontoppidan H: Effect of mechanical ventilation with end inspiratory pause on blood-gas exchange. *Anesth Analg* 1976; 55:122–130.
22. Gabel JC, et al: Intermittent mandatory ventilation. *South Med J* 1977; 70:274–276.
23. Goldfarb MA, et al: Tracking respiratory therapy in the trauma patient. *Am J Surg* 1975; 129:255–258.
24. Gordon E: Management of acute head injuries by controlled ventilation, in Arias A, et al (ed): *Recent Progress in Anaesthesiology and Resuscitation*. Amsterdam, Excerpta Medica, 1975, no 347, 1974.
25. Goris RJ, et al: Improved survival of multiply injured patients by early internal fixation and prophylactic mechanical ventilation. *Injury* 1982; 14:39–43.
26. Gracey DR, Divertie MB, Howard FM Jr: Mechanical ventilation for respiratory failure in myasthenia gravis: Two-year experience with 22 patients. *Mayo Clin Proc* 1983; 58:597–602.
27. Haraguchi Y, et al: Treatment of postoperative respiratory distress syndrome. *Resuscitation* 1981; 9:331–343.
28. Hedenstierna G: The effect of respiratory frequency on pulmonary function during artificial ventilation: A review. *Acta Anaesthesiol Scand* 1976; 20:20–31.
29. Hewlett AM, Platt AS, Terry VG: Mandatory minute volume: A new concept in weaning from mechanical ventilation. *Anaesthesia* 1977; 32:163–169.
30. Higgs BD, Bevan JC: Use of mandatory minute volume ventilation in the perioperative management of a patient with myasthenia. *Br J Anaesth* 1979; 51:1181–1184.
31. Hooper RG, Browning M: Acid-base changes and ventilator mode during maintenance ventilation. *Crit Care Med* 1985; 13:44–45.
32. Ibanez J, Raurich JM, Moris SG: A simple method for measuring the effect of PEEP on functional residual capacity during mechanical ventilation. *Crit Care Med* 1982; 10:332–334.
33. Jenkins J, Lynn, A, Edmonds J, et al: Effects of mechanical ventilation on cardiopulmonary function in children after open heart surgery. *Crit Care Med* 1985; 13:77–80.
34. Jones PW: Hyperventilation in the management of cerebral oedema. *Intensive Care Med* 1981; 7:205–207.
35. Johansson H: Effects on breathing mechanics and gas exchange of different inspiratory gas flow patterns in patients undergoing respiratory treatment. *Acta Anaesthesiol Scand* 1975; 19:19–27.
36. Kanak R, Fahey PJ, Vanderwarf C: Oxygen cost of

breathing: Changes dependent upon mode of mechanical ventilation. *Chest* 1985; 87:126–127.

37. Kirby RR: Intermittent mandatory ventilation in the neonate. *Crit Care Med* 1977; 5:18–22.

38. Kirby RR, et al: Cardiorespiratory effects of high positive end-expiratory pressure. *Anaesthesiology* 1975; 43:533.

39. Klein MT, Moyes DG: Ventilation monitors and alarms. *Afr Med J* 1985; 67:310–341.

40. Klein EF Jr: Weaning from mechanical breathing with intermittent mandatory ventilation. *Arch Surg* 1975; 110:345–347.

41. Kondo T, et al: Measurement of functional residual capacity and pulmonary carbon monoxide diffusing capacity during mechanical ventilation with PEEP. *Tokai J Exp Clin Med* 1982; 7:561–573.

42. Laaban JP, et al: Influence of caloric intake on the respiratory mode during mandatory minute volume ventilation. *Chest* 1985; 87:67–72.

43. Larny M: Techniques of ventilatory therapy in the adult respiratory distress syndrome (ARDS). *Acta Anaesthesiol Belg* 1982; 33:243–257.

44. Laver MB: The pulmonary response to trauma and mechanical ventilation: Its consequences on hemodynamic function. *World J Surg* 1983; 7:31–41.

45. Leventhal SR, Orkin FK, Hirsh RA: Prediction of the need for postoperative mechanical ventilation in myasthenia gravis. *Anesthesiology* 1980; 53:26–30.

46. Lindahl S: Influence of an end inspiratory pause on pulmonary ventilation, gas distribution, and lung perfusion during artificial ventilation. *Crit Care Med* 1979; 7:540–546.

47. Lindahl S, Kugelberg J, Okmian L: The circulatory response to specific ventilatory patterns using a tidal volume ventilator. *Acta Anaesthesiol Scand* 1979; 23:370–378.

48. Luce JM: The cardiovascular effects of mechanical ventilation and positive end-expiratory pressure. *JAMA* 1984; 252:807–811.

49. MacDonnell KF, et al: Comparative hemodynamic consequences of inflation hold, PEEP, and interrupted PEEP: An experimental study in normal dogs. *Ann Thorac Surg* 1975; 19:552–560.

50. Margand PM, Chodoff P: Intermittent mandatory ventilation: an alternative weaning technic. *Anesth Analg* 1975; 54:41–44.

51. Mathru M, Rao TL, Venous B: Ventilator-induced barotrauma in controlled mechanical ventilation versus intermittent mandatory ventilation. *Crit Care Med* 1983; 11:359–361.

52. Morgan BC, Crawford EG, Guntheroth WG: The hemodynamic effect of changes in blood volume during intermittent positive pressure breathing. *Anesthesiology* 1965; 30:297.

53. Morgan WL, et al: The hemodynamic effects of intermittent pressure respiration. *Anesthesiology* 1966; 27:584.

54. Mushin WW, Rendell-Baker L, Thompson PW: *Automatic Ventilation of the Lungs*. Oxford, Blackwell Scientific, 1980.

55. Norlander O: New concepts of ventilation. *Acta Anaesthesiol Belg* 1982; 33:221–234.

56. Picado C, et al: Mechanical ventilation in severe exacerbation of asthma: Study of 26 cases with six deaths. *Eur J Respir Dis* 1983; 64:102–107.

57. Popovich J, Jr: The physiology of mechanical ventilation and the mechanical zoo: IPPB, PEEP, CPAP. *Med Clin North Am* 1983; 67:621–631.

58. Rarey KP, McCrae CR: A high flow system for intermittent mandatory ventilation. *Respir Care* 1976; 21:985–987.

59. Rasanen J, Nikki P, Heikkila J: Acute myocardial infarction complicated by respiratory failure. The effects of mechanical ventilation. *Chest* 1984; 85:21–28.

60. Rasanen J, Nikki P: Respiratory failure arising from acute myocardial infarction. *Ann Chir Gynaecol* 1982; 71:43–47.

61. Richardson JD, Adams L, Flint LM: Selective management of flail chest and pulmonary contusion. *Ann Surg* 1982; 196:481–487.

62. Robotham JL, Scharf SM: Effects of positive and negative pressure ventilation on cardiac performance. *Clin Chest Med* 1983; 4:161–187.

63. Santesson J: Oxygen transport and venous admixture in the extremely obese: Influence of anaesthesia and artificial ventilation with and without positive end-expiratory pressure. *Acta Anaesthesiol Scand* 1976; 20:387–394.

64. Schuster DP, Klain M, Snyder JV: Comparison of high frequency jet ventilation to conventional ventilation during severe acute respiratory failure in humans. *Crit Care Med* 1982; 10:625–630.

65. Schackford SR, Virgilio RW, Peters RM: Selective use of ventilatory therapy in flail chest injury. *J Thorac Cardiovasc Surg* 1981; 81:194–201.

66. Shinozaki T, et al: Comparison of high frequency lung ventilation with conventional mechanical lung ventilation. Prospective trial in patients who have undergone cardiac operations. *J Thorac Cardiovasc Surg* 1985; 89:268–274.

67. Sjostrand UH, et al: Conventional and high-frequency ventilation in dogs with bronchopleural fistula. *Crit Care Med* 1985; 13:191–193.

68. Turner E, et al: Metabolic and hemodynamic response to hyperventilation in patients with head injuries. *Intensive Care Med* 1984; 10:127–132.

69. Tyler DC, Cheney FW: Comparison of positive end-expiratory pressure and inspiratory positive pressure plateau in ventilation of rabbits with experimental pulmonary edema. *Anesth Analg* 1979; 58:288–292.

70. Venus B, Jacobs HK, Mathru M: Hemodynamic responses to different modes of mechanical ventilation in dogs with normal and aspirated lungs. *Crit Care Med* 1980; 8:620–627.

71. Vincken W, Cosio MG: Clinical applications of high frequency jet ventilation. *Intensive Care Med* 1984; 10:275–280.

72. Vuori A, Jalonen J, Laaksonen V: Continuous positive airway pressure during mechanical and spontaneous ventilation. Effects on central haemodynamics and oxygen transport. *Acta Anaesthesiol Scand* 1979; 23:453–461.

73. Yeston NS, Graserger RC, McCormick JR: Severe combined respiratory and myocardial failure treated with high-frequency ventilation. *Crit Care Med* 1985; 13:208–209.

Cardiopulmonary Resuscitation

Mary E. Watson, Ed.D., R.R.T.

The importance of beginning CPR immediately cannot be overstated. Clinical death occurs at the time the heart stops, but there is a period of time in which the heart may be restarted. Brain death will occur within minutes of the arrest if cardiac compressions are not initiated and oxygen delivered through artificial ventilation. Cardiac arrest is defined as the cessation of cardiac output or a reduction of cardiac output to a point where it is ineffective in providing oxygenated blood to the organs which leads to death if not treated successfully. A respiratory arrest is defined as the cessation of breathing, and, if not treated, will lead to a cardiac arrest.

Early recognition of inadequate ventilation and circulation allows time for intervention so that an arrest is prevented. CPR situations occur less often in hospitals where patients are intubated electively in the presence of an unstable cardiac rhythm, when the PO_2 and spontaneous ventilation are inadequate, or when the unstable patient requires stressful procedures.[25, 26] Intervention procedures for these patients at risk should include locating them where they can be adequately monitored and where CPR can be promptly initiated. Other problems in the critically ill patients that precipitate arrests and should be corrected are electrolyte imbalance and hypotension.

The survival rate reported in the literature for patients requiring cardiopulmonary resuscitation (CPR) varies from 5% to 56%.[7, 17, 25, 26] The likelihood of survival may be dependent on the patient's fitness prior to the arrest, the underlying illness, the place where the arrest occurs, the efficiency and duration of resuscitation, and the patient's condition after resuscitation.[26] Metabolic or respiratory acidosis before the arrest is associated with a low survival rate. The mortality is also high for patients who have pneumonia, renal failure, acute stroke accompanied by a neurological deficit, and those who have hypotension secondary to intrinsic myocardial failure or sepsis.[26] Reports have also indicated that the chance for survival is better if the arrest occurs in the intensive care unit or the emergency room.[17, 25, 26] The best survival rate has been seen in patients who have ventricular fibrillation as opposed to asystole, have had a recent myocardial infarction without prearrest hypotension or cardiac failure, and are resuscitated for less than 15 minutes.[7, 17, 25, 26]

The team approach is a method that has been shown to increase the survival of patients who have required CPR.[36] There should be a qualified designated "STAT" team on duty 24 hours a day. The team may vary depending on the type and size of the hospital, but it should include a cardiologist, anesthesiologist, internist or other staff fellow, respiratory care practitioner, and a nurse. Also, the pharmacist has been shown to be a valued member of the CPR team in progressive hospitals. Support for the role of the pharmacist on the CPR team is in the areas of organization and recording of medications, speed and accuracy of medication preparation and labeling, as well as providing current drug information.[36] Often it is not clear who the charge person is in a CPR situation, especially in large teaching hospitals. Designating leaders of the CPR teams can eliminate some confusion during an emergency situation. Clearly delineating who the charge person is, defining the staff roles, and periodically reinforcing these responsibilities will help maximize the team effort.[47]

CARDIOPULMONARY RESUSCITATION TRAINING

Everyone working in the hospital should be trained in basic life support. If a non–health professional in the hospital witnesses an arrest, it is critical that the person know how to initiate a "code" call and begin CPR. In many situations, unsuccessful attempts are the result of time delays. CPR initiated soon after cardiac arrest substantially increases the long-term survival rate of victims and decreases the possibility of neurological damage.[6, 37, 41]

There are several intervention procedures that may increase the success of resuscitation attempts within the hospital. Improvements in CPR training for hospital personnel and periodic retraining is important. CPR procedures must be reviewed and practiced periodically for maximum retention. Deliberate overtraining in the initial basic life support class has resulted in satisfactory skills retention for at least 1 year.[52]

Maintaining skills requires opportunities for review and practice, even for those practitioners regularly involved with CPR. However, motivating physicians, nurses, and respiratory care practitioners to attend review sessions is often a problem. Including some advanced cardiac life support techniques and creativity in designing the training sessions may overcome this issue. For example, role playing or videotapes where health professionals deliberately make mistakes in CPR situations can be used as a technique for correcting problems.

A resuscitation committee within the hospital can be designated for the purpose of reviewing and maintaining resuscitation records, assuring the continuing competence of the health care workers, and making changes in CPR policies when appropriate. The committee should also assure that a postarrest conference be held after each CPR situation. This is important whether the CPR was successful or not. Each resuscitation attempt is unique and postarrest conferences can be useful in reinforcing successful techniques as well as identifying and correcting problems occurring during the CPR procedure.

Maximal performance during CPR may also depend on the organization and maintenance of the crash carts. "Crash carts" should be standardized throughout the hospital including the location of each item on the cart. They should include medications and supplies necessary for at least the first 10 minutes of resuscitation.[47] The cart should not include any unnecessary equipment or supplies. A method should be established for stocking and checking the cart. Sealing the cart will assure that no one takes the supplies. A protocol should also be provided for nursing, respiratory therapy, and medical personnel to familiarize themselves with the organization of the cart. The respiratory therapy department is responsible for assuring the presence and proper function of the equipment needed for an emergency intubation and a manual resuscitator capable of delivering 100% oxygen.

PROTOCOL FOR CARDIOPULMONARY RESUSCITATION

The American Heart Association recommends a specific protocol for treating an unwitnessed arrest outside the hospital.[44] The inexperienced person should follow the protocol strictly. Some steps can be done simultaneously by the experienced health care practitioner. The protocol also forms the basis for dealing with arrests occurring in the hospital.

Establishing Unresponsiveness

Unresponsiveness should be established by shaking the patient and shouting at a level that would cause arousal if the patient were conscious. There are many situations in which the unresponsiveness of the patient is obvious, and a call for help should be done simultaneously.

Open the Airway

The patient's airway should be opened by the head-tilt/chin-lift method. This is accomplished by placing one hand on the victim's forehead and applying firm backward pressure with the palm to tilt the head back. The fingers of the other hand are placed under the bony part of the lower jaw near the chin and lifted to bring the chin forward and the teeth almost to occlusion (Fig 11–1). Caution should be taken not to injure or increase an injury to the cervical spine. This maneuver should lift the tongue off the back of the throat opening the airway. In some situations, this may be all that is required to restore breathing. For example, the tongue can fall back and obstruct the airway in an unconscious patient due to relaxation of the upper airway muscles.

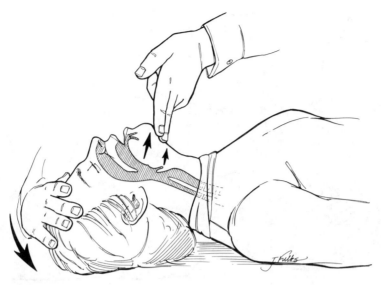

FIG 11–1.
Opening the airway.

Opening the airway can allow breathing for these patients.

If the head tilt method of opening the airway is unsuccessful, the jaw thrust is accomplished by placing the fingers behind the angles of the jaw and displacing the mandible forward while tilting the head backward (Fig 11–2). The position that opens the airway must be maintained at all times.

Establishing Breathlessness

Apnea is confirmed by positioning the ear over the patient's nose and mouth. In this position, the chest is observed for a rising and falling motion and air flow is felt during the expiratory phase (Fig 11–3). Assisted breathing should begin immediately for the patient who is apneic or obstructed.

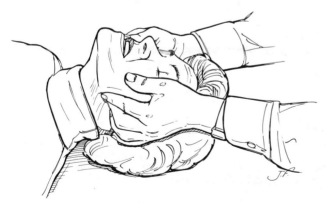

FIG 11–2.
Jaw thrust method for opening the airway.

Mouth-to-Mouth Breathing

The technique of mouth-to-mouth breathing should be used in the absence of a manual resuscitator. The airway is kept open by the head-tilt/chin lift method. The other hand is used to pinch off the nostrils while continuing to exert pressure on the patient's forehead (Fig 11–4). Two full breaths are given in 1 to 1½ seconds to allow enough time to provide good chest expansion. The rescuer should take a breath after each ventilation with a volume of approximately 800 ml for an adult victim. If the airway is patent and air flow is assured, breathing should continue every 5 seconds for an adult. The same technique is used for an older child.

For an infant, a seal is made over the nose and the mouth and two slow breaths (1 to 1½ seconds per breath) are given, with a pause between each breath. The volume will depend on the size of the child and should be limited to the amount of air needed to cause the chest to rise. Breathing should continue every 3 seconds for an infant.

During mouth-to-mouth ventilation, the most common cause of resistance to ventilation is improper positioning of the head. Therefore, if the airway is obstructed, the head should be repositioned and mouth-to-mouth ventilation should be attempted again. Mouth-to-mouth breathing results in an F_{IO_2} of approximately 0.16 which would produce a P_{AO_2} tension of 80 mm Hg.[42] Shunting, ventilation-perfusion mismatching, and a low cardiac output in the code patient will result in a low Pa_{O_2}.

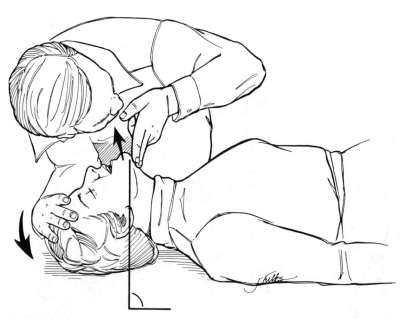

FIG 11–3.
Confirming apnea.

Therefore, a manual resuscitator capable of delivering 100% oxygen should be used as soon as possible.

Oropharyngeal Airways

Oropharyngeal airways will best facilitate manual resuscitation via a face mask when an endotracheal tube is not in place. They are useful in preventing upper airway obstruction caused by prolapse of the tongue in the unconscious patient.

They are inappropriate for patients who are conscious and have a gag reflex because stimulation of the oropharynx could potentially cause vomiting and aspiration. Therefore, the oropharyngeal airway should be removed immediately as the patient shows signs of returning consciousness. The insertion of the oropharyngeal airway is accomplished by opening the mouth, turning the airway upside down while placing it against the tongue. The airway is turned as it is introduced into the oropharynx

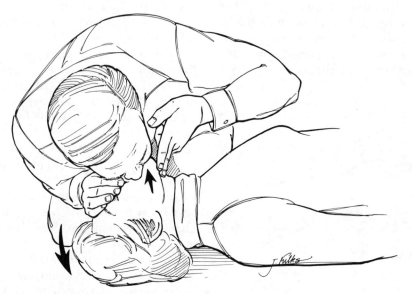

FIG 11–4.
Mouth-to-mouth resuscitation.

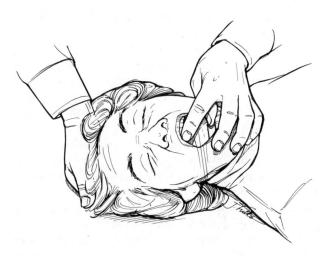

FIG 11–5.
Cross-finger technique.

alongside the tongue. This maneuver pulls the tongue forward, maintaining an open position of the upper airway.

In the situation where the mouth will not open readily, the cross-finger technique should be used. The thumb is placed on the patient's lower teeth and the index finger on the upper teeth. Upward pressure by the index finger and downward pressure by the thumb should force the mouth open (Fig 11–5). The oropharyngeal airway can then be inserted.

There are a variety of oropharyngeal airways available for clinical use (Fig 11–6). They consist of a hollow tube which allows a pathway for breathing and for pharyngeal suctioning. They are made with a rigid material at the point where the patient's teeth could clamp. The rigid material is used to prevent the patient from occluding the tube.

Circulatory Inadequacy

Circulatory inadequacy is determined by palpating the carotid artery in the adult patient (Fig 11–7). This artery is the most accessible for the respiratory care practitioner who is maintaining the airway. The femoral artery is also a common alternative for establishing circulatory adequacy, but it is not as easily accessible. If a pulse is absent, external cardiac compressions should be initiated immediately.

The apical pulse is auscultated to determine circulatory inadequacy for infants and small children in the hospital situation. The stethoscope bell is placed over the heart, below the nipple line, slightly left of the patient's sternum (Fig 11–8).

Patient Positioning

The patient should be positioned supine to allow the maximum blood flow to the brain during cardiac compressions. Even when compressions are performed properly, cardiac output is reduced to approximately 25% to 30% of normal. If the head is elevated, blood flow to the brain will not be ade-

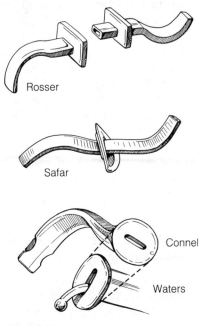
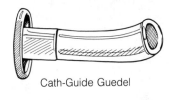
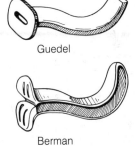

Rosser

Cath-Guide Guedel

Safar

Guedel

Connel

Waters

Berman

FIG 11–6.
Various types of oropharyngeal airways.

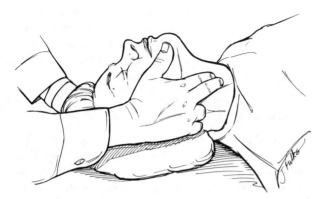

FIG 11–7.
Palpation of the carotid pulse.

quate. Elevation of the legs may also improve cardiac output by enhancing venous return.

For external cardiac compressions to be effective, the patient must be on a firm surface. If a cardiac board is not readily available, the backs of some hospital beds are designed to easily detach for this purpose. The alternative would be any firm surface available, such as a tray placed under the back of the patient. Cardiac compressions should not be delayed while waiting for this support.

Technique for External Cardiac Compressions

External cardiac compressions are performed on the lower half of the adult sternum, above the xiphoid process. The tip of the xiphoid is felt by the

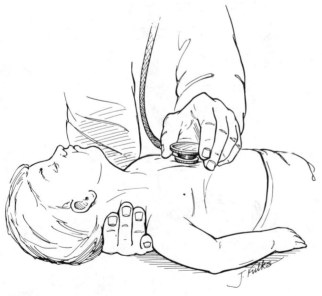

FIG 11–8.
Auscultation of the heart rate of an infant.

fingers on one hand and the heel of the opposite hand is placed on the lower half of the sternum about 1 to 1½ in. away from the tip of the xiphoid (Fig 11–9). The hand that determined the position of the xiphoid is then put on top of the other hand and the fingers may be interlocked. Arms are kept straight with the shoulders directly over the sternum (Fig 11–10). For an adult, pressure is exerted downward enough to depress the sternum 1½ to 2 in. at a rate of 80 to 100 times per minute. The position of compressions is critical for effectiveness; therefore, the hands must never be removed from the chest during relaxation. However, pressure must be completely removed on the upward stroke of compressions. Compressions are done in conjunction with artificial ventilation. The ratio of compressions to ventilation is 5:1 with a pause for ventilation for 1 to 1½ seconds.

Switching

When the two people performing CPR want to switch, they must do so without serious interruption of the 5:1 sequence. The person performing the compressions initiates the switch by indicating that a switch will take place at the end of the next 5:1 sequence. After giving the breath, the person performing the ventilations moves into position to give compressions. The person giving the compressions moves to the head and checks the pulse after giving the fifth compression. If there is no pulse, CPR is continued.

For the short time that the health care practitioner may be performing CPR alone, a ratio of compressions to ventilation should be maintained at 15:2. The compressions are done at a rate of 80 to 100 per minute. When a second person becomes available to assist with CPR, that person should check the pulse to assure that a correct diagnosis has been made. When the carotid artery is palpated, he calls out "stop compressions" and checks for the pulse. If a pulse is absent, two-man CPR is continued.

Cardiopulmonary Resuscitation for Infants and Children

The cardiac compression technique for small children is similar to that of adults. The heel of only one hand is placed over the midsternum, and compressions are at a rate of 80 to 100/min depressing the sternum 1 to 1½ in. depending on the size

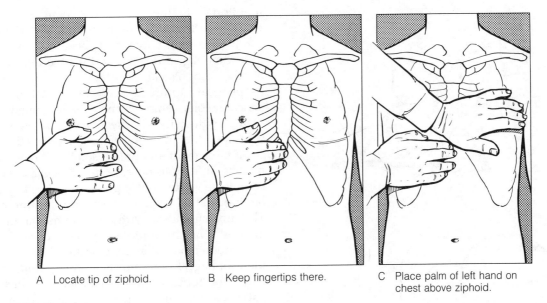

A Locate tip of ziphoid.   B Keep fingertips there.   C Place palm of left hand on chest above ziphoid.

FIG 11–9.
Hand position for cardiac compressions: **A,** locate tip of xiphoid. **B,** measure two fingerwidths from tip xiphoid. **C,** place heel of hand over lower half of sternum above xiphoid.

of the child. A breath is delivered after every 5 compressions.

The tips of the middle and index fingers are used to compress the midsternum of an infant ½ to 1 inch. The rate should be maintained at 100 per minute with a breath given every five compressions. The back of the hand can provide a firm surface for effective compressions with infants and small children (Fig 11–11).

ARTIFICIAL AIRWAYS

Esophageal Obturators

A cardiac arrest victim may be admitted to the emergency room with an esophageal obturator in place. The obturator consists of a mask attached to a cuffed tube (Fig 11–12). The mask is placed tightly around the nose and mouth to provide a seal (Fig 11–13). This airway is inserted into the esophagus rather than the trachea and is designed so that the distal end is sealed. Air from a manual resuscitator is delivered to the laryngeal area through holes in the tube. The tube is cuffed to prevent gastric inflation and regurgitation. The advantage of using an esophageal obturator is thought to be its easy placement by inexperienced personnel because no visualization of the vocal cords is required for its introduction.[40]

The esophageal obturator presents problems that make it inferior to the endotracheal tube.[48] The

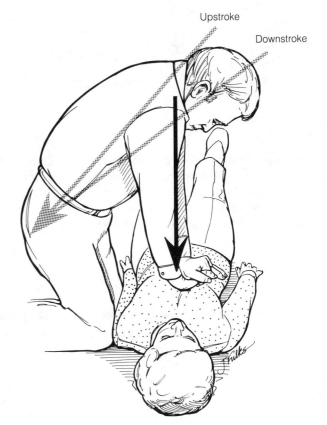

Upstroke

Downstroke

FIG 11–10.
Arm position for cardiac compressions.

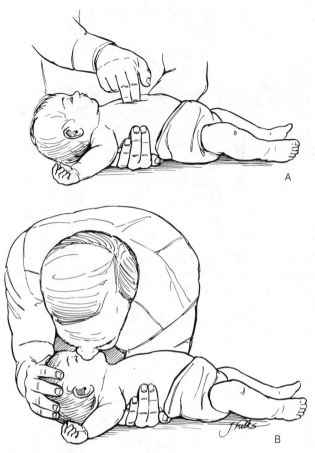

FIG 11–11.
CPR for infants.

endotracheal tube is the emergency airway of choice and can be successfully placed in patients without complications by trained health professionals.[32] The obturator should only be used when no person trained in endotracheal intubation is available. Close

monitoring in the emergency room is required to recognize the critical complications related to its use.

Fatal complications have been reported to occur from esophageal rupture and inadvertent placement of the esophageal obturator into the trachea.[49] Esophageal rupture is suspected by the presence of subcutaneous emphysema, pneumomediastinum, pleural effusion, and chest pain. Placement of the tube into the trachea is recognized by absence of chest movement and breath sounds.[40] However, this may be difficult to observe in the obese patient, and sounds generated by air going into the stomach may be transmitted to the chest and misinterpreted.[54] The tube should be withdrawn immediately if signs indicate it has been placed in the trachea.

Another potential complication related to using the esophageal obturator is vomiting and aspiration when the tube is removed. When the unconscious patient is admitted to the emergency room with an esophageal obturator in place, an endotracheal tube should be inserted before the obturator is removed.[42] If the patient has become conscious and is breathing spontaneously, the cuff of the obturator is deflated and the obturator removed. Precautions should be taken to prevent aspiration. The patient's head is turned to the side and suction equipment should be available. Also, a nasogastric tube can be inserted to decompress the stomach before removing the obturator.

Endotracheal Intubation

The respiratory care practitioner should learn the skill of endotracheal intubation. There are many hospitals where the primary responsibility for emergency intubation belongs to the respiratory thera-

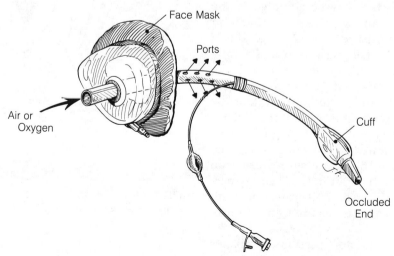

FIG 11–12.
Esophageal obturator.

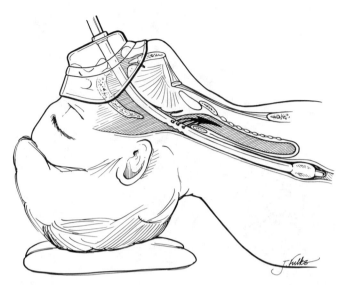

FIG 11–13.
Esophageal obturator.

pist. In other hospitals, the therapist performs intubation when he is the most experienced person available, for example, during the night shift at a community hospital when an anesthesiologist is not present. In situations where the respiratory therapist does not actually perform the intubation, he or she has the responsibility of assisting the physician during the procedure. Therefore, the respiratory care practitioner must be familiar with the preparation, equipment, and procedure for intubation.

Laryngoscopes and Blades

Laryngoscopes are instruments designed to facilitate tracheal intubation. They consist of two parts; the handle and a detachable blade (Fig 11–14). The handle contains batteries which conduct electrical current to light the bulb located near the end of the blade. The handle is designed to accommodate both adult size and pediatric size blades. However, smaller handles for pediatric intubation are available for those who prefer a smaller grip.

Straight and curved blades, in several sizes, are commonly used (see Fig 11–14). The straight blade is designed to allow the tip of the blade to lift the epiglottis during intubation to expose the vocal cords. This blade has the advantage of being long enough to accommodate a child's epiglottis, which is difficult to elevate with a curved blade. There is the possibility of dental damage in situations where pressure is put on the upper incisors during the procedure. The design of the curved blade partially prevents this hazard if used properly. The curve of the blade conforms to the shape of the tongue, and the

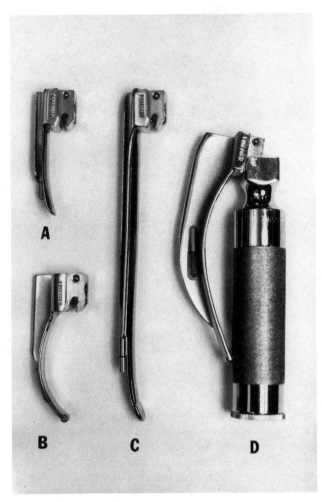

FIG 11–14.
Laryngoscope blades: Straight pediatric (A), curved pediatric (B), straight adult (C), and curved adult (D, attached to handle).

tip of the blade is between the epiglottis and the base of the tongue. The tongue is lifted by the laryngoscope blade and the epiglottis is pulled anteriorly. This procedure exposes the vocal cords so that the tube can be placed (Fig 11–15).[5]

The respiratory therapist should take the responsibility to assure that both types of blades are available on the emergency carts throughout the hospital. The equipment check should include assuring that the bulbs on the blades are functional.

Endotracheal Tubes

Several sizes of endotracheal tubes should be available to accommodate a variety of patients. Tube sizes are designated according to internal diameter (ID) and a size 7- or 8-mm tube is appropriate for most adults. A rough guideline for endotracheal tube size in children can be produced by the for-

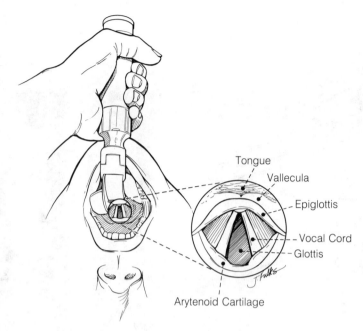

FIG 11–15.
Visualization of vocal cords with laryngoscope.

mula: ID(mm) = age in years.[11] The tubes should have the standard 15/22-mm fittings that attach to a mask or manual resuscitator. Table 11–1 indicates the recommended sizes for endotracheal tubes and suction catheters for newborns through adult patients. The tubes should be cuffed for adults and older children and uncuffed for infants and small children.

The American National Standards Z-79 Committee has suggested standards for endotracheal tubes and cuffs.[14] These standards do not prohibit the

manufacture or use of tubes not conforming to the standards. However, ANSI standards are considered by the medical community to be important in delivering safe care to patients.

The Z-79 stamped on tracheal tubes indicates the manufacturer has used a cell culture technique specified by the ANSI Z-79 Committee for Anesthesia Equipment, to establish that the material used for the device is nontoxic. The IT on the tube stands for implantation tested, which indicates that the tube has undergone testing using a rabbit muscle implantation and that the material is free from tissue reaction. The package should include the ID size (internal diameter) near the right corner of the package. The tube itself should be marked oral or nasal. If it is smaller than 6.0 mm ID, the actual outside diameter in millimeters should also be shown.[14]

The most common material used for tracheal tubes is polyvinylchloride (PVC).[14] The advantages of this material are that it is flexible to mold at body temperature and it is nontoxic so that no tissue reaction should occur. Sterilization of artificial airways made with PVC require the same precautions as other devices made with PVC. Tubes that are labeled "gamma-radiation sterilized" should not be resterilized because of the risk of toxic levels of ethylene chlorohydrin formation. The package of the tracheal tube should suggest the method of sterilization unless resterilization is prohibited by the manufacturer.

TABLE 11–1.

Recommended Sizes for Endotracheal Tubes and Suction Catheters*

AGE	ENDOTRACHEAL TUBE (INTERNAL DIAMETER), mm	SUCTION CATHETERS, F
Newborn	3.0	6
6 mo	3.5	8
18 mo	4.0	8
3 yr	4.5	8
5 yr	5.0	10
6 yr	5.5	10
8 yr	6.0	10
12 yr	6.5	10
16 yr	7.0	10
Adult (F)	8.0–8.5	12
Adult (M)	8.5–9.0	14

*From Burton GG, Hodgkin JE: *Respiratory Care: A Guide to Clinical Practice*, ed 2. New York, JB Lippincott Co, 1984. Used with permission.

Tracheal tubes should be stored in a round container with a 14-in. diameter to maintain their required curved shape when not in use and should be relatively resistant to agents used in chemical cleansing and sterilization.[14] The packaging at a slight curve allows the tube to be easily introduced into the trachea.

Although there are a variety of endotracheal tubes available for clinical use, those meeting the Z-79 standards incorporate the same components (Fig 11–16). The bevel is the slanted end of the tracheal tube and faces left when viewed from the concave aspect. It is located at the distal end and is 45 degrees in relation to the long axis. The inflating tube provides a route for inflating the cuff and a place for monitoring cuff pressures. The pilot balloon is fitted to the inflating tube and indicates cuff inflation. The cuff itself is the inflatable sleeve that is located at the distal end of the tube, which provides a seal between the tube and the trachea. This allows ventilation, prevents aspiration, and positions the tube in the trachea. The cuff length ranges from 20 mm in a 5.0 mm ID tube to 40 mm in an 11.0 mm ID tube. The length of the tube distal to the cemented end of the cuff should be less than 13 mm except in tubes smaller than 5 mm in diameter, where it should be 5 to 6 mm.[14]

The most commonly used tracheal tubes incorporate a high-volume low-pressure cuff. They are designed so that a minimum amount of pressure is exerted on the trachea while providing a seal between the tube and the trachea. This type of tube decreases the risk of inhibiting capillary blood flow which may lead to tracheal necrosis and stenosis. High pressures on the tracheal wall are also associated with tracheoesophageal fistulas, which can be prevented with low-pressure cuffs. However, even cuffs designed to be low pressure can exert high pressure on the trachea if too much air is inserted. Intracuff pressures must be monitored frequently to assure that they are maintained at a minimal occluding volume.

The proper size tube for intubation must be chosen. If the tube is too large, pressure necrosis on the trachea is a hazard, even with small amounts of air in the cuff. If the tube is too small, more air will be required to inflate the cuff. Also, suctioning may not be as effective because the suction catheter used for small tubes must also be smaller. Table 11–1 suggests specific size tubes according to the age of the patient. One size smaller or one size larger should be considered for individual variations.

Endotracheal Intubation Procedure

The equipment necessary for oral-tracheal intubation should be on every emergency cart and be checked frequently. The equipment should include a manual resuscitator capable of delivering 100% oxygen; masks in a variety of sizes; suction equipment including a large tonsil suction tip to clear the airway of mucus, blood, or vomitus; a variety of endotracheal tubes; laryngoscope with different size straight and curved blades; a flexible metal stylet and Magill forceps to aid insertion.

The head, neck, and shoulders should be positioned so a straight line is possible between the open mouth and the glottis. A small towel placed under the head may facilitate the proper alignment which is referred to as the "sniffing position" (Fig 11–17).

The blade is attached to the laryngoscope and it is held in the left hand. The blade is inserted on the right-hand side of the mouth and the tongue is

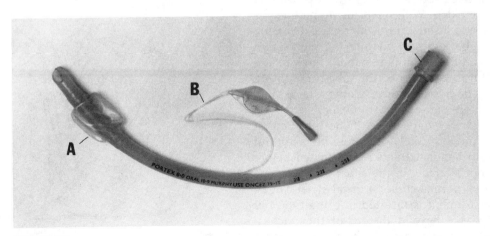

FIG 11–16.
Oral endotracheal tube: *A,* cuff. *B,* pilot tube for inflating cuff. *C,* 15/22 mm connector.

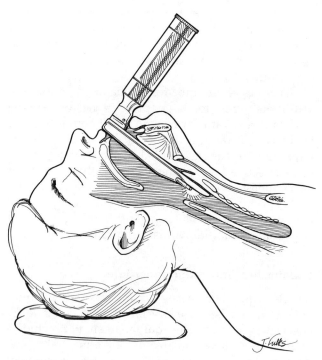

FIG 11–17.
Adult laryngoscope with straight blade.

moved to the left as the blade is brought to the midline. The blade is advanced forward along the surface of the tongue with a slight lifting pressure until the tip of the epiglottis is visualized.[5] Contracting the forearm muscles as opposed to the upper arm muscles helps to assure the pressure is not exerted on the front teeth.

The primary landmarks of intubation are the epiglottis and the arytenoid cartilages. When these structures are recognized, the vocal cords and the opening of the glottis are known.[46] The esophageal opening can also be seen so that incorrect placement of the tube is avoided. With the blade in midline position, the tube is inserted into the right side of the mouth. The tube is advanced into the glottis and through the vocal cords in one smooth motion. Repeatedly trying to jab or poke the tube through the glottis should be avoided since glottic edema may develop, making subsequent intubation attempts more difficult, if not impossible. If the tube cannot be placed within 30 seconds, it should be taken out and the patient ventilated and reoxygenated before another attempt is made. In the situation where the tube has lost its normal curve, a metal stylet can be used. This instrument is inserted into the tube but should not project beyond the tip of the tracheal tube or it could cause damage to the tracheal tissue.

Immediately after the tube is placed, the cuff is

inflated and a stethoscope is used to assure that the tube is in the trachea. The manual resuscitator is connected to the endotracheal tube adapter and ventilation continued. Breath sounds are evaluated bilaterally. The stethoscope should be placed under each axilla to assure bilateral breath sounds. Placement of the tube in the right main-stem bronchus is suspected if breath sounds are heard on the right side of the chest and are absent on the left side. When this situation is present, the cuff is deflated and the tube pulled out 1 to 2 cm or until bilateral breath sounds are heard. Placement of the tube in the esophagus is suspected when breath sounds are not heard in either lung and air flow is heard over the epigastrium during manual ventilation. When this situation occurs, the cuff is deflated and the patient is extubated. The patient is reoxygenated via the manual resuscitator and mask before reintubation is attempted.

When proper placement of the tube is determined, it must be secured in position. Marking the tube at the point where it meets the corner of the mouth will assist in reevaluating the tube position. The tube is taped in place to prevent inadvertent extubation or problems with the tube going forward into the right main-stem bronchus. There are a variety of acceptable techniques available for securing the tube. Cloth tape tied around the tube and secured behind the neck or adhesive tape secured to the face using benzoin so that the adhesive is not lost are commonly used methods (Fig 11–18). In addition, there are a variety of commercially available endotracheal tube holders or harnesses available for securing tubes (Fig 11–19). Whichever method is used to secure the tube, correct positioning must be constantly monitored.

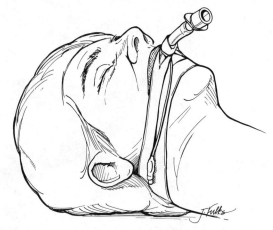

FIG 11–18.
Securing the endotracheal tube.

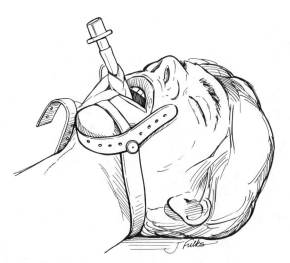

FIG 11–19.
Endotracheal tube harness.

A chest x-ray will confirm proper tube placement when the emergency situation has passed.[5, 11] The tip of the tube should be located at least 2 cm above the tracheal bifurcation.

Pediatric/Neonatal Intubation

Pediatric and neonatal patients should be positioned by placing a towel under the neck. The neck should be extended slightly for straight alignment of the airway. The patient should be oxygenated with a pediatric or neonatal manual resuscitator. The proper size blade is attached to the laryngoscope and it is placed in the left hand. Infants and small children have a relatively large epiglottis which may require a straight blade to lift it out of the way. The blade is inserted into the center of the mouth and the tongue is moved to the left side. The blade is advanced into the base of the tongue, and the larynx is observed by lifting the laryngoscope and blade. Suctioning may be necessary, and then the tube is inserted along the right side of the blade and through the vocal cords. An uncuffed tube is used for infants because the cricoid cartilage forms the narrowest part of the airway and acts as a seal. Immediately the lungs are auscultated to determine correct placement. Bilateral breath sounds should be heard under the axillae. If breath sounds are evident on the right but not the left, the tube should be pulled back slightly until bilateral breath sounds are auscultated. The tube is then secured using tape or a commercially available endotracheal tube holder. When the emergency situation is over, a chest x-ray is taken to confirm tube position.[5]

Emergency Cricothyrotomy

An emergency cricothyrotomy is indicated when upper airway obstruction cannot be relieved and an endotracheal tube cannot be inserted.[31, 46] The problem may result from aspiration of a foreign object or other causes of upper airway obstruction such as laryngeal edema, epiglottitis, or trauma. This situation is evident when mouth-to-mouth, mouth-to-nose, and ventilation with a manual resuscitator does not result in lung inflation. If repositioning of the airway and pushing the mandible forward does not relieve obstruction and an endotracheal tube still cannot be placed, a cricothyrotomy is done. A cricothyrotomy is the procedure of choice in emergency situations because the cricothyroid membrane is easily located and it is the safest point of entry.[46] This portion of the airway is thin and relatively avascular which limits the risk of hemorrhage. The chance of vocal cord damage is also minimal because the membrane is below the cords. The cricothyroid space is large enough to place at least a 6 mm tracheal tube for ventilation.

The patient is positioned so the neck is fully extended and the larynx is prominent. The thyroid cartilage is located and the finger is moved downward until the cricoid cartilage is palpated. The cricoid is a ridged structure just below the thyroid cartilage. A vertical, midline incision is made between the two cartilages. The edges of the incision are separated and the membrane is cut horizontally just above the cricoid cartilage (Fig 11–20). A tube is then inserted to maintain an open airway.[5, 31]

A cricothyrotomy should take less than a minute to complete, and the most experienced person available should perform this procedure. However, the respiratory therapist should thoroughly understand the emergency techniques so they may be performed safely and successfully in a life-threatening situation. An alternative to making an incision into the membrane is puncturing it with a large bore needle (14- to 16-gauge). This procedure can be done easily by inexperienced therapists and may be lifesaving while waiting for a physician to take charge. Needle puncture allows easy access to the airway but has limited effectiveness for ventilation. Therefore, an incision is made and a tracheal tube inserted as soon as possible.

Transtracheal Jet Ventilation

Transtracheal jet ventilation may be a temporary alternative to a cricothyrotomy or tracheotomy for

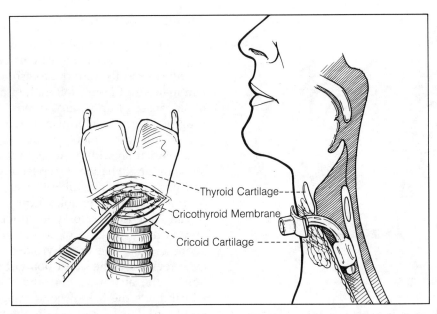

FIG 11–20.
Emergency cricothyrotomy.

emergency ventilation.[31, 42] This procedure requires the cricothyroid membrane be punctured with a needle-catheter attached to a syringe. The needle is directed caudually at a 45-degree angle while negative pressure is maintained with the syringe. The return air indicates that the trachea has been entered. The catheter is then advanced and its hub is attached to an oxygen delivery device. Intravenous tubing is extended from the catheter hub to an oxygen flowmeter open to 15 L/min. A side hole cut near the distal end of the tubing is occluded by a finger during inspiration. Inflation is continued until the chest rises and then passive expiration is allowed (Fig 11–21). Transtracheal cannulation is quick and relatively

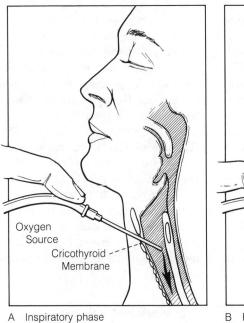
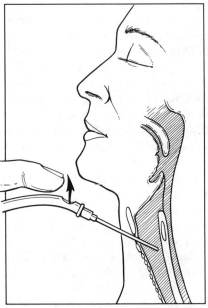

A Inspiratory phase

B Passive expiration

FIG 11–21.
Transtracheal jet ventilation.

atraumatic. Possible complications are local bleeding, subcutaneous or mediastinal emphysema, and esophageal injury from incorrect catheter placement.[31]

Emergency Tracheotomy

A tracheotomy is not usually indicated in an emergency situation because there are more risks associated with the procedure compared to a cricothyrotomy.[5, 45] Tracheotomy is indicated, however, when upper airway obstruction cannot be relieved and a cricothyrotomy is not elected. The procedure must be done under conditions that are as controlled as possible to decrease the risk factors.

Ideally an endotracheal tube will be in place first so that the tracheotomy can be done electively. In this situation, the respiratory therapist can continue to oxygenate and ventilate the patient while an incision into the trachea is made. As the tracheal tube is inserted the therapist deflates the cuff and withdraws the endotracheal tube. The cuff of the tracheal tube is immediately inflated and manual ventilation continued. During this procedure, ventilation is only interrupted for a couple of breaths.

Immediate Tracheostomy Complications

The tracheostomy tube should not be left in place longer than required for airway maintenance because of the associated complications. Complications from long-term tracheotomies (more than 24 hours) include tracheitis, wound infections, innominate artery rupture, stomal stenosis, and cuff complications.[5, 45] There are several complications that can occur during the tracheostomy procedure or during the first few hours that follow.[5, 45] The respiratory care practitioner may be the first person to be aware of these complications. Therefore, continuous monitoring of the patient is required.

During the procedure, a major vessel can be severed, especially if the tracheostomy is done in an emergency situation. Even small amounts of bleeding should not be ignored. Any amount of bleeding could indicate that a substantial hemorrhage has occurred and the patient may have aspirated large quantities of blood.

Severe hypotension and cardiac arrest occurs more often when the procedure is done under less than optimal conditions. These problems can result from vagal response and hypoxia during the procedure. Therefore, an endotracheal tube should be placed first whenever possible. This would allow effective oxygenation and ventilation to be continued during the tracheostomy procedure.

Laryngeal nerve damage can also occur during the tracheostomy procedure. The laryngeal nerves are located between the trachea and the esophagus. The damage occurs when the incision is made more toward the lateral wall of the trachea rather than anteriorly. If both nerves are injured, vocal cord paralysis may result. A tracheoesophageal fistula occurs if the incision is made into the posterior wall. This complication is serious if aspiration of gastric contents results. If an endotracheal tube is in place first a tracheoesophageal fistula is less likely to occur.

MANUAL RESUSCITATORS

A variety of manual resuscitation units are currently available (Figs 11–22 to 11–24). These units are used to support the ventilation of patients who have a respiratory or cardiopulmonary arrest. These units should have the capability of performing under a variety of conditions to meet the needs of the emergency situation for which they are being used.

Manual resuscitation units consist of a self-inflating bag, an air intake valve, a nonrebreathing valve, an oxygen inlet nipple, and a high-oxygen reservoir attachment. One end of the nonrebreathing valve connects to the bag and the other end is connected to the patient's tracheal tube or face mask. The self-inflating bag is compressed by the operator and the nonrebreathing valve directs gas from the bag to the patient as the exhalation port closes. When the operator releases the bag, the exhaled gas is directed through the exhalation port. The bag reinflates through a one-way air inlet valve opening directly into the bag. The air inlet valve is part of the nonrebreathing valve in some units (Fig 11–25) and is part of the valve at the bottom of other units (Fig 11–26).

In units where the air intake valve is part of the nonrebreathing valve, higher oxygen concentrations can be delivered to the patient by placing an adapter around the valve with a reservoir attached. Oxygen accumulates in the adapter and reservoir and allows oxygen to flow into the bag during reinflation. When the air intake valve is at the bottom of the bag, an oxygen reservoir is attached there for oxygen accumulation. Oxygen flows into the bag as the air intake valve opens during the expiratory phase reinflating the bag.

During a cardiac arrest situation, it is important to administer the highest oxygen concentration pos-

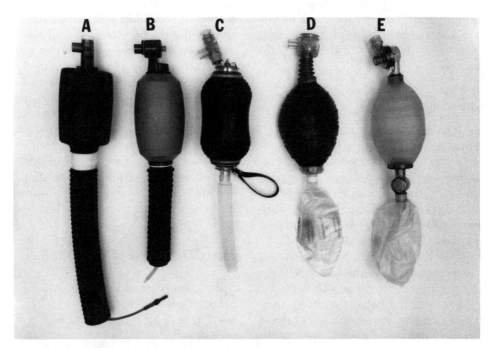

FIG 11–22.
Adult manual resuscitators with oxygen reservoirs attached: Hope 2 *(A)*, PMR 2 *(B)*, Ambu MS 30 *(C)*, Air Viva *(D)*, Laerdal Silicone *(E)*.

sible. The American Heart Association recommends that a manual resuscitator should be capable of delivering 100% oxygen.[42] The American Society for Testing and Materials (ASTM) has recommended that manual resuscitators be capable of delivering at least 85% oxygen at a minute ventilation of 12 L/min (600 ml × 12/min) with an oxygen flow of 15 L/min. However, 85% oxygen may not be adequate to treat a cardiopulmonary arrest, and there are several manual resuscitators available that will deliver

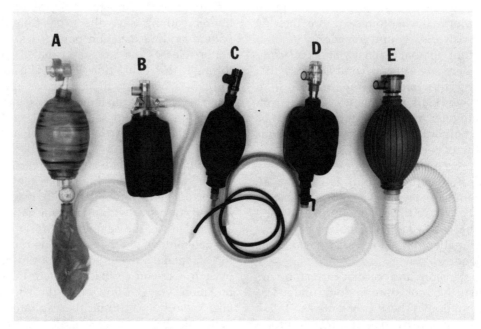

FIG 11–23.
Adult manual resuscitators with oxygen reservoirs attached: Laerdal *(A)*, Hope 1 *(B)*, Penlon *(C)*, Ambu *(D)*, Vitalograph *(E)*.

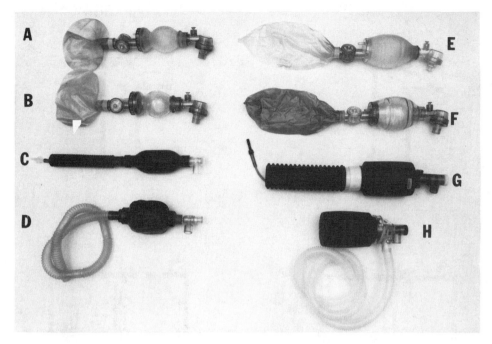

FIG 11–24.
Infant manual resuscitators with oxygen reservoirs attached: Laerdal silicone *(A)*, Laerdal *(B)*, Penlon *(C)*, Ambu *(D)*. Pediatric manual resuscitators with oxygen reservoirs attached: Laerdal silicone *(E)*, Laerdal *(F)*, Hope 2 *(G)*, Hope 1 *(H)*.

greater than 85% oxygen. The respiratory therapy practitioner has the responsibility to know the capabilities and limitations of the manual resuscitators currently available and to assure the delivery of high oxygen concentration during a cardiopulmonary arrest.

ASTM Standards for Manual Resuscitators

The ASTM Committee on F-29 on Anesthetic and Respiratory Equipment has recommended standards to establish minimum performance and safety requirements for manual resuscitators.[4] The standards are important because they can be used as criteria for selecting safe and effective manual resuscitators. Although there are several standards, the following is a description of those that are thought to be most important for selecting a manual resuscitator to be used during a cardiopulmonary arrest.

The resuscitator should be capable of delivering at least 85% oxygen at an O_2 flow of 15 L/min with the high oxygen reservoir attached with a specified minute ventilation pattern. The device should also be designed to prevent valve malfunction at an oxygen flow of 30 L/min. This standard is important because high flow rates have been reported to jam the non-rebreathing valve.[33] The result is that the valve sticks in the inspiratory position, preventing exhala-

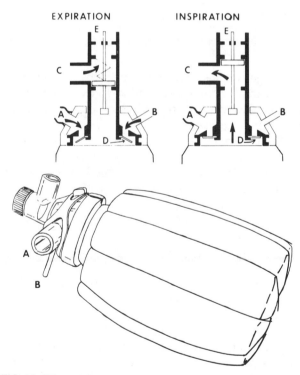

FIG 11–25.
Design of Hope 1 manual resuscitator: Blount adapter *(A)*, oxygen inlet *(B)*, patient connector *(C)*, gas intake valves *(D)*.

EXPIRATION

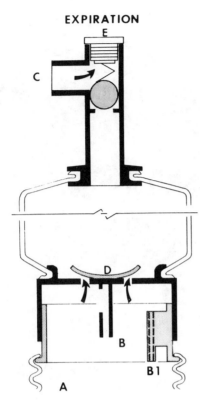

INSPIRATION

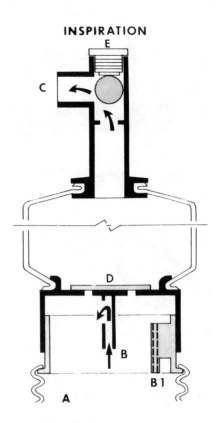

FIG 11–26.
Design of Hope 2 manual resuscitator: Blount adaptor *(A)*, oxygen inlet when reservoir is not attached *(B)*, oxygen inlet when reservoir is attached *(B1)*, patient connector *(C)*, gas intake valve *(D)*, exhalation port *(E)*.

tion which can lead to barotrauma. This problem can occur with the older Ambu model NR resuscitator, but the newer Ambu resuscitators are designed to prevent this problem.

When disabled by vomitus, the valve should be capable of being restored to proper function within 20 seconds. This is important during a cardiac arrest situation because the patient often vomits.

The patient connector of the resuscitator should have a 15-mm female/22-mm male adapter for connection to a tracheal tube or face mask. This standard is important because all tracheal tubes have the same size adapter; without a compatible connection, manual resuscitation cannot be accomplished. The resuscitator should also be designed to facilitate effective operation by one person when used with a face mask to provide adequate ventilation. This recommendation is important because the first few minutes of a cardiac arrest are critical, and the respiratory care practitioner must maintain effective ventilation and oxygenation using a face mask before tracheal intubation occurs.

The ASTM committee also recommends that the resuscitator be capable of complying with pressure limit requirements and minute ventilation requirements after being dropped 1 m onto a concrete surface. This recommendation is important because if the resuscitator is dropped during a CPR situation, ventilation and oxygenation should not be interrupted while waiting for another resuscitator. If the adult resuscitator has a pressure limit system, it should be capable of being overridden. The pediatric and neonatal resuscitators have a mandatory pressure relief system with an opening pressure of 40 cm H_2O. These pressures should not be exceeded under the conditions of ventilation, but an override mechanism may be provided. The override mechanism, however, must be designed so that its operating mode is readily apparent to the user.[28]

Although all the criteria described are important when choosing a manual resuscitator for CPR, the first consideration should be delivered oxygen capability. Table 11–2 indicates the delivered oxygen concentration in adult manual resuscitators with reservoirs attached when delivering a tidal volume of 600 ml at a rate of 12/min with an oxygen flow of 15 L/min. This table illustrates that the Penlon and the Hope 1 were not capable of delivering 85% oxygen

TABLE 11–2.

Delivered Oxygen Concentration and Dead Space for Adult Manual Resuscitators

RESUSCITATORS	WITH RESERVOIR, F_{IO_2}	WITHOUT RESERVOIR, F_{IO_2}	DEAD SPACE, ML
Ambu MS 30	1.00	0.95	10.2
Laerdal Silicone	1.00	0.36	11.4
Laerdal	1.00	0.37	8.0
Hope 2	0.99	0.41	9.8
Ambu R	1.00	0.40	14.0
PMR 2	0.96	0.35	7.4
Air Viva	0.90	0.37	32.6
Vitalograph	0.89	0.32	38.0
Penlon	0.80	0.43	11.9
Hope 1	0.71	0.65	10.7

and therefore should not be used in CPR situations. The best choices for manual ventilation during CPR are those resuscitators capable of delivering 100% oxygen.

Table 11–3 indicates the delivered oxygen concentration of pediatric and neonatal manual resuscitators. All of the resuscitators are capable of delivering 100% oxygen with the reservoirs attached, with the exception of the Hope 1 pediatric model. Therefore, the Hope 1 should not be used during CPR. Also, pediatric models may require the pressure relief valve to be overridden to achieve 100% oxygen.

All of the resuscitators listed in the tables are capable of functioning at a flow of 30 L/min and are capable of maintaining proper function when the valve is disabled by vomitus. They have a 15/22-mm adapter for connection to a tracheal tube mask, are functional after the drop test, and meet the pressure limit requirements discussed above.

TABLE 11–3.

Delivered Oxygen Concentration for Neonatal/Pediatric Manual Resuscitators

RESUSCITATOR	WITH RESERVOIR, F_{IO_2}	WITHOUT RESERVOIR, F_{IO_2}
Ambu (Neonatal)	1.00	0.93
Hope 1 (Pedi)	0.75	0.48
Hope 2 (Pedi)	1.00	0.49
Laerdal (Pedi)	1.00	0.47
Laerdal Silicone (Pedi)	1.00	0.46
Laerdal (Neonatal)	1.00	0.71
Laerdal Silicone (Neonatal)	1.00	0.68
Penlon (Neonatal)	1.00	NA

Increasing Oxygen Delivery of Manual Resuscitators

Some manual resuscitators deliver very low oxygen concentrations without the reservoirs attached, and should not be used without them.[9, 10, 19] Table 11–2 indicates that the Ambu MS 30 is the only manual resuscitator capable of delivering above 85% oxygen without the reservoir attached. The design of the air inlet on the MS 30 creates a vortex effect that allows the resuscitator to deliver a high F_{IO_2} without the reservoir attached. The oxygen whirls around the inlet chamber of the valve in a circular motion and limits the amount of air entrained. The design of this valve makes the Ambu MS 30 a good choice for CPR situations if there is any doubt that personnel using the resuscitator will attach an oxygen reservoir.

Increasing the oxygen flow to manual resuscitators will increase delivered oxygen concentration.[9, 10, 19] However, it is not necessary to increase the oxygen flow above 15 L/min with most manual resuscitators. Several studies have reported that some valves stick in the inspiratory position at high flows which can prevent exhalation.[9, 15, 33] The result could be barotrauma. The resuscitators listed in Tables 11–2 and 11–3 were shown to function effectively even at high flow rates. However, practitioners should be aware that valve malfunction may occur with some manual resuscitators, and make it a practice to turn the flowmeter only to 15 L/min.

The minute ventilation pattern will also effect delivered oxygen concentration.[9, 10, 15, 16, 19, 22] Higher F_{IO_2} has been reported to occur with decreasing minute ventilation. Lower tidal volumes result in less room air and more oxygen being drawn into the bag during exhalation which increases the oxygen concentration delivered on the next breath. Slow bag reinflation has also been shown to increase the delivered oxygen concentration.[21] This is accomplished by slowly releasing the self-inflating bag so there is a 3- to 4-second expiratory time. This maneuver allows more oxygen and less room air to flow into the bag.

EXTERNAL HEART MASSAGE

Mechanical Devices

Devices that mechanically compress the sternum are limited to use with adult patients (Fig 11–27). Their safety and effectiveness has not been demonstrated in children or infants. The manual chest

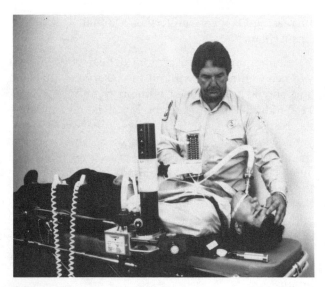

FIG 11–27.
Mechanical device for compressing the sternum. (Courtesy of Dixie USA, Houston.)

compressors should provide an adjustable stroke volume of 1½ to 2 in. Some studies have shown that mechanical compressors can be superior to manual chest compressions in producing higher mean arterial pressures and they have produced a survival rate at least comparable to that of manual chest compressions.[38, 50] They have the advantage of minimal mechanical breakdown. However, if the compressor head shifts positions or if the device becomes loosened, the plunger will not compress the chest adequately.

The automatic chest compressors are pneumatically powered. They are mounted on a backboard and can be adjusted to vary the depth of compressions as well as the relaxation ratio. They are also capable of automatic ventilation of the lungs and the ratio of compressions to ventilations can be adjusted. These devices produce an acceptable electrocardiograph tracing and do not have to be turned off to defibrillate.

Chest compressors have the advantage of eliminating fatigue and variability in technique during cardiopulmonary resuscitation. This may be especially important during prolonged resuscitations. However, if they are not positioned properly or if they deviate from position, they will not be effective and complications such as fractured ribs, sternal fractures, or lacerations of the lung and liver can occur.[20, 42]

VENTRICULAR FIBRILLATION

Ventricular fibrillation represents clinical death; therefore, it requires immediate attention or biological death will occur within minutes. This arrhythmia is the result of chaotic twitching of the ventricles which produce fibrillation waves of varying amplitude and shape. The fibrillating heart is not capable of producing a pulse or blood pressure, therefore the cardiac output drops to zero. Ventricular fibrillation may be caused by a variety of clinical situations such as a myocardial infarction, drug toxicity, hypoxia, hypothermia, or acid-base and electrolyte imbalances. Often the patient will first experience another arrhythmia which can be treated to prevent ventricular fibrillation. The critically ill patient should constantly be monitored so that arrhythmias resulting in decreased perfusion can be treated appropriately (Fig 11–28).

Defibrillation

Precordial Thump
The American Heart Association currently recommends one precordial thump in patients with monitored ventricular fibrillation and in witnessed cardiac arrests if a defibrillator is not available. A thump may also be used in patients with asystole or marked bradycardia with hemodynamic instability.[42] To administer a precordial thump, the fist is raised with the ulnar side down, 8 to 12 in. above the midsternum. A single, quick, sharp blow is delivered, and then CPR is begun.

Electrical Conversion
If the precordial thump is not effective in converting ventricular fibrillation, electrical defibrillation should be initiated immediately. The longer cardiac arrest is permitted to continue without CPR, the more difficult it is to successfully defibrillate.[34] The optimal amount of electrical energy has not been established and may vary significantly for individual situations. However, the American Heart Association recommends that an initial defibrillation of approximately 200 W-sec for adults. The initial dose recommended for a child is 2 W-sec/kg.[42] If unsuccessful, that energy dose should be repeated twice. Then, if 4 W-sec/kg is unsuccessful, attention should be toward correcting acidosis, hypoxia, and hypothermia.[42]

To prepare for defibrillation, the main switch is

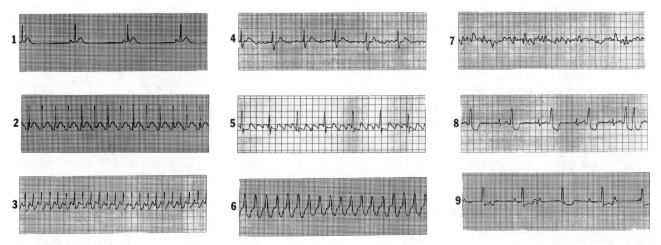

FIG 11–28.
Cardiac arrhythmias: bradycardia *(1)*, sinus tachycardia *(2)*, paroxysmal tachycardia *(3)*, atrial fibrillation *(4)*, atrial flutter *(5)*, ventricular tachycardia *(6)*, ventricular fibrillation *(7)*, premature ventricular contractions *(8)*, and third-degree heart block *(9)*.

turned on and the electrode paste is placed on the paddles. The entire surface of both paddles should be completely covered or the current will not be maximally conducted and the patient may sustain burns.[30] The defibrillator is then charged to 200 W-sec for an adult and less for a child, depending on their size. The person charging the paddles should state clearly that the "paddles are charged." Holding the hand grips only, the paddles are placed on the chest. One paddle is placed over the right sternal border at the second intercostal space and the other over the apex of the heart, below the patient's left nipple. Ventricular fibrillation is verified by observing the ECG monitor. The person holding the paddles has the responsibility of making a visual check that no one is in contact with the patient or the bed. All persons must stand back from the bed to avoid receiving a fatal shock. When everyone is cleared, the person defibrillating states, "Stand back. I am going to defibrillate on 3—1, 2, 3." On 3, the buttons of both paddles are depressed. The ECG machine is observed to determine the effect of defibrillation. CPR should be continued if the patient still does not have an effective cardiac rhythm. If ventricular fibrillation still exists, the procedure is repeated immediately. The initial energy level is maintained the second time or increased to 300 W-sec for the adult patient. If the second attempt is not effective, the defibrillator is increased to 360 to 400 W-sec with effective CPR continued between attempts.[30, 42]

There are four mechanical factors that influence the success of defibrillation.[8] The size of the paddles is one consideration. The large paddles result in a lower impedance, which may improve the success of defibrillation. The electrode placement is also of critical importance. One paddle is placed over the apex of the heart. If the second paddle is placed directly over the sternum, greater impedance will result which decreases the success of defibrillation. Time should not be taken to place the paddles in the anterior-posterior position in an emergency situation even though current that is delivered directly through the myocardium may be more effective than the transverse defibrillation.

The conducting gel used in defibrillation may influence the success rate. The gel pads currently on the market are less messy, but they may have a higher impedance compared to other conducting material. Therefore, the electrode gels are recommended to lessen impedance during defibrillation. However, if too much conductive gel is used, a short circuit between the paddles can cause a drop in the amount of current delivered to the heart, and defibrillation will not be successful.

The number of previous shocks also influences the effectiveness of defibrillation. Successive defibrillation attempts have been demonstrated to decrease impedance, resulting in higher delivered current, without increasing the voltage on the defibrillator.[8]

There are also several physiological factors that may cause ineffective defibrillation. One important factor is time delay. Chances for survival decrease with the duration of fibrillation. Inadequate CPR resulting in hypoxia, acidosis, and hypercarbia or patient conditions such as valvular heart disease, massive myocardial infarction, cardiac tamponade, pulmonary emboli, severe respiratory disease, hemorrhage, drug toxicity, or hypothermia may cause ineffective defibrillation. If every attempt to defibrillate is not successful, drug therapy should begin to improve some of the influencing factors, and then defibrillation may be successful. The administration of lidocaine, procainamide, or bretylium tosylate may be useful in treating fibrillation that is refractory to countershock.[18, 53]

THE OBSTRUCTED AIRWAY

Sudden Choking

Most airway obstruction situations are foreign body obstructions which occur while eating. However, many cases of sudden choking are due to cardiac ischemia that simulates food impaction. Differentiating between these two emergencies can be important for successful management. In both situations, the victim clasps his neck or upper chest because of pain, panic, and constriction of that area. In the case of complete foreign body obstruction most patients do not lose consciousness immediately but are unable to speak, breathe, or cough. If the victim is becoming cyanotic, this means there is hypoxemia, which may indicate respiratory obstruction. This situation requires further attempts at dislodging the obstruction. Circulatory failure is indicated by pallor as opposed to frank cyanosis.[29]

Foreign bodies that cause partial obstruction result in some ability to ventilate. Varying degrees of retraction, agitation, respiratory noises, and activity of the accessory muscles will be evident. If there is good air exchange, a strong cough may force the foreign body out of the airway. A normal cough is superior to any of the artificially induced coughs. Therefore, if a choking victim can speak or breathe and is coughing, intervention is unnecessary and potentially dangerous.[23]

Partial obstruction with poor air exchange or the presence of cyanosis requires immediate intervention. Poor air exchange is indicated by a weak, ineffective cough, high-pitched noises during inspiration, and use of accessory muscles. When these signs occur, the management protocol is the same as with a complete airway obstruction. Emergency maneuvers to relieve airway obstruction are designed to generate positive intrathoracic pressure to expel a foreign body from the trachea.

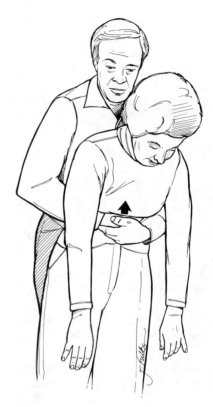

FIG 11–29.
Performing the Heimlich maneuver.

Heimlich Maneuver

The maneuver recommended to relieve airway obstruction is the Heimlich maneuver (Fig 11–29). This maneuver exerts upward subxiphoid pressure with the fist. The rescuer puts both arms around the victim from the back and encircles the upper abdomen. One fist is grasped with the other hand and placed thumb side against the victim's abdomen between the waist and the rib cage. Each thrust given should exert force inward and upward. If the victim becomes unconscious, this maneuver can be done by placing one hand against the upper abdomen with the second hand on top applying force inward and upward.

Chest Thrust

Another maneuver to relieve airway obstruction is a chest thrust. This maneuver is used in special situations, such as pregnancy or extreme obesity. To perform a chest thrust, the rescuer's arms encircle the victim and one fist is placed thumb side on the midsternum. The other hand grasps the fist, and four backward thrusts are given. If the victim is unconscious, the hand position is the same as for applying closed chest cardiac compressions.

Complications of Abdominal Thrusts

The complications of abdominal thrusts are abdominal trauma including pneumoperitoneum, laceration or rupture of the stomach, fractured ribs, and regurgitation. Also, a possible danger in young children is that of liver laceration.[51] Therefore, abdominal thrusts should be limited to the older child and the adult.

Finger Sweeps

Finger sweeps of the oropharynx should also be avoided in the young age group to prevent pushing the foreign body back and increasing the obstruction. Only if the foreign body is visualized should it be removed with the finger in a small child. Finger sweeps may be effective in removing a foreign body in the older child or an adult. To perform this technique, the index finger is inserted to the base of the tongue. A hooking action is used to dislodge the object. A Kelly clamp or Magill forceps may be useful if the object is visable. A laryngoscope may help to permit direct visualization.

Recommended Sequence for the Adult

The Heimlich maneuver should be applied as soon as airway obstruction has been identified. This maneuver is continued until the airway is cleared or the patient becomes unconscious. When the patient becomes unconscious, he should be positioned supine with the airway open using the technique previously described. Two breaths are given, and, if unable to ventilate, the jaw lift is used and an attempt to remove the obstruction with a finger sweep, Kelly clamp, or Magill forceps is made. Also, suctioning the upper airway may be helpful in removing the obstruction.

If the obstruction is still not relieved, six to ten Heimlich maneuvers are performed and the sequence repeated. Positive pressure breathing between other attempts at removing the obstruction is important because it may help relieve the obstruction. Also, if the obstruction has been partially relieved, some air flow may be lifesaving. Advanced life support techniques used to open the airway are initiated as soon as skilled professionals are available. Time is critical because complete obstruction of the airway for longer than 5 minutes will cause death.

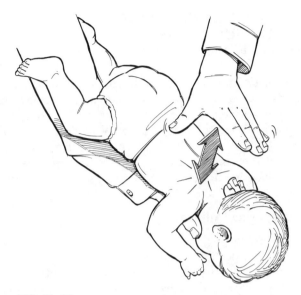

FIG 11–30.
Treatment of the choking child.

Neonatal and Pediatric Considerations

The literature indicates ongoing controversy over which maneuver is the optimal one. The Heimlich maneuver is recommended for the child as it is for the adult. Six to ten thrusts are repeated rapidly until the obstruction is relieved. However because of the potential intra-abdominal injury from the subdiaphragmatic thrusts in patients younger than age 1 year, a combination of back blows and chest thrusts is recommended.[42] It may be that the combination of back blows and manual thrusts is more effective than either technique alone.[24]

The position for delivering back blows to the choking infant is to place the infant over an arm with the head lower than the body (Fig 11–30). Four back blows are given with the heel of the hand between the infant's shoulder blades. If four back blows do not relieve the obstruction, the infant should be rolled over facing upward with the head lower than the trunk. Four chest thrusts are delivered rapidly in the same manner as external cardiac compressions but at a slower rate. Several attempts may be necessary to relieve the obstruction. Blind finger sweeps are to be avoided, but suctioning may relieve the obstruction in the hospital situation. CPR incorporating advanced techniques is initiated as with adults.

DRUG THERAPY DURING CARDIOPULMONARY RESUSCITATION[20, 30, 42]

An IV route for the administration of drugs and fluids is essential to managing advanced cardiac life support. In emergency cardiac care situations, IV fluids are used to keep open an IV line for drug administration. Crystalloid or colloid solutions may benefit the patient who requires volume expansion. The following drugs are commonly used during CPR.

Epinephrine (Adrenalin)

Indications
The indications for epinephrine are as follows: ventricular asystole, to convert fine ventricular fibrillation to coarse fibrillation; to increase mean arterial pressure (MAP) and cardiac output, in hypotensive states and in electromechanical dissociation.

Drug Action
The alpha-adrenergic activity increases systemic vascular resistance (SVR) and MAP. The beta-adrenergic activity enhances the contractile state of the heart, increases heart rate, and stimulates spontaneous contractions.

Dosage and Routes of Administration
The usual adult dose is 0.5 to 1.0 mg (5 to 10 ml of a prepackaged 1:10,000 solution) given IV during resuscitation efforts every 5 minutes. The usual dose for a child is 0.1 ml/kg of 1:10,000 dilution. If an IV cannot be established quickly, 1 mg (10 ml of a 1:10,000 solution) of epinephrine can be instilled into the tracheobronchial tree via the endotracheal tube and will be rapidly absorbed. Intracardiac injection is used only if the IV or intratracheal routes of administration fail to produce a response because of the invasiveness of the procedure. Epinephrine should not be added directly to a bicarbonate infusion since catecholamines may be partially inactivated by an alkaline solution.

Adverse Reactions and Hazards
Epinephrine increases myocardial oxygen demand, therefore it is potentially hazardous if given in the presence of ischemic heart disease and acute myocardial infarction. Hazards of intracardiac injection include coronary artery laceration, cardiac tamponade, pneumothorax and the need to interrupt CPR during the period of injection.

Atropine

Indications
Atropine is indicated in sinus bradycardia accompanied by hemodynamic compromise such as severe hypotension or frequent ventricular ectopic beats. Also, it is useful in bradycardia when the cardiac output is severely reduced. Atropine may also be beneficial in high-degree AV block at the nodal level and in ventricular asystole.

Drug Action
Reduces vagal tone and enhances the rate of sinus node discharge and improves AV conduction.

Dosage and Routes of Administration
The usual dose is 1.0 mg given IV and repeated in 5 minutes if asystole persists. For bradycardia, the dose is 0.5 mg every 5 minutes not exceeding 2.0 mg. The usual dose for a child is 0.01 to 0.03 mg/kg not to exceed 0.4 mg. Atropine is also well absorbed via the endotracheal tube.

Bretylium (Bretylol)

Indications
Bretylium is indicated in ventricular tachycardia and fibrillation which is unresponsive to lidocaine, procainamide, and defibrillation. The cardiovascular actions include the initial release of catecholamines initially on injection followed by postganglionic adrenergic blocking action which often induces hypotension.

Dosage and Routes of Administration
The usual dose is by an IV bolus of 5 mg/kg followed by defibrillation. The dose can be doubled and repeated at 15 to 30 minutes until a maximum dose of 30 mg/kg has been reached. In recurrent ventricular tachycardia, 5 to 10 mg of bretylium can be diluted to 50 ml and 5 to 10 mg/kg injected IV over 8 to 10 minutes then as a continuous infusion at a rate of 1 to 2 mg/min.

Isoproterenol

Indications
Isoproterenol is indicated in bradycardia resulting from a heart block not responsive to atropine and cardiogenic shock resulting in electromechanical dissociation.

Drug Action

This is a synthetic catecholamine related to epinephrine with pure beta-adrenergic receptor agonist qualities. It has potent iontropic and chronotropic properties that cause an increase in cardiac output by increasing myocardial contractility and heart rate.

Dosage and Routes of Administration

The usual adult dose is 1 mg of isoproterenol, which is added to 500 ml of 5% dextrose in water to yield a concentration of 2 μg/ml; 2 to 20 μg/min of isoproterenol can be given to increase the heart rate above 60/min. The usual dose for a child is 0.1 to 0.5 mg/kg/min and titrate to desired effects.

Adverse Reactions and Hazards

Isoproterenol increases myocardial oxygen demand. Therefore, it is potentially hazardous if given in the presence of ischemic heart disease and acute myocardial infarction.

Lidocaine

Indications

Lidocaine is indicated for ventricular arrhythmias such as premature ventricular contractions and ventricular tachycardia, especially those following a myocardial infarction.

Drug Action

Lidocaine slows myocardial conduction, suppresses ventricular ectopic beats, and increases the electrical stimulation threshold of the ventricle during diastole, thus exerting an antidysrhythmic effect.

Dosage and Routes of Administration

Lidocaine is only administered as a bolus in the cardiac arrest situation. The usual dose is an IV bolus of 1 mg/kg given every 8 to 10 minutes if necessary for a total of 3 mg/kg. An infusion of 2 to 4 mg/min should be initiated after successful resuscitation. The usual dose for a child is 0.5 to 1.0 mg/kg every 20 to 60 minutes and titrated at 0.05 to 0.15 mg/kg/min.

Adverse Reactions and Hazards

Excessive doses can produce myocardial and circulatory depression. Seizures, twitching, or obtundation are observed in toxicity. No more than 200 to 300 mg of lidocaine should be administered in 1 hour. It is of no value in cardiac asystole. If symptoms of toxic effect are noted, the dosage should be decreased at once.

Dobutamine (Dobutrex)

Indications

Dobutamine is indicated in electromechanical dissociation and refractory pump failure, particularly caused by temporary depression of ventricular function and myocardial contractility.

Drug Action

Dobutamine increases cardiac output by its direct beta-adrenergic action and directly increases myocardial contractility. It produces little systemic arterial constriction at usual dose levels.

Dosage and Routes of Administration

The usual dose range for Dobutamine is 2.5 to 10 μg/kg/min.

Adverse Reactions and Hazards

When Dobutamine is administered in excess doses of 20 μg/kg/min, tachycardia or other dysrhythmias may occur. Therefore, optimal use requires hemodynamic monitoring.

Procainamide

Indications

Procainamide is indicated when dysrhythmias are refractory to lidocaine.

Drug Action

The action of procainamide is similar to lidocaine. It slows myocardial conduction, suppresses ventricular ectopic beats, and increases the electrical stimulation threshold of the ventricle during diastole, therefore exerting an antidysrhythmic effect.

Dosage and Routes of Administration

The usual dose of procainamide is 50 mg IV every 5 minutes until the arrhythmia is suppressed, hypotension occurs, the QRS is widened by 50%, or until a total loading dose of 1 gm is reached. Maintenance dose is 1 to 4 mg/min. In an emergency situation, up to 20 mg/min may be administered to a total dose of 1 gm.

Adverse Reactions and Hazards

Hypotension is a problem if procainamide is given too rapidly. Therefore, ECGs must be monitored during administration. Blood levels of procainamide must be monitored in patients with renal failure and patients receiving a constant infusion of more than 3 mg/min for more than 24 hours.

Dopamine (Intropin)

Indications

Dopamine is used to correct hemodynamic imbalances present in shock due to myocardial infarctions.

Drug Action

Dopamine is chemically similar to norepinephrine. Mesenteric and renal vessels are dilated in doses that do not affect mean arterial pressure or heart rate (1 to 2 μg/kg/min). At doses of 2 to 10 μg/kg/min, it has beta-adrenergic effects that result in increased cardiac output, and above 10 μg/kg/min it has alpha effects that increasingly constrict peripheral vessels and increase systemic vascular resistance. At doses above 20 μg/kg/min, the alpha action may reverse the dilation of renal and mesenteric vessels.

Dosage and Routes of Administration

The usual dose is by IV, and the initial dose may vary from 2 to 5 μg/kg/min. The infusion is increased until the desired response is observed; 200 mg of dopamine may be mixed in 500 ml of 5% dextrose in water to yield an infusion of 400 μg/ml. Monitoring of left ventricular filling pressure, cardiac output, and peripheral resistance will help obtain optimal dosage. The usual dose for a child is 2 to 20 μg/kg/min and monitor for effects.

Adverse Reactions and Hazards

High doses of dopamine may result in tachydysrhythmias or an undesirable degree of vasoconstriction. Accordingly, the dose should be increased gradually while monitoring for the desired response. Also, the drug should not be added to sodium bicarbonate since it is inactivated in alkaline solutions.

Digitalis

Indications

Digitalis is useful in decreasing the ventricular rate in the presence of arterial flutter, fibrillation, or supraventricular tachycardia.

Drug Action

Digitalis increases myocardial contractility (a positive inotropic effect). It also enhances vagal effects on the atrioventricular node, decreasing the ventricular rate in the presence of rapid atrial fibrillation.

Dosage and Routes of Administration

The usual dose is a loading dose of 1 mg of digoxin in divided oral or IV doses. Maintenance dose is 0.125 to 0.375 mg/day.

Adverse Reactions and Hazards

There is a narrow margin between therapeutic dose and toxic effects. Dysrhythmias are seen if digitalis toxic response occurs, especially in the patient who has hypokalemia.

Norepinephrine

Indications

Norepinephrine is indicated in patients with severe hypotension and low total peripheral resistance.

Drug Action

The vasoconstrictor action results in elevation of SVR and MAP. Cardiac output may increase or decrease depending on the blood pressure, the state of the left ventricle, and reflex responses such as carotid baroreceptor mediated cardiac slowing. It produces a slightly more rapid blood pressure response than other catecholamines, including dopamine.

Dosage and Routes of Administration

The usual dose is 8 mg of norepinephrine in 500 ml of 5% dextrose in water or saline as the solution is infused continuously. Blood pressure monitoring is required. The usual dose for a child is started at 0.1 μg/kg/min and titrated to obtain the desired effect.

Adverse Reactions and Hazards

Prolonged administration can result in ischemic tissue damage, contraindicated if hypotension is due to hypovolemia. Norepinephrine should not be administered in the same IV line as alkaline solutions, which may inactivate it. Cautious use of this agent is important with ischemic heart disease because of the increase in myocardial oxygen requirement.

Sodium Nitroprusside (Nipride)

Indications

Nipride may be useful in treating congestive heart failure caused by acute myocardial infarction and to decrease myocardial work in patients with hypertension and acute ischemic heart disease.

Drug Action

Nipride is a direct peripheral vasodilator which decreases SVR and increases cardiac output in patients with congestive heart failure. Hemodynamic monitoring is important when giving this drug to the patient with pump failure caused by a myocardial infarction. Arterial blood pressure may fall and left ventricular filling pressure should not be allowed to drop below 15 to 18 mm Hg.

Dosage and Routes of Administration

The usual dose is a 50-mg vial of sodium nitroprusside, which is added to 250 ml of dextrose in water for IV infusion. The usual dose for a child starts at 0.5 μg/kg/min with the effect usually seen at 1 to 10 μg/kg/min.

Adverse Reactions and Hazards

Nipride is metabolized to cyanide, which is a toxic substance.

POSTARREST DRUGS

Diuretics

Indications

Diuretic therapy may be indicated in the postarrest treatment of cerebral edema and the treatment of pulmonary edema.

Drug Action

Furosemide (Lasix) reduces left ventricular end diastolic volume and inhibits the reabsorption of sodium in the proximal and distal tubules and the loop of Henle. Lasix also has a venodilating effect with patients who have pulmonary edema. However, for patients with chronic heart failure, there may be a transient vasoconstrictor effect. The vasodilator effects occur after IV administration; diuresis occurs later, within 5 minutes, peaks at 30 minutes and lasts several hours.

Dosage and Routes of Administration

The usual dose for treatment of pulmonary edema when using furosemide (Lasix) is 0.5 to 1.0 mg/kg injected slowly IV. The usual dose for a child is 1 mg/kg of furosemide.

Nitroglycerin

Indications

Nitroglycerin is the treatment of choice for acute angina pectoris. In the emergency cardiac care set-ting it may be indicated in congestive heart failure or unstable angina.

Drug Action

Nitroglycerin decreases left ventricular end-diastolic volume and relaxes smooth muscles, particularly vascular smooth muscle. When taken sublingually, it is effective in relieving angina pain within minutes. The effect lasts up to 30 minutes.

Dosage and Routes of Administration

The usual dose is one tablet administered sublingually and may be repeated at 3- to 5-minute intervals (up to three tablets) if the pain is not relieved. The IV dose is 10 μg/min and can be increased in 5- to 10-μg/min increments according to the response.

Adverse Reactions and Hazards

Hypotension may occur, which may exacerbate ischemia. Hemodynamic monitoring is required when nitroglycerin is administered by the IV route.

Morphine Sulfate

Indications

Morphine sulfate is used in the treatment of pain, including pain accompanying myocardial infarction and pulmonary edema.

Drug Action

Morphine has an analgesic action, decreases venous return by pooling blood peripherally, decreases myocardial oxygen demand, decreases systemic vascular resistance.

Dosage and Routes of Administration

The usual dose is 2 to 5 mg IV every 5 to 30 minutes until the desired response is seen.

Adverse Reactions and Hazards

Respiratory depression may occur or hypotension especially in volume-depleted patients. Administering morphine in small IV increments reduces these problems.

Sodium Bicarbonate

The 1986 American Heart Association standards did not recommend sodium bicarbonate as a first-line drug during CPR.[42] Laboratory and clinical data have indicated that bicarbonate does not improve the ability to defibrillate or improve survival rates. Bicarbonate inhibits the release of oxygen, induces hyperosmolarity and hypernatremia, produces paradoxical acidosis due to production of carbon dioxide, exacerbates central venous acidosis, and may inactivate simultaneously administered catecholamines. After defibrillation, compressions, intubation, ventilation, and other drug therapies have been given, bicarbonate can be given at the discretion of the team leader, but it is not recommended.

Dosage

When bicarbonate is used, 1 mEq/kg is given and no more than half the dose every 10 minutes. Bicarbonate comes in ampules of 44.6 or 50 mEq of sodium salt. In the postarrest phase, bicarbonate administration should be guided by blood gas analysis.

COMPLICATIONS OF CARDIOPULMONARY RESUSCITATION

Improper Performance of Cardiac Compressions

Liver Lacerations

Compression of the xiphoid process can cause laceration of the liver that can lead to severe internal bleeding. The risk of this problem can be minimal if time is taken to locate the correct position for cardiac compressions. The xiphoid process extends downward over the upper abdomen and finding the correct position above it will decrease the possibility of its lacerating the liver. This may be the most common complication of cardiac compressions in infants and children.

Rib Fractures

Rib fractures and costochondral separation can occur if the compressions deviate from midline or if pressure with the fingers is put on the rib cage. Interlocking the fingers will help to avoid this. Also, between compressions the heel of the hand should remain on the chest. This will help prevent excessive compression of the rib cage or the costochondral cartilages. Even when compressions are being done correctly, there is still a possibility of causing fractured ribs or sternum. The broken ends of the ribs can in turn cause laceration of the lung. Elderly patients and patients on chronic steroids are the most susceptible. If cracking of the ribs is felt or heard, the compressor should check his hand position and continue to compress (since the alternative is death of the patient).[42]

Fat Emboli

The formation of fat emboli is another complication of closed chest massage and may occur without evidence of overt fractures.[42] Compressing bones such as the rib cage and sternum may lead to microfractures within the medulla of the ribs and sternum and an increase in marrow pressure. Fat may enter the venous circulation from the marrow. Cerebral fat emboli may be considered a cause of mental deterioration following CPR.

Improperly Performed Compressions

Improperly performed chest compressions may lead to less than optimal cardiac output, causing inadequate blood flow to the brain. Compressions that are smooth, regular, and uninterrupted provide the best cardiac output and reduce injury. Also, the correct amount of pressure to depress the sternum will help to optimize cardiac output.[42]

Regurgitation and Aspiration

Regurgitation and aspiration of gastric contents may occur during CPR. A cuffed endotracheal tube in the airway will help to prevent aspiration. Also, a clear transparent mask is preferred over a solid color anatomical mask so that regurgitation occurring before intubation can be observed. If the abdomen is observed to be rising during ventilation with a manual resuscitator and mask, the airway should be repositioned. If regurgitation does occur, the head should be turned to the side and the airway suctioned. Continuous pressure on the abdomen during CPR should be avoided. If epigastric pressure is being employed ideally, a gastric tube should be inserted first and connected to suction. This may be necessary since overdistention of the stomach can cause a decrease in venous return and cardiac output. Also, the gastric pressure may decrease ventilation by compressing the lungs.

Gastric Trauma

There are several documented cases of gastric trauma complicating external cardiac massage and mouth-to-mouth resuscitation.[2] Some cases have occurred in which death was shown to be the direct result of gastric lacerations occurring during CPR. Improper support of the jaw and high inflation pressures contribute to producing the gastric distention. Air enters the stomach during ventilation when the upper airway is obstructed at the level of the pharynx. This is related to improper positioning of the airway and requires higher inflating pressures. Gastric lacerations can in turn be produced. To minimize gastric lacerations and ruptures, the following are recommended: early intubation, chest compressions performed with the least amount of pressure required for effective circulation, stomach decompression by nasogastric suction, lower insufflation pressures, proper position of the patient's head, elimination of pressure on the patient's upper abdomen, and careful assessment of chest motion following endotracheal intubation. Gastric rupture should be considered a possibility in the postresuscitation period when signs indicate acute blood loss.[2, 35, 39]

Pneumothorax and Hemothorax

A pneumothorax may occur during CPR from high pressures and high volumes being delivered to the lung. A pneumothorax may also result from laceration of the lung from a rib fracture during CPR or from a penetrating foreign object. In these situations, a hemothorax may complicate the pneumothorax. During CPR a pneumothorax is suspected when increasing pressures are required to ventilate the lung. A shift of the trachea and mediastinum to the opposite side may be observed if a tension pneumothorax has developed. A chest x-ray would confirm the diagnosis, but is not appropriate during CPR. If manual ventilation becomes increasingly difficult and is ineffective, a chest tube should be inserted to relieve the pneumothorax and/or hemothorax. A large bore needle can relieve a pneumothorax if a chest tube cannot be inserted immediately.

Infectious Diseases

Mouth-to-mouth resuscitation carries the risk of transmitting infectious diseases. Cutaneous tuberculosis, meningococcal infections, and hepatitis B have been reported.[1] Meningococcal infection is particularly important because it can be rapidly fatal. Therefore, it has been recommended that those exposed to patients with meningococcal infections be given the chemoprophylaxis of rifampicin, sulfadiazine, or minocycline. It is also suggested that those exposed to menigococcal infections be admitted to the hospital, started on penicillin and discharged in 2 days if no symptoms develop and the blood cultures are sterile.[1]

Interruption of CPR

Interruption of CPR causes cardiac output and blood pressure to drop to zero. Therefore, CPR should not be interrupted for more than 5 seconds.[42] The exception to this rule is for endotracheal intubation which can take between 15 and 30 seconds. If the tube cannot be placed within that time, the procedure should be stopped and the patient reoxygenated.

When moving a patient up or down a stairway, CPR may be interrupted for up to 30 seconds. In this situation, a plan is made for moving quickly to a certain place on the next stair level where CPR can then be continued until another move is planned. If a patient is being transported from one hospital to another, stabilization should be assured before transfer. Also, a resuscitation team capable of delivering advanced life support should accompany the patient on transport.

Evaluation of Effectiveness of CPR

Determining the adequacy of ventilation during CPR involves inspection, auscultation, and attention to changes in inflation pressure. During artificial ventilation, the chest should rise and fall symmetrically. Auscultation of the lungs should reveal bilateral breath sounds. If breath sounds are heard over the right lung and not on the left side, the endotracheal tube should be repositioned as previously described.

Only manual resuscitators capable of delivering 100% oxygen should be used during CPR. The adequacy of oxygenation is determined by arterial blood gas analysis in addition to observation of the skin color. The mucous membranes should be inspected for central cyanosis and the nailbeds and ear lobes inspected for peripheral cyanosis. If cyanosis persists during CPR and arterial blood gases show an inadequate Po_2, the respiratory care practitioner should check the manual resuscitator for proper function and assure that an adequate oxygen flow is being used. If the manual resuscitation bag is refilling very slowly, the liter flow may be too low or the air intake valve may only be partially opening.

During external heart massage, a pulse should be felt with each compression. The carotid or femoral pulse is palpated in the older child or adult to determine the effectiveness of circulation. The brachial pulse is checked in the neonate. The respiratory therapist who is maintaining the airway should periodically check for a pulse. If a palpable pulse is not being produced, the person performing compressions should evaluate the position and technique.

The adequacy of cerebral circulation is reflected in the reactivity of the pupils, level of consciousness, and the presence of movement and spontaneous respirations. Within 1 to 2 minutes from the onset of circulatory arrest, the pupils become nonreactive.

Pupils that remain fixed and dilated for longer than 30 minutes, deep unconsciousness, and absence of respirations indicate a poor prognosis but are not absolute in every case. A pupil that is constricted or reacts to light indicates a satisfactory cerebral state.

Specific criteria for ceasing CPR cannot be standardized. Each CPR situation involves variables related to clinical, ethical, and psychological circumstances. However, cardiopulmonary resuscitation should be continued until it is determined that the cardiovascular system is unresponsive. Unusual circumstances such as hypothermia in children may require longer periods of resuscitation. Complete recovery has occurred in hypothermic patients after prolonged unconsciousness and 2 to 4 hours of resuscitation.[3]

Hypothermia

Interrupted circulation can occur without permanent brain damage in the presence of hypothermia because low temperatures reduce body and cerebral oxygen requirements. At a body temperature of 20°C, the ischemic tolerance of the brain increases approximately tenfold as compared to normothermic conditions. Therefore, in hypothermic situations, CPR should be vigorous and prolonged, even when the patient demonstrates symptoms indicating irreversible damage.

At temperatures below 27°C, the patient will be motionless and pulseless, with fixed dilated pupils.[3] At 25°C, ventricular fibrillation may appear spontaneously, and at 20°C, the heart will be in cardiac standstill. Resuscitation efforts should include maintaining adequate circulation, ventilation, and oxygenation, minimizing additional heat loss, restoring normal body temperature, and homeostasis. Methods available for rewarming include: peritoneal irrigation, gastrointestinal rewarming, extracorporeal blood rewarming, airway rewarming, and diathermy. There is much controversy over which method

should be used and how fast the rewarming should occur.[27] However, it is agreed that resuscitation should never be terminated before the patient has rewarmed.

RESUSCITATION IN THE DELIVERY ROOM

At the time of delivery, secretions should be suctioned from the baby's mouth and nose with a bulb syringe. When the umbilical cord is cut, the baby is dried with a warm towel to reduce heat loss. The baby should then be put in a well-lighted warm resuscitation area and evaluated using the Apgar score (Table 11–4).

Monitoring by Apgar Score

An Apgar score between 0 and 3 indicates that the infant is severely depressed and ventilation is required.[13] A manual resuscitator capable of delivering 100% oxygen is used to deliver between 20 to 50 breaths/min. The baby is also suctioned as needed. Intubation is indicated if the baby does not respond or if the baby is less than 32 weeks' gestation.[12] A size 3.0 to 3.5-mm tracheal tube is used to intubate and ventilation maintained at an inflating pressure of 20 to 30 cm H_2O. Cardiac compressions should be started if the heart rate is below 60 and appropriate drug therapy begun. An umbilical artery catheter is placed for monitoring blood pressure, blood gases, and for administering fluids. To assess cardiac compressions, the umbilical artery blood pressure is monitored and the brachial blood pressure palpated. Small or midsize pupils indicate adequate perfusion and oxygenation.[13]

An Apgar score of 4 to 6 indicates a moderately depressed newborn. The infant should be suctioned as needed and kept warm and dry. Oxygenation and ventilation with a manual resuscitator is started.

TABLE 11–4.

Apgar Score Chart

CATEGORY	0	1	2
Color	Blue, pale	Body—pink; extremities—blue	Body and extremities pink
Heart rate	Absent	Below 100	Above 100
Respiratory effort	Absent	Slow, irregular	Regular, strong
Reflex	No response	Grimace	Cry, cough, sneeze
Muscle tone	Flaccid	Strong extremity flexing	Active, well-flexed

Stimulation of the infant is done by tapping the feet or rubbing the back.

An Apgar score of 7 to 10 indicates a normal or slightly depressed newborn in whom general routine care is given. The baby is suctioned as required and kept warm and dry in a proper thermal environment. The skin temperature should be maintained at 35° to 36.5°C.

A reassessment of the baby should be done at 5 minutes. If the Apgar score is less than 6 at 5 minutes, arterial blood gas analyses are done. Hypoxia and acidosis are assessed and the baby treated accordingly. Respiratory acidosis can be corrected with a manual resuscitator.

Meconium Aspiration

Babies born through meconium are often normal at birth but may develop severe respiratory distress 6 to 12 hours after delivery. This presents a special danger because meconium pneumonitis has a mortality of 20% to 35%.[12] To decrease the morbidity and mortality from meconium pneumonitis, the following procedure has been recommended.[12, 43] If meconium is present in the trachea at birth, as much as possible should be removed by suctioning. The infant should be intubated with a 3.0-mm tube immediately. The tube should be suctioned, removed, and inspected for meconium. If meconium is present, a clean endotracheal tube is inserted and suctioning continued until there is no evidence of meconium. Gastric suctioning is also done after the trachea has been cleared. Newborn resuscitation should be continued as long as there is hope for a positive neurological outcome. Close observation and appropriate cardiopulmonary monitoring is continued following resuscitation.

Postarrest Period

The period immediately following a successful resuscitation can be a critical one. Patient evaluation and monitoring during this time are essential. The endotracheal tube should be evaluated to determine that it is placed correctly and is secure. A chest x-ray is done to verify tube placement and to diagnose complications that may have occurred during CPR.

The secretions suctioned from the patient should also be evaluated and the patient treated accordingly. Pink, frothy secretions indicate pulmonary edema and frank red blood may indicate varying degrees of hemorrhage requiring further evaluation. Suctioning of gastric contents indicates that aspiration occurred during CPR. When this is suspected, good endotracheal toilet is important including bronchoscopy in some situations. The patient should be monitored for secondary infections since they are seen in 25% to 45% of the cases in which aspiration has occurred. The signs to watch for are an increase in temperature, new or extending infiltrates after 36 to 48 hours, increased leukocytosis, increased hypoxia, or unexplained clinical deterioration. Steroids are often given to treat aspiration pneumonitis.

Oxygen is given following CPR to reverse hypoxia or maintain an adequate P_{O_2}. Signs of inadequate tissue perfusion are evaluated, including hypotension, cool extremities, poor capillary refill, and acidosis. Urine output is a valuable index to determine the adequacy of peripheral perfusion. An hourly urine output of less than 0.5 cc/kg should be viewed as a medical emergency.

Mechanical ventilation is usually indicated in the postarrest phase for at least the first 24 hours. It is always indicated for the patient who has not regained spontaneous respirations. Also, mechanical hyperventilation can be used to decrease intracranial pressure during the postarrest period.

The appropriate drug therapy will help to decrease the incidence of a second arrest. Careful ECG monitoring is critical and the patient treated accordingly. Intravenous lidocaine is given to the patient who had ventricular tachycardia or ventricular fibrillation. Atropine is given intravenously to the patient in bradycardia. Diuretics may be used to relieve cerebral or pulmonary edema.

REFERENCES

1. Achong MR: Infectious hazards of mouth to mouth resuscitation. *Am Heart J* 1980; 100:759–761.
2. Aguilar JC: Fatal gastric hemorrhage: A complication of cardiopulmonary resuscitation. *J Trauma* 1981; 21:537–545.
3. Althaus U, Aeberhard P, Schupbach P, et al: Management of profound accidental hypothermia and cardiopulmonary arrest. *Ann Surg* 1982; 195:492–495.
4. American Society for Testing and Materials Committee on Manual Resuscitators: *Standard for Minimal Performance and Safety Requirements for Resuscitators Intended for use on Humans.* Philadelphia, American Materials Testing Society, 1984.
5. Applebaum EL, Bruce DL: *Tracheal Intubation.* Philadelphia, WB Saunders Co, 1976.
6. Babbs C, Winslow E, Ritter G: Knowledge gaps in CPR: Synopsis of a panel discussion. *Crit Care Med* 1980; 8:181.

7. Baldwin M, Iverson RL: Cardiopulmonary resuscitation: Does it work? *Indiana Med* 1984; 77:246–248.

8. Bander JJ: Cardiac arrest-defibrillation. *Topics in Emergency Medicine.* Aspen Publication, 1979.

9. Barnes TA, Watson ME: Oxygen delivery performance of four adult resuscitation bags. *Respir Care* 1982; 27:139–146.

10. Barnes TA, Watson ME: Oxygen delivery performance of old and new designs of Laerdal, Vitalograph and AMBU adult manual resuscitators. *Respir Care* 1983; 28:1121–1128.

11. Beamer WC, Prough DS: Technical and pharmacologic considerations in emergency translaryngeal intubation. *Ear Nose Throat J* 1983; 62:11–20.

12. Biehl D: Resuscitation of the newborn at delivery. *Can Anaesth Soc J* 1983; 30:94–97.

13. Blodgett D: *Manual of Pediatric Respiratory Care Procedures.* Philadelphia, JB Lippincott Co, 1982.

14. Caldwell SL, Sullivan KN: Artificial airways, in Burton GG, Hodgkin JE (eds): *Respiratory Care: A Guide to Clinical Practice,* ed 2. Philadelphia, JB Lippincott Co, 1984, pp 493–521.

15. Carden E, Bernstein M: Investigation of the nine most commonly used resuscitator bags. *JAMA* 1970; 212:589–592.

16. Carden E, Freidman D: Further studies of manually operated self-inflating resuscitator bags. *Anesth Analg* 1977; 56:202–206.

17. Debard ML: Cardiopulmonary resuscitation: Analysis of six years experience and review of the literature. *Ann Emerg Med* 1981; 10:408–416.

18. Dronen SD: Antifibrillatory drugs: The case for bretylium tosylate. *Ann Emerg Med* 1984; 13:805–807.

19. Eaton JM: Medical technology: Adult manual resuscitators. *Br J Med* 1984; 31:67–70.

20. Ellis PD, Billings DM: *Cardiopulmonary Resuscitation—Procedures for Basic and Advanced Life Support.* St Louis, CV Mosby Co, 1980.

21. Emergency Care Research Institute: Manual resuscitators. *Health Devices* 1979; 8:133–146.

22. Fitzmaurice MW, Barnes TA: Oxygen delivery performance of three adult resuscitation bags. *Respir Care* 1980; 25:928–933.

23. Greensher J, Mofenson HC: Aspiration accidents: Choking and drowning. *Pediatr Ann* 1983; 12:747–752.

24. Greensher J, Mofenson HC: Emergency treatment of the choking child. *Pediatrics* 1982; 70:110–112.

25. Hamelberg W: Twenty-five years experience with cardiopulmonary resuscitation. *Ohio State Med J* 1984; 80:482–483.

26. Hanson GC: Cardiopulmonary resuscitation: Chances for success (editorial). *Br Med J* 1984; 288:1324–1325.

27. Harnett RM, Pruitt JR, Sias FR: A review of the literature concerning resuscitation from hypothermia: I. The problem and general approaches. *Aviat Space Environ Med* 1983; 54:425–434.

28. Hirschman AM, Kravath RE: Venting vs ventilating. A danger of manual resuscitation bags. *Chest* 1982; 82:369–370.

29. Howells TH: Disaster at the dining table. *Br Med J* 1984; 289:510–511.

30. Huszar RJ: *Emergency Cardiac Care.* Bowie, Md, Robert J Brady Co, 1974.

31. Iserson K, Sanders AB, Kaback K: Difficult intubations: Aids and alternatives. *Am Fam Phys* 1985; 31:99–112.

32. Jacobs LM, Berrizbeitia LD, Bennett B, et al: Endotracheal intubation in the pre-hospital phase of emergency medical care. *JAMA* 1984; 250:2175–2177.

33. Klick J, Bushnell L, Bancroft M: Barotrauma: A potential hazard of manual resuscitators. *Anesthesiology* 1978; 49:363–365.

34. Kouwenhoven WB: The development of the defibrillator. *Ann Intern Med* 1969; 71:449.

35. Krause S, Donen N: Gastric rupture during cardiopulmonary resuscitation. *Can Anaesth Soc J* 1984; 31:319–322.

36. Ludwig DJ: The pharmacist as a member of the CPR team: Evaluation by other health professionals. *Drug Intell Clin Pharm* 1983; 17:463–465.

37. Lund I, Skulberg A: Cardiopulmonary resuscitation by lay people. *Lancet* 1976; 2:702–704.

38. McDonald JL: Systolic and mean arterial pressures during manual and mechanical CPR in humans. *Ann Emerg Med* 1982; 11:292–295.

39. McDonnell PJ, Hutchins GM, Hruban RH, et al: Hemorrhage from gastric mucosal tears complicating cardiopulmonary resuscitation. *Ann Emerg Med* 1984; 13:230–233.

40. Michael TA, Gordon AS: The oesophageal obturator airway: A new device in emergency cardiopulmonary resuscitation. *Br Med J* 1980; 281:1531–1534.

41. Murphy RJ: Citizen cardiopulmonary resuscitation training and use in a metropolitan area: the Minnesota Heart Survey. *Am J Pub Health* 1984; 74:513–515.

42. National conference on standards for cardiopulmonary resuscitation and emergency cardiac care. *JAMA* 1986; 255:2841.

43. Ostheimer GW: Newborn resuscitation. *Clin Obstet Gynecol* 1981; 24:653–658.

44. Patrus RJ, Goren CC: The precordial thump: An adjunct to emergency medicine. *Heart Lung* 1983; 12:61–64.

45. Price HC, Postma DS: Tracheostomy. *Ear Nose Throat J* 1983; 62:11–20.

46. Roven AN, Clapham MB: Cricothyroidotomy. *Ear Nose Throat J* 1983; 62:68–75.

47. Schade J: An evaluation framework for code 99. *Q Rev Bull* 1983; 9:306–309.

48. Smith JP, Balazs IB, Aubourg R: A field evaluation of the esophageal obturator airway. *J Trauma* 1983; 23:317–321.

49. Smith JP, et al: The esophageal obturator: A review. *JAMA* 1983; 250:1081–1084.

50. Taylor GI, Rubin R, Tucker M: External cardiac compressions: A randomized comparison of mechanical and manual techniques. *JAMA* 1978; 240:644–646.

51. Torrey SB: The choking child—a life threatening emergency. *Clin Pediatr* 1983; 22:751.

52. Tweed WA, Wilson E, Isfeld B: Retention of cardiopulmonary resuscitation skills after initial overtraining. *Crit Care Med* 1980; 8:651–653.

53. White RD: Antifibrillatory drugs: The case for lidocaine and procainamide. *Ann Emerg Med* 1984; 13:802–804.

54. Yauncey W, Wears R, Kamajian G: Unrecognized tracheal intubation: A complication of the esophageal obturator airway. *Ann Emerg Med* 1980; 9:18–20.

SUGGESTED READING

Airway Management

Berminger G, Forrete M: Adult manual resuscitators. *Curr Rev Respir Ther* 1979; 1:115–119.

Boidin MP: Mechanical ventilators for emergency medical care using a manual resuscitator. *Acta Anaesth Belg* 1984; 35:43–51.

Carden E, Hughes T: An evaulation of manually operated self-inflating resuscitation bags. *Anesth Analg* 1975; 54:133–138.

Day RL, Crehn ES, Dubois AB: Choking: The Heimlich abdominal thrust vs. back blows: An approach to measurement of inertial and aerodynamic forces. *Pediatrics* 1982; 70:113–119.

Doren N, Tweed WA, Dashfsky S, et al: The esophageal obturator airway: An appraisal. *Can Anaesth Soc J* 1983; 30:194–200.

Emergency Care Research Institute: Evaluation-manually operated infant resuscitators. *Health Services* 1973; 2:240–248.

Emergency Care Research Institute: Evaluation-manually operated resuscitators. *Health Services* 1971; 1:13–17.

Emergency Care Research Institute: Evaluation-manually operated resuscitators. *Health Services* 1974; 3:164–176.

Gordon BD, Terranova GJ: Heimlich maneuver in cold-water drowning. 1981; 45:775–776.

Greensher J, Mofenson HC: Emergency treatment of the choking child. *Pediatrics* 1982; 70:110–112.

Harrison RR, Maull KI: Keanan RL, et al: Mouth-to-mask ventilation: A superior method of rescue breathing. *Ann Emerg Med* 1982; 11:74–76.

Heimlich HJ: First aid for choking children: Back blows and chest thrusts cause complications and death. *Pediatrics* 1982; 70:120–125.

Le Bouef L: 1980 assessment of eight manual resuscitators. *Resp Care* 1980; 25:1136–1142.

Melker R, Cavellaro S, Krischer J: One rescuer CPR—a reappraisal of present recommendations for ventilation. *Crit Care Med* 1981; 9:423.

Priano L, Ham J: A simple method to increase the F_{DO_2} of resuscitator bags. *Crit Care Med* 1978; 6:48–49.

Redick L: Hand-operated self-inflating resuscitation equipment: A re-evaluation. *Anesth Analg* 1971; 50:554–556.

Redick L, Dunbar R, MacDougall D, et al: An evaluation of hand-operated self-inflating resuscitation equipment. *Anesth Analg* 1970; 49:28–32.

Sainsbury DA, Davis R, Walker MC: Artificial ventilation for cardiopulmonary resuscitation. *Med J Aust* 1984; 141:509–511.

Steinbach B, Carden E: 1973 assessment of eight adult resuscitators bags. *Resp Care* 1975; 20:69–76.

Vottery B: Hand-operated emergency ventilation devices. *Heart Lung* 1972; 1:2–6.

White R, Gilles B, Polk B: Oxygen delivery by hand operated emergency ventilation devices. *J Am Coll Emerg Phys* 1973; 2:2–5.

Complications

Adler SN, Klein RA, Pellecchia C, et al: Massive hepatic hemorrhage associated with cardiopulmonary resuscitation. *Arch Intern Med* 1983; 143:813–814.

Dohi S: Post cardiopulmonary resuscitation pulmonary edema. *Crit Care Med* 1983; 11:434–437.

Dryden GE, Benz J, et al: Efficiency studies: Aspiration, chest injury and prone CPR. *J Indiana State Med Assoc* 1983; 76:269–270.

Evans RD: Gastric rupture as a complication of cardiopulmonary resuscitation: Report of case and review of literature. *J Am Osteopath Assoc* 1981; 80:830–831.

McLaren CA, Robertson C, Little K: Missed orthopaedic injuries in the resuscitation room. *J R Coll Surg Edinb* 1983; 28:339–401.

Nagel EL, Fine EG, Krischner HP, et al: Complications of CPR. *Crit Care Med* 1981; 9:424.

Powner DJ: Cardiopulmonary resuscitation-related injuries. *Crit Care Med* 1984; 12:54–55.

Young CD: Esophageal perforation associated with combined use of the thumper resuscitator and esophageal airway. *South Med J* 1983; 76:322–324.

Defibrillation and Drug Therapy

Abstracts of the Fourth Purdue Conference on Cardiac Defibrillation and Cardiopulmonary Resuscitation: Purdue University. *Med Instrum* 1981; 15:319–328.

Cotoi S: Precordial thump and termination of cardiac transient tachyarrhythmias. *Am Heart J* 1981; 101:675–677.

Ewy GA: Recent advances in cardiopulmonary resuscitation and defibrillation. *Curr Probl Cardiol* 1983; 8:1–42.

McCabe JB, Ventriglia WJ, Anstadt GL, et al: Direct mechanical ventricular assistance fibrillation. *Ann Emerg Med* 1983; 12:739–744.

McIntyre KM, Lewis AJ (eds): *Advanced Cardiac Life Support*. Dallas, American Heart Association, 1981.

Patros RL, Goren CC: The precordial thump: An adjunct to emergency medicine. *Heart Lung* 1983; 12:61–64.

Tacker WA: Some research needs in defibrillation and CPR. *Med Instrum* 1983; 17:21–22.

Weaver WD, Copass MK, Bufi D, et al: Improved neurological recovery and survival after early defibrillation. *Circulation* 1984; 69:943–948.

SECTION III

Respiratory Care Equipment

Equipment for Mixed Gas and Oxygen Therapy

Jeffrey J. Ward, M.Ed., R.R.T.

The objectives of this chapter are to provide information on equipment and techniques used to provide medical gas therapy. Clinicians should have an understanding of the rationale for use of supplemental oxygen, carbon dioxide–oxygen, and helium-oxygen therapy; Chapter 5 should be prerequisite reading. Of special importance are the basics of oxygen transport, recognition of signs and symptoms of hypoxemia, indications for therapy, physiologic effects of oxygen and carbon dioxide, and recognition of the potential hazards during administration. Supplemental oxygen and carbon dioxide should be considered as "drugs." Helium is used for its low-density physical properties, helium being physiologically inert.

Medical gas therapy begins with the initial assessment of the patient. As orders are written, one needs to choose from a variety of equipment systems. Cylinders, regulators, bulk pipelines, flowmeters, and a host of administration devices can bewilder the providers of gas therapy. Safe and appropriate care requires knowledge of both equipment and pathophysiology. Problems due to either an untoward response to the drug, unsuitability of equipment, or a technical problem may arise during therapy. A background in both areas is required to provide competent medical gas therapy.

HISTORICAL NOTE: DISCOVERY OF OXYGEN AND CARBON DIOXIDE

The ancient records note that the Chinese and Greeks believed that the air contained a substance that was required for life. Little was done until 1500 A.D. when Leonardo da Vinci found that animals required something in the atmosphere to sustain life. In 1660 Robert Boyle suggested that combustion of a flame and respiration both required a common substance in air. About that same time Evangelista Toricelli and Blaise Pascal were working on relationships of atmospheric pressure, and the barometer was developed. In 1670 Robert Hook, working with Boyle, surmised that the primary purpose of respiratory movements was to provide a fresh supply of air to the lungs.

Instead of building on the work by Boyle and others of that time, George Stahl proposed a chemical theory he called the "phlogiston theory." According to Stahl, air supported combustion by "taking up" the phlogiston given off by the burning object.

During the late 1700s a number of investigators almost simultaneously discovered oxygen and carbon dioxide. Discovery involves (1) preparation of the pure gas, (2) identification of its significance as oxidant and supporter of combustion, plus (3) the recognition that oxygen related to respiration in animals. In 1771 Swedish apothecary Carl Scheele heated magnesium oxide (MnO_2) with concentrated sulfuric acid (H_2SO_4), generating oxygen (Fig 12–1). Apparently understanding the significance of his finding, he did communicate by letter to others working in this area in 1773. Until 1962 it was believed that Scheele did not publish his finding until 1777, in his *Chemical Treatise on Air and Fire*. However, a summary of Scheele's work was published by Torbern Bergman in 1775, but printed in June of 1774, 3 months before England's Joseph Priestly

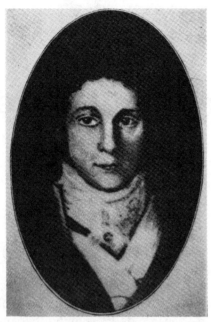

FIG 12–1.
Carl Wilhelm Scheele (1742–1786), Swedish apothecary, is credited with the first synthesis of oxygen. (From *Pharm Sci* 1931; 20:1061. Reproduced by permission.)

made his discovery of oxygen in August 1774 (Fig 12–2). Being a true phlogiston man, he named oxygen "dephlogisticated air." Scheele called oxygen "fire air."[22]

In France Antoine Lavoisier published details of his finding on oxygen in 1775 (Fig 12–3). Although a moot point, Scheele appears to have priority for the

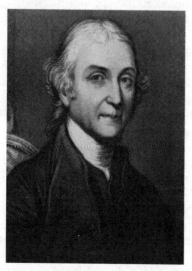

FIG 12–2.
Joseph Priestly (1733–1804), British discoverer of oxygen. (Courtesy of Wellcome Institute for the History of Medicine, London.)

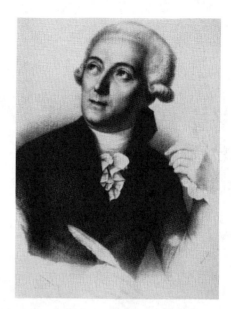

FIG 12–3.
Antoine Laurent Lavoisier (1743–1794), French scientist, explained the true nature of combustion and respiration. (Courtesy of Wellcome Institute for the History of Medicine, London.)

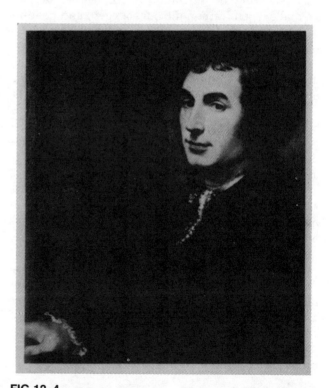

FIG 12–4.
Joseph Black (1728–1799) investigated carbon dioxide and showed that it was produced during respiration. (From Guerlac H: Joseph Black and fixed air: A bicentenary retrospective with some new or little known material. *Isis* 1957; 48:152. Reproduced by permission.)

TABLE 12–1.

Physical Characteristics*

	OXYGEN	AIR	CARBON DIOXIDE	HELIUM
Symbol	O_2	Air	CO_2	He
Molecular weight	31.999	28.975	44.01	4.003
Percent by mole	20.946	—	0.0335	—
Partial pressure (ATPD†)	158 torr	—	0.25 torr	0.000524
Density at 21°C and 1 atm viscosity	1.326 kg/m^3	1.2 kg/m^3	1.833 kg/m^3	0.1656 kg/m^3
Viscosity poise	201.8×10^{-6}	182.7×10^{-6}	148×10^{-6}	194.1×10^{-6}
Specific gravity at 21°C	1.1049	1	1.52	0.138
Boiling point at 1 atm	−297.3°F (−183°C)	−317.8°F (−194.3°C)	−29	−452.0°F (−268.9°C)
Freezing point at 1 atm	−361.1°F (−218.4°C)	−357.2 to −312.4°F (−216.2 to −191.3°C)	—	‡
Critical temperature	−181.4°F (−118.6°C)	−221.2°F (−140.7°C)	87.9°F (31.1°C)	−450.2°F (−267.9°C)
Critical pressure	731.4 psia§ (5,043 kPa, absolute)	547 psia (3,770 kPa, absolute)	1070.6 psia (7,382 kPa, absolute)	3 psia (227 kPa, absolute)
Triple point	−361.8°F (at 0.022 psia)	—	−69.9°F at 60 psig‖ (416 kPa)	—
Sublimation temperature (1 atm)	—	—	−109.3°F (−78.5°C)	—
Solubility (v/v) H$_2$O at 0°C	0.0489	0.0292	0.90	0.0086
Color	Colorless	—	Colorless	Colorless
Odor	Odorless	—	Odorless	Odorless
Taste	Tasteless	—	Taste?	Tasteless
Flammability	Support combustion	Nonflammable	Nonflammable	Nonflammable

*Adapted from Gilbert DL: Cosmic and geophysical aspects of the respiratory gases, in Fenn WO, Rahn H (eds): *Handbook of Physiology.* Washington, DC, American Physiological Society, 1964, vol 1, pp 153–157.
†ATPD = ambient temperature and pressure dry.
‡Will not solidify at 1 atm −458°F (−272°C) and 25 atm, or 367.7 pounds per square inch (psi) (2,335 kPa, absolute).
§Psia = pounds per square inch absolute.
‖Psig = pounds per square inch gauge.

actual discovery. Of greater interest is the fact that these three researchers nearly simultaneously and independently came to similar conclusions. Lavoisier, however, reported disproof of the phlogiston theory. In contrast, Priestly and Scheele both believed their work supported Stahl's beliefs. In 1780 he published that "respiration is a combustion . . . similar to the combustion of charcoal," with knowledge of oxygen as a participant in the two processes. Lavoisier also renamed the gas "oxygen," or "acid generator."[22, 89, 92]

Joseph Black is credited with the discovery of carbon dioxide (Fig 12–4). Black heated limestone and found that it lost weight due to loss of "fixed air." He discovered that this same substance was produced when charcoal was burned and when beer fermented. Actually Black's work was a rediscovery of Jean Baptiste van Helmont's work performed 100 years earlier (Fig 12–5). Black believed that his work with carbon dioxide did not relate to the phlogiston theory.[89]

PHYSICAL AND CHEMICAL CHARACTERISTICS AND SOURCES OF MEDICAL GASES

Oxygen

Pure oxygen can be compared with air, carbon dioxide, and helium (Table 12–1). Oxygen's concentration in the atmosphere is 20.94%. It remains constant to an altitude of 60 miles (96.5 km) above sea level. Changes in total and partial pressure of oxygen will decrease at higher altitude and increase below sea level or hyperbaric conditions (Table 12–2). The following formula using Dalton's law will determine oxygen's portion of the total atmospheric gas pressure:

$$P_{O_2} = (P_B)F_{I_{O_2}}$$

where

P_B = barometric pressure (mm Hg or torr)
P = partial pressure (mm Hg or torr)

F = fractional concentration
I = inspired.

Thus, at sea level

$$P_{O_2} = (760)0.2094$$
$$= 159.14 \text{ mm Hg, or torr.}$$

Although the fraction of oxygen does not change in our atmosphere, the partial pressure will vary considerably. On Mount Everest the partial pressure is only 37.4 mm Hg, and the equivalent oxygen fraction is only 0.06. When one is going below sea level, 1 atm is added for each 33 ft (10 m) of sea water. Therefore, for a diver 66 ft below sea level (or in a hyperbaric chamber) the partial pressure of oxygen would be 477 mm Hg and the equivalent oxygen fraction 0.63.

The equivalent oxygen concentration at altitude can be determined using the following formula: For example, for Denver, Colorado:

Equivalent $F_{I_{O_2}}$ (air at altitude)

$$= \frac{P_B \text{ at altitude (dry)}}{P_B \text{ at sea level (dry)}} \times F_{I_{O_2}} \text{ (at sea level)}$$
$$= \frac{600 \text{ torr}}{760 \text{ torr}} \times 0.21$$
$$= 0.17.$$

The atomic weight of oxygen is 16 and the gram molecular weight is 32 gm/mole. There is some difference in proportion of atomic and molecular oxygen with altitude. At about 20 km, photodissociation produces atomic oxygen. Also there is an increase in ozone. Each reaches its maximum concentration at 30 km (0.003%) and 90 km (7%), respectively. Radiation strips off an electron from atomic oxygen, producing ionized species O^+ and O^{++}. However, the atomic form is quite reactive, and oxygen commonly exists in molecular form.[95]

Oxygen is interesting in its molecular bonding characteristics. Figure 12–6, A shows an oxygen atom with its eight electrons. The outer 2p orbit of

TABLE 12–2.

Partial Pressures of Oxygen With Alterations in Altitude*

ALTITUDE		ATMOSPHERIC PRESSURE				EQUIVALENT
FT	M	ATM	PSI	MM HG	P_{O_2}	$F_{I_{O_2}}$
300,000	99,435	7.3×10^{-6}	1.1×10^{-4}	0.0035	1.1×10^{-4}	1.4×10^{-7}
200,000	60,957	3.2×10^{-4}	4.6×10^{-3}	0.24	5×10^{-2}	6.6×10^{-5}
100,000	30,478	0.011	0.155	8.0	1.7	2.2×10^{-3}
90,000	27,430	0.017	0.250	12.9	2.7	3.6×10^{-3}
80,000	24,382	0.027	0.403	20.8	4.3	5.7×10^{-3}
70,000	21,334	0.044	0.649	33.6	7.0	9.2×10^{-3}
60,000	18,287	0.071	1.05	54.1	11.3	0.015
50,000	15,239	0.115	1.69	87.4	18.3	0.038
40,000	12,191	0.191	2.72	140.6	29.4	0.049
30,000	9,143	0.296	4.36	225.7	47.3	0.062
25,000	7,619	0.372	5.46	282.0	59.1	0.078
20,000	6,096	0.460	6.76	348.8	73.1	0.096
15,000	4,572	0.566	8.29	428.6	89.8	0.118
10,000	3,048	0.690	10.11	522.9	109.5	0.144
5,000	1,524	0.835	12.23	623.3	132.3	0.174
Sea level		1.00	14.7	760.0	159	0.2095
Below sea level						
33		2.00	29.4	1520.0	318	0.419
66		3.0	44.1	2280.0	477	0.628
99		4.0	58.8	3040.0	636	0.838
132		5.0	73.5	3800.0	795	1.047
165		6.0	88.2	4560.0	954	1.257
198		7.0	102.9	5320.0	1113	1.466
231		8.0	117.6	6080.0	1272	1.676
264		9.0	132.3	6840.0	1431	1.885
297		10.0	147.0	7600.0	1590	2.095

*From Dittmer PS, Grebe RW (eds): *Handbook of Physiology*. Philadelphia, WB Saunders Co, 1958. Used by permission.

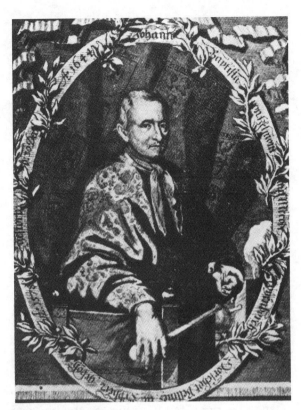

FIG 12–5.
Jean Baptiste von Helmont (1577–1644) discovered the gas sylvestre, carbon dioxide. (From Helmont JB: *Dageraed oft Nieuwe Opkomst der Geneeskunst.* Amsterdam, 1659. Reproduced by permission.)

the L shell has "room" for six electrons, but only four are filled. In its molecular form (Fig 12–6,B), the 2p orbit stability is achieved by "filling" the orbit, by each atom sharing one of its electrons. In addition, the outermost orbit is occupied by two electrons, one from each atom. This outer orbit configuration provides the basis for the paramagnetic susceptibility or quality of oxygen. Oxygen has the ability to intensify the force of a magnetic field. It is the only naturally occurring gas with this characteristic, which is used as the basis for the design of one type of gas analyzer.[5]

Another physical quality of oxygen that is important to providers of therapy is the density and viscosity. Density is of great importance when oxygen is administered through orifices (e.g., flowmeters), and viscosity affects laminar flow through tubes according to Poiseuille's law. Critical velocity (an index of turbulent flow) and flow through orifices depend to a greater degree on density than viscosity. The equation for calculating density is shown below.

Density of a gas
$$= \frac{\text{Atomic or gram molecular weight}}{\text{Number of L/mole of gas}}.$$

For example,

$$\text{Density of oxygen} = \frac{32 \text{ gm/mole}}{22.4 \text{ L/mole}} = 1.43 \text{ gm/L}.$$

Oxygen is less dense than carbon dioxide, but air and helium are significantly less dense than oxygen. The differences in viscosity are not as significant. Pure oxygen and helium are nearly identical in viscosity values, and carbon dioxide is the lowest. These physical properties must be taken into consideration when designing flowmeters and explains why switching to different gas mixtures may require recalibration of flowmeters.

Since we are ultimately interested in gases dissolving into body fluids, gas solubility should be reviewed. Henry's law states that at a constant temperature, gases will dissolve into fluid and exert a tension (or escaping tendency) proportional to the pressure above the fluid and coefficient of solubility. The Bunsen solubility coefficient for oxygen dissolving into plasma at 37°C is 0.023 ml of O_2/ml of plasma at 760 mm Hg. A commonly used coefficient to determine the amount (content) of oxygen dissolved in *blood water* is computed as follows[87]:

Solubility coefficient for O_2
$$= \frac{0.023 \text{ ml of } O_2}{760 \text{ mm Hg}} \times 100 \text{ ml of blood}$$
$$= 0.003 \text{ ml of } O_2/\text{mm Hg/dl}.$$

Example: If a patient's Pa_{O_2} is 90 mm Hg, how many milliliters of O_2 will be dissolved in 100 ml of the patient's arterial blood (100 ml = 1 dl)?

1 ml of O_2 dissolved
$$= 90 \text{ mm Hg} \times 0.0031 \text{ ml/mm Hg/dl}$$
$$= 0.27 \text{ ml/dl}.$$

When Graham's law is applied to oxygen and carbon dioxide to determine diffusion rates in a gas mixture, the results are relatively comparable. A light gas diffuses faster than a heavy gas. Graham's law states that gases diffuse at rates that are inversely proportional to the square roots of their molecular weights:

$$\frac{\text{Diffusion rate for } CO_2}{\text{Diffusion rate for } O_2} = \frac{\sqrt{32 \text{ gm/mole}}}{\sqrt{44 \text{ gm/mole}}}$$
$$= \frac{5.6}{6.6}.$$

A

B

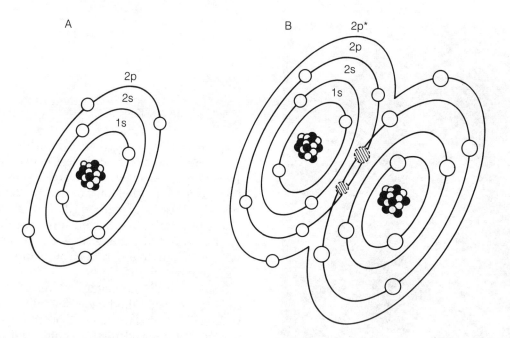

FIG 12–6.
A, atomic oxygen showing unfilled electrons in the K + L shells. **B,** molecular oxygen showing the sharing of two electrons in the

2s subshell but two in the P + L shell unshared. The incomplete L shell provides the basis of oxygen's paramagnetic susceptibility.

When diffusion rates between gas, fluids, and tissues, are compared, Graham's and Henry's laws are applied. Partial pressure gradient and solubility coefficients are also significant factors:

$$\frac{\text{Diffusion rate for } CO_2}{\text{Diffusion rate for } O_2}$$

$$= \frac{\text{solubility coefficient } CO_2}{\text{solubility coefficient } O_2} \times \frac{\sqrt{O_2}}{\sqrt{CO_2}}$$

$$= \frac{0.592 \text{ ml } CO_2/\text{ml/mm Hg}}{0.024 \text{ ml } O_2/\text{ml/mm Hg}} \times \frac{\sqrt{32 \text{ gm/mole}}}{\sqrt{44 \text{ gm/mole}}}$$

$$= \frac{21}{1}.$$

Therefore, carbon dioxide diffuses 21 times more rapidly between alveoli and pulmonary capillaries than oxygen. Oxygen's normal physical state is a gas. However, most hospitals and some patients have liquid supplies. Oxygen will stay in liquid form only if its temperature is kept below $-183°C$, its boiling point. The temperature above which oxygen gas could not be converted back to a liquid, regardless of pressure applied, is the *critical temperature*, $-118°C$. The pressure required to convert gaseous oxygen back to a liquid at the critical temperature, or the critical pressure, is 716 psi.

Sources of Supplemental Oxygen

Oxygen is produced in nature by the photosynthetic process. Chlorophyll in plants traps radiant energy and converts carbon dioxide and water into glucose and oxygen. Laboratory or commercial manufacture of oxygen can take place using four methods: (1) heating metallic oxides, (2) electrolysis, (3) fractional distillation, and (4) filtration by membrane or molecular sieve.

Scheele and Priestly generated oxygen by heating metallic oxides of mercury, silver, or barium. The following formula demonstrates the chemical reaction:

$$2 \text{ HgO} \xrightarrow{\text{Heat}} 2 \text{ Hg} + 2 \text{ O}_2.$$

Since water is 33% oxygen by volume and 88% by weight, it can be a source of oxygen in a laboratory. The process is termed *electrolysis* and occurs by passing an electric current through water (with a trace of acid to improve conduction). Oxygen can be collected in a glass chamber above the anode. Hydrogen is obtained at the cathode.

The most common commercial source of oxygen and complex technique is termed *fractional distillation of air*, or the *Joule-Kelvin method*. It utilizes the different boiling points of the constituents of air in the production of liquid oxygen. This process was first done commercially in 1907 by Linde. The following is a simplified explanation of three basic steps of *fractional distillation*:

1. *Purification of air.* Filtered air is first compressed to 1,500 psi, then further to 2,000 psi. During each pressurization, the heat built up by molecular compaction is eliminated by water cooling heat exchangers. The cooling process extends below the freezing point of water, which removes water vapor.

2. *Liquefaction.* Liquid ammonia is used to cool the purified air to approximately $-40°F$ ($-40°C$), which removes any remaining water vapor. The cooling is now extended to $-265°F$ ($-160°C$) and compression to 200 psi. Further lowering of temperature is next accomplished by releasing the compressed gas into a relative vacuum. Molecules lose kinetic energy, causing the temperature to drop, which causes partial liquefaction.

3. *Distillation.* The liquid air is allowed to flow down vertically stacked distillation columns. Nitrogen boils off the top as it descends down the column, and the gas increases its pure oxygen content as it reaches the bottom. Near the base the oxygen-rich liquid is reboiled, releasing rare gases, such as argon and krypton, because they have lower boiling points than oxygen (Fig 12–7).[7]

The most recent devices used to make oxygen for medical purposes are called *oxygen concentrators.* This term is somewhat generic in that there is con-

centration, but the devices themselves are actually sieves that filter out molecules other than oxygen. The most common is the molecular sieve or pressure swing absorbent method (Fig 12–8,A). A vacuum draws room air into cylinders packed with crystallized zeolite, a silicate with ion exchange properties. The air is compressed (100–300 psi) and N_2 filtered (i.e., absorbed by the zeolite). The process is reversed by the depressurization phase, which causes the crystals to release the nitrogen as exhaust. The final concentration of oxygen varies among manufacturers as well as the flow setting exiting the sieve. Most concentrators can deliver 90% to 95% oxygen in the 1 L/min range but fall to 80% to 90% when run at flows of 2 to 5 L/min. The increasing concentration of argon causes a decrease in F_{IO_2}.[24]

Membrane oxygen concentrators utilize a set of plastic polymer membranes through which air is filtered (Fig 12–8,B). A pump provides the pressure gradient across the membrane cells. Oxygen and water vapor are more permeable than nitrogen and move through the system to be collected. These concentrators are less popular commercially because they can produce only 30% to 40% oxygen. However, the concentration is less subject to reduction as flow is increased.[24]

Carbon Dioxide

Under normal atmospheric conditions carbon dioxide gas has a concentration of 0.03% by volume. Since it is a by-product of human and animal metabolism and carbonaceous fuels, the concentration may increase in certain environments. The current Occupational Safety and Health Act (OSHA) standards for maximal allowable concentration is 0.5% for 8 hours of continuous exposure or 3% carbon dioxide over a 10-minute period.[28] In carbon dioxide/oxygen therapy, commonly a concentration of 5% is used for short periods (about 10 minutes), during which the patient is carefully monitored. Actually high CO_2 levels can displace air, the former being 1.5 times heavier (see Table 12–1).

In gaseous form, carbon dioxide is relatively nonreactive, is nontoxic, and will not support combustion. However, when carbon dioxide is dissolved in water, carbonic acid (H_2CO_3) is formed, which is corrosive to metals. These characteristics lend themselves to nonmedical use in carbonated beverages, in food preservation, in refrigeration, and as a fire extinguishing agent. Solid carbon dioxide (dry ice) ex-

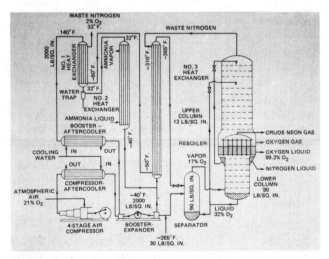

FIG 12–7.
Schematic of fractional distillation plant for the production of liquid oxygen from air. (Courtesy of Union Carbide Corporation, Linde Division, Indianapolis.)

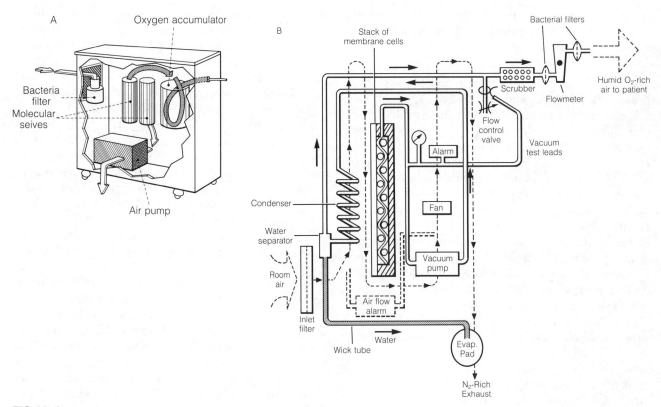

FIG 12–8.
A, molecular sieve oxygen concentrator. (Courtesy of DeVilbis Company, Toledo.) **B,** membrane-type oxygen concentrator. (Courtesy of Oxygen Enricher Company, Schenectady, N.Y.)

ists at temperatures below its triple point of $-69°F$ and at a pressure above 60.4 psi. At temperatures below its triple point and 1 atm pressure, dry ice will sublime into a gas without passing through liquid phase, as when dry ice is seen "smoking." Carbon dioxide also has a low thermal conductivity, which allows dry ice to remain relatively stable.[28]

Cylinders of CO_2 commonly contain both liquid and gas if the temperature is below 31°C with pressures above 60 psi. This possibility requires that cylinders be weighed to determine the quantity of remaining gas. This phenomenon does not occur with medical mixtures of 95%/5% and 90%/10% oxygen–carbon dioxide. There is significant difference in the density and viscosity of carbon dioxide when compared with oxygen or air (see Table 12–2). Accurate metering of gas through tubes and orifices must be corrected if a device calibrated for the specific concentration of CO_2 is not used.

Sources of Carbon Dioxide

Carbon dioxide in an unrefined form is obtained from combustion of coal, coke, natural gas, oil, steam hydrocarbon reformers, lime kilns, the fermentation process, and natural springs. Refining removes carbon monoxide, hydrogen sulfide, nitric acid, water, and other impurities. For medical purposes the purity is 99.5% or better. Three types of carbon dioxide are available: type 1 (cylinders at ambient temperatures), type 2 (liquid at subambient temperatures), and type 3 (solid carbon dioxide).[28]

Helium

Helium is the second lightest element in the atmosphere (see Table 12–1). It is considered a rare gas, having a concentration of only 5 ppm. Helium is chemically inert, nontoxic, tasteless, and nonflammable. Helium is used in respiratory care as a diagnostic gas in closed circuit analysis of lung volume and for its low-density properties in treating airway obstruction.[31] Commercially helium is used as a nuclear reactor coolant, in cryogenic research, as a shield in arc welding, in silicon and germanium crystal growing atmosphere, in lighter than air craft, and in breathing mixtures in deep water diving.[28]

Sources of Helium

Natural gas containing up to 2% helium is found in wells in the southern United States. Other wells are located in Saskatchewan, Canada and near the Black Sea. Helium/oxygen, or heliox, is potentially life saving in emergency application, although somewhat expensive compared with other medical gases mixtures, and not used frequently.

Discussion of correcting for the low-density characteristics of medical mixtures (80%/20% and 70%/30% He-O_2) to allow use on non-helium-calibrated variable orifice flowmeters will follow when those devices are detailed. It should be noted, however, that there is little benefit when 60%/40% heliox is used because the density of that mixture approximates that of pure oxygen.[28]

SYSTEMS FOR GAS STORAGE AND DISTRIBUTION

The manufacture and storage of oxygen was done on a small scale prior to 1868. Each provider used chemical methods for oxygen production and "fresh" gas was collected in a rubber bag for administration. In England Barth was the first to use a hand pump to compress the chemically generated oxygen into a copper cylinder at around 450 psi (Fig 12–9).[69]

Today medical gases are made available to medical consumers in portable cylinders, bulk (liquid) cylinders (Fig 12–10), and fixed liquid systems that feed pipelines for gas supply. Because of the potential hazards to the general public during transportation and to handlers and patients, a fairly complex array of regulating and recommending agencies have become involved. Each group provides extremely detailed information, specifications, regulations, and safety procedures (Table 12–3).[80, 84, 85]

The standards for construction and vessel safety are established by the ASME. They may appear quite complex, because there are actually two systems portrayed. System A is the primary supply, and system B is the reserve, or backup, supply. Liq-

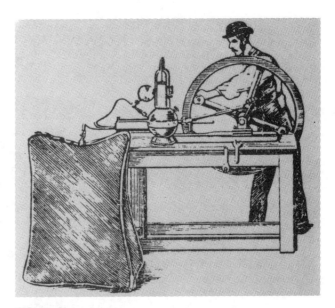

FIG 12–9.
Barth (England) was the first to compress chemically generated oxygen into copper cylinders. (From Leigh JM: The evolution of the oxygen therapy apparatus. *Anaesthesia* 1974; 29:462–485. Reproduced by permission.)

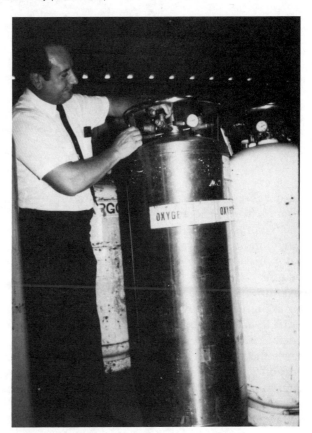

FIG 12–10.
Portable liquid bulk cylinder.

TABLE 12–3.

Governmental and Nongovernmental Agencies That Regulate or Determine Standards by Their Legal Authority

REGULATING BODY	ACTIVITY/RESPONSIBILITY
GOVERNMENTAL AGENCIES	
Department of Transportation (DOT) inspection (prior to 1970, Interstate Commerce Commission, ICC)	Compressed gas cylinder specification and inspection
Department of Health and Human Services (HHS) (formerly Department of Health, Education and Welfare), Food and Drug Administration	Purity levels of medical gases
HHS, Bureau of Medical Devices	Classify, provide standards and regulate medical devices
Federal Department of Labor, OSHA	Occupational safety related to medical gases
NONGOVERNMENTAL AGENCIES	
Compressed Gas Association (CGA)	Specifications, recommendations in manufacture and safety systems
National Fire Protection Association (NFPA)	Codes and safety recommendations for storage of flammable/oxidizing gases
International Standards Organization (ISO)	Standards related to technical standards for manufacture
American National Standards Institute (ANSI) and its Z-79 Committee	Coordination of standards for health devices (anesthesia, ventilatory equipment, adaptors, artificial airways, humidifier and nebulizers)
Association for the Advancement of Medical Instrumentation (AAMI)	Education and standards related to a wide range of biomedical equipment
American Society of Mechanical Engineers (ASME)	Standards for liquid gas bulk reservoir

uid oxygen is transported to the facility by truck or rail and filled at location 1 (Fig 12–11). To provide positive pressure within the system, liquid oxygen is drawn off at locations 6 and 7, where a pressure regulator and vaporizer reintroduce gaseous oxygen to the tank. The atmosphere warms the liquids as they pass through the vaporizer, which increases the internal pressure. The liquid oxygen is continually vaporizing and fed into the liquid pipeline in an economizer circuit at location 4. The main liquid supply leaves the tank and is led to the main vaporizers and location 9. Following the vaporizers, gas flows to the main supply regulators, a primary and backup, location 11, 11a, and 11b (see Fig 12–11). A pressure relief valve will vent off pressure if the pressure exceeds the normal level, 55 psi, by 50%, or 80 psi.

A reserve supply of another liquid bulk system may be used (see Fig 12–11,B). Some facilities would need only a bank of large gas cylinders, in that the NFPA requires that the reserve supply be equal to 1 day's normal supply need. In the diagram, it is a parallel design to the main unit. Besides acting as a backup, it also continuously adds a small amount of gas as normal vaporization occurs. Check valves (one-way valves) prevent any leaks in either system from inadvertently draining the other.[6]

Incidents involving bulk oxygen systems are not rare. Far too often maintenance is not done in a preventive manner, or poor communication between maintenance and the respiratory therapy department leads to problems. Once an oxygen system abruptly stops, there is major emergency. Oxygen loss in the operating room or critical care unit must be quickly corrected with cylinder gas. However,

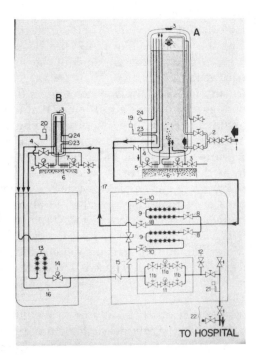

FIG 12–11.
Schematic of main and reserve liquid oxygen reservoirs. (From Bancroft ML, du Moulin GC, Hedley-Whyte J: Hazards of hospital bulk oxygen delivery systems. *Anesthesiology* 1980; 52:504–510. Reproduced by permission.)

that response will usually be slow unless prior protocol has been established. Separate alarms to alert personnel to problems in a bulk system traditionally consist of the following:

1. Low liquid level in either primary or reserve systems.
2. Reserve in use following a switchover when the main supply falls to approximately 85 psi.
3. Main supply line pressure variations exceed −20%.

A report of incidents of a 500-bed hospital noted fairly numerous problems when the hospital's bulk system was followed for 1 year. The following were of most significance[7]:

1. False alarms due to calibration drift of pressure sensors.
2. Excessive depletion of the reserve supply because of pressure imbalance between the main and reserve supply.
3. Failure of the vacuum seal on the reserve supply.

4. Inappropriate manipulation of supply valves.
5. Leakage due to ruptured piping and around valves.
6. Failure of monitoring personnel to notify appropriate service personnel.
7. Occlusion of pressure sensors with foreign substance.

Other serious problems have occurred because of connecting internal pipelines to the wrong gas or error in filling the bulk tank itself. Finally, high winds, tornadoes, earthquakes, and fires are potentially catastrophic to liquid medical gas systems.

Miniature versions of a hospital bulk liquid system are available for use in homes or where a portable supply is needed. Commercial units are the Linde Walker (Union Carbide) and the Liberator (Cryogenics Associates) shown in Figure 12–12. The basic design is identical to larger units except that the pressure within the vessel is less (20 to 50 psi). A major advantage of these systems is that a small, portable reservoir can be transfilled from the main unit. Patients who can ambulate only with continuous oxygen are liberated from having to use small cylinders with limited volume.

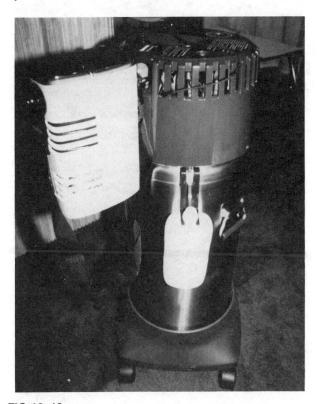

FIG 12–12.
Home liquid oxygen reservoir and portable reservoir.

Pipeline Supply Systems

Bulk medical gas liquid reservoirs or banks of compressed gas cylinders can provide a source for multiple supply outlets in medical facilities. These outlets for one or a number of different medical gases offer convenience and prevent safety problems and significant human resource needs related to cylinders. The plumbing of a hospital or clinic with gas is regulated by the NFPA. They provide numerous guidelines and regulations for construction, materials specifications, and maintenance.[83-85] A *continuous system* uses one source, namely, the large liquid reservoir, and the reserve (cylinder bank or second liquid). The reserve is used only if the main unit fails or is depleted (Fig 12–13,A). The *alternating system* is used with a pair of compressed gas cylinder banks or portable liquid reservoirs. They are filled on an alternating use schedule (Fig 12–13,B). Check valves prevent gas from draining any limb of the system if a leak occurs in another area.

Once any type of supply system enters the facility, it divides into a labyrinth of pipes that are sent to all locations requiring a gas source. Engineers utilize different diameter pipe to maintain a fairly constant pressure of ±50 psi, independent of the distance from the main inlet. A system of zoning or partitioning off branches of the system is required. *Zone valves* are strategically installed to allow isolation of outlets in specific areas (Fig 12–14) to stop gas flow for repair or in case of a fire. However, provision should be made for patients dependent on the medical gas prior to being closed. The zone system must be mapped out to understand what areas may be affected.

Problems that do occur appear in pipeline systems appear to be largely preventable if regulations are followed. Seamless type K or L copper or brass pipe, secured by independent supports, should be used. All fittings and their soldered or brazed connections must be carefully inspected to test for leaks. A special cleaning procedure is required for new or modified systems to remove bits of flux, corrosion, or rust. Each gas system is individually tested to confirm its capability by charging it to 1.5 times its working pressure for 24 hours. If a new section is added to an existing system, multiple measurements must be made to confirm the proper gas is connected to the specific labeled outlet. Errors have occurred and are similar to a patient receiving the wrong drug because of improperly labeled syringe. It can be the source of litigation and unsatisfactory publicity if one gives critically ill patients carbon dioxide or nitrous oxide, thinking it oxygen. Each gas source is termed a *station outlet*. There are numerous types of connectors to provide access to the gas, most common are the *quick connect* style. The NFPA and CGA regulations have caused the development of noninterchangeable gas connectors incorporating automatic shut-off valves. Most manufacturers have some sort of plunger that is inserted into a spring-loaded station outlet (Fig 12–15,A). Normally the male connector is held in place until a button or collar is activated to allow release. Adapters that allow different types of outlet connectors to be used are available (Fig 12–15,B). Also, many of the connectors are color coded similar to cylinders, and all have the specific gas type printed on them.

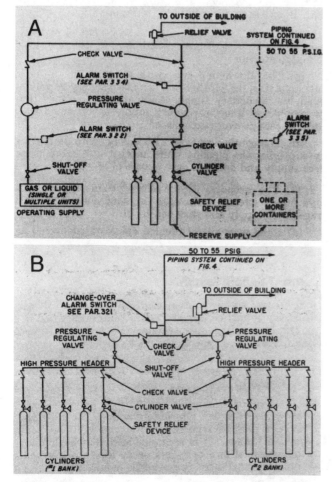

FIG 12–13.
A, schematic of bulk oxygen supply with cylinder reserve. **B,** schematic of two banks of high-pressure cylinders. One manifold system functions as the reserve. (From *NFPA 56F-1983, Standard for Nonflammable Medical Gas Systems.* Quincy, Mass, National Fire Protection Association, 1983. Reproduced by permission.)

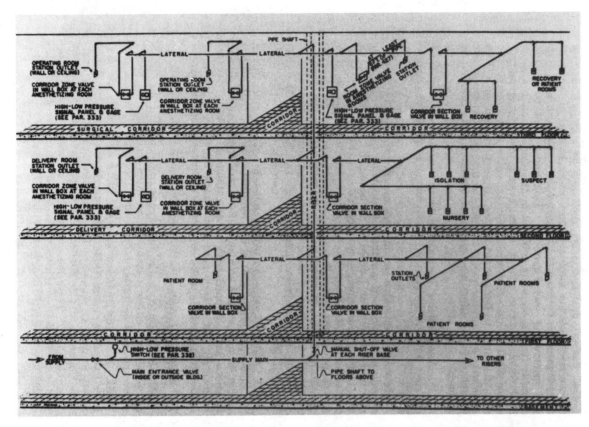

FIG 12–14.
Schematic of medical gas piping through a hospital. Zone valves and check valves isolate areas. (From *NFPA 56F-1983, Standard for Nonflammable Medical Gas Systems.* Quincy, Mass, National Fire Protection Association, 1983. Reproduced by permission.)

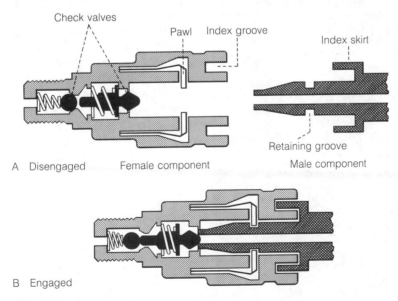

FIG 12–15.
Quick-connect medical gas wall outlets showing different styles of allowing immediate gas access, secure fixing of appliance, and leak-free operation. **A,** disengaged. **B,** engaged.

Sources of Compressed Air

Piped medical compressed air is commonly incorporated into medical gas systems for use in certain areas such as the operating room and intensive care units. Blended mixtures of air and oxygen are required for many ventilators and other devices using oxygen-air blenders. Various designs of large compressors are available, but the piston type appears to be the industrial standard. A pressure-sensitive switch senses pressure levels and turns the compressor on and off to maintain line pressures of 50 psi. Normally a holding reservoir is incorporated into the system to provide a ready supply and prevent the compressor from being run all the time. In large institutions, it is common to have two compressors that alternate, prolonging compressor life.[27] Smaller versions are also available for hospital or home use that requires a portable air compressor (Fig 12–16).

Since the source of these systems is the hospital ambient air, humidity can cause considerable condensation. It is important that a compressed air system incorporate condensers to scavenge water during cooling after the gas is warmed during the compression phase. Water trap drains must be religiously maintained to prevent wet air from fouling flowmeters and ventilators. The federal specifications BB-A-1034 for source II grade C breathing air permits a maximum of 0.3 mg/L for total water content. Inline dessicant dryers or filters may also be needed, especially in humid summer months.[27, 38]

Medical Gas Cylinders

As early as the 1890s, cylinders were used to store compressed oxygen and nitrous oxide for "therapeutic" gas during seances.[70] Cylinders continue to be used substantially in medical care today in spite of piped gas supply systems. Properly handled, they are quite safe, and small cylinders offer portability to provide patients with gas during transport or ambulation. Today the cost of cylinder gas is quite reasonable; however, the cylinders themselves are expensive. These containers are carefully regulated because of their potential hazard if gas under considerable pressure is suddenly released or if flammable or gases that augment combustion are involved in a fire.

Oxygen cylinders are constructed of high-quality alloy steel and usually spun into shape while the steel is still hot. A 3A designation indicates non-heat-treated and 3AA heat-treated steel. Aluminum cylinders have become popular in the recent past because their weight is one half that of steel cylinders. They are also labeled 3AA since they too have a working pressure of 2,015 psi. However, if aluminum cylinders are exposed to high temperatures (more than 400°F [204°C]), the metal loses its elastic properties and is more subject to rupture than steel.

The DOT requires that all cylinder gas contents be identified by label, and unlabeled cylinders should be returned to the vendor. In addition, the cylinder itself is identified by stampings on the front and back shoulders below the cylinder valve (Fig 12–17).[28]

The DOT and the CGA offer the following general rules for safe handling of high-pressure gas cylinders[26]:

1. No petroleum-based lubricants should come in contact with cylinder valves, regulators, high-pressure gas hoses, or fittings.
2. Never use open flames to detect leaks, but use solutions of a leak detector or soapy water.
3. Never interchange regulators that are not

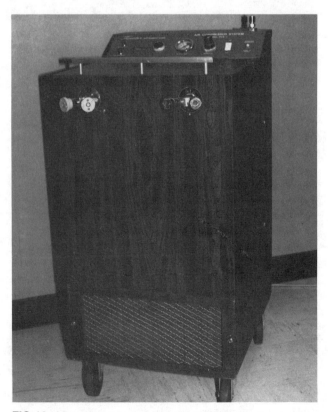

FIG 12–16.
Portable air compressor.

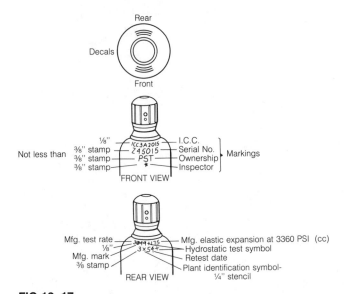

FIG 12–17.
High-pressure medical gas cylinder stampings and their significance.

intended for use with that specific gas or gas blend.

4. Open valves on cylinders or regulators slowly to allow dissipation of heat. Valves should be opened fully for use.
5. Unlabeled cylinders should be returned to the vendor.
6. Cylinders should not be subjected to temperatures exceeding 54.4°C or put in areas with flames or sparks.
7. Do not attempt to modify or repair cylinders.
8. Cylinder valves should remain in the closed position when not in actual operation.
9. Cylinder valve caps (found on larger cylinders) should remain on when in storage or when being transported.
10. Do not drop cylinders, and move them only with suitable carts with capability of securing the cylinder via chain.

The following are guidelines from the NFPA regarding proper storage of high pressure medical gas cylinders[84]:

1. Cylinders should be stored in locations that meet NFPA standards with regard to physical construction and materials. The area should be cool, dry, and well ventilated.
2. Full and empty cylinders should be stored in

separate areas to prevent confusion as to their status.
3. Flame-resistant wall partitions should be used.
4. Large cylinders should be restrained from being knocked over by chain or other style of physical restraint.
5. Cylinder areas should be locked to prevent unauthorized use or tampering.

Cylinder manufacturers have given letter code designations to indicate the size, and therefore potential gas capacity (Table 12–4). The most common sizes are the H or K and the E cylinders (Fig 12–18). Those sizes with letter designation AA through E are used a great deal because they are relatively portable sources of medical gas and also are found in the operating room for anesthetic gases and in the laboratory for calibration gases. This group employs a yoke style connection to mount regulators on the cylinder valve (Fig 12–19,A). A hand-tightening screw forces the yoke inlet into the cylinder valve outlet, with a plastic ring gasket providing a leakproof seal. Manufacturers have agreed on a system of varying the position of the pins for various types of gas so that only regulators for that gas can be mounted. Larger cylinders utilize different threads, sizes of connecting nipples, and thread direction to guard against misconnection (Fig 12–19,B).

Using different colored paint is another method of identifying cylinder gases used in the United States and Canada (Table 12–5).[26]

Cylinders are tested and checked for their integrity every 5 years for 3A and 3AA high-pressure containers unless the markings are following by a star, in which case they are tested every 10 years. All aluminum cylinders are inspected every 5 years.

TABLE 12–4.

Medical Gas Cylinder Code Designations, Specifications, and Capacities*†

LETTER DESIGNATION	DIMENSION, IN	WEIGHT LB	VOLUME CU FT/L
D	4.2 × 20	7	12.6/356
E	4.2 × 30	9	22/622
M	7 × 47	27	21.9/1,337
G	8.5 × 55	100	186/5,260
H or K	9 × 55	132	244/6,900
Scuba	7 × 21	29	45/1,270

*From Compressed Gas Association: *Handbook of Compressed Gases*, ed 2. New York, Van Nostrand Reinhold Co, 1981. Used by permission.
†Cylinder pressures at 70°F. Capacities and dimensions may vary slightly among manufacturers.

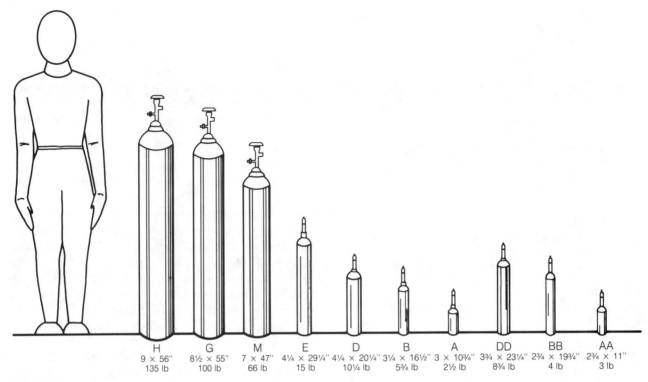

FIG 12–18.
Letter designation and approximate dimensions of high-pressure medical gas cylinders.

The owner of the cylinder is required to follow DOT standards for cylinder inspection[28]:

1. Visual inspection of external and internal surfaces to detect arc burns, dents, bulging, gouges, rust, or corrosion. Loose scale should be removed from the cylinder interior.

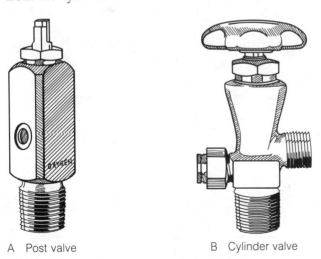

A   Post valve

B   Cylinder valve

FIG 12–19.
A, small yoke-style valve *(AA–E)*. **B,** large-size American standard cylinder valve *(M–H)*.

2. Hammer or dead ring testing (upon each refilling) to detect any dampening of the normal 2- to 3-second ring when struck with a hammer. If dampening occurs, fire damage, corrosion, or oil or water contamination should be suspected.

3. Hydrostatic testing involving immersing a cylinder in a special water jacket container, both filled with water. An initial water level is noted when the water-filled cylinder is under no pressure (Fig 12–20). Water pressure is increased to an excess of 3,000 psi, and the water that the expansion displaced is measured. Loss of the *compliance* of the steel or aluminum is a sign of aging. The elastic expansion information is stamped following the test along with date and inspector's mark.

Filling a gas cylinder from another gas cylinder, usually portable cylinders from larger ones, is called *transfilling*. This procedure is in contrast to the practice of most medical gas vendors who use large stores, usually liquid, to fill a group of cylinders at once. Transfilling has met with some resistance, and some older publications (e.g., the CGA) forbade the practice by hospital or nonprofessional workers. Problems occur because of the tremendous energy release as gas passes from the full to empty cylinder,

TABLE 12–5.

Color Code for Medical Gas Cylinders

GAS	UNITED STATES	CANADA
Oxygen	Green	White
Nitrogen	Black	Black
Carbon dioxide	Gray	Gray
Air	Yellow or black	White or black
Helium	Brown	Brown
Carbon dioxide/oxygen	Gray top/green bottom if less than 7% CO_2 (reverse if > 7%)	Gray/white
Helium-oxygen	Green top/brown bottom if helium 80% (reverse if <80%)	White/brown
Nitrous oxide	Blue	Blue
Cyclopropane	Orange	Orange
Ethylene	Red	Red
Oxygen/nitrogen	Green/black	White/black

*Adapted from Compressed Gas Association: *Characteristics and Safe Handling of Medical Gases*, pamphlet P-1. Arlington, Va, Compressed Gas Association, 1965. Used by permission.

causing heat. In addition, there is risk of contamination of gas. Labels and inspection of the cylinder being transfilled must be in accordance with DOT standards. They suggest using a gas control unit to (1) isolate the supply cylinder, (2) limit the filling rate to 200 psi/min, and (3) offer calibrated pressure gauges on the cylinder being filled. They also suggest that the system be mounted on a wall or installed on a portable cart.[29]

Other than the commonly used E cylinder with 620 to 682-L capacity and the D with up to 406-L capacity, there has been application of the scuba type of cylinder. This cylinder, used for recreational underwater diving, is capable of holding 45 cu ft, or 1,270 L, of oxygen (Fig 12–21). The scuba cylinder has approximately twice the capacity of the E cylinder and is shorter and wider. Some institutions have found them useful for mechanical ventilation transport within hospitals and in areas without pipeline supply. Racks under carts and small box transport carts can be custom made to secure the round-bottomed cylinders. Since they normally are filled with compressed air, owners must label them and paint them green for use in oxygen therapy.

Duration of Cylinder Gas Flow

Providers of gas therapy cannot always expect a pipeline outlet to be readily available, and cylinders must be used in transport or emergency medical situations. Therefore, knowledge of how much gas is remaining or how many minutes per hour are left at a certain flow must be calculated. The need to use a

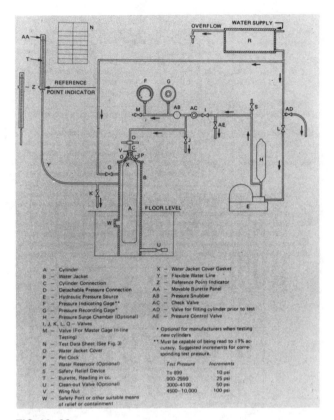

FIG 12–20.
Schematic of water jacket hydrostatic cylinder testing system. (From Compressed Gas Association: *Handbook of Compressed Gases*, ed 2. New York, Van Nostrand Reinhold Co, 1981. Reproduced by permission.)

combination of English and metric units to calculate the volume of gas can cause errors.

A key piece of information is the factor used to convert from cubic feet (cylinder units) to liters (patient administration units): 1 cu ft = 28.3 L.

Next it is necessary to find a conversion factor for each cylinder size that will allow pressure to be equated to available liters of gas (Table 12–6):

$$\text{Conversion Factor} = \frac{\text{cu ft in full cylinder} \times 28.3 \text{ L}}{\text{psi of full cylinder}}.$$

$$\text{Conversion Factor E cylinder} = \frac{22 \text{ cu ft} \times 28.3 \text{ L}}{2,200 \text{ psi}}$$

$$= 0.28 \text{ L/psi}.$$

The final steps are to compare the flow needed with the volume of gas in the cylinder, thereby determining how long the cylinder will last before needing to be replaced.

Example: How long will a one-half full E cylinder at 2 L/min flow last?

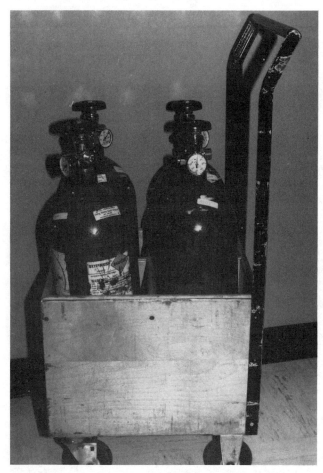

FIG 12–21.
Scuba cylinders for oxygen shown in transport cart.

Minutes remaining

$$= \frac{\text{Cylinder pressure} \times \text{conversion factor}}{\text{Flow rate}}$$

$$= \frac{1,100 \text{ psi} \times 0.28 \text{ L/psi}}{2 \text{ L/min}}$$

$$= 154 \text{ minutes, or } 2.6 \text{ hours.}$$

Cylinder-Indexed Connections and Other Safety Systems

In an effort to prevent mistaken administration of therapeutic gases, a complex system of connection devices is employed. A large part of the system involves access to the cylinder valve. The most common high-pressure type of valve is the direct-acting style (Fig 12–22). As the operator opens or closes the outer stem or valve wheel, the screwlike movement is reflected in the opening or closing of the area immediately above the valve seat. It is, in essence, a

TABLE 12–6.

Cylinder Duration Factors

SIZE	FACTOR (L/PSIG)
D	0.16
E	0.28
M	1.36
G	2.14
H or K	3.14
Scuba	0.58

Assuming 2,200 psig (full cylinder) at 70°F:

$$\text{Factor} = \frac{\text{cu ft (full)} \times 28.3 \text{ L/cu ft}}{\text{Pressure in full cylinder (psig)}}.$$

$$\text{Duration (minutes)} = \frac{\text{Actual gauge pressure} \times \text{factor}}{\text{Flow (L/min)}}.$$

needle valve in which a needle-like projection or, in this case, a valve plunger is moved by the threads, away or toward the valve seat.

In addition to the valve itself, a safety valve is incorporated in the body of the valve. If a cylinder is exposed to heat that raises its internal pressure to 1.5 times its working pressure (normally 2,025 psi) or is directly exposed to fire, a valve will open and vent the gas. This response will prevent the explosive release if the cylinder wall bursts. Some valves use a *rupture disk*–fusible metal plug or a combination of the disk and the plug. Wood's metal is commonly used for the fusible plug material. It is an alloy of bismuth, lead, cadmium, and tin. It will yield to pressure when the temperature reaches 208°F (97.8°C) to 220°F (104°C). Copper is used as fragible disk material.

The outlets of the cylinder's valves are manufactured so that only regulators or other connectors specific for that gas or mixture can be connected. The American Standards Association specified indexing for the connections, and the CGA publishes these industrial standards. A series of numbers indicate details such as diameter of the threaded outlet, number of threads per inch, and whether it's right- or left-hand threaded. Left-handed threads are reserved for gases such as carbon monoxide, hydrogen, pure helium, and mixtures with less than 20% oxygen (toxic gases, or those not capable of supporting life).

Recently the CGA and the DOT have implemented new connection standards for *laboratory gases*. In the past, cylinder valve to regulator intergas connectors were available. The so-called *cheaters* allowed one regulator to be used on almost any mixture. Because of the danger involved in this practice, the CGA 504 or 500 series connections have been developed.

Small cylinders (AA through E) that use the yoke and post-type of valve use the Pin Index Safety System (Fig 12–23,A). As long as the pins remain in place, regulators not specific for that gas cannot be attached (Fig 12–23,B).

Practitioners who work with medical gas systems must also be familiar with the Diameter Index Safety System (DISS). The CGA system is based on the diameter of threaded gas connections that will be subjected to 200 psi or less. Hence, the fittings from medical gas regulators, flowmeters, oxygen concentrators, and interconnecting *high-pressure hoses* have specific-diameter threaded connections. There is a generic DISS size that allows connecting a bubble humidifer or nebulizer to many of these devices that use either air or oxygen (Fig 12–24). When two gases are used on a single piece of equipment, such as an oxygen-air blender, the DISS connections have different sizes (Fig 12–25).

Regulators (Pressure-Reducing Valves)

Gas pressure regulators or reducing valves are used throughout medical gas pipeline systems and with high-pressure gas cylinders. They are required to step down pressures to levels that manufacturers have designed or calibrated for specific working pressures, such as 50 psi. Regulators also modulate the large span of pressure decay as a cylinder is exhausted of gas. If gas was administered from a cylinder with only a needle valve type of device, the operator would have to make frequent adjustments to open the valve slightly, or flow would decrease as the pressure dropped (Fig 12–26).

Theory of Operation

The principle of regulator design and operation can be simply explained by a playground teeter-totter. By varying the distance of the lever arms, either side of a balance point, a lighter child can be balanced by a heavy one. In regulators, instead of varying lengths or lever arms, the size of two different surface areas, are each exposed to different gas pressures (Fig 12–27). The technique is also known as the Pascal principle.

A cylinder's high gas pressure (Pc), is balanced by a lower regulated pressure (Pr) because the area subjected to the high pressure (A_1) is very small compared with the area (A_2) of a flexible diaphragm (Fig 12–28). As A_1 opens, gas fills a chamber, and it can exert force on only one side, the diaphragm A_2. Pr is an indication of the level of reduced pressure.

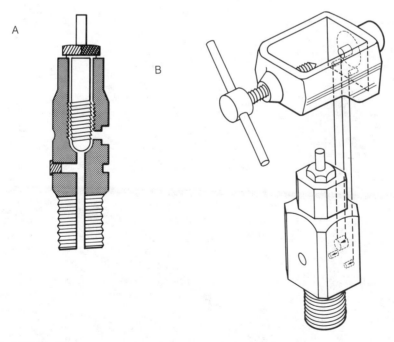

FIG 12–22.
A, cross section of small yoke-type cylinder valve. **B,** yoke connector showing regulator inlet and pin safety system.

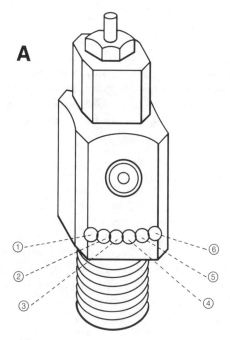

A

B

Gas	Index hole position
O_2	2-5
O_2/CO_2 (CO_2 not over 7%)	2-6
He/O_2 (He not over 80%)	2-4
C_2H_4	1-3
N_2O	3-5
$(CH_2)_3$	3-6
He/O_2 (He over 80%)	4-6
O_2/CO_2 (CO_2 over 7%)	1-6
Air	1-5

FIG 12–23.
A, diagram of Pin Index Safety System pin position. **B,** table showing pinhole positions for various medical gas combinations.

V represents a needle valve or on/off valve, allowing gas to flow from the regulator. The following expression explains the balance of forces (note: pressure = force/unit area, and force = pressure × unit area):

$$Pc \times A_1 = Pr \times A_2.$$

If one solves for Pr, the reduction pressure is equal to the ratio of valve seat/diaphragm areas and the level of the pressure in the cylinder:

$$Pr = \frac{A_1}{A_2} \times Pc.$$

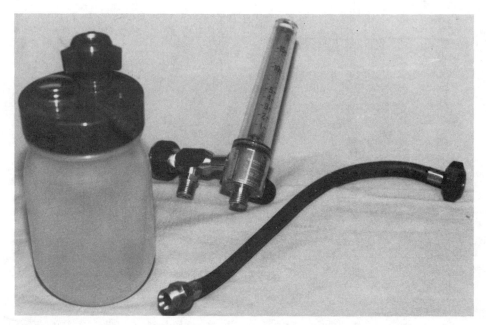

FIG 12–24.
Gas appliances showing DISS threaded connections.

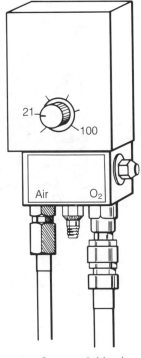

A   Oxygen-air blender
     with DISS fittings

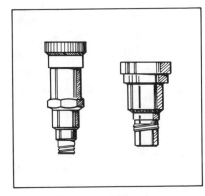

B   Quick-connect fittings

FIG 12–25.
Air/oxygen blender showing inlet connections for air and oxygen **(A)** and quick-connect
fittings **(B)**.

Therefore, if the valve seat is very small and the diaphragm is made quite large (producing a small number), there will be a substantial reduction in cylinder pressure.

Example 1: What is the reduction in cylinder pressure (Pr)?

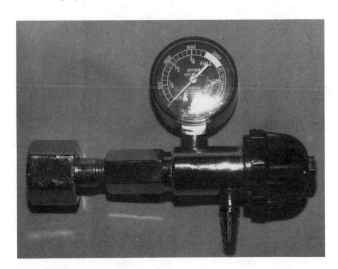

FIG 12–26.
Simple needle valve and cylinder pressure gauge.

Given
  Pc = 2,200 psi
  A_1 = 2 mm^2
  A_2 = 4 mm^2

$$Pr = \frac{2 \text{ mm}^2}{4 \text{ mm}^2} \times 2,200 \text{ psi}$$
$$= 1,100 \text{ psi.}$$

Example 2: What is the reduction in cylinder pressure (Pr)?

Given
  Pc = 2,200 psi
  A_1 = 1 mm^2
  A_2 = 44 mm^2

$$Pr = \frac{1 \text{ mm}^2}{44 \text{ mm}^2} \times 2,200 \text{ psi}$$
$$= 50 \text{ psi.}$$

There are limits to areas that can be used because of the flexibility of metal diaphragms. One improvement is to add a spring S_1 to counteract the forces in the reduction chamber R pressing on the diaphragm (Fig 12–29). The balance of forces now reads:

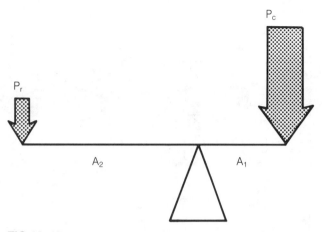

FIG 12–27.
Basic principle for pressure reduction using different-sized areas to interact with pressure sources.

$$(Pc \times A_1) + S_1 = Pr \times A_2.$$

Another problem in the primitive regulator is modulating the effects of decreasing cylinder pressure on the reduction pressure. Using a spring with substantial force helps minimize the variation. The main spring is preset in regulators that need only deliver gas as a certain pressure. Others are made adjustable by turning a screw connection that compresses or relaxes the spring. Since the adjustment could be completely relaxed when not in use, some gas could escape through the nozzle. A sealing spring S_2 is normally added to prevent gas flow if S_1 is slack (Fig 12–30).

Direct-acting regulators have components arranged relative to a balance, so that the cylinder pressure will tend to open the nozzle valve seat. In

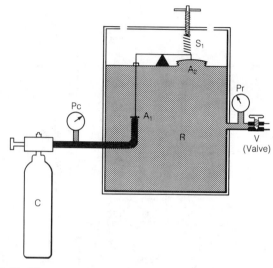

FIG 12–29.
Spring S_1 is added to act against pressure in the reduction chambers.

this type, as the cylinder pressure decays, the reduction pressure would also tend to drop. Another type, the *indirect-acting design*, reverses the connection between the valve seat and the diaphragm when compared with the former design (Fig 12–31). This change in balance causes the cylinder contents to tend to close the valve seat against the nozzle of high-pressure gas. The result is that in the indirect style, cylinder content decay will result in slight increases in reduction pressures. Solving for the reduction pressures yields the following equation:

$$Pr = (S_1 - S_2) - Pc(A_1/A_2).$$

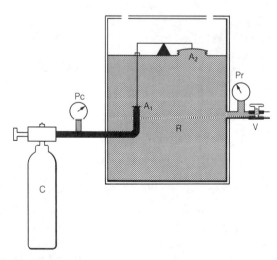

FIG 12–28.
Schematic of simple regulator (see text).

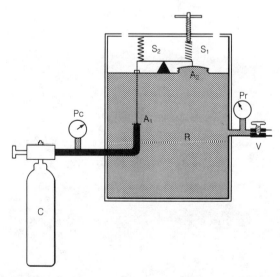

FIG 12–30.
Spring S_2 is added as a sealing spring when gas flow is not needed.

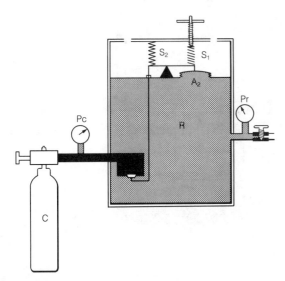

FIG 12–31.
Indirect-acting regulator.

Those who have operated regulators will have noticed a slight difference in regulated pressure when the gas is passing through the system versus when the outlet valve is closed. This difference is known as the *static increment*.

Contemporary regulators do not exactly resemble the simplified diagrams I have presented. With a contemporary version of the direct-acting design, when the outlet valve is closed, the sealing spring keeps the valve seat against the nozzle outlet (Fig 12–32,A). Flow is initiated when the main spring is displaced downward by the screw mechanism, displacing a *valve thrust pin,* moving the valve opening. Therefore, gas at a reduced pressure will slip out the valve and into the reduction chamber, increasing pressure on the diaphragm. An equilibrium is reached as the diaphragm is displaced and the connection begins to restrain the opening of the nozzle.

With the contemporary version of the indirect-acting regulator, the valve thrust pin operates differently than the direct style. In addition to the sealing spring, the cylinder pressure tends to cork the valve nozzle. As the thrust pin is displaced when the main spring is compressed, more and more gas can slip by the thrust pin and the walls of the shaft in which it moves (Fig 12–32,B).

Because of the high pressures to which the components of a regulator are subjected, manufacturers build in pressure relief valves or devices. Usually there is one for each stage of the regulator. Normally increased pressure in the regulator chamber tends to close the nozzle that holds pressure constant. However, if debris or a mechanical failure prevents this

normal valve closure, the device connected to that regulator could be exposed to higher pressure than normal. Also, rupture of metallic parts may discharge shrapnel toward the operator or patient.

There are two basic types of regulator relief systems. The most obvious is the external spring-loaded kind with an adjustable stud. It connects the reduction chamber and the atmosphere. Adjustment is made with an Allen wrench. Leak detector solution is placed over the safety valve, and the wrench loosens the spring until it begins to leak gas. At that point it is advanced so that the bubbles cease (Fig 12–33).

An internal pressure relief system utilizes a separate spring located in the vicinity of the main spring. When pressures exceed safe levels, it allows the diaphragm to lift away from the regulator chamber body, thus releasing the gas (Fig 12–34). It is not easily adjustable. Premature leakage usually indicates a faulty or dirty diaphragm sealing gasket or the spring itself is tired. Relief pressures for either type of relief valve are set in the 140- to 200-psi range.

Another necessary component of a pressure regulator are the gauges that indicate the pressure remaining in the cylinder and that which is measured in the reduction chamber. Not all regulators require the latter unless they are the adjustable type. The gauges operate by distorting a crooked, dead-ended compliant metal tube. The straightening, reflecting higher pressure is referred by a connecting rod to a set of gears. They turn an indicator needle on a calibrated background scale. Different ranges of pressure reading can be designed by varying the compliance of the metal (Fig 12–35).

Because of the various applications of cylinder gases, there are several different options for regulators and outlets. For a regulator used to operate a respirator, only a DISS or quick-connect outlet is needed. However, if the gas must also be measured, a flowmeter can be permanently attached.

Regulators are subject to certain problems and require periodic maintenance. O rings, springs, diaphragms, and diaphragm-sealing gaskets do wear out with use. However, the point of greatest stress is at the valve seat and nozzle. Cylinder gas is normally quite clean and should not be the source of debris to clog or block valve seat operation. A cylinder valve should be cracked to blow away dust and other contaminants before it is connected to a regulator. Threaded blanks that replicate a cylinder outlet can seal the inlet of the regulator and be mounted on a wall to protect the units from damage while not

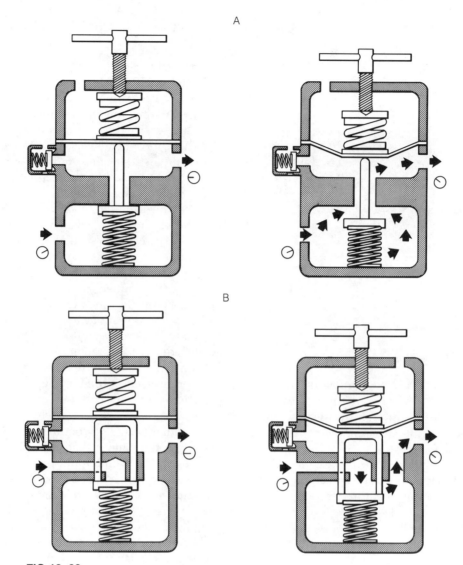

FIG 12–32.
A, contemporary direct regulator. **B,** indirect regulator.

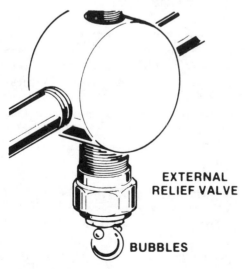

EXTERNAL RELIEF VALVE

BUBBLES

FIG 12–33.
External spring tension pressure relief valve.

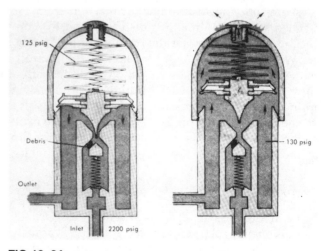

125 psig

Debris

Outlet

Inlet   2200 psig

130 psig

FIG 12–34.
Internal (double-spring) pressure relief valve. (Courtesy of Puritan-Bennett Corporation, Overland Park, Kansas.)

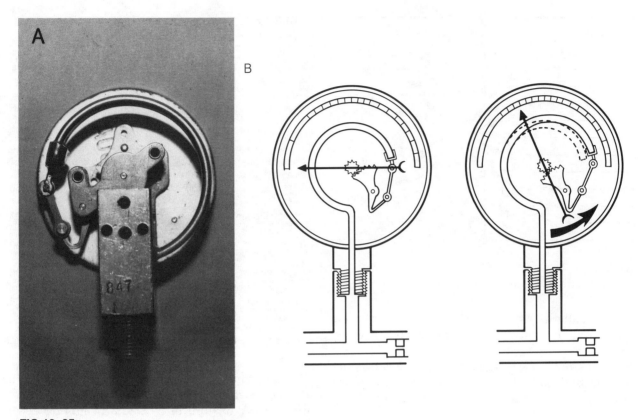

FIG 12–35.
A, Pressure gauge *(back view)* showing crooked tube and gearing. **B,** same gauge (front view) showing how tube "straightening" is translated to alter the needle position.

in use. Most regulator gauges will not withstand a drop from the height of a large cylinder. If dropped, the regulator should not be used until inspected. Petroleum-based lubricants should not be used with regulators or cylinder connections due to fire hazard when oxygen is used. Leaky threaded connections should be sealed with Teflon tape or similar substance. Following the use of a regulator, the reduction chamber should be depressurized by first closing the cylinder valve then venting the remaining gas. Unqualified personnel should not attempt to service regulators because they require special tools, such as torque and bonnet wrenches, and a jig to hold the body in a vise.

Flowmeters

Flowmeters have previously been mentioned during the discussion on regulators as devices to permit release of gas and metering of the volume per time unit. The indication of flow is done indirectly by various techniques, or, simply assumed, all variables (i.e., regulated pressure) are kept constant. Since gas administration is analogous to drug therapy, flowmeters can be compared with parenteral drip systems or infusion pumps. The major designs of flowmeters will be reviewed with regard to the physical principles, which, if understood, will help operators recognize potential inaccuracies.

Physical Principles Related to Orifices

An orifice can be fixed in its diameter or variable, such as diameter being changed by opening or closing a needle valve. The type of flow seen with a fixed-orifice device may be turbulent or laminar dependent on certain variables (Fig 12–36). The following four principles are used to describe the behavior of gases flowing through a fixed orifice:

1. Reynold's number (N_R) is used to predict the type of flow pattern that will result for any given flow and tube or orifice. It is the ratio of the force of momentum within the fluid (gas) to the force of viscous friction:

$$N_R = \frac{\text{density} \times \text{velocity} \times \text{radius}}{\text{viscosity}}$$

Reynold's number is dimensionless yet gives an indication whether the flow will be laminar (<2,000) or turbulent (>4,000). Intermediate values will have

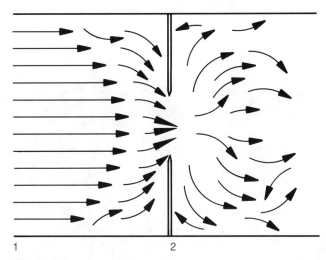

FIG 12–36.
Gas flow (turbulent) through an orifice.

TABLE 12–7.
Densities of Therapeutic Medical Gases*

GAS	PERCENTAGE	DENSITY	√DENSITY	DIFFUSIBILITY RELATIVE TO PURE OXYGEN
Helium	100	0.179	0.432	
Air	100	1.293	1.135	
Oxygen	100	1.429	1.182	
Oxygen-nitrogen	40/60	1.321	1.105	
Helium-oxygen	80/20	0.429	0.655	
Helium-oxygen	70/30	0.554	0.745	
Oxygen	100		1.135	0.960
Air	100		1.182	
Oxygen-nitrogen	40/60		1.135	1.027
Air	100		0.105	
Helium-oxygen	80/20		1.135	1.743
Air	100		0.655	
Helium-oxygen	80/20		1.182	1.805
Oxygen	100		0.655	
Helium-oxygen	70/30		1.182	1.586
Oxygen	100		0.745	

*Adapted from Egan DF: Therapeutic uses of helium. *Conn Med* 1967; 31:355.

a mixed pattern. As a general rule density plays a greater role in orifices, and viscosity dominates in tubes.[33]

2. The flow of gas through an orifice is proportional to the square root of the pressure difference across the orifice, that is, the head of pressure[33]:

$$\dot{V} \propto \sqrt{P_1 - P_2}$$

If a source of pressure applied to the proximal side of the orifice is increased or decreased, the flow will change respectively. The pressure on the distal orifice in most medical gas situations will approximate atmospheric pressure. However, if the gas appliance attached to the orifice increases P_2 by impeding flow, the $P_1 - P_2$ relationship will be distorted and the flow decreased proportionally.

3. Flow through an orifice will be proportional to the square of the diameter of the opening. If pressures at P_1 and P_2 are constants, the flow will vary exponentially as the opening is increased or decreased.[33]

$$\text{Flow} \propto (\text{diameter})^2$$

4. Flow through an orifice will be proportional to the inverse of the square root of the density of the gas. If pressure and the diameter are constant, flow will increase with lower-density gases and vice versa[33]:

$$\text{Flow} \propto \frac{1}{\sqrt{\text{density}}}$$

The relationship is important to consider when gases whose density varies substantially from air or oxygen are administered, helium/oxygen mixtures being the most significant (Table 12–7).

Example: A mixture of 80%/20% helium-oxygen is being substituted in a flowmeter calibrated for oxygen. The flow of pure oxygen was 10 L/min. What will be the flow of heliox if no changes are made to the orifice diameter or gas inlet pressures?

80%/20% He-O_2 density

$$= \frac{0.80 \, (\text{GMW He}) + 0.20 \, (\text{GMW } O_2)}{22.4 \text{ L}}$$

$$= \frac{0.80 \, (4 \text{ gm}) + 0.20 \, (32 \text{ gm})}{22.4 \text{ L}} = 0.43 \text{ g/L}$$

$$O_2 \text{ density} = \frac{1.00 \, (\text{GMW } O_2)}{22.4 \text{ L}}$$

$$= \frac{1.00 \, (32 \text{ gm})}{22.4 \text{ L}} = 1.43 \text{ gm/L}$$

Actual flow

$$= \text{indicated flow} \times \frac{\sqrt{\text{Density for which calibrated}}}{\sqrt{\text{Density of alternate gas}}}$$

$$= 10 \text{ L/min} \times \frac{\sqrt{1.43}}{\sqrt{0.43}}$$

$$= 10 \text{ L/min} \times \frac{1.20}{0.66}$$

$$= 18 \text{ L/min}.$$

Therefore, for each liter of oxygen previously flowing through the orifice, 1.82 L of heliox will now exit. The actual flow of the 80%/20% He-O$_2$ mixture is 18 L/min even though the flowmeter (calibrated for O$_2$) will indicate a lower value.

Temperature changes affect the viscosity and density of a gas. Although the effect is slight, density of a gas varies proportionally with the absolute pressures. Flowmeters used at significantly different altitudes may require correction. A rough approximation of the error involved has been calculated to be about 1% for each 1,000 feet (304 m) of variance from sea level. The equation is as follows:

$$\text{Actual flow} = \text{Indicated flow} \times \frac{\text{Barometric pressure at sea level}}{\text{Actual barometric pressure}}$$

Fixed Orifice and Constant Pressure

The most basic flowmeter is commercially known as a *flow restrictor*. It is a carefully machined orifice attached to a 50-psi gas source. There are no adjustments and no gauges (Fig 12–37). They are of value when a fixed flow is required, a specific gas is always used, and the pressure source is stable. The most common use is in home oxygen concentrators. Other applications would be in emergency resuscitation packs where a compact, lightweight device can be used to provide relatively high flows to a bag-mask-valve system. Because there is no way to indicate to the operator what the actual flow is, flow restrictors must be periodically checked by calibration flowmeter or volume vs. time spirometer. However, they are quite stable and have no moving

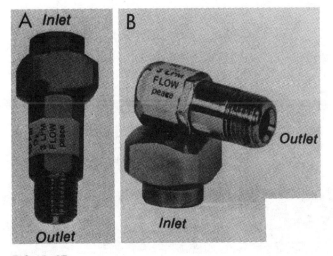

FIG 12–37.
A and **B,** fixed-orifice flow restrictors. (Courtesy of Peace Medical, East Hanover, N.J.)

parts. Multiple fixed–orifice flowmeters are an extension of the basic unit, with several restrictors in combination. The operator can make a selection by rotating a knob that directs gas to that orifice. Although more expensive, it offers a variety of therapeutic flows (Fig 12–38).

Fixed Orifice and Variable Pressure

The term *Bourdon gauge flowmeter* is clinically used to describe a fixed orifice placed distal to an adjustable pressure regulator (Fig 12–39). In this design, the operator can manually increase or decrease the pressure at the orifice (P$_1$). Therefore, flow will vary as previously described. The gauge referred to in the term Bourdon gauge is simply the compliant crooked tube used to record pressures in cylinders (see Fig 12–35). Manufacturers recalibrate the gauge to reflect the flow change due to the pressure change proximal to the orifice. Accurate flow indication is assured unless the density of the gas is different than designed, or impedance to gas flow out of the orifice causes an increase in distal pressure (P$_2$). In clinical practice, placing an administration appliance that has an orifice smaller than that in the flowmeter will distort the P$_1$ − P$_2$ relationship, and the crooked tube will be distended out of proportion to the actual flow. Therefore, the flow will be indicated to be higher than actual. Pneumatic nebulizers are an example of such a device that should not be used with a Bourdon gauge if accurate indication of flow rate is necessary.

Bourdon gauges are commonly used on medical gas cylinders for transport and when masks or nasal cannulas are used. The flowmeters are handy because there is some knowledge of flow (in contrast to flow restrictors), and they can be read correctly without being held in a vertical (gravity-dependent position).

Variable Orifice and Constant Pressure

The most common type of flowmeter in medical gas administration incorporates a needle valve to allow adjustment of desired flows and a hollow tube with an indicator device. The terms *Thorpe tube* and *rotameter* are commonly used to refer to this basic design. The use of rotameter often implies the use of a bobbin instead of a spherical-type flow indicator. Rotameters are often used in administration of anesthetic gases, which require greater accuracy in flow indication.

However, the needle valve itself is the critical component of this type of device, and the flow indicator merely reflects the level of gas flow. The

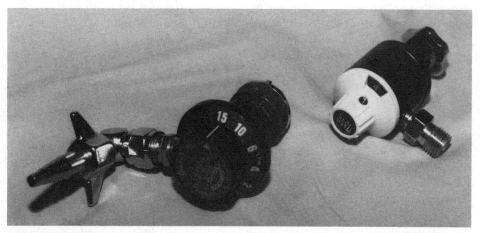

FIG 12–38.
Adjustable-orifice flow restrictors.

physics involved in the flow indicator is quite complex. It relates to Reynold's number, density and viscosity of gas, and Stokes' law of gravitational sedimentation. Factors that govern the position of the indicator are not attributable to Bernoulli's law, which some publications report. Detailed reviews are available for interested readers.[41,47,48]

Up to this point the positioning of the needle valve has not been discussed. In clinical use, the most common type positions the float tube between the inlet pressure source and the needle valve (Fig 12–40). This type is called a *pressure-compensated flowmeter*. Internal pressure changes within the float tube are not affected if the operator attaches an appliance (e.g., nebulizer) with an orifice smaller than that set by the needle valve. Adding a large downstream impedance, in essence, is like reducing the diameter of the flowmeter's own needle valve. The

actual flow is slowed, and the float will change to a new equilibrium of forces but at a lower level. The operator will be correctly informed of the actual output flow. The physical relationships above and below the float were altered from the previous conditions but not distorted.

Pressure compensated flowmeters will indicate actual flow unless:

1. The source gas pressure varies from 50 psi.
2. The flowmeter is set to deliver a higher flow than is available from its gas source.
3. The float tube is not set in the vertical position.

If an operator is not able to determine if a flowmeter is pressure compensated by examination, a simple test can be performed. With the needle valve

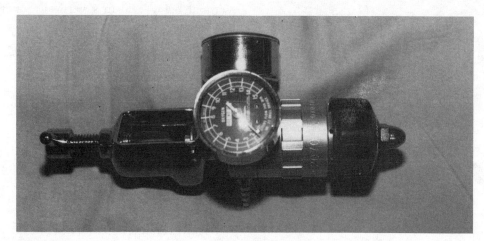

FIG 12–39.
Bourdon-style high-pressure regulator. One gauge indicates cylinder pressure, the other liters per minute flow.

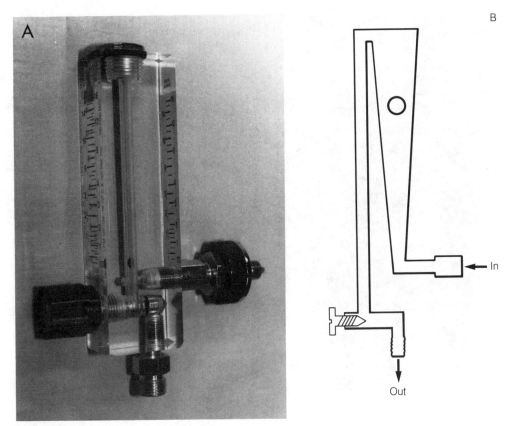

FIG 12–40.
A, compensated Thorpe-style flowmeter. **B,** gas flows up the measuring tube, then down to the adjustable needle valve.

closed, it is connected to the pressure source and then the gas is activated. If the ball jumps, it indicates this design, because the gas has to pass through the indicator tube before it reaches the needle valve (see Fig 12–40).

In the past *non-pressure-compensated flowmeters* were commonly used. They are still used for laboratory or industrial applications. The difference in design is the placement of the indicator tube distal to the needle valve (Fig 12–41). Although a subtle change, the pressure and other physical factors above and below the float will be distorted if a smaller orifice, such as a nebulizer, is applied. It will elevate the pressure above the float and distort the head of pressure relationship that the manufacturer has calculated. It can result in a depression of the float, incorrectly underestimating the actual flow.

Some non-pressure-compensated flowmeters are used clinically (see Fig 12–42). This one is designed to deliver low flows, providing only 1 L full scale, and is used for chronic obstructive pulmonary disease patients quite sensitive to higher flows of oxy-

gen. There are no problems in accurate indication of flows as long as low-impedance appliances, such as bubble humidifiers and nasal cannulas, are used.

When ball-type float flowmeters are used, the center of the ball should be read against the background scale. The operator should read the scale with his eye on the same level to eliminate error due to parallax. Although Thorpe tube flowmeters are usually quite accurate, they should be checked by another flowmeter initially and periodically when in service. The handiest method is to connect the clinical flowmeter to a calibration flowmeter designed for this purpose. They are available as electronic devices or are very accurate float tube flowmeters themselves (Fig 12–43). The flows over several different settings on the clinical unit should be identical to that on the calibration unit. Another approach is to let a flowmeter fill a volume displacement type of spirometer, commonly found in pulmonary function laboratories. Since flow is volume per time, flow can be read out directly or calculated as the slope of the tracing on a kymographic recording.

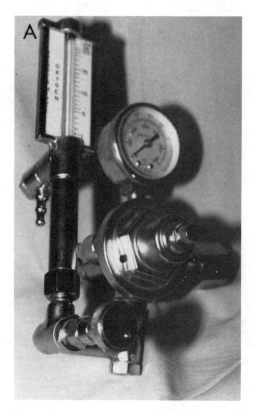

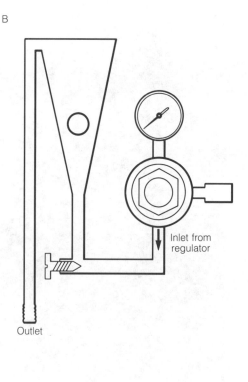

FIG 12–41.
A, noncompensated Thorpe tube flowmeter and regulator combination. **B,** schematic of gas flow.

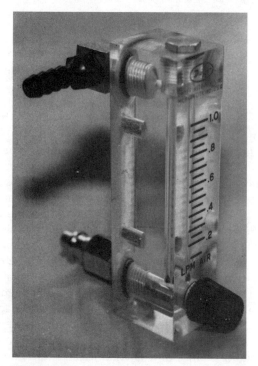

FIG 12–42.
Noncompensated *low-flow* (0–1 L/min) flowmeter.

If a flowmeter is found to read differently than its actual output, it should be serviced. Fouled sintered metal inlet filters, leaky O rings, and broken float tubes are components that can result in inaccuracy. Needle valve seats are the most common area for wear. Needle valves should be closed before the units are connected to gas sources to avoid additional wear.

Traditionally clinical flowmeters have been scaled from 0 to 15 L/min. Need for more accurate reading of low flows fostered development of 0 to 5 L/min units and also some with dual or expanded scales for more accurate low-flow reading. Most flowmeters also have a *flush position* beyond the calibrated range. There is no industrial standard, but most can provide greater than 60 L/min. High-flow systems requiring actual metering have caused some manufacturers to develop 0 to 75 L/min Thorpe tubes. They are popular in continuous positive airway pressure (CPAP) systems or with oxygen-air blenders. Dual high-flow air and oxygen flowmeters can set the F_{IO_2} as well as guarantee adequate total flows to exceed patient's inspiratory flow demands (Fig 12–44).

think and use algebra. The following will hopefully correct the latter problem:

The first premise:

Fraction of gas x

$$= \frac{\text{Volume of gas } x \text{ in the system}}{\text{Total volume of all gas in the system}}.$$

This relationship can be expanded into a generic mixing equation that can be used to mix oxygen and air or any other substance:

$$F_x(\dot{V}_a + \dot{V}_b) = F_x(\dot{V}_a) + F_x(\dot{V}_b)$$

The total volume of gas equals $(\dot{V}_a + \dot{V}_b)$; it is assumed that x can be found in both $\dot{V}_a$ and $\dot{V}_b$; F_x equals the fraction of gas x in a volume. A common application is mixing oxygen and air. The equation can be rewritten:

$$F_{IO_2}(\dot{V}_{O_2} + \dot{V}_{air}) = F_{IO_2}(\dot{V}_{O_2}) + F_{IO_2}(\dot{V}_{air})$$

Because the F_{IO_2} of pure oxygen and air is 1.0 and 0.21, respectively, the equation is simplified further:

$$F_{IO_2}(\dot{V}_{total}) = \dot{V}_{O_2} + 0.21(\dot{V}_{air}) \qquad [1]$$

With a parallel equation dealing only with volume of gas, any gas mixing problem can be solved. Several clinical examples follow to illustrate equations 1 and 2.

$$\dot{V}_{total} = \dot{V}_{O_2} + \dot{V}_{air} \qquad [2]$$

Example 1: Solving for the proportion (ratio) of air to oxygen to obtain a desired F_{IO_2}, what is the air/O_2 ratio for an F_{IO_2} of 0.60?

$$F_{IO_2}(\dot{V}_{total}) = \dot{V}_{O_2} + 0.21(\dot{V}_{air}) \qquad [1]$$

$$0.6(\dot{V}_{total}) = \dot{V}_{O_2} + 0.21(\dot{V}_{air})$$

Since the conventional expression for air/O_2 ratio is $x:1$, substitute 1 for $\dot{V}_{O_2}$:

$$0.6(\dot{V}_{total}) = 1 + 0.21(\dot{V}_{air})$$

To eliminate two unknowns, substitute equation 2 for $\dot{V}_{total}$:

$$0.6(1 + \dot{V}_{air}) = 1 + 0.21(\dot{V}_{air})$$

$$0.6 + 0.6(\dot{V}_{air}) = 1 + 0.21(\dot{V}_{air})$$

$$0.39(\dot{V}_{air}) = 0.4$$

$$\dot{V}_{air} = 1.03$$

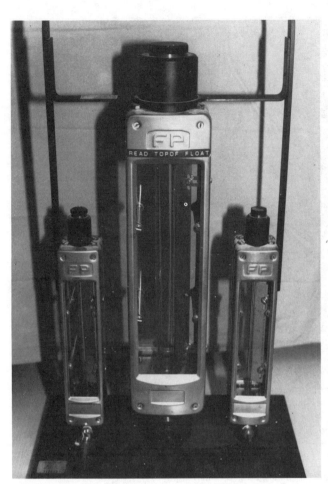

FIG 12–43.
Bank of three calibration flowmeters.

Oxygen-Air Blending and Proportioners

Precise delivery of oxygen fractions is required to supply therapeutic levels of oxygen and hopefully avoid complications. Several methods exist for control of F_{IO_2} and delivery of an adequate flow to meet inspiratory demands. One method is use of a jet-type nebulizer or *Venturi system* with internal mixing of room air with a stream of oxygen. Dilution devices cannot be reliably used with mechanical ventilators and often do not deliver the variety of concentrations and flows that are possible with true oxygen-air blenders, or proportioners, or dual air-oxygen flowmeters.

Dual Air-Oxygen Flowmeters

Dual flowmeters are the simplest and most economical method to deliver a specific F_{IO_2} and total flow. Applications include intermittent mandatory ventilation (IMV) and CPAP systems. The only drawback is that the medical gas provider must

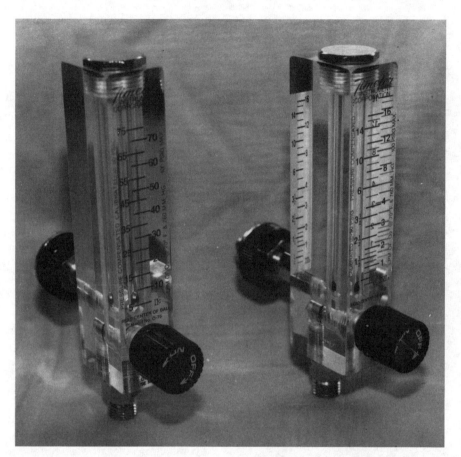

FIG 12–44.
Pressure-compensated flowmeters, ranges 0–75 L/min *(left)* and 0–16 L/min *(right)*.

Therefore, the air/O_2 ratio for F_{IO_2} of 0.60 equals 1.03:1. (See Table 12–8 for common air/O_2 ratios listed by desired F_{IO_2}.)

Example 2: Solve for F_{IO_2} knowing the flows of air and oxygen. For example, what is the F_{IO_2} if $\dot{V}O_2$ equals 10 L/min and $\dot{V}_{air}$ equals 30 L/min?

$$F_{IO_2}(\dot{V}_{total}) = \dot{V}O_2 + 0.21(\dot{V}_{air})$$

$$F_{IO_2}(\dot{V}_{total}) = 10 \text{ L/min} + 0.21(30 \text{ L/min})$$

$$F_{IO_2}(40 \text{ L/min}) = 10 \text{ L/min} + 6.3 \text{ L/min}$$

$$F_{IO_2} = (16.3 \text{ L/min} \div 40 \text{ L/min}) = 0.41$$

Example 3: Solve for $\dot{V}O_2$ and $\dot{V}_{air}$ to give a specific F_{IO_2} and a required total output required to match the patient's needs. For example, if the clinician estimates the patient needs 40 L/min and the F_{IO_2} ordered is 0.70, at what level should the O_2 and air flowmeters be set?

$$F_{IO_2}(\dot{V}_{total}) = \dot{V}O_2 + 0.21(\dot{V}_{air}). \qquad [1]$$

(Since $\dot{V}_{total} = \dot{V}O_2 + \dot{V}_{air}$, $\dot{V}_{air} = \dot{V}_{total} - \dot{V}O_2$)
Substitute for $\dot{V}_{air}$:

$$F_{IO_2}(\dot{V}_{total}) = \dot{V}O_2 + 0.21(\dot{V}_{total} - \dot{V}O_2)$$

$$0.70(40 \text{ L/min}) = \dot{V}O_2 + 0.21(40 \text{ L/min} - \dot{V}O_2)$$

$$28 \text{ L/min} = \dot{V}O_2 + 8.40 \text{ L/min} - 0.21(\dot{V}O_2)$$

$$19.6 \text{ L/min} = 0.79(\dot{V}O_2)$$

$$25 \text{ L/min} = \dot{V}O_2$$

Since

$$\dot{V}_{air} = \dot{V}_{total} - \dot{V}O_2,$$

$$\dot{V}_{air} = 40 \text{ L/min} - 25 \text{ L/min}$$

$$= 15 \text{ L/min}$$

TABLE 12–8.

Air/Oxygen Ratios to Achieve Specific Fractions of Oxygen

F_{IO_2}	AIR/O_2
0.24	25.1:1
0.25	18.75:1
0.30	7.78:1
0.35	4.64:1
0.40	3.17:1
0.45	2.29:1
0.50	1.72:1
0.55	1.32:1
0.60	1.02:1
0.65	0.79:1
0.70	0.61:1
0.75	0.46:1
0.80	0.34:1
0.85	0.23:1
0.90	0.145:1
0.95	0.065:1

The general mixing equation can be solved for each of its components. Instead of algebraic skills, a good memory can help:

$$F_{IO_2} = \frac{\dot{V}_{O_2} + 0.21(\dot{V}_{air})}{\dot{V}_{total}} \quad [2]$$

$$\dot{V}_{O_2} = \frac{\dot{V}_{air}(F_{IO_2} - 0.21)}{1 - F_{IO_2}} \quad [3]$$

$$\dot{V}_{air} = \frac{\dot{V}_{O_2}(1 - F_{IO_2})}{F_{IO_2} - 0.21} \quad [4]$$

$$\dot{V}_{total} = \frac{0.79\,(\dot{V}_{O_2})}{(F_{IO_2} - 0.21)} \quad [5]$$

The previous equations will function well with dual flowmeter applications. Practitioners may prefer to use nomograms to reach an answer (Figs 12–45 and 12–46).[109]

All purpose nebulizers can be combined with air and oxygen flowmeters to create F_{IO_2} values not available on the devices themselves. On many units it is not possible to deliver F_{IO_2} values of less than 0.35 to 0.40 when the nebulizer is powered by oxygen. However, the nebulizer can be run on air to generate the aerosol, and a separate oxygen flow can be connected to the system (usually into the top of the nebulizer).[17]

The following equation is a further development of the general mixing equation for this specific application:

$$\dot{V}_{O_2} = \dot{V}^s_{air} \times \left(\frac{0.79\,(F_{IO_2}^D - 0.21)}{(F^s_{IO_2} - 0.21)(1 - F^D_{IO_2})} \right)$$

$\dot{V}^s_{air}$ = Flow of air into nebulizer

$F^D_{IO_2}$ = Desired F_{IO_2}

$F^s_{IO_2}$ = Dilution setting on nebulizer.

Example: If a nebulizer is set on 0.40 dilution and the air flowmeter equals 10 L/min, how much supplemental oxygen should be added to produce a F_{IO_2} of 0.25?

$$\dot{V}_{O_2} = 10 \times \frac{0.79(0.25 - 0.21)}{(0.4 - 0.21)(1 - 0.25)}$$
$$= 10 \times 0.22$$
$$= 2.2 \text{ L/min}$$

It should be noted that air-oxygen systems should always be checked with an oxygen analyzer. Although the equations are valid, errors in calculations and inaccurate equipment may affect the F_{IO_2}.

Oxygen-Air Blenders (Proportioners)

Oxygen-air blenders, or proportioners, provide a convenient compact device to premix by dialing in a specific oxygen concentration (Fig 12–47). They are commonly used to mix gas for mechanical ventilators (e.g., Siemens-Elema Servo 900 ventilator models and the Sechrist infant ventilators), continuous-flow CPAP systems, add-on IMV systems, heart-lung bypass machines, and controlled F_{IO_2} oxygen therapy.

Manufacturers offer different styles that generally relate to the flow output needs. Low-flow blenders are most accurate at low-flow applications requiring less than about 20 L/min. High-flow blenders must be accurate in providing controlled F_{IO_2} levels at flows in the 80 to 100 L/min range.

Oxygen-air proportioners receive each gas separately from a pipeline or compressed gas cylinder. Ideally the supply pressures of both gases are nearly equal, usually 50 psi. Because clinically nearly equal pressure does not always occur, blenders have internal pressure regulating systems (Fig 12–48). Air and oxygen enter the blender and pass through check valves. Then gas flows through spool-shaped valves separated by a flexible diaphragm. They lower and balance the inlet pressures. This process should produce similar pressures for air and oxygen. If that is the case, a dual orifice needle valve controls the proportion of each gas flowing out of the orifices. For higher concentrations, the valve would simulta-

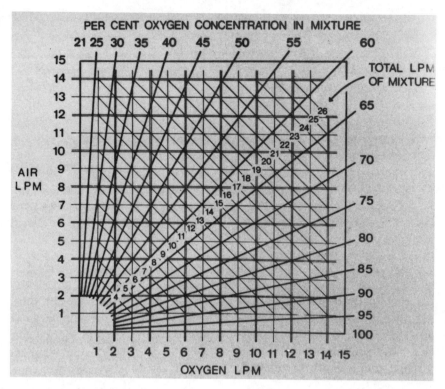

FIG 12–45.
Nomogram to rapidly compute air/oxygen proportions for flows from 1–26 L/min. (From Yost LC, Barnhard WN, Kaiman A, et al: Oxygen air blending nomogram for medium and high flow rates. *Respir Care* 1977; 22:607–609. Reproduced by permission.)

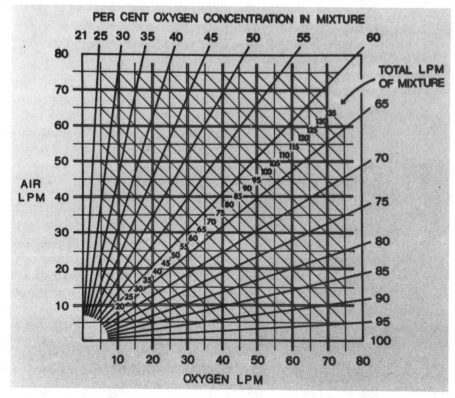

FIG 12–46.
Nomogram for computing air/oxygen mixtures for flows from 20–135 L/min. (From Yost LC, Barnhard WN, Kaiman A, et al: Oxygen air blending nomogram for medium and high flow rates. *Respir Care* 1977; 22:607–609. Reproduced by permission.)

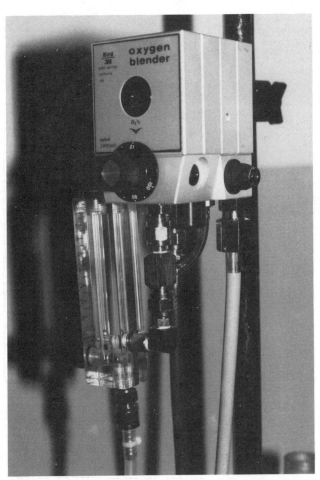

FIG 12–47.
Air/oxygen blender shown with high-flow flowmeter attachment.

neously open for more oxygen flow as it decreased air flows. However, the reader should see that if the pressure gradient across the orifices is different, the valve will be fooled. Therefore, when inlet pressures of either gas drop below a certain point or differ too much, accurate mixing cannot be guaranteed. Blender manufacturers have built-in alarm systems and, in some, pressure gauges. The Bird blender demonstrates how loss of pressure from one gas allows a flow of the remaining gas to move past a spring-loaded-valve and reach a reed valve audio alarm (see Fig 12–48,A).

Clinical Use and Troubleshooting.—A recent report evaluated commercially available medical oxygen-air blenders against ECRI criteria. The investigators found that all blenders were quite accurate when both inlet pressures were 50 psi. High-flow blenders tend to be inaccurate at low flow rates and low-flow blenders inaccurate at high flow rates.

Some of the high-flow units were not able to meet the 80 L/min criteria.[36]

Units should be able to mix with an accuracy of ±3% over a F_{IO_2} range of 0.21 to 1.00. All blenders should be checked by properly calibrated oxygen analyzers when initially placed in a breathing system and periodically thereafter. With an in-line analyzer, an operator should be able to adjust the concentration within 1% over the 21% to 35% range and 5% in the 40% to 100% range.

One of the most common problems involves contamination of one gas supply because of retrograde flow from the other source. The higher pressure gas can flow into the opposing gas lines if check valves fail. Contaminates from gas lines can prevent pressure valves from sealing properly. Corrosion due to moisture and particulate matter can build up and restrict flow or prevent sealing of check valves. Routine inspection cleaning or replacement of inlet sintered metal filters and use of water trap filters should help this problem. In more serious cases, more complex filter systems may be required.[36]

High-Flow Generator

A modern version of an oxygen-driven air-entrainment device is based on the Venturi tube. Commercially known as *Down's flow generator*, it was initially designed to be incorporated in a mask CPAP system. In contrast to other entrainment devices (e.g., all-purpose nebulizer), this unit was designed to provide gas at high flows. Continuous positive airway pressure systems must meet patient's inspiratory flow demand to maintain the therapeutic threshold pressure in the system.

Two styles are currently available: a fixed F_{IO_2} and a model that can adjust flow and F_{IO_2} (Fig 12–49,A). The fixed F_{IO_2} unit delivers an oxygen concentration of approximately 0.33 at 100 L/min when the output is unrestricted. However, with downstream resistance of 15 cm H_2O/L/sec, the total output falls and the F_{IO_2} increases to 0.37. Both units can be connected to an oxygen flowmeter or directly to a 50-psi DISS outlet.

The adjustable flow generator provides a F_{IO_2} of 0.3 to 1.0 and maintains output flows of 100 L/min. This is in contrast to the all-purpose nebulizer, which decreases output flow as the F_{IO_2} increases. In that unit the flow of incoming oxygen stays constant, and the amount of the entrained air is manipulated by changing orifices. The flow generator's F_{IO_2} adjustment manipulates oxygen inlet flows (Fig 12–49,B). As the oxygen enrichment control needle valve is opened, more oxygen passes through a side

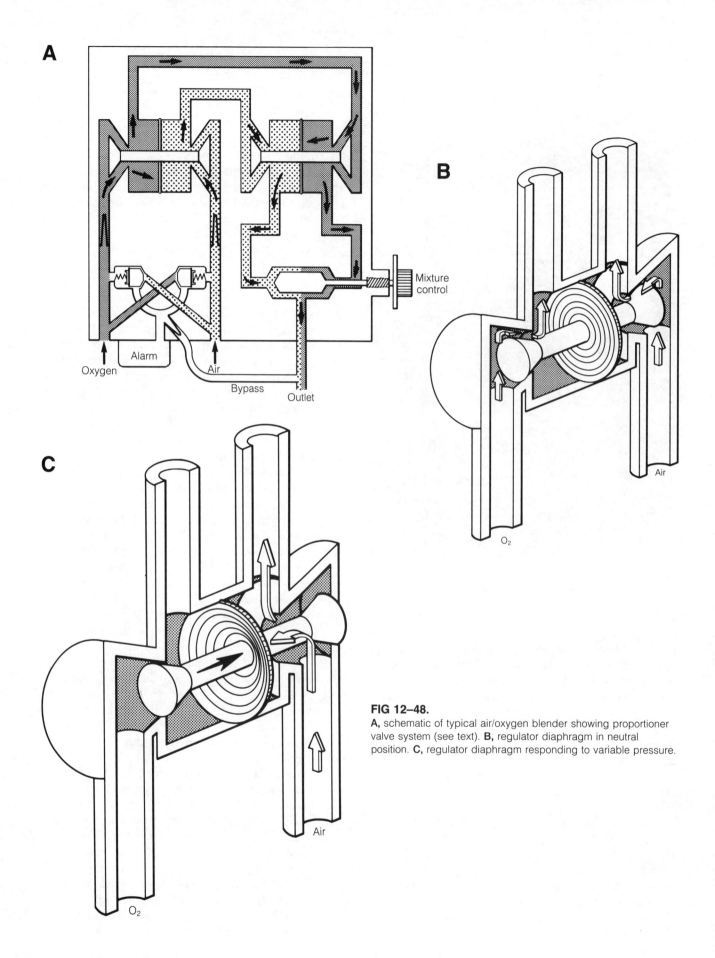

FIG 12–48.
A, schematic of typical air/oxygen blender showing proportioner valve system (see text). **B,** regulator diaphragm in neutral position. **C,** regulator diaphragm responding to variable pressure.

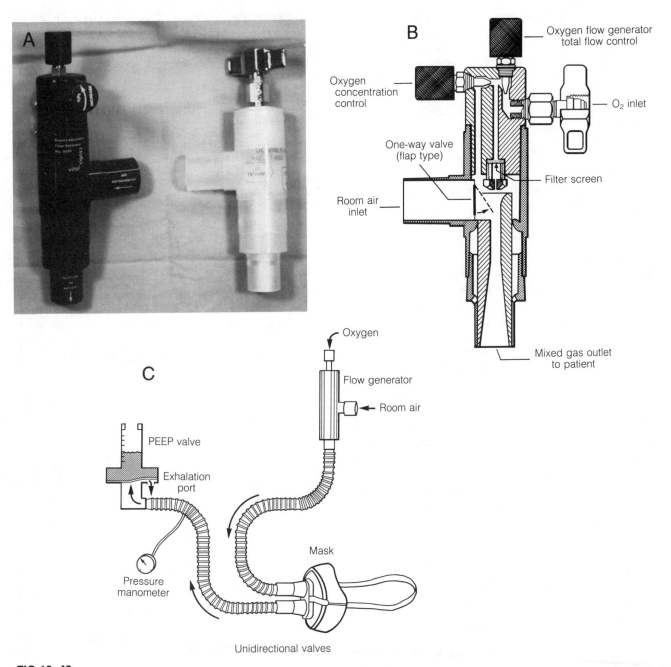

FIG 12–49.
A, Down's flow generators. Fixed flow and F_{IO_2} *(right)* and adjustable F_{IO_2} *(left).* **B,** schematic of adjustable flow generator (see text). **C,** flow generator used with mask-applied CPAP system. (Courtesy of Vital Signs Corporation, Totowa, N.J.)

channel, avoiding the channel that goes to the Venturi jet. By shifting greater proportions of source oxygen away from the jet, the F_{IO_2} increases. Higher flows of pure oxygen compensate for lesser amounts of entrained room air. The needle valve at the top of the flow tube controls the total amount of source oxygen into the system. It is adjusted to supply the appropriate total flow of mixed gas into a CPAP system. Flow ideally should be high enough to mini-mize drops in the system pressure during the most rapid inspiratory efforts of the patient. However, total flows must be adjustable to accommodate ventilation ranges of infants to adults. With a 15 cm H_2O CPAP system pressure, maximum flow from the unit is greater than 75 L/min.[105]

It would appear that the flow generator's application is not limited to only mask-applied CPAP systems (Fig 12–49,C). This same system may also be ideal to provide humidified oxygen to patients at a low or high FI_{O_2} who have inspiratory demands greater than a Venturi mask or all-purpose nebulizer can deliver. For example, asthmatics whose bronchospasm is adversely affected by bland aerosol may do better with a humidifier but may still need a high-flow device to match a high inspiratory flow requirement.

AMBIENT OXYGEN THERAPY EQUIPMENT

The goal of ambient (nonhyperbaric) oxygen therapy devices applied to the face or artificial airway is to elevate the oxygen partial pressure in the inspired gas. The increase in the partial pressure of inspired oxygen (PI_{O_2}) is accomplished by increasing the factor multiplied the barometric pressure (PB).

$$PI_{O_2} = (PB - PH_2O)FI_{O_2}$$
$$149.7 \text{ mm Hg} = (760 - 47)0.21$$

It should be noted that this gas is considered to be humidified and warmed to body temperature. Therefore the water vapor tension (PH_2O) must be subtracted. The effect of elevating the PI_{O_2} directly influences the partial pressure of oxygen in the alveolar gas (PA_{O_2}). By increasing the head of oxygen pressure across the alveolar capillary membranes, the arterial oxygen tension (Pa_{O_2}), should increase. This then can hopefully compensate for defects in oxygen transport that can be expressed as an increased gradient between alveolar and arterial oxyen levels, ($P(A-a)_{O_2}$). The normal $P(A-a)_{O_2}$ on room air is approximately 10 mm Hg.[79] The following is an estimate of PA_{O_2} that assumes a normal diet and metabolism (R = respiratory quotient = $\dot{V}_{CO_2}/\dot{V}_{O_2}$) and a normal level of carbon dioxide in the alveolar gas. This is clinically measured as the arterial carbon dioxide tension (Pa_{CO_2}), which should closely reflect the level in the average alveoli.

$$PA_{O_2} = (PB - PH_2O)FI_{O_2} - Pa_{CO_2}(FI_{O_2} + \frac{1 - FI_{O_2}}{R})$$

$$PA_{O_2} = (760 - 47)0.21 - 40\left[0.21 + \frac{(1 - 0.21)}{0.8}\right]$$

$$= 149.73 - 40(0.21 + 0.99)$$

$$= 149.73 - 48$$

$$= 101.73 \text{ mm Hg.}$$

The reader may see abbreviated versions of the alveolar oxygen equation. They may present a simpler calculation but are inaccurate if the patient is breathing supplemental oxygen.[56,72]

Correcting Hypoxemia Secondary to Hypoventilation

When patients hypoventilate, increased alveolar carbon dioxide (PA_{CO_2}) causes a displacement of oxygen partial pressure in the alveoli. A larger number for PA_{CO_2} must then be subtracted from the potential oxygen pressure, causing a lower value for PI_{O_2}. However, increased supplemental oxygen can raise the FI_{O_2}, and the PA_{O_2} can be elevated sufficiently to compensate for elevated Pa_{CO_2}. The following examples illustrate the concept:

Example: A drug overdose patient with hypoventilation has a Pa_{CO_2} of 80 mm Hg and a Pa_{O_2} of 44 mm Hg. What is the estimated PA_{O_2}?

$$PA_{O_2} = (PB - PH_2O)FI_{O_2} - Pa_{CO_2}\left[FI_{O_2} + \frac{1 - FI_{O_2}}{R}\right]$$

$$= (760 - 47)0.21 - 80\left[0.21 + \frac{1 - 0.21}{0.80}\right]$$

$$= 149.73 - 95$$

$$= 54 \text{ mm Hg.}$$

Assuming a normal oxygen tension loss or gradient from alveolar gas to arterial blood ($P(A-a)_{O_2}$) of 10 mm Hg, one would estimate the arterial oxygen at 44 mm Hg:

$$Pa_{O_2} = PA_{O_2} - P(A-a)_{O_2}$$

$$= 54 - 10$$

$$= 44 \text{ mm Hg.}$$

Example: If 30% oxygen is given to the patient with a Pa_{CO_2} of 80 mm Hg, what is the estimated PA_{O_2}? What is the estimated Pa_{O_2}?

$$PA_{O_2} = (PB - PH_2O)FI_{O_2} - Pa_{CO_2}\left[FI_{O_2} + \frac{1 - FI_{O_2}}{R}\right]$$

$$= (760 - 47)0.30 - 80\left[0.30 + \frac{1 - 0.30}{0.80}\right]$$

$$= 213.9 - 94$$

$$= 120 \text{ mm Hg.}$$

Assuming the same $P(A-a)_{O_2}$ of 10 mm Hg, the estimated Pa_{O_2} would be 110 mm Hg. The effect of oxygen administration on the alveolar oxygen tension can be estimated for variable levels of arterial carbon dioxide tension (Table 12–9).

TABLE 12–9.

Effect of Pa_{CO_2} and FI_{O_2} on PA_{O_2}*

Pa_{CO_2}	FI_{O_2}					
	0.21	0.28	0.35	0.50	0.80	1.0
	PA_{O_2}, MM HG					
20	126	176	226	333	549	693
40	102	152	203	311	528	673
60	78	129	180	289	507	653
80	54	105	157	266	486	633
100	30	82	133	243	465	613
120	6	58	110	221	444	593

*Assumptions: P_B = 760 mm Hg; P_{H_2O} = 47 mm Hg; and R = 0.8.

Improving Hypoxemia With Increased $P(A-a)O_2$

In the presence of lung or heart disease (or both), several types of problems can result in hypoxemia apart from increases in Pa_{CO_2}. The following are the classic categories of hypoxemia that result in an increased $P(A-a)O_2$ and would result in depressed arterial oxygen tensions during normal air breathing:

1. Increased mismatching of pulmonary blood to pulmonary ventilation, decreasing the efficiency of gas exchange
2. Increased shunting of blood through pulmonary, vascular or cardiac areas, bypassing functioning ventilated alveoli
3. Increased defect in diffusion across the alveolar capillary membrane

The net improvement in Pa_{O_2} when supplemental oxygen is given to a patient with one or more of these problems is quite variable.[81] It depends on the category and severity of the problem. Those patients with predominant shunt will not respond well to increasing FI_{O_2}. When given 100% oxygen, those with sizable shunts usually do not increase Pa_{O_2} beyond 400 mm Hg. Patients with predominant $\dot{V}/\dot{Q}$ mismatching and diffusion defect normally achieve 400 mm Hg or more, although the response may be slow. Normal subjects given 100% oxygen can achieve a Pa_{O_2} of more than 500 mm Hg.[110]

Hypoxic conditions produced by lack of hemoglobin anemia or lack of functional hemoglobin (e.g., carboxyhemoglobinemia) can be helped by supplemental oxygen. What hemoglobin is present and functioning can be saturated to its fullest. The net positive effect is governed by the severity of the primary problem. However, supplemental oxygen also provides a therapeutic action of accelerating the "displacement" of carbon monoxide from hemoglobin.

Hypoxias produced by inadequate cardiac output primarily depend on the degree of perfusion inadequacy. The goal of oxygen therapy during periods of low cardiac output is to maximize the blood's oxygen content. If lack of oxygen to the myocardium is the cause of low cardiac output, oxygen therapy has a more direct role in therapy. Increasing the Pa_{O_2} in the areas of good $\dot{V}/\dot{Q}$ matching cannot *supersaturate* hemoglobin to overcompensate for poorly saturated blood from shuntlike areas (Table 12–10). Quantitative indices to describe the severity of hypoxemias and separate them in categories are useful to those evaluating oxygen therapy. For example, hypoventilation causing hypoxemia can be separated from shunt and other lung disorders by calculating the $P(A-a)O_2$. Other indices commonly used in clinical practice are Pa_{O_2}/PA_{O_2} and Pa_{O_2}/FI_{O_2} ratios (see Appendix B).

Classifying Oxygen Therapy Equipment

Oxygen therapy devices are commonly grouped by classification. The purpose is to assist providers of therapy in understanding the capabilities and limitations of their equipment. The following describe the most popular classification systems:

1. *Low-flow or variable-performance equipment.* Supply oxygen at a fixed flow that is only a portion of all inspired gas. As ventilatory demands change, variable amounts of room air will dilute the oxygen flow.

TABLE 12–10.

Pa_{O_2} (mm Hg) at Various FI_{O_2} Demonstrating Shunt Effect*

FI_{O_2}	PERCENT SHUNT						
	5	10	15	20	25	30	50
	Pa_{O_2}, MM HG						
0.21	95	80	65	60	55	50	42
0.35	150	110	85	65	57	52	45
0.40	185	180	90	70	65	60	47
0.60	315	235	160	105	75	65	52
0.80	460	360	265	180	110	70	55
1.00		475	400	290	170	100	60

*From Benetar SR, Hewlett AM, Nunn JF: The use of iso-shunt lines for control of oxygen therapy. *Br J Anaesth* 1973; 45:711. Used by permission.

2. *High-flow or fixed-performance equipment.* Supply all inspired gas at a preset F_{IO_2}. Generally the performance is not affected by variations in patient ventilatory demands or patterns.

Variable-Performance Equipment

Nasal Catheter.—Since its introduction in 1907 and use during World War I, the catheter is essentially unchanged in its design. Its therapeutic benefits were noted in treating victims of war gas inhalation (Fig 12–50,A). The catheter is humble in its technology. It consists of a soft plastic tube with small outlet holes at the distal tip (Fig 12–50,B). It is available in various sizes, usually outside diameter (O.D.) French (F), for a range of patient sizes. An adult would use F 12–14 and pediatric patients F 8–10. It is usually connected to an oxygen flowmeter with a bubble humidifier. Small-bore connecting tubing is used. The catheter is lubricated with water-soluble material prior to insertion to reduce or prevent adherence to mucosal surfaces. Patency of the distal outlets should be confirmed prior to insertion.

Placement.—The catheter is inserted into either external naris and along the floor of the nasal cavity. It is designed to be inserted to just behind the uvula in the oropharynx. This procedure produces mild discomfort in all patients. It can be complicated if there is nasal pathologic condition or the catheter is inserted upward, injuring the nasal turbinates. A defect in the blood clotting mechanism would be a contraindication since catheter insertion may cause

nasal bleeding. Deviated septums, severe mucosal congestion, and nasal polyps may prevent passage of the catheter. The alternative nare may be considered or a different appliance used altogether. The catheter can be secured by tape to the external nose.

The appropriate distance to pass the catheter into the nose can be determined by two techniques. Direct vision can be used to locate the catheter. After the catheter is advanced into the nose, the conscious patient can open his or her mouth, and with the tongue depressed, the catheter can be visualized with a light as it emerges from behind the uvula. It should be pulled back to a position where it just disappears behind that structure.

The nasal catheter can also be inserted blindly. The appropriate distance estimate can be determined by measuring the length from the nose to the external ear. Insertion for that distance should place the catheter in the approximate location. The catheter should be changed periodically (e.g., every 8 hours) to prevent secretions from encasing the catheter, causing problems on removal.

Performance.—Nasal catheters are best suited to provide a low F_{IO_2}. They appear to be most useful with patients breathing with stable, low rates and normal or small tidal volumes. Actual delivered F_{IO_2} will be substantially influenced if there is profound hypoventilation or hyperventilation. Also, the amount of *open-mouth breathing* will potentially vary the balance of room air and oxygen. The literature varies greatly regarding the actual performance of

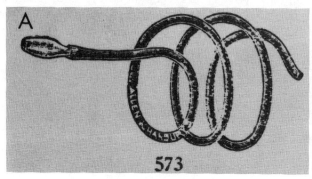

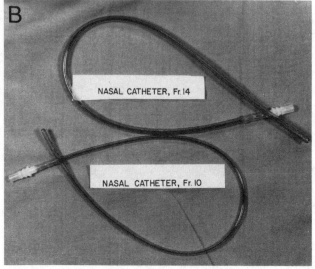

FIG 12–50.
A, vintage oxygen inhaler with glass mouthpiece. (From Leigh JM: The evolution of the oxygen therapy apparatus. *Anaesthesia* 1974; 29:462–485. Reproduced by permission.) **B,** two sizes of contemporary nasal oxygen catheters.

catheters. Some have reported values as high as 69% to 82% at flow rates in the 6 to 10 L/min range.[67] However, the researchers admitted problems in measurement due to gas streaming from the catheter to the measuring device. Other investigators have reported much lower values (Table 12–11).[45] Because of the ability of the nasal catheter to be firmly secured in position, and since infants require lower flow rates than adults, catheters have been favorably used in pediatric practice.[52] Nasal catheters have several positive and negative factors that should be considered before being used to administer oxygen therapy (Table 12–12).

Complications and Troubleshooting.—The two major problems deal with insertion and removal and with catheter positioning. As has been mentioned, trauma to the nasal area can occur if the catheter is forced into a blocked nasal passage. Nosebleeds may occur at this point or on removal if the catheter adheres to mucosal surfaces.

The other major concern is oxygen being passed down the esophagus if the catheter is placed or migrates distally. Patients should be assessed initially to observe for gulping movements or epigastric distention. The stomach filling with oxygen can potentially lead to gastric rupture or at least mechanical resistance to diaphragm descent.

Blockage of the connecting tubing or catheter itself can occur if water particles collect and block gas flow to the patient. Alternative devices should be considered if problems occur. If the patient begins to profoundly change his or her ventilatory pattern, arterial blood gas analyses or noninvasive oximetry should be used to titrate flows to attain therapeutic levels.

Nasal Cannulas.—The application of oxygen to the external nose was first done by Barth in 1871 using a hand-held ivory nostril piece. In 1929 Barach

TABLE 12–11.

F_{IO_2} Achieved With Nasal Catheters*

OXYGEN FLOW RATE, L/MIN	F_{IO_2} (WITH NORMAL VENTILATION)
2	0.21
3	0.23
5	0.24
10	0.31
15	0.44

*Adapted from Gibson RL, Comer PB, Beckham RW, et al: Actual tracheal oxygen concentrations with commonly used oxygen equipment. *Anesthesiology* 1976; 44:71–74.

TABLE 12–12.

Advantages and Disadvantages of Nasal Catheters for Oxygen Therapy

Advantages
Patients are able to speak and eat.
They can be securely fastened to the face and are less subject to patient manipulation.
They are a simple nonclaustrophobic appliance.
They can be used for unconscious-obtunded adults and infants.

Disadvantages
Insertion is technically difficult and timely.
Insertion and removal can cause discomfort and trauma.
Nasal pathology may prevent insertion.
They require frequent changing.
Gastric insufflation or rupture may occur if they are placed too far into the oropharynx.
Changing ventilation patterns affect the delivered F_{IO_2}.
Assessment of F_{IO_2} can be estimated only by hypopharyngeal sampling with an oxygen analyzer.
Drying of the oropharynx can occur at higher flows.

developed a dual nasal catheter and later a forked metal cannula.[69] Today the nasal cannula is a blind-ended soft plastic tube with either an over-the-ear elastic or lariat with under-the-chin adjustment. Both designs are sized for adult and pediatric patients (Fig 12–51). Cannulas are connected to the flowmeter and bubble humidifer with small-bore tubing.

Variations in Cannula Design.—Cannulas were combined with spectacle frames in the past (Fig 12–52), and modern versions can be found (Fig 12–53). Because oxygen usually flows continuously, approximately 80% of the oxygen is wasted. The proportion of inspiratory time vs. expiratory time varies. Also there is a certain amount of dead space gas in each tidal volume. In the past, valved storage systems and reservoir bags were used in an effort to hold oxygen during the expiration time period (Fig 12–54). Recently this concept has returned primary to lower the cost of oxygen for long-term patients.[98]

A *mustache cannula* and *pendant storage device* are contemporary versions of the storage bag idea (Figs 12–55 and 12–56). The former can store 20 ml of oxygen. Devices with a small reservoir volume have the disadvantage of decreasing F_{IO_2} at higher flow rates (e.g., >4 L/min). In clinical practice, the savings were about 50% at flow rates of 3 to 4 L/min. Cosmetically, the mustache appearance may not appeal to patients.[103] The pendant reservoir holds 40 ml of oxygen and 20 ml in a conduit leading to a standard-appearing cannula. Patients probably find its appearance more acceptable because the pendant

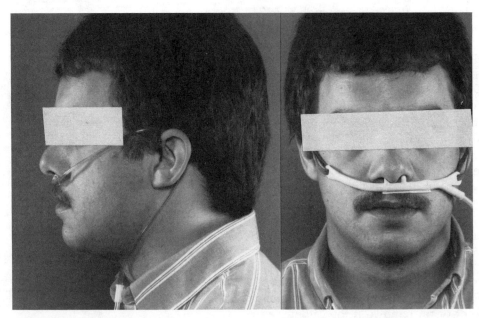

FIG 12–51.
Two styles of contemporary oxygen cannulas: lanyard **(A)** and elastic headband **(B).**

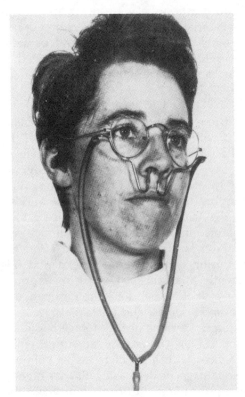

FIG 12–52.
Old oxygen cannula mounted on spectacles. (From Leigh JM: The evolution of the oxygen therapy apparatus. *Anaesthesia* 1974; 29:462–485. Reproduced by permission.)

is away from the face. It can achieve similar supplemental oxygen performance compared with a standard nonstorage cannula but at a reduced flow rate.[103]

Another attempt to reduce oxygen costs used a demand valve approach (Fig 12–57). One design, using a fluidic valve senses inspiration at the patient's nose. The *demand cannula* then initiates a puff of oxygen quite rapidly. The size of the bolus can be adjusted. A battery-powered system is incorporated

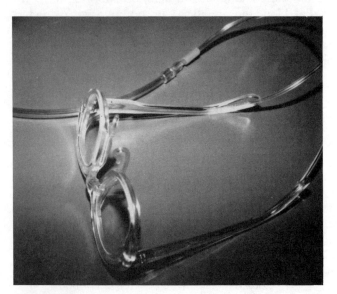

FIG 12–53.
Contemporary "oxygen spectacles."

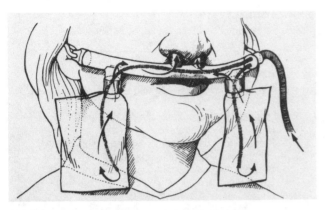

FIG 12–54.
Old nasal cannula with reservoir bags. (From Tiep BL, Belman M, Mittman C, et al: A new pendant storage oxygen-conserving nasal cannula. *Chest* 1985; 87:381–383. Reproduced by permission.)

with a standard cannula. A 67% to 71% savings has been reported.[77] However, relatively high costs for demand cannulas and potential technical problems are disadvantages that should be considered.[2, 3, 15]

Placement.—The nasal cannula can rapidly and comfortably be placed on most patients. The elastic headband or ear lariat should be adjusted to hold the prongs in the nares and not allow twisting or kinking. Care must be taken to prevent pressure sores on the ears, cheeks, and nose.

Performance.—When patients are breathing "normally," the F_{IO_2} of tracheal gas during cannula breathing can be analyzed (Table 12–13).[44, 94] However, each patient will be different. Those pro-

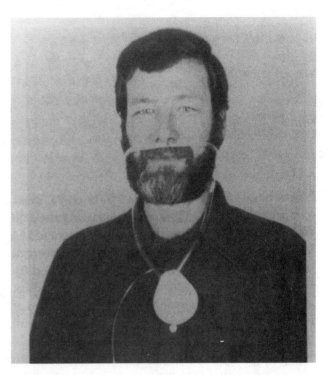

FIG 12–56.
Pendant reservoir cannula of Barach, circa 1960. (From Leigh JM: The evolution of the oxygen therapy apparatus. *Anaesthesia* 1974; 29:462–485. Reproduced by permission.)

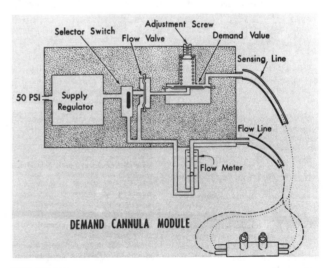

FIG 12–57.
Schematic of demand valve device for nasal cannula. (From Anderson WM, Ryerson G, Block AJ: Evaluation of an intermittent demand nasal oxygen flow system with a fluidic valve (abstract). *Chest* 1984; 86:313. Reproduced by permission.)

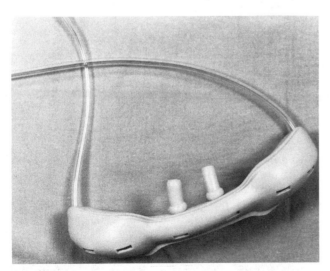

FIG 12–55.
Contemporary storage cannula mustache.

TABLE 12–13.

F$_{IO_2}$ Achieved With Nasal Cannulas

OXYGEN FLOW RATE, L/MIN	TRACHEAL F$_{IO_2}$
1*	0.23 ± 0.06
2*	0.24 ± 0.06
3*	0.25 ± 0.06
4*	0.26 ± 0.06
10†	0.35–0.46
15†	0.44–0.60

*Adapted from Schacter EN, Littner MR, Luddy P, et al: Monitoring of oxygen delivery systems in clinical practice. *Crit Care Med* 1980; 8:405–409.
†Adapted from Gibson RL, Comer PB, Beckham RW, et al: Actual tracheal oxygen concentrations with commonly used oxygen equipment. *Anesthesiology*. 1976; 44:71–74.

TABLE 12–14.

Advantages and Disadvantages of Nasal Cannulas for Oxygen Therapy

Advantages
They are easy to place.
They are comfortable, allowing speech and eating.
Low-oxygen concentration needs are easily met.
They are nonclaustrophic.
There is potential for oxygen saving, using units that save oxygen during expiration.
They are relatively nonobtrusive (improves compliance).

Disadvantages
There are variable F$_{IO_2}$ levels if the patient has a variable respiratory pattern.
High flows tend to dry and irritate nasal mucosa.
They are limited to low to moderate F$_{IO_2}$.
They can cause pressure sores on the nose and face.
Cannula tubing can be blocked by kinking or by water in the connecting tubing.

foundly gasping or with high breathing frequencies will have reduced inspired oxygen concentrations.

Potentially higher concentrations can be obtained in the 40% to 50% range when flows of 6 to 8 L/min are used. Higher flows should be done for only short periods of breathing. In addition, there is a greater tendency for problems of irritation and drying of the nasal mucosa.

The nasal cannula is one of the most commonly ordered devices to provide supplemental oxygen probably because many patients need only low levels of oxygen, it is easy to use, and usually is quite comfortable. Some patients with COPD who tend to hypoventilate with high oxygen concentrations, yet are hypoxemic on room air, usually do well with the cannula at 1 to 2 L/min or less. Patients on long-term oxygen therapy most commonly use the cannula.[90] The nasal cannula, similar to other oxygen therapy devices, has several advantages and disadvantages that should be reviewed (Table 12–14).

Troubleshooting.—Actual flow from the distal prongs should be confirmed by feeling for gas flow. Absent or low flows should prompt the operator to check (1) flowmeter accuracy, (2) twisted cannula, (3) or leaky humidifier bottle seal. Most humidifiers are equipped with audible pop-off valves to alert of an obstruction that builds up sufficient pressure, about 40 mm Hg.

Gauze padding can be added to protect pressure points on the ears or over the cheekbones. Cannula patients who become tachypneic or change their tidal volume should be evaluated by blood gas analyses or ear or finger oximeters. The flow to the cannula may have to be reset to achieve desired blood levels. Some patients should use alternative devices if blood levels are critical and the patient appears to require higher oxygen concentrations. Fixed-performance or high-flow systems may be more appropriate for a COPD patient who is in distress but who tends to hypoventilate at concentrations higher than 30%. Blender, dual oxygen-air flowmeters, or Venturi masks should be used with the high-flow systems. Some clinicians also combine a cannula with an oxygen mask (e.g., aerosol face mask) in an attempt to provide high flow rates with greater F$_{IO_2}$ reliability.[32, 45]

Transtracheal Oxygen Catheters.—Instead of using the nasal or oral route, the trachea has been used for low-flow supplemental oxygen. Dead space is minimized by this technique, allowing an F$_{IO_2}$ to be maintained with lower flow rates than with a cannula.

Equipment Placement and Performance.—A small metallic catheter is surgically placed through the tracheal cartilage (Fig 12–58). Initial placement is recommended for 60 to 90 days, but long-term replacement periods have not been established or proved efficacious.[55] Transtracheal catheters have been described as having an overall oxygen savings of 54% to 59%. Performance is comparable with the nasal cannula but at reduced oxygen flow rates.

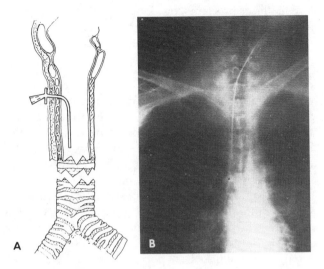

FIG 12–58.
Transtracheal catheters. **A,** drawing of lateral view of neck showing placement. **B,** chest radiograph of catheter in place. (From Heimlich HJ: Respiratory rehabilitation with transtracheal oxygen system. *Ann Otol Rhinol Laryngol* 1982; 91:643–647. Reproduced by permission.)

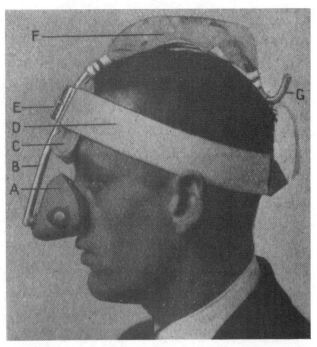

FIG 12–59.
Nasal oxygen mask with hat reservoir, circa 1938. (From Ward JJ, Gracey DR: Arterial oxygen values achieved by COPD patients breathing oxygen alternatively via nasal mask and nasal cannula. *Respir Care* 1985; 30:250–255. Reproduced by permission.)

The major application of the transtracheal catheter is related to long-term oxygen therapy for outpatients. Lower cost and lack of a conspicuous device on the face are the main advantages. Complications of hemoptysis, subcutaneous emphysema, and infection have been noted. Therefore, the surgical aspects are of most concern. If the tracheal catheter fails, a backup standard catheter should be available. In addition, if a fixed-flow restrictor was being used, a device to give higher flow must be used.[55, 64, 67]

Nasal Mask.—The first "nasal-only" mask appeared in 1938 with a hatlike reservoir and headband (Fig 12–59). About the same time a nasal inhaler with under the chin reservoir was an option of the B-L-B oronasal mask (Fig 12–60).[18] Currently, a nasal mask is available in the United States (Fig 12–61) and Great Britain (Fig 12–62).

Placement and Performance.—The current nasal masks are either attached by over-the-ear lariat or headband strap. Either device should be fastened so the lower edge of the mask gently rests on the upper lip, surrounding the external nose. These newer masks do not provide a significant reservoir for oxygen. The nasal masks have been shown to provide supplemental oxygen equivalent to the nasal cannula under low-flow conditions for patients at rest.[54, 106]

The primary advantage of the nasal mask appears to be patient comfort. Sores can develop around the external nares of long-term cannula wearers. The nasal mask should be considered under these circumstances, especially if pain reduces patient compliance in wearing the oxygen device.

Troubleshooting.—The nasal mask is subject to similar technical problems as the cannula—malpositioning, water in the tubing, and limited $F_{I_{O_2}}$ range. Blocked nasal passages and unstable breathing patterns may require an alternative device.

Oxygen Masks.—*Simple Mask.*—This nonreservoir mask is commonly a disposable lightweight plastic device that covers both nose and mouth (Fig 12–63). The face seal is normally not fitted with any special system to ensure a leak-free system. Also, there are no valves as in older versions of this mask (Fig 12–64). Thus, the patient receives a mixture of pure oxygen and room air, depending on oxygen flow and breathing pattern. Exhaled air exits through holes in the side of the mask or between the face and mask. Oxygen enters the mask from the flowmeter and bubble humidifier via small-bore tub-

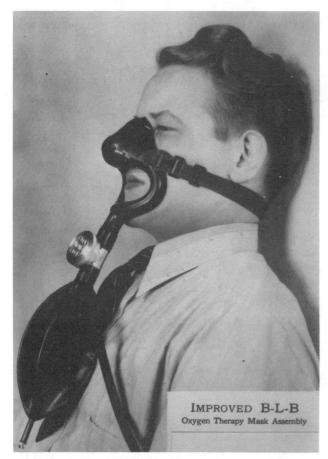

FIG 12–60.
B-L-B nasal oxygen mask with reservoir. (From Ward JJ, Gracey DR: Arterial oxygen values achieved by COPD patients breathing oxygen alternately via nasal mask and nasal cannula. *Respir Care* 1985; 30:250–255. Reproduced by permission.)

ing. Some brands of the simple mask connect tubing to a standard tapered fitting; others have a small room air–entrainment hole at the connection.

The body of the mask functions as a reservoir for both oxygen and expired carbon dioxide. Therefore, a minimal flow of oxygen to the mask must be provided to purge carbon dioxide from the mask's dead space. Without adequate flow the mask increases anatomic dead space and may lead to an elevation of arterial carbon dioxide tension.

Placement.—Most masks are fastened to the patient's face by adjustment of an elastic headband. Some manufacturers provide a malleable metal nosebridge adjustment device. It usually allows a better fit of the mask over the nose. Those applying masks must secure a tight seal but not cause facial pressure sores at the mask edges, especially where they pass over cheek bones. Periodic massage to tender areas

is usually appreciated by patients. Wearing a mask for long periods is uncomfortable and hot. Speech is muffled and drinking and eating difficult.

Performance.—The amount of oxygen enrichment of the inspired air depends on mask volume, pattern of ventilation, and the oxygen flow to the mask. It is very difficult to predict specific concentrations at certain flows. An estimate of 35% to 50% can usually be achieved in the 6 to 10 L/min flow range. The concentration will usually be higher in those with slow rates and small tidal volumes.[66, 91]

The simple mask seems best suited to patients who require higher levels of oxygen than what a cannula will provide but need this therapy for only short periods (Table 12–15). Examples would be emergency medical transport of a trauma victim, as interim therapy in the emergency room, prior to specific care, or in the postoperative recovery area.

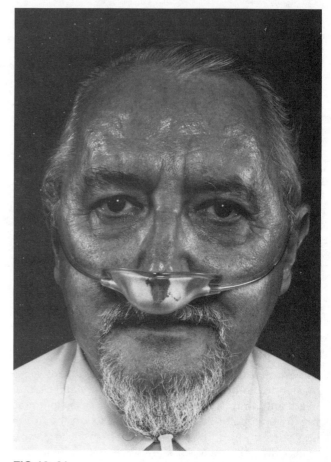

FIG 12–61.
American nasal oxygen mask. (From Ward JJ, Gracey DR: Arterial oxygen values achieved by COPD patients breathing oxygen alternately via nasal mask and nasal cannula. *Respir Care* 1985; 30:250–255. Reproduced by permission.)

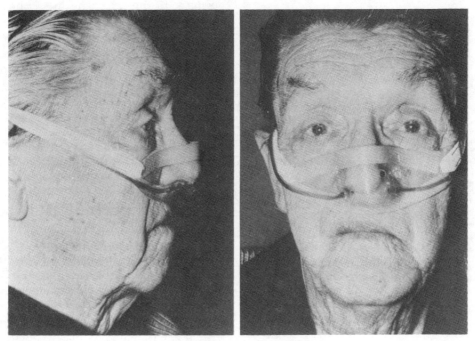

FIG 12–62.
British nasal oxygen mask. (From Harvey JE, Schlecht BJ, Grant LJ, et al: A new nasal oxygen mask. *Br J Dis Chest* 1983; 77:376–380. Reproduced by permission.)

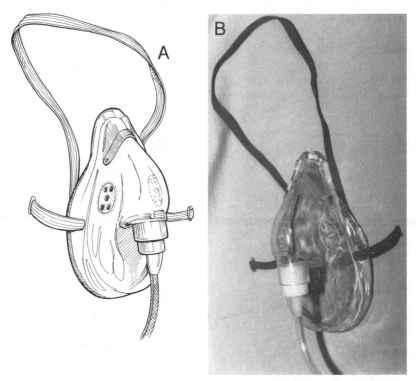

FIG 12–63.
A, drawing of contemporary nonreservoir mask. **B,** photograph of same mask.

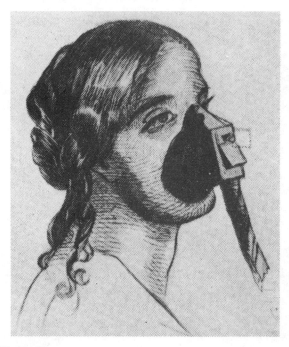

FIG 12–64.
Nonreservior oxygen mask with flap for exhaled gas, circa 1847.
(From Leigh JM: The evolution of the oxygen therapy apparatus.
Anaesthesia 1974; 29:462–485. Reproduced by permission.)

Troubleshooting.—The problems of mask dead
space have been mentioned as well as those associated with mask pressure on facial skin. There also is
potential for worsening the extent of aspiration if a
patient vomits while a mask is in position. Those applying the mask to unconscious victims or to profoundly hypoxic obtunded patients should not strap

TABLE 12–15.
Advantages and Disadvantages of Simple Masks for
Oxygen Therapy

Advantages
They supply moderate oxygen concentrations, estimated
at 30% to 40%.
They are simple, easy to apply.
They offer better humidification than cannulas or
catheters.
High flows are possible without undue mucosal irritation
or drying.
Disadvantages
They are relatively uncomfortable for extended periods.
Mask dead space requires minimal flow to keep flushed.
They are claustrophobic and hot.
There is potential for aspiration (risk greatest with
unconscious patients).
It is difficult to estimate $F_{I_{O_2}}$ and to maintain constant
oxygen concentration in patients with variable
breathing patterns.

the mask to the face. The mask should be held in
place or just set on the face.

The simple mask is not the device of choice for
patients with severe respiratory disease who are
profoundly hypoxemic and have rapid breathing.
Blood gases or oximetric measurements should be
used to titrate oxygen flow rates to provide therapeutic levels on patients assessed to have moderate
hypoxemia.

Reservoir Mask.—Incorporating some type of
gas reservoir with a mask was an early adaptation
for clinical therapy (Fig 12–65). Haldane and others
developed fairly sophisticated-looking systems by
the end of World War I (Fig 12–66). The B-L-B oronasal mask was the standard in the 1940s (Figs 12–
60 and 12–67). An interesting design involved a gas
mask and a football bladder (Fig 12–68).[69]

Currently two types of reservoir masks are commonly used: the disposable partial rebreathing mask
and the nonrebreathing mask. Both are usually
lightweight transparent plastic devices with plastic
under-the-chin reservoirs. Typically the bags hold
less than 1 L (600–800 ml). On first glance, there appears to be only slight differences (Fig 12–69).

The concept behind the partial rebreather is that
the patient can have some oxygen on demand during inspiration beyond that in the mask and coming
from the flowmeter. In addition, during the initial
phase of exhalation, some of the expired gas can be
used to refill the bag. Since the initial expiratory gas

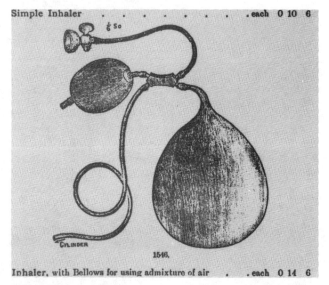

FIG 12–65.
Reservoir oxygen inhaler, circa 1914. (From Leigh JM: The evolution of the oxygen therapy apparatus. *Anaesthesia* 1974; 29:462–485. Reproduced by permission.)

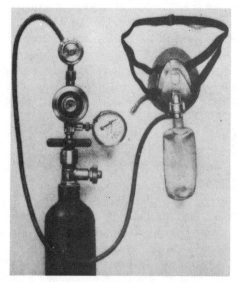

FIG 12–66.
Haldane's oxygen mask and reservoir, circa 1919. (From Leigh JM: The evolution of the oxygen therapy apparatus. *Anaesthesia* 1974; 29:462–485. Reproduced by permission.)

is very low in CO_2, as it is dead space gas, it is worthy to be contributed to the reservoir bag. The oxygen inlet is usually placed at the bag-mask connection or the neck.

The nonrebreather uses the same basic system as the other but incorporates flap-type valves between the bag and mask and the exhalation ports. Oxygen is directed to the bag side of the mask valve connection by small-bore tubing. Some system must be provided to allow room air to enter the mask in

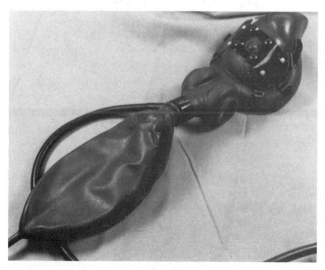

FIG 12–67.
B-L-B oxygen mask and reservoir system.

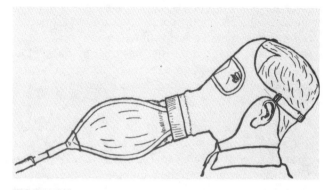

FIG 12–68.
Full-face oxygen mask and reservoir, circa 1919. (From Leigh JM: The evolution of the oxygen therapy apparatus. *Anaesthesia* 1974; 29:462–485. Reproduced by permission.)

case of a failure of the oxygen supply. Some masks leave one exhalation port open. Those that have both exhalation ports valved have a spring valve at the neck of the bag that opens with subatmospheric pressure on the patient's side.

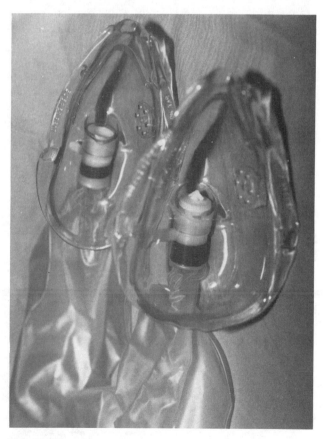

FIG 12–69.
Contemporary reservoir oxygen masks: partial rebreathing *(left)* and nonrebreathing *(right)* (see text).

Placement.—Both types of mask are placed on the patient's face with some attention to a good facial seal. A metallic strip allows a fair nose-bridge seal. Elastic straps hold the mask to the face. However, leaks are common, and room air will enter during brisk inspiratory flows, even when the bag contains gas.

Performance.—Because of the lack of a good sealing system and a substantially large reservoir, both masks are considered variable performance devices. They can provide higher inspired concentrations than the simple mask. Neither type can provide close to 100% oxygen unless the patient has a slow shallow breathing pattern. The key factor to successful application of the masks is to maintain an adequate flow of oxygen, thus assuring a full reservoir bag. Operators should not be afraid to use high flow rates. The reservoir bags should not fully deflate during a peak inspiratory effort.

The well-fitted partial rebreathing mask should provide approximately 35% to 60% oxygen when flow rates are in the 6 to 10 L/min range.[66] The nonrebreathing masks can produce oxygen concentrations slightly higher, 57% to 70% when used on normal subjects.[18] There is a variable amount of room air dilution depending on mask valve function and ventilatory demand. Valves on these masks are simple rubber flaps and may not function perfectly, especially when wet (Table 12–16).

Both masks appear to be indicated for patients suspected of significant hypoxemia who are spontaneously breathing, such as a victim of a heart attack or carbon monoxide exposure.

Troubleshooting.—General problems of mask therapy have been mentioned. These masks are subject to those related to facial seals and aspirations.

TABLE 12–16.

Advantages and Disadvantages of Reservoir Masks for Oxygen Therapy

Advantages
Relatively moderate to high concentrations:
Partial rebreathing, 35%–60%
Nonrebreathing, 57%–70%
Inexpensive, disposable, easily applied
High oxygen flows possible
Disadvantages
Relatively uncomfortable for long periods
Lack of good seals, permitting room air dilution
Unable to estimate precise oxygen concentration
Variable performance dependent on breathing pattern
Potential for aspiration

Blood gases are normally used to adjust flows to achieve therapeutic levels. However, profound changes in minute ventilation will require an adjustment of oxygen flow. Profoundly dyspneic patients with gasping respiration may be better suited with a fixed-performance, high-flow oxygen system. Because of the high oxygen concentrations possible, those COPD patients who have a tendency to hypoventilate with a high $F_{I_{O_2}}$ should be carefully observed.

Fixed-Performance Devices

Although the following devices offer the potential for a constant $F_{I_{O_2}}$, it may not always occur. These situations must be recognized, or clinicians may be misled in thinking the patient is receiving a specific concentration of oxygen. There are limits to the ability of each system to maintain its fixed-performance characteristics.

Anesthesia Bag-Mask-Valve Systems.—The basic design of this device is similar to the partial rebreathing and nonrebreathing oxygen masks previously reviewed. The basic difference deals with the more competent components. The reservoir bag consists of a 1- or 2-L anesthesia bag with a tail piece gas inlet. The masks used are those designed for ventilation purposes and have good facial sealing characteristics. In addition, most respiratory therapy and anesthesia departments have a supply of different styles and sizes to fit different patients.

The valve systems may vary (Fig 12–70). A simple spring-loaded valve can be used if opened sufficiently to allow exhaust of exhaled carbon dioxide by the relatively high flows of incoming gas. Flow to the reservoir bag must be kept quite high so that the bag does not deflate substantially. The operator may have to frequently adjust the oxygen flow and spring tension to respond to changing breathing patterns or demands. A unidirectional gas flow can also be used. Two one-way valves, one directing reservoir gas to the mask and the other exhaled gas from the mask, prevent rebreathing.

Placement.—The face mask is carefully fitted to the patient's face to provide a comfortable leak-free seal. The mask is usually held on the patient's face by personnel providing therapy. This system is not to be used casually. There is a great risk of aspiration because of the mask seal. Straps to hold the mask on the face should be used only if there is low risk of aspiration in conscious cooperative patients. Spon-

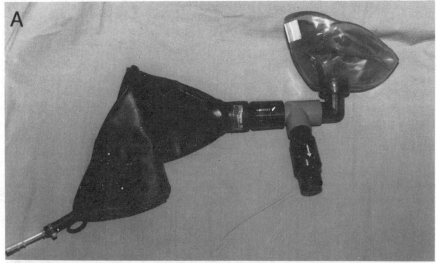

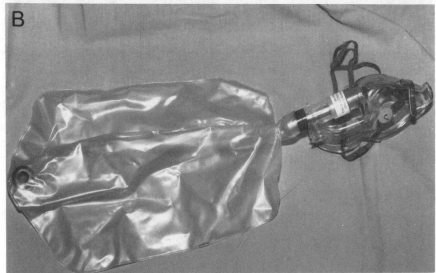

FIG 12–70.
A, nonrebreathing oxygen system using *resuscitation mask*, anesthesia bag reservoir, and one-way valve (see text). **B,** disposable nonrebreathing bag and large reservoir.

taneously breathing patients who have an endotracheal or tracheostomy tube can breathe from this system because they use standard 15/22-mm inside diameter/outside diameter fittings.

Performance.—Both designs can provide 100% oxygen or other specific gas mixtures such as CO_2/O_2 or He/O_2. Patients are allowed to breathe only the contents of the reservoir if the mask seal is tight. Operators must remember that gas flow to the bag must be in excess of the normal minute ventilation to accommodate for any increases in demand (Table 12–17).

Troubleshooting.—Although transparent masks allow inspection of the oropharynx, a primary concern for clinicians is aspiration. Patients who are receiving this therapy device are often quite ill. Operators must be able to immediately remove the mask. Nasogastric suction is helpful and minimizes the risk. However, sealing the mask with a nasogastric tube in place is more difficult.

Failure to maintain an adequate oxygen supply in the reservoir and inlet flow is another concern. Since room air breathing is prevented by valve systems, patients can suffocate if they exhaust the gas supply or if it is interrupted. When in doubt, the

TABLE 12–17.

Advantages and Disadvantages of Anesthesia
Bag-Mask-Valve Systems

Advantages

They can provide 100% oxygen or other gas
  mixture. All inspired gas comes from the
  reservoir bag.
Mask styles and sizes and different reservoir
  volumes can adapt to various patients.

Disadvantages

They are uncomfortable, claustrophobic, heavy,
  and hot.
The mask often must be held in place.
The risk of aspiration is significant.
One-way valves can offer resistance to breathing.
Water must be drained from the bag if humidity
  devices are used.

oxygen flow should be increased. Any excess will
pass out the valves. The spring-loaded valve must
be adjusted properly. If the valve is not opened, the
reservoir will pressurize, and the patient will be at
risk for gastric insufflation or pneumothorax.

Air-Entrainment Venturi Masks.—The concept
in air-entrainment masks is somewhat different than
the nondisposable reservoir and mask. The goal is to
flood the area around the nose and mouth with a
high flow of gas with a constant $F_{I_{O_2}}$. It was first

used by Barach in supplying greater than 40% oxygen in the early 1940s. The gases premixed by a jet
entraining a specific ratio of room air were held in a
reservoir and made available to a mask.[12, 13]

In 1960 Campbell developed an entrainment
mask to provide low concentrations of oxygen with
high flow rates to remove exhaled gas. The systems
were designed to exceed the patient's peak inspiratory flow rate with an overflow of premixed gas. The
original mask design had a large volume device with
many small exhaust holes (Fig 12–71).[19]

Today most masks are based on Campbell's design (Fig 12–72). Commercially they are known as
Venturi masks or high air flow with oxygen-entrain-
ment (HAFOE) systems. The former term is incorrect as a description of how room air is actually
brought into the system. Instead of the jet creating a
zone of lower pressure to suck air in, the air is
drawn in by viscous shearing forces (Fig 12–73).[94]
The exact physics do not alter the clinical use of the
mask with patients. The basic design requires that
the flow to the patient be greater or at least equal to
their demands at any time. The greatest flow rates
are required by tachypneic and gasping patients.
Therefore, formulas to estimate required flow rates
have been developed to assist the clinician (Table
12–18). Such calculation should be kept in perspective and not delay implementation of therapy. The

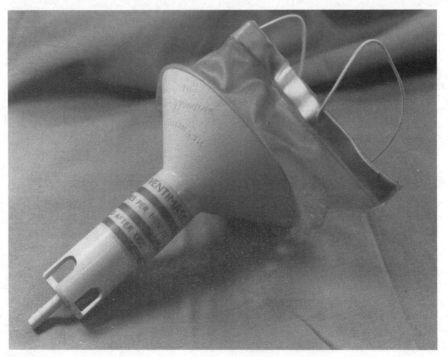

FIG 12–71.
Original Venturi mask designed by Campbell in 1960.

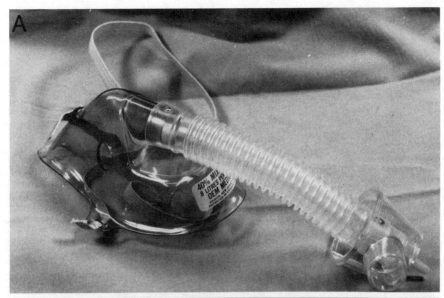

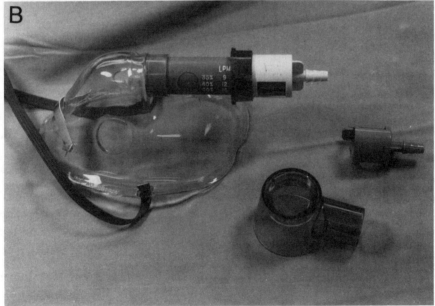

FIG 12–72.
Contemporary Venturi masks: fixed $F_{I_{O_2}}$ model **(A)** and variable $F_{I_{O_2}}$ model **(B).**

formulas in Table 12–18 are presented to give an idea of normal inspiratory peak flows and those of patients in distress.[104]

Placement.—Entrainment masks are commonly light-weight disposable devices. The mask-face seal is not tight fitting. Usually there is a jet device to which the mask is attached, sometimes by a length of large-bore tubing. The mask is placed on the face in a similar fashion to other masks and attached by elastic band.

Oxygen is directed to the jet by small-bore tubing from flowmeter and bubble humidifier. Higher humidity may be needed, because bubble humidifiers do not add much water to the total gas flow. An air-driven aerosol nebulizer can direct aerosol into a Venturi mask by attaching its wide-bore tubing to a cuplike adapter surrounding the entrainment ports.

The masks are no less comfortable than others previously discussed. They are not as good for long-term oxygen therapy as the cannula, for example.

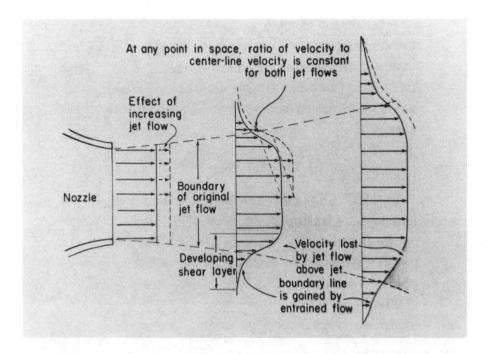

FIG 12–73.
Diagram describing physics of entrainment (see text). (From Scacci R: Air entrainment masks: Jet mixing is how they work; the Bernoulli and Venturi principles are how they don't. *Respir Care* 1979; 24:928–931. Reproduced by permission.)

Performance.—The oxygen concentration developed in an air-entrainment mask depends primarily on the oxygen flow and the mixing ratio of the jet system. Manufacturers have developed both fixed F_{IO_2} and adjustable selections over a large range. Most manufacturers give instructions for the operator to set a certain flow of oxygen. However, they should be considered the low limits that can be exceeded if the patient requires higher flows.[100] Most masks can be run on a wider range of flows and still maintain F_{IO_2} within a 1% to 2% range of accuracy.

Others can vary up to 6%.[60, 65, 68, 76, 101, 104] The oxygen flow can be varied from the manufacturer's specifications if the patient situation indicates.

When oxygen flow rates recommended by manufacturers are used, total flows may not be adequate for patients with rapid inspiratory flows, especially with masks designed to deliver an F_{IO_2} above 30% (Table 12–19). However, in spite of published data describing this fact, the masks are commonly misused.[42, 43] Some researchers have suggested that there will be further dilution at the patient's face in spite of adequate flows. The gas flows from the jet are subjected to high acceleration by patient's inspiration. Patients with short inspiratory times, smaller I/E ratios, and larger tidal volumes will tend to have lower tracheal oxygen concentrations than found in-

TABLE 12–18.
Calculation of Required Flow Rates*

PATIENT	$(V_T \times f)$	t_I, SEC	I/E RATIO	MEASURED $\dot{V}_{max}$, L/MIN	CALCULATED $\dot{V}_{max}$, L/MIN Eq1	Eq2
Normal	(470 × 15)	2.00	1:1.5	28	21	22
COPD	(613 × 11)	1.43	1:3.8	39	20	40
Respiratory distress	(668 × 14.4)	0.71	1:5.8	73	29	89

$$\dot{V}_{max} = 3 \times \dot{V}_E \qquad [1]$$

$$\dot{V}_{max} = \frac{\pi \times V_T}{2 \times t_I} \times 60 \qquad [2]$$

*V_T = tidal volume; f = respiratory frequency; t_I = inspiratory time; I/E = inspiratory/expiratory ratio; $\dot{V}_{max}$ = maximum inspiratory flow; $\dot{V}_E$ = expired volume per minute.

TABLE 12–19.
Comparison of Oxygen Input Flow and Total Flow From Air-Entrainment Masks

F_{IO_2}	INPUT FLOW RECOMMENDED BY MANUFACTURERS, L/MIN	TOTAL FLOW, L/MIN
0.24	4	97
0.28	6	68
0.30	6	54
0.35	8	45
0.40	12	50
0.50	12	33

side the mask.[21] Without this knowledge, calculations and decisions regarding therapy may be misdirected because of false assumptions. Campbell has complained about masks that are more "modern" versions of his original unit. He objects to the small mask volume and very large exhaust holes in the mask. The oxygen flows that may have been appropriate to Campbell's larger volume–containing design may not be sufficient for the smaller masks.[20, 43]

The air-entrainment masks are a logical choice for patients whose hypoxemia cannot be controlled on lower F_{IO_2} devices such as the cannula (because of increases in breathing frequency, tidal volume, or both). Patients with COPD who tend to hypoventilate with a moderate F_{IO_2} are candidates for the Venturi mask. Hypoventilation usually occurs when they have an exacerbation of their bronchitis and appear in the emergency room in distress.

Severe asthmatics who are hyperventilating may require supplemental oxygen. The air-entrainment mask works well because it can deal with high inspiratory flows and does not involve particulate water aerosol. The latter can produce further bronchospasm by an irritant effect (Table 12–20).

Troubleshooting.—Clinicians providing oxygen therapy by air-entrainment mask therapy should be aware of the previously mentioned problems involving the mask itself. A technical problem can occur if the entrainment ports are obstructed by the patient's hands, bed sheets, or water condensate. All attempts should be made to keep the mask on the face constantly. Interruption in the oxygen is a serious problem in patients with borderline blood gases.

Direct analysis of the F_{IO_2} a patient is receiving from an air-entrainment mask is possible but difficult to do accurately. Placement of an analyzer probe in the mask is not as accurate as hypopharyngeal sampling. It is not necessary to make direct measurements on the majority of patients. Correlating blood gases with some index of inspiratory flow demand, such as breathing rate, should allow clinicians to know when to suspect that the patient's demands may not be met by the mask's flow. Inlet oxygen flows may need to be increased. However, under extremes of breathing rate, the actual inspired gas will have a lower F_{IO_2} than that provided by the mask.

Air-Entrainment Nebulizers.—Large-volume or *all-purpose nebulizers* have been used in respiratory therapy for many years to provide bland mist therapy with some control of the F_{IO_2} of the output gas. These units are discussed in detail in Chapter 13. Their air-entrainment abilities will be reviewed, not their aerosol-producing properties. There are several advantages and disadvantages that should be reviewed before air-entrainment systems are used (Table 12–21).

Both disposable and permanent nebulizers use an adjustable dilution setting device to vary F_{IO_2} at fixed setting points (e.g., 40%, 70%, and 100%) or are continuously adjustable from 30% to 100%. The inlet flows are limited by the orifice diameter to allow only 15 L/min when the driving pressure is 50 psi. Nebulizers may be connected directly to DISS

TABLE 12–20.

Advantages and Disadvantages of Air-Entrainment Masks

Advantages
High flows allow the device to meet inspiratory demands of patients with fast rates and large tidal volumes.
They supply relatively consistent F_{IO_2} as patients change ventilation demands when using the lower F_{IO_2} masks.
Low F_{IO_2} models (0.3) are well suited to COPD patients who tend to hypoventilate with higher concentrations.
An air-driven aerosol generator can be added to the system to improve water content of the inspired gas.
Disadvantages
They are relatively uncomfortable.
High flows can cause drying if only a bubble humidifier is used.
Entrainment ports may be occluded, increasing F_{IO_2}.
They may give a false sense of security when a fixed-performance device is used if the total flows do not meet the patient's inspiratory flow demands.

TABLE 12–21.

Advantages and Disadvantages of Air-Entrainment Aerosol Nebulizer Systems

Advantages
They combine bland mist therapy with oxygen delivery (adequate humidity for patients with artificial airways).
Air-entrainment aerosol devices are varied to adapt to various patient situations (e.g., mask, tent, or Briggs adapter).
Dilution devices have multiple settings or continuous dilution setting options.
Actual analysis of F_{IO_2} is not difficult.
Disadvantages
Limitations to oxygen inlet flows prevent adequate total flows to patients with higher inspiratory flow demands. This limitation is most significant at higher F_{IO_2} levels.
Practitioners often incorrectly assume patients are receiving gas with a constant known F_{IO_2}.
Aerosol particles tend to cause bronchospasm in patients with hypersensitive airways (asthma).

outlets without a flowmeter to attain maximum flows, but it means that on the 100% setting with no air entrainment, the peak inspiratory flow is 15 L/min. Only patients breathing at slow rates and small tidal volumes will receive close to 100%. As the FI_{O_2} is reduced, more and more room air is entrained, increasing the total flow output. Knowledge of the air/oxygen ratio and the input flow rate of oxygen allows the total outflow to be calculated:

Example: Given a large-volume nebulizer set on 40% and driven by an oxygen flow rate of 15 L/min, what is the total flow to the patient?

1. The air/O_2 ratio for 40% is 3.17:1. Therefore, air flow will be 3.17 × 15 L/min, or 48 L/min.
2. $\dot{V}_{total} = \dot{V}_{air} + \dot{V}_{O_2}$
   $= 48 + 15$
   $= 63$ L/min.

Severely dyspneic patients may not have their inspiratory needs met by this system. To make matters more complex, air-entrainment nebulizers commonly give a slightly higher FI_{O_2} than the preset value. The increased FI_{O_2} is the result of the resistance to the output flow caused by patient tubing. Thus, less room air is drawn into the system, the FI_{O_2} increases, and the total flow decreases. On a 40% setting, nebulizers may actually provide an FI_{O_2} of 45% to 50%.[37, 82] With an increased FI_{O_2} comes a lower air/O_2 entrainment ratio, so the total flows would be lower than calculated. The settings for higher concentrations are severely flow limiting. When input flow is 15 L/min, the total flows at 60%, 70%, and 100% would be 30, 24.5, and 15 L/min, respectively. High FI_{O_2} settings should be used only with stable patients who have normal inspiratory flow demand.

Placement.—Nebulizer systems can be applied to the patient with many different devices. The *aerosol mask, tracheostomy collar, face tent,* and *T piece* or *Briggs adapter* can all be used by attaching a large-bore tubing to the nebulizer. All of these attachments provide an open system that freely vents inspiratory and expiratory gases around the patient's face or out a distal port of a Briggs adapter on an endotracheal tube (Fig 12–74). They also allow patients to easily breathe in room air. Although suffocation is unlikely, delivery of gas with a consistent FI_{O_2} is even less likely. Aerosol masks are placed on patients in a similar fashion to other masks. Tracheostomy collars are placed around patient's necks and loosely cover the tracheostomy. Face tents are placed with the lower edge under the chin with a head strap option. Briggs adapters can be simply attached to endotracheal tubes. It is common practice to use either a reservoir bag prior to the T or a reservoir tube on the distal side of the T to provide a larger volume of gas that can be available to match peak inspiratory flows. It has been proposed that up to 200 ml of distal reservoir may be added to 40% aerosol systems, run at 15 L/min, without risk of rebreathing carbon dioxide.[52]

Performance.—Performance of air-entrainment aerosol systems in providing FI_{O_2} and adequate total flows have been discussed (Table 12–22). There are several lessons learned from the previous data. First, increasing the FI_{O_2} by decreasing entrainment ratios does not guarantee a specific oxygen concentration will be provided. Second, the highest input flow settings should be used. Third, patients with rapid breathing rates (high inspiratory flow rates) are not guaranteed a specific oxygen concentration at FI_{O_2} settings greater than 0.40.

In an effort to correct for an inadequate output flow from a nebulizer system, some clinicians connect two or three units in parallel, which may appear to help but does not solve the problem. As additional nebulizers and tubing are added, the resistance to gas flow increases and there is interference with air entrainment. Thus, simply adding another nebulizer does not guarantee the patient will receive the desired FI_{O_2}. Measurement of hypopharyngeal oxygen concentrations during inspiration, when normal subjects breathed with an aerosol device and face tent, found similar data to that of investigators who studied air-entrainment masks (Table 12–23). Simply supplying adequate flows may not solve the problem. They suggested that the position-

TABLE 12–22.

Performance Characteristics of Air-Entrainment Aerosol Systems*

FI_{O_2} SETTING (DILUTION)	f, BREATHS/MIN	O_2 FLOW, L/MIN	HYPOPHARYNGEAL FI_{O_2}
0.40	14	8	0.42
0.40	40	14	0.39
0.60	14	8	0.47
0.60	40	14	0.47
1.00	14	8	0.54
1.00	40	8	0.41
1.00	40	14	0.54

*Adapted from Schacter EN, Littner MR, Luddy P, et al: Monitoring of oxygen delivery systems in clinical practice. *Crit Care Med* 1980; 8:405–409.

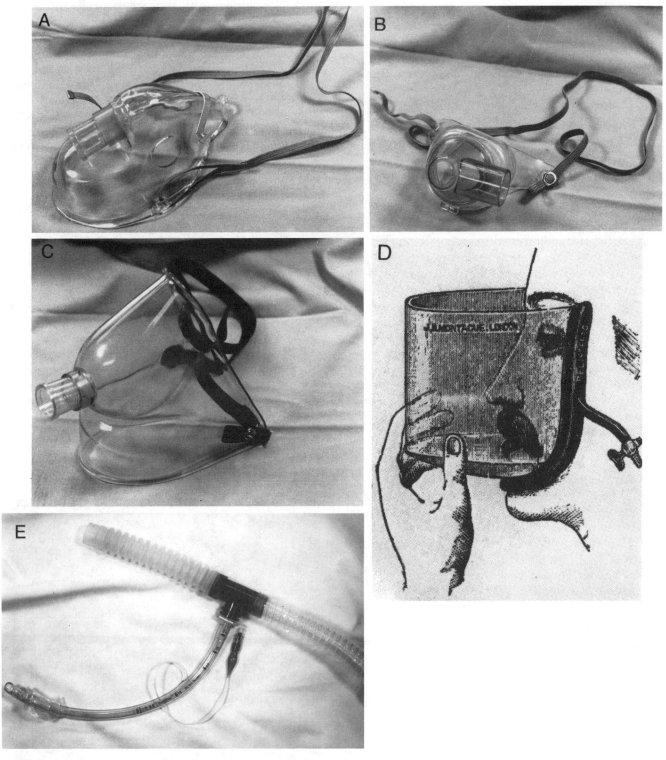

FIG 12–74.
Various masks for use with aerosol or high-flow gas delivery systems. **A,** aerosol face mask. **B,** tracheostomy collar. **C,** face tent. **D,** open face tent originally used for nitrous oxide, circa 1899. **E,** Briggs adapter, or T-piece. (From Leigh JM: The evolution of the oxygen therapy apparatus. *Anaesthesia* 1970; 25:210–222. Reproduced by permission.)

TABLE 12–23.

Hypopharyngeal $F_{I_{O_2}}$ With Single- and Double-Aerosol Nebulizer Systems*

$F_{I_{O_2}}$ SETTING	SINGLE-NEBULIZER $F_{I_{O_2}}$	DOUBLE-NEBULIZER $F_{I_{O_2}}$
0.40	0.33	0.34
0.50	0.35	0.38
0.60	0.39	0.42
0.70	0.42	0.47
1.00	0.47	0.54

*From Monast RL, Kay W: Problems in delivering desired oxygen concentrations from jet nebulizers to patients via face tents. *Respir Care* 1984; 29:994–1000. Used by permission.

ing of the face tent may act to entrain room air about the patient's face, causing secondary dilution.[82]

Lower concentrations than 0.40 may be delivered to patients at adequate flows by running a nebulizer on air and injecting oxygen from a separate flowmeter or by combining an air-driven with an oxygen-powered unit in parallel.[34]

Troubleshooting.—The major concern of those applying air-entrainment aerosol therapy with controlled $F_{I_{O_2}}$ is that the system is providing adequate flow. The mist can be used clinically like a tracer to allow some idea of adequacy of flow rate. In a T piece, if the visible mist exiting the distal port obviously disappears during inspiration, the flow should be increased.

Another concern in clinical practice is that excess water in the tubing collects and can obstruct gas flow completely or offer increased resistance to flow. The latter may increase the $F_{I_{O_2}}$ above the desired setting.

Patients should be assessed carefully if they worsen on an aerosol system. It may be an adverse response to the particulate water, causing bronchospasm in susceptible patients.

Oxygen-Air Blender Systems.—Dual air-oxygen flowmeters or air-oxygen blenders are commonly used for simple oxygen administration or with CPAP and IMV systems. They have a major advantage in providing very consistent $F_{I_{O_2}}$ in contrast to some air-entrainment devices. In addition, the total flow to the patient can be independently set to exceed patient needs up to 100 L/min.

Open masks, such as an aerosol mask, or well-fitted nonrebreathing system masks may be applied with blenders. Usually a heated humidifier is used

instead of an aerosol nebulizer. It poses an advantage for asthmatics sensitive to aerosol particles.

Oxygen Hoods.—Although many of the devices previously described have pediatric-sized variations, such as cannulas and masks, many young infants and neonates will not tolerate facial appliances. Oxygen hoods cover only the head, allowing access to the infant's lower body and still permit use of a standard incubator or radiant warmer (Fig 12–75). The hood is ideal for relatively short-term oxygen therapy for newborns and inactive infants. However, for mobile infants requiring long-term therapy, for example, the nasal cannula or tracheostomy collar afford greater mobility.

Normally oxygen and air are premixed by a blending device and passed through a heated humidifier since many nebulizers approach danger limits for noise levels (65 dB), and cold gas can induce an increase in oxygen consumption.[14] Hoods come in different sizes to accommodate a variety of infants. Some are simple plexiglass boxes; others have elaborate systems for sealing the neck opening. There is no attempt to completely seal the system, since a constant flow of gas is needed to remove carbon dioxide. In practice, flows in the range of 10 to 15 L/min are adequate for a majority of patients.[70]

Performance.—The concentration of oxygen the infant will breathe is related to the device providing the oxygen. Normally dual air-oxygen flowmeters or

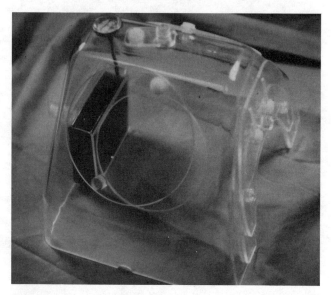

FIG 12–75.
Infant oxygen hood. Thermometer and sound-reducing sponge in place.

blenders are used. Flow should be set to guarantee a flushing effect to remove carbon dioxide. When 100% oxygen is used, there can be a layering effect, with highest concentrations at the bottom of the hood depending on hood design and gas flows. Continuous oxygen analysis is required for hood systems. Analysis should be made at several different locations in the hood.

Troubleshooting.—Because of the simplicity of the device, there are no real problems if the hood is sized sufficiently large for the infant's head. The danger of hypoxemia or complications from oxygen justify the use of alarm systems that can alert personnel to dangerously high or low $F_{I_{O_2}}$. Often transcutaneous oxygen monitors or pulse oximetry are also used.

Incubators.—Incubators have been used commonly to provide a humid, neutral thermal environment for infants, especially those born prematurely (Fig 12–76). Supplemental oxygen systems have been incorporated into incubators but often have difficulty maintaining a specific $F_{I_{O_2}}$. Because of the relatively large internal volume, maintaining a constant $F_{I_{O_2}}$ often cannot be achieved. Opening incubator access ports will allow dilution of accumulated oxygen. A better system is to use a hood and incubator. Some manufacturers of incubators have installed systems to limit the flow of oxygen into the chamber. In theory it was to prevent oxygen concentra-

tions of more than 40%, which were likely to cause opthalamologic complications such as retrolental fibroplasia. A red paddle on the back of the incubator had to be elevated to allow increased flows. It was a warning to staff that potentially hazardous concentrations were being administered.

Oxygen Tents and Aerosol Enclosures.—In the 1920s there were developments to provide supplemental oxygen to the environment surrounding the patient similar to an incubator. Oxygen rooms with elaborate air conditioning systems were made in some hospitals (Fig 12–77). In 1926, Barach published information on an oxygen tent that had the ability to remove carbon dioxide (soda lime) and excess heat (ice) (Fig 12–78).[8]

Tents continued to be used for oxygen administration into the 1950s. The major problems were difficulties in controlling the consistency of the $F_{I_{O_2}}$ and attaining levels higher than 0.50. Oxygen flows of 12 to 15 L/min were generally used with tents to deliver oxygen.

Tents are still commonly used in pediatric respiratory care for patients with problems such as croup and cystic fibrosis. Normally a high-output aerosol generator is used to provide a high humidity environment. A detailed discussion can be found in Chapter 13. Supplemental oxygen can be supplied to aerosol tents if the patients require correction of hypoxemia in addition to bland mist therapy. The most common technique is to run the aerosol generators on oxygen and adjust the $F_{I_{O_2}}$ by manipulating the

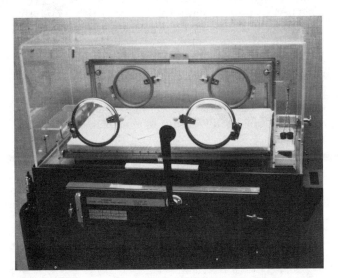

FIG 12–76.
Infant incubator. The paddle shown in the raised position indicates that relatively high $F_{I_{O_2}}$ may be given by the inlet device on the isolette.

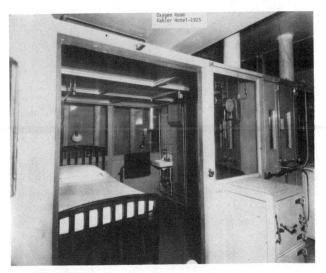

FIG 12–77.
Oxygen room in Kahler Hotel, Rochester, Minn., circa 1925.

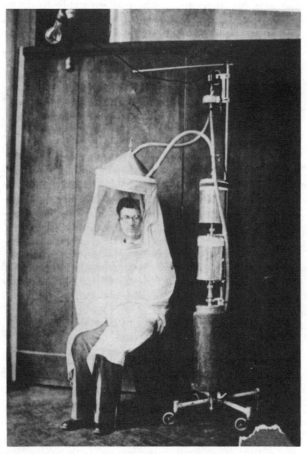

FIG 12–78.
Barach's oxygen tent, circa 1926. Metal canisters contained soda lime and ice. (From Barach AL: Symposium—inhalation therapy historical background. *Anesthesiology* 1962; 23:407–421. Reproduced by permission.)

amount of room air that is entrained. Units can also be run on air with oxygen titrated into the system to produce a moderate F_{IO_2}. Like the tent, it is difficult to consistently control the oxygen concentration.

Troubleshooting.—The most publicized problem with oxygen tents or aerosol tents with supplemental oxygen is fire hazard. Static charge sparks, nurse call devices, and electric appliances are all potential fire starters if the spark generates enough heat energy above its flash or ignition temperature. Other problems deal with elimination of patient's body heat. Elaborate refrigeration systems have been developed along with open top tents that allow heat to rise. Finally, inadequate oxygen concentrations in aerosol enclosures will develop if children place teddy bears or other toys in the gas outlets or inlets that recirculate gas.

HYPERBARIC OXYGEN THERAPY

Hyperbaric oxygen therapy involves administration of gas at an increased atmospheric pressure. Patients are placed inside a chamber that can be pressurized to several times normal atmospheric pressure, 760 mm Hg. Hyperbaric oxygen therapy has had a variable presence in medicine over the years. Currently it is receiving renewed enthusiasm for therapy (Table 12–24).[99,110] Treatment of recreational or occupational decompression sickness does not necessarily involve use of supplemental oxygen. The goal is to increase the oxygen dissolved in the blood, using Henry's law. Treatment of the *bends* (nitrogen coming out of solution in the joints of the body) has never been questioned.

Equipment

There are generally two types of chambers: the fixed multiplace unit and the portable single patient unit. The multiplace chambers are enclosed rooms built into treatment facilities (Fig 12–79). Some are designed for simple decompression treatment for 4 to 12 subjects. Others are sophisticated technically and have full operating room facilities for a surgical team. Such facilities are generally expensive, have elaborate gas plumbing systems, and are located regionally near a coast or large lakes.

The single, or monoplace, chambers are somewhat portable and allow therapy for one patient (Fig 12–80,A) or patient with an attendant (Fig 12–80,B). These devices resemble a small submarine and can be adapted to any facility. A sliding stretcher system allows loading the patient into the chamber.[53]

Patients who require 100% oxygen in a multiplace chamber usually breathe via tight-fitting face masks and bag reservoir. In monoplace units, the entire chamber is filled with oxygen, eliminating the

TABLE 12–24.
Indications for Hyperbaric Oxygen Therapy

Gas gangrene
Cyanide poisoning
Carbon monoxide poisoning
Ischemic tissue transplants
Chronic osteomyelitis
Body or inhalational burns
Air embolism
Severe acute anemia or hemorrhage
Facilitation of cardiac surgery in cyanotic heart disease
Decompression sickness

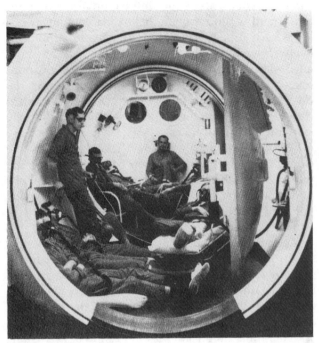

FIG 12–79.
Multiplace hyperbaric oxygen chamber. (From Davis JC, Hunt TK: *Hyperbaric Oxygen Therapy.* Bethesda, Md, Undersea Medical Society, 1977. Reproduced by permission.)

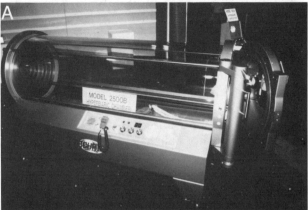

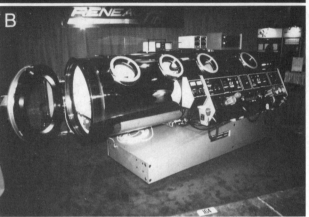

FIG 12–80.
Single-person (**A**) and two-person (**B**) portable hyperbaric oxygen chambers. (Courtesy of Sechrist Corporation, Anaheim, Calif., and Reneau, Inc, Stafford, Tex.)

need for a mask. Some units constantly purge themselves of gas as fresh oxygen enters. Others recycle all or a portion of the gas by removing carbon dioxide and water vapor. All hyperbaric chambers can adjust internal pressure up to at least 3 atm (3 × 760 = 2,280 mm Hg). Most current protocols require oxygen breathing with intermittent periods of air breathing to prevent oxygen toxicity. Exact treatment protocols for specific disease problems have been proposed by the Underwater Medical Society. The duration of the dive, oxygen concentration, atmospheric pressure level, and frequency of therapy may all be varied. Specifically trained personnel are required to maintain controls and calculate decompression stops using tables prepared for these purposes.[30, 53] Several problems related to working with hyperbaric pressures must be understood by clinicians before they administer oxygen in these chambers (Table 12–25).

Troubleshooting

Inability to attain pressure or loss of pressure during therapy should prompt operators to check seal facings or O rings. Air filters must be carefully maintained as well as frequent evaluation of gas

concentrations. Also, the treatment area should be as dust free as possible.[30, 53]

Manufacturers provide careful instructions for checking out a chamber's functions before a dive as well as maintenance procedures. Analysis of oxygen

TABLE 12–25.

Common Problems in Hyperbaric Oxygen Therapy

Access to patients in single chambers is limited.
Monoplace chambers may seem claustrophobic.
There is an electrical fire hazard with high oxygen levels.
The tympanic membrane may rupture when middle ear pressure cannot be equalized (myringotomies may be required).
Air-filled cavities may rupture if there are lung problems (e.g., emphysematous blebs, cysts).
The air volume in endotracheal or tracheostomy tube cuffs may be altered.
Intravenous bottles must be vented to pressure changes, or plastic should be used.
Microbial decontamination requires careful cleaning of chambers with nonflammable solutions.

---

concentrations should be made prior to and during therapy.

Topical Hyperbaric Oxygen Therapy

Although total body hyperbaric therapy with oxygen has been documented as successfully promoting wound healing, toxic side effects can occur. Application of the pressurized oxygen only on the affected body area or limb has received moderate attention. Topical hyperbaric therapy has been used in treating body ulcers of various origins and decubitus ulcers.[39,99]

Small clear plastic chambers have been used to enclose a limb or cover a small area. Seals allow pressure (low compared with hyperbaric chambers) to be maintained but allow a constant flushing of the enclosure. Disposable polyethylene bags have also been used since they eliminate cleaning and cross-infection problems. Although various levels of success with therapy have been reported, there are still questions on whether this form of treatment can develop significantly high oxygen tensions in body tissues.[57]

HELIUM-OXYGEN THERAPY

Since Barach established the value of low-density gas therapy in 1934, helium-oxygen mixtures have had an important, yet limited, role in medicine.[9] Other than its uses in industry and deep sea diving, there are a number of therapeutic rationales for heliox therapy:

1. In anesthetic practice, pressures needed to ventilate patients with small diameter endotracheal tubes can be substantially reduced (halved) when an 80%/20% mixture is used.[74]
2. Treatment of obstructive airway diseases vary: (a) Patients with upper airway lesions causing acute distress are ventilated prior to definitive, usually surgical, therapy[9, 10, 71]; and (b) Chronic obstructive lung disease patients (emphysema-bronchitis) have reductions in airway resistance that lead to a decrease in functional residual capacity and CO_2 excretions.[9, 10, 23, 49, 63, 101]

The theme here appears to be *aggressive conservative therapy* to hopefully avoid intubation and mechanical ventilation if possible. The clinical acceptance and guidelines for this therapy are not firm.

Some patients who require intubation also show improvement when receiving heliox via ventilator.

Barach used a simple mouthpiece to administer heliox breathing mixtures as well as a tight-fitting mask. The latter was used with heliox, using continuous positive pressure through the breathing cycle.[10] In any breathing system, a tightly sealed closed system is required, because helium will easily leak through small holes.

Nonintubated patients may receive therapy via close-fitting mask and reservoir bag. Another option would be a demand valve combined with a well-fitting mask. The disposable nonrebreathing mask is not well suited because of its loose-fitting face seal and mask holes.

Accurate flows are not needed in administering He/O_2 mixtures. The objective when using a reservoir bag and mask is to keep the reservoir bag nearly full at all times. The precise flow is not ordered but the needle valve is adjusted to meet the breathing demands.

Helium is premixed with oxygen in several standard mixtures. They are available in large-sized compressed gas cylinders. The most popular mixtures are the 80%/20% and 70%/30% helium-oxygen. Table 12–26 lists the relative density of each blend compared with oxygen.

For those needing accurate flow corrections, most companies who make calibration flowmeters will provide formulas or nomograms to allow accurate reading of low-density gases.[40, 41, 48] Others may want to invest in flowmeters specifically designed to correctly indicate the accurate flow. An estimate can be made by multiplying the level indicated on an oxygen flowmeter by the relative density compared with oxygen.

CARBON DIOXIDE GAS THERAPY

Historical Review

In the past (30 years), carbon dioxide therapy was commonly used for its pharmacologic effects. Today therapeutic applications are quite limited or

TABLE 12–26.

Relative Density of Helium-Oxygen Blends Compared With Oxygen

GAS MIXTURE	DENSITY, GM/L	DENSITY RELATIVE TO OXYGEN
80%/20% He/O_2	0.429	1.805 times less dense
70%/30% He/O_2	0.554	1.586 times less dense

controversial. This section will function as a historical review and will provide examples of therapeutic applications for increased carbon dioxide fraction in the inspired gas. Carbon dioxide therapy has several dangerous side effects, and efficacy remains unproved in many of the following applications:

1. Treatment of syncopal attacks caused by hysterical hyperventilation, causing decreased blood carbon dioxide tensions (hypocarbia). Five percent carbon dioxide in oxygen was used or rebreathing into a paper bag or tubing reservoir. Advantages of the gas was more rapid response.[78,110]

2. To stimulate ventilation in patients who are predisposed or having signs of atelectasis. It was an indirect approach to encourage patients to take deep breaths. Mechanical or nonmechanical methods to cause sustained inspiration with breath hold (e.g., intermittent positive pressure breathing, chest physical therapy maneuvers, incentive spirometry) appear to attack the primary problem more directly.

3. Treatment of hiccoughs (singulus) occasionally successful but mechanisms unknown. No more than 5% CO_2 is normally used.[110]

4. To terminate seizures (petit mal) by decreasing brain excitability. Five percent carbon dioxide in oxygen was recommended.[107]

5. Used as part of the treatment of carbon monoxide poisoning, in which 3% to 7% carbon dioxide in oxygen was used. In theory it increases the overall ventilation and facilitates the unloading of carbon monoxide from hemoglobin.[110] However, carbon dioxide can compound the acidosis if the victim has a significant lactic acidosis secondary to tissue hypoxia. Victims also often complain about headaches following therapy.

6. During cardiopulmonary bypass, use of low concentrations (3%) to prevent total body CO_2 washout.[73]

7. To improve regional blood flow by dilating vessels in the brain. Low concentrations (5% in oxygen) have been used to treat impending ophthalmic artery occlusion or prophylaxis for developing stroke. Although total blood flow may increase, perfusion to ischemic areas is probably not increased or may decrease.[80]

8. Treatment of neuropsychiatric disorders by inducing seizure activity with 30% CO_2. This approach has been abandoned because of the side effect of a significant acidosis.[110]

9. Use of CO_2 to facilitate uptake or elimination of potent volatile anesthetic agents. However, elimination of the drugs from the brain is not dependent on ventilation.[74]

Therapy Application

Because the expired air normally has an increased carbon dioxide fraction, rebreathing that gas can provide CO_2 gas therapy. The paper bag is the simplest device. The *Adler Rebreather* and *Dale-Schwarz Tube* have been commercial adaptations.

Administration of specific mixtures of carbon dioxide can be provided by premixed high-pressure gas cylinders. Regulators that attach to the cylinder valves must be specific for the concentration used. The most common are 5%/95% CO_2/O_2 and 7%/93% CO_2/O_2. Concentrations greater than 10% are available but are not used because of the risk of rapid development of side effects.

Administration devices for CO_2/O_2 gas therapy include the disposable nonrebreathing mask with reservoir and the well-fitted mask with reservoir. Administration times are normally limited to fairly short periods of 5 to 15 minutes.

Problems

Toxic manifestations of carbon dioxide must be recognized by those administering therapy. Patients must be carefully monitored for pulse, respiratory rate, blood pressure, and mental state. Significant changes in any of the aforementioned items should prompt the discontinuance of the therapy. Higher concentrations cause more rapid onset and more severe symptoms and signs. Normally, pulse rate and rate and depth of breathing all increase. Blood pressure usually increases, but the response is quite varied depending on the cardiovascular system and sympathetic nervous system response. Mental state can be depressed, ultimately resulting in convulsions, coma, and then death. When mask therapy is used, the potential for aspiration should be a concern.

GASEOUS OXYGEN ANALYSIS

When accurate analysis of oxygen concentrations can be performed, it should be done as part of safe therapy protocol. Analysis is routinely performed in infant oxygen hoods, incubators, mechanical ventilators, anesthetic circuits, and some fixed-performance oxygen administration devices (e.g., aerosol-entrainment T-piece). Dual air-oxygen flowmeters and blenders should always be checked to confirm desired oxygen concentrations. Monitoring can consist of spot sample, periodic, or continuous monitoring with high-low limit alarms.

Monitoring drug therapy is commonly done by comparing blood level and patient response to the amount given. This objective process allows a scientific approach. Medical gas therapy patients should be considered no differently. Gas analysis can often identify errors in gas concentrations and prevent harmful side effects. Some analyzers can be connected to recorders, which can document trends over long periods of time. Three methods have been commonly used to measure oxygen concentration. They are usually designated by terms that refer to their method of analysis:

1. Paramagnetic analyzer (Pauling meter)
2. Thermoconductivity analyzer (Wheatstone bridge)
3. Electrochemical cells (electrodes)
   a. Polargraphic
   b. Galvanic cell (fuel cell)

Paramagnetic Analyzer

Linus Pauling and associates developed an analyzer based on the physical principle that oxygen's electron shell configuration causes it to exhibit magnetic qualities. Increasing the oxygen level intensifies the magnetic field around a permanent magnet. Pauling termed it the "paramagnetic susceptibility" of oxygen.[88] Other common gases are diamagnetic. Paramagnetic gases, like iron filings, line up parallel to magnetic flux lines between north and south poles. Diamagnetic gases do not exhibit such properties.

In the United States, Beckman is the only manufacturer of this type of oxygen analyzer. They place a small hollow glass dumbbell filled with a specific concentration of oxygen and nitrogen between poles of a permanent magnet. The dumbbell is suspended on a quartz thread so that it can rotate in response to slight changes in the intensity of the magnetic field (Fig 12–81). The relative positive of the dumbbell changes with increases and decreases in the oxygen within the magnetic field. The position is measured by a light beam reflected on a mirror attached to the quartz thread. The light is then cast on a translucent scale. The analyzers are calibrated at sea level so that the device, which is actually responding to the partial pressure of oxygen, can be read out in percent oxygen. If at a different barometric pressure

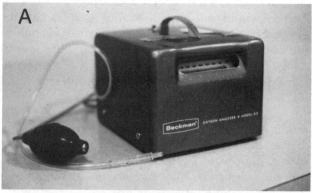

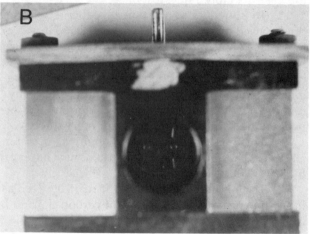

FIG 12–81.
A, Beckman model D-2 oxygen analyzer. **B,** close-up of gas-filled dumbbell suspended in the magnetic field.

(i.e., altitude), the ratio that follows can correct to give the proper F_{IO_2}. The partial pressure reading will always be correct.

$$\text{Actual \%} = \frac{\text{Indicated \%} \times 760 \text{ mm Hg}}{\text{Actual barometric pressure}}$$

Correction for water vapor pressure is not required because the gas to be analyzed is passed through a dessicant prior to entering the magnet chamber. The paramagnetic analyzer is less frequently used because of its relative expense to buy and service and because it can make only static spot analysis. Its advantages are a simple principle of operation and safety when used with flammable gases.

Thermoconductivity Analyzer

The principle behind these analyzers is that increasing oxygen concentrations (relative to nitrogen) dissipates greater heat from metallic resistors. By forming a Wheatstone bridge of four wire resistors, changes in the resistance correlates to the concentration of oxygen. Only one resistor is subjected to the gas to be analyzed. Since the bridge is calibrated on room air and 100% oxygen, unknown samples can be measured. Thermoconductivity analyzers actually measure concentration, not partial pressure of oxygen.[5]

OEM and Mira analyzers were previously manufactured in the United States but are no longer being made (Fig 12–82). Although inexpensive and rugged, they could only analyze a static spot sample. Flammable measuring areas posed a fire hazard. Also, samples with significant difference from a nitrogen and oxygen mixture alters accuracy because of different heat-dissipating properties.[4]

Polarographic and Galvanic Cell Analyzers

Electrochemical cells similar to batteries, also called *electrodes,* are available in two different forms. Both utilize the principle that increasing partial pressure of oxygen causes an increase in a chemical reaction that results in electrical activity. Both polarographic and galvanic cell analyzers have the advantage that they can measure gas samples continuously, thus allowing built-in high-low oxygen alarms. Instead of drawing a gas sample into measuring chamber, like the Beckman and Mira, the electrochemical cells are in a probe that can be placed in a gas environment. Either analog or digital readouts give percent or $F_{I_{O_2}}$, although partial pressure is actually analyzed.

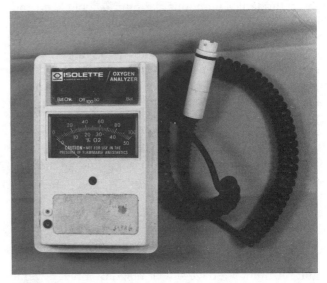

FIG 12–83.
Polarographic oxygen analyzer.

Galvanic and polarographic units produce a current flow by reducing oxygen. Oxygen molecules pass through a special membrane into an electrolyte solution. As more oxygen migrates to a charged (0.5-V) cathode, an increasing number of electrons are generated. The power to charge the cathode of a polarographic analyzer comes from a separate battery supply (Fig 12–83). Four electrons are exchanged for the reduction of the oxygen molecule, and four hydroxyl ions are formed. The material for

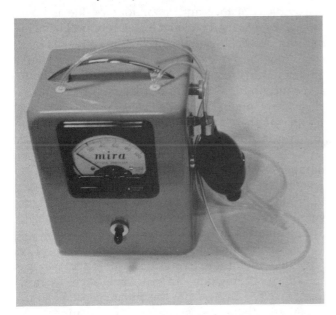

FIG 12–82.
Mira thermoconductivity oxygen analyzer.

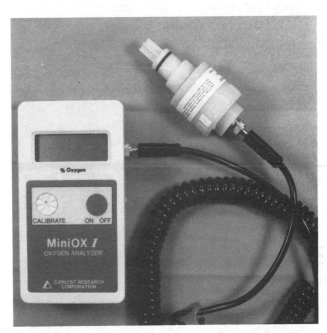

FIG 12–84.
Galvanic or fuel cell oxygen analyzer.

the cathode is commonly platinum or gold, and the anode is silver-silver chloride. Polarographic units must be carefully maintained with regard to adequacy of the batteries, the potassium chloride (KCl) electrolyte solution, and the integrity of the membrane. These analyzers have a relatively rapid response time in responding to changing oxygen partial pressures. Galvanic cells are nearly identical to the polarographic design (Fig 12–84). Oxygen molecules are reduced at a gold cathode and move to a lead anode through a *hydroxide*, cesium hydroxide (CsOH) electrolyte solution. The cathode is charged not by an external battery but one built into the sensor itself.[1]

The entire sensor-battery combination has a life span and must be replaced periodically. These electrodes tend to last longer than sensors on polarographic units but have slower response time. Several other considerations should be reviewed before galvanic and polarographic gas analyzers are placed into clinical use (Table 12–27). Clinicians who use

TABLE 12–27.

Considerations for Clinical Use of Galvanic Cell or Polarographic Gas Analyzers

1. Operators must be diligent in confirming that the batteries or galvanic sensors are up to required voltage specifications. Most units have a battery check mode.
2. Operators must routinely calibrate sensors on room air and 100% oxygen. Analyzers are generally accurate to within ± 3% oxygen. No barometric corrections are needed unless the sensor is placed in a closed high-pressure ventilator circuit with positive end-expiratory pressure (PEEP).
3. Nitrous oxide and halothane can also be reduced at cathodes and mistakenly interpreted as oxygen, which will distort the indicated O_2 level to falsely high.
4. Analyzer sensor probes should be placed in gas circuits prior to (proximal) humidification devices. Since most analyzers are calibrated on dry gas, saturated gas will dilute the gas sample and interpret it as a lower concentration of oxygen. The following example illustrates:
   Dry Oxygen:

   $$\text{Measured } \% = \frac{(760 - 0)}{760}1.0 \times 100 = 100\%.$$

   Saturated 100% oxygen at 37°C (P_{H_2O} = 47 mm Hg):

   $$\text{measured} = \frac{(760 - 47)}{760}1.0 \times 100 = 94\%.$$

   This phenomenon can cause confusion and suspicion that the oxygen-blending system or analyzer itself is malfunctioning.
5. Analyzers with standby settings should be left in that mode between analyses to minimize warm-up time.
6. To maximize sensor life:
   a. Remove electrodes from high oxygen atmospheres when not actually analyzing gas.
   6. Keep shorting bars on galvanic cells if taken out of the analyzer.

oxygen analyzers should consult the technical material with their specific unit.

GUIDELINES TO DIRECT RATIONAL MEDICAL GAS THERAPY

It is not possible or appropriate to advise practitioners on the selection of specific medical gas therapy equipment and method of application for each patient problem. Guidelines will be suggested to direct the selection process and modify the therapy based on patient response. The simple algorithm in Figure 12–85 diagrams the decision-making process and parallels the text narrative.

At some point the decision is made that a patient has a problem that oxygen or other medical gas may assist in treating (see Fig 12–85,A). Either there is a suspicion based on clinical circumstances or specific signs or symptoms suggest hypoxemia or hypoxia. Sometimes laboratory data (e.g., blood gases) reveal a surprise problem. The many factors related to oxygen transport tend to make the decision-making process more complex. In summary, there may be problems in:

1. Ventilation (removal of CO_2)
2. Oxygen content of arterial blood (e.g., hemoglobin, gas tensions, saturation levels, oxyhemoglobin dissociation curve position)
3. Local perfusion

A complete history and laboratory profile is commonly absent when patients have acute problems indicating medical gas therapy. Clinical signs and symptoms may be the only guides. As a general guideline, it is usually safer to provide liberal flows and concentrations than to restrict oxygen. There are always exceptions, but side effects are usually less significant than profound brain damage secondary to hypoxia. In the past there was undue emphasis on withholding oxygen because of a relatively small number of COPD patients with chronic hypercarbia. They may hypoventilate when given enough oxygen to produce a Pa_{O_2} above 60 to 65 mm Hg. Having to ventilate a patient is a problem but can be managed if the patient is carefully monitored.

Following the initial assessment, patients can be separated into those requiring hyperbaric therapy and those needing only ambient medical gas therapy (see Fig 12–85,B). Usually the situations demanding hyperbaric therapy are obvious, or treatment involves a planned event. Severe carbon monoxide

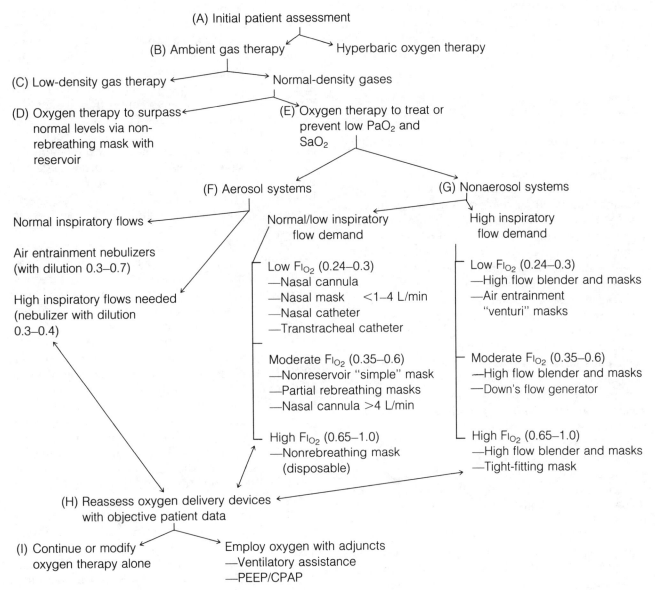

FIG 12–85.
Guidelines for medical gas therapy.

poisoning can be treated with hyperbaric therapy if there is immediate access to a chamber.[16]

The initial assessment may provide information that the cause of the dyspnea or hypoxemia is due to acute asthma, worsening chronic bronchitis or emphysema, or obstructed upper airway. If this diagnosis is confirmed, helium-oxygen therapy (see Fig 12–85,C) is an option for their care. Heliox breathing may buy time while more definitive therapy is being made ready, or pharmacologic agents can take effect.

The next decision for those receiving ambient oxygen therapy is related to the concentration of ox-

ygen needed to surpass normal levels, or to the treatment or prevention of abnormally low oxygen tensions or saturations (see Fig 12–85,D). Examples are victims of carbon monoxide poisoning, absorption of air pockets (pneumothorax), and recent postmyocardial infarction victims.

History and laboratory data may not be immediately available for many patients, especially those arriving in the emergency room. Oxygen should be applied immediately based on empiric judgment. A room air blood gas is quite valuable if it can be obtained without significant delay. Besides assisting with the diagnosis, arterial blood data can be used to select the type of oxygen concentration needed. The room air blood gas can be compared with an estimate of normal based on the patient's age. The following equations will allow an estimate for clinicians:

Normal (supine) = 103.5 − 4.2 (age) ± 4 mm Hg.
Normal (sitting) = 104.2 − 0.27 (age) ± 4 mm Hg.

Generally patients' PaO_2 should be maintained above 60 mm Hg with a saturation near 90%.

Applying a specific oxygen therapy system should now be based on the apparent FI_{O_2} need and the inspiratory flow requirement. High-flow or fixed-performance devices allow more consistent levels with patients who have rapid respiratory rates or gasping respiratory patterns (see Fig 12–85,E). Those with normal breathing can usually receive low-flow or variable-performance systems.

Further discrimination should be used to rule out or involve aerosol delivery devices to provide oxygen (see Fig 12–85,F). Aerosol may be part of gas therapy for treatment of secretion retention. Asthmatic patients may develop bronchospasm, in which case blender-humidifier systems or Venturi devices may be advised. In addition, patients requiring FI_{O_2} greater than 0.60 who have high inspiratory flows will probably exceed the output from the nebulizer. Oxygen analysis should be performed so that blood gases may be correlated with the FI_{O_2}. The FI_{O_2} should be titrated to achieve desired blood levels.

The options for patients with normal inspiratory flow requirements are those commonly used (position G, Fig 12–85). Again, aerosol therapy modes may be ruled out if bronchospasm is a concern or if it develops during therapy. Specific low-flow devices should be selected with several factors in mind. Patient comfort, perceived duration of therapy, and blood levels needed should all be considered. Because analysis of inspired oxygen concentrations is somewhat difficult, arterial blood analysis, noninvasive methods may assess therapeutic goals. Pulse oximetry and transcutaneous oxygen monitoring can provide valuable information, especially in documenting trends. However, they do have limitations that should be recognized.[86]

As patients begin to respond to oxygen therapy, inspiratory flow and breathing rates may decrease, and blood oxygen levels should increase. The converse may also occur. Those administering initial therapy should carefully observe patients and modify therapy as new information (physical signs and blood data) dictate (see Fig 12–85,H). Those who show signs of bronchospasm should be removed

from aerosol systems. Uncomfortable facial masks should be replaced with more comfortable nasal cannulas. Toxic levels are a concern, and FI_{O_2} should be reduced when possible below 0.60. Certain COPD patients may develop increased arterial CO_2 tensions if given excessive oxygen fractions. Careful reduction of flow rates or oxygen concentration should be performed with knowledge of PaO_2.

A number of clinical researchers have been interested in applying various mathematical relationships to help estimate new FI_{O_2} values to produce desired blood levels in patients. Various approaches have been used: the PaO_2/FI_{O_2} ratio,[62] $P(A-a)O_2$ (nomogram),[61] and PaO_2/PAO_2 ratio[25,46,58,75] and nomogram.[50,96]

Each application makes certain assumptions and has limitations. Their value is in lending a quasi-scientific approach, which may reduce frequent blood gas analysis and hit-or-miss guesswork.[59] (For further information on the use of these mathematical equations, refer to Appendix B.)

Oxygen therapy alone may not correct hypoxemia, hypoxia, or both in all patients (see Fig 12–85,I). Patients with profound hypercapnia with hypoxemia must frequently receive ventilatory assistance. Positive end-expiratory pressure or CPAP may be needed to augment oxygen inhalation. The type of primary cardiopulmonary or hematologic disorder will determine the potential response to oxygen. Those with large right to left shunts, for example, will not show dramatic improvement in PaO_2 regardless of the FI_{O_2} applied.

It should be noted that the schematic presentation in Figure 12–85 does not function as a complete decision-making tool. Other authors have provided similar algorithms.[32] Each patient should be treated as a special case and these guidelines used to suggest reasonable approaches.

REFERENCES

1. Adams AP, Hahn CE: *Principles and Practice of Blood-Gas Analyzers.* Morris Plains, General Diagnostics, 1979.
2. Anderson WM, Ryerson G, Block AJ: Evaluation of an intermittent demand nasal oxygen flow system with a fluidic valve [abstract]. *Chest* 1984; 86:313.
3. Auerback D, Flick MR, Block AJ: A new oxygen cannula system using intermittent-demand nasal flow. *Chest* 1978; 74:38–44.
4. Bageant RA: Oxygen analyzers. *Respir Care* 1976; 21:410–416.
5. Bageant RA: Accuracy of oxygen analyzers [letter]. *Respir Care* 1978; 23:742–743.

6. Bancroft ML, du Moulin GC, Hedley-Whyte J: Hazards of hospital bulk oxygen delivery systems. *Anesthesiology* 1980; 52:504–510.

7. Bar ZG: Predictive equation for peak inspiratory flow. *Respir Care.* 1985; 30:766–770.

8. Barach AL: New oxygen tent. *JAMA* 1926; 87:1213.

9. Barach AL: Use of helium as a new therapeutic gas. *Proc Soc Exp Biol Med* 1934; 32:462.

10. Barach AL: The therapeutic use of helium. *JAMA* 1936; 107:1273–1280.

11. Barach AL: Symposium—inhalation therapy historical background. *Anesthesiology* 1962; 23:407–421.

12. Barach AL, Eckman M: A mask apparatus which provides high concentration with accurate control of the percentage of oxygen in the inspired air and without accumulation of carbon dioxide. *Aviat Med* 1941; 12:39.

13. Barach AL, Eckman M: A physiologically controlled oxygen mask apparatus. *Anesthesiology* 1941; 2:421.

14. Beckham RW, Mishoe SC: Sound levels inside incubators and oxygen hoods used with nebulizers and humidifiers. *Respir Care* 1982; 27:33–40.

15. Block AJ: Intermittent flow oxygen devices—technically feasible, but rarely used [editorial]. *Chest* 1984; 86:657–658.

16. Boutros AR, Hoyt JL: Management of carbon monoxide poisoning in the absence of a hyperbaric chamber. *Crit Care Med* 1976; 4:144–147.

17. Brower SM, Durham MP: A nomogram for oxygen-air mixing in oxygen therapy. *Respir Care* 1972; 17:177–180.

18. Boothby WM, Lovelace WR, Uihlein A: The B.L.B. oxygen inhalation apparatus: Improvements in design and efficiency by studies on oxygen percentages in alveolar air. *Proc Mayo Clin* 1940; 15:194–206.

19. Campbell EJM: A method of controlled oxygen administration which reduces the risk of CO_2 retention. *Lancet* 1960; 1:12.

20. Campbell EJM, Gebbie T: Masks and tent providing controlled oxygen concentrations. *Lancet* 1966; 1:468.

21. Canet J, Sanchis J: Performance of a low flow O_2 venturi mask: Diluting effects of the breathing pattern. *Eur J Respir Dis* 1984; 65:68–73.

22. Cassebaum H, Schufle JA: Schelle's priority for the discovery of oxygen. *J Chem Ed* 1975; 52:442–444.

23. Chan Yeung M, Abboud R, Ming ST, et al: Effect of helium on maximal expiratory flowrate in patients with asthma before, and during induced bronchoconstriction. *Am Rev Respir Dis* 1976; 113:433–443.

24. Chusid EL: Oxygen concentrators. *Int Anesthesiol Clin* 1982; 20:235–247.

25. Cohen A, Taeusch HW Jr: Usefulness of the arterial/alveolar oxygen tension ratio in the care of infants with respiratory distress syndrome. *Respir Care* 1983; 28:169–173.

26. Compressed Gas Association: *Characteristics and Safe Handling of Medical Gases.* Pamphlet P-1. Arlington, Va, Compressed Gas Association, 1965.

27. Compressed Gas Association: *Compressed Air for Human Respiration.* Pamphlet G-7. Arlington, Va, Compressed Gas Association, 1976.

28. Compressed Gas Association: *Handbook of Compressed Gases,* ed 2. New York, Van Nostrand Reinhold Co, 1981.

29. Compressed Gas Association: *Transfilling of High Pressure Gaseous Oxygen to be used for Respiration.* Pamphlet P-25. Arlington, Va, Compressed Gas Association, 1981.

30. Davis JC, Hunt TK: *Hyperbaric Oxygen Therapy.* Bethesda, Md, Undersea Medical Society, 1977.

31. Despas PJ, Leroux M, Macklem PT: Site of airway obstruction in asthma as determined by measuring mid-expiratory flowrate breathing air and a helium-oxygen mixture. *J Clin Invest* 1972; 51:3235–3243.

32. Don H: *Decision Making in Critical Care.* St Louis, CV Mosby Co, 1985, pp 102–103.

33. Duffin J: *Physics for Anaesthetists.* Springfield, Ill, Charles C Thomas, Publisher, 1976.

34. Durham M, Miller WF: Controlled oxygen administration with adequate humidification. *Inhal Ther* 1969; 14:87–90.

35. Emergency Care Research Institute: Oxygen analyzers for breathing circuits. *Health Devices* 1983; 12:183–197.

36. Emergency Care Research Institute: Oxygen-air proportioners. *Health Devices* 1985; 14:263–284.

37. Farney RJ: Oxygen therapy: Appropriate use of nebulizers. *Am Rev Respir Dis* 1977; 115:567–570.

38. Fink JB, Lopez A, Mahlmeister MJ: Blender and ventilator failure associated with hospital grade compressed air [abstract]. *Respir Care* 1985; 30:893.

39. Fischer BH: Treatment of ulcers on the legs with hyperbaric oxygen. *J Dermatol Surg Oncol* 1975; 1:55–58.

40. Fischer and Porter Company: *Theory of the Flowrater.* FP no 98-A. Warminster, Pa, Fischer and Porter Co, 1947.

41. Fisher and Porter Company: *Variable Area Flowmeter Handbook.* Warminster, Pa, Fisher and Porter Co, 1982, vol 2, pp 1021–1022.

42. Friedman SA, Weber B, Briscoe WA, et al: Oxygen therapy—evaluation of various air-entraining masks. *JAMA* 1974; 228:474.

43. Fulmer JD, Snider GL (chrm): *ACCP-NHLBI national conference on oxygen therapy. Chest* 1984;86:234–247.

44. Gibson RL, Comer PB, Beckham RW, et al: Actual tracheal oxygen concentrations with commonly used oxygen equipment. *Anesthesiology* 1976; 44:71–74.

45. Gilbert DL: Cosmic and geophysical aspects of the respiratory gases, in Fenn WO, Rahn H (eds): *Handbook of Physiology.* Washington, DC, American Physiological Society 1964, vol 1, pp 153–157.

46. Gilbert R, Keighley JF: The arterial/alveolar oxygen tension ratio: An index of gas exchange applicable to varying oxygen concentrations. *Am Rev Respir Dis* 1974; 109:142–145.

47. Gilmont R, Maurer PW: A generalized equation for

rotameters with special floats. *Instruments Control Systems* 1961; 34:40–41.

48. Gilmont R, Roccanova BT: Low-flow rotameter coefficient. *Instruments Control Systems* 1966; 39:35–37.

49. Grape B, Channin E, Tyler JM: The effect of helium and oxygen mixture on pulmonary resistance and emphysema. *Am Rev Respir Dis* 1960; 81:823–829.

50. Gross R, Israel RH: A graphic approach for prediction of arterial oxygen tension at different concentrations of inspired oxygen. *Chest* 1981; 79:311–315.

51. Guilfoile T, Dabe K: Nasal catheter oxygen therapy for infants. *Respir Care* 1981; 26:35–39.

52. Gura D, Saidman LJ: Alveolar oxygen and carbon dioxide concentrations during simulated breathing through a T-piece. *Crit Care Med* 1974; 2:11–16.

53. Hart GB, Kindwall EP: Hyperbaric chamber clinical support: Monoplace, in Davis JC, Hunt TK (eds): *Hyperbaric Oxygen Therapy.* Bethesda, Md, Undersea Medical Society, 1977, pp 41–46.

54. Harvey JE, Schlecht BJ, Grant LJ, et al: A new nasal oxygen mask. *Br J Dis Chest* 1983; 77:376–380.

55. Heimlich HJ: Respiratory rehabilitation with transtracheal oxygen system. *Ann Otol Rhinol Laryngol* 1982; 91:643–647.

56. Helmholz HF Jr: The abbreviated alveolar air equation. *Chest* 1979; 75:748.

57. Heng MC, Pilgrim JP, Beck FW: A simplified hyperbaric oxygen technique for leg ulcers. *Arch Dermatol* 1984; 120:640–645.

58. Hess D: Prediction of the change in PaO_2 [letter]. *Crit Care Med* 1979; 7:568–569.

59. Hess D, Maxwell C: Which is the best index of oxygenation—$P(A-a)O_2$, PaO_2/PAO_2 or PaO_2/FIO_2 [editorial]? *Respir Care* 1985; 30:961–963.

60. Hill SL, Barnes PK, Hollway T, et al: Fixed performance oxygen masks: An evaluation. *Br Med J* 1984; 288:1261–1263.

61. Hoover DM, Moore P: A mathematical model for prediction of room air PaO_2 using the alveolar-arterial oxygen pressure gradient on 40% oxygen [abstract]. *Respir Care* 1979; 24:1202–1203.

62. Horovitz JH, Carrico CJ, Shires T: Pulmonary response to major injury. *Arch Surg* 1974; 108:349–355.

63. Ishilcawa S, Segal MS: Re-appraisal of helium-oxygen therapy on patients with chronic obstructive pulmonary disease. *Ann Allergy* 1973; 31:536.

64. Kirilloff LH, Dauber JH, et al: Nasal cannula and transtracheal delivery of oxygen [abstract]. *Chest* 1984; 87:313.

65. Klein EF, Mon BK, Mon MJ: Oxygen accuracy with Venturi nebulizer systems [abstract]. *Crit Care Med* 1979; 7:186.

66. Kory RC, Bergmann JC, Sweet RD, et al: Comparative evaluation of oxygen therapy technique. *JAMA* 1962; 179:123–128.

67. Leger P, Gerard M, Mercatillo A, et al: Transtracheal catheter for oxygen therapy of patients requiring high oxygen flows [abstract]. *Respiration* 1984; 46(suppl 1):103.

68. Leigh JM: Variation in performance of oxygen therapy devices. *Anaesthesia* 1970; 25:210–222.

69. Leigh JM: The evolution of the oxygen therapy apparatus. *Anaesthesia* 1974; 29:462–485.

70. Lough MD, Doershuk CF, Rawson JE: *Newborn Respiratory Care.* Chicago, Year Book Medical Publishing Co, 1979, pp 131–135.

71. Lu T, Ohmura A, Wong KC, et al: Helium-oxygen in treatment of upper airway obstruction. *Anesthesiology* 1976; 45:678–680.

72. Martin L: Abbreviating the alveolar gas equation: An argument for simplicity. *Respir Care* 1985; 30:964–967.

73. Mathewson HS: Drug capsule: Carbon dioxide: Therapeutic for what? *Respir Care* 1982; 27:1272–1273.

74. Mathewson HS: Drug capsule: Helium—who needs it? *Respir Care* 1982; 27:1400–1401.

75. Maxwell C, Hess D, Shefet D: Use of the arterial/alveolar oxygen tension ratio to predict FIO_2 needed for a desired PaO_2. *Respir Care* 1984; 29:1135–1139.

76. McPherson SP: Oxygen percentage accuracy of air-entrainment masks. *Respir Care* 1974; 19:658.

77. Mecikalski M, Shigeoka JW: A demand valve conserves oxygen in subjects with chronic obstructive pulmonary disease. *Chest* 1984; 86:667–670.

78. Meduna LJ: Alterations of neurotic pattern by use of CO_2 inhalation. *J Nerv Ment Dis* 1948; 108:373–379.

79. Mellemgard K: $PA-aO_2$ in normal man. *Acta Physiol Scand* 1966; 67:10.

80. Meyer JS, Fukuucni Y, Shimazu K: Abnormal hemispheric blood flow and metabolism in cerebrovascular disease: II. Therapeutic trials with 5% CO_2 inhalation, hyperventilation and intravenous infusion of THAM and mannitol. *Stroke* 1972; 3:157–167.

81. Mithoefer JC, Keighley JF, Karetzky MS: Response of the arterial PO_2 to oxygen administration in chronic pulmonary disease. *Ann Intern Med* 1971; 64:328–335.

82. Monast RL, Kay W: Problems in delivering desired oxygen concentrations from jet nebulizers to patients via face tents. *Respir Care* 1984; 29:994–1000.

83. National Fire Protection Association: *Respiratory Therapy.* NFPA no 56B. Quincy, Mass, National Fire Protection Association, 1973.

84. National Fire Protection Association: *Bulk Oxygen Systems.* NFPA no 50. Quincy, Mass, National Fire Protection Association, 1974.

85. National Fire Protection Association: *Storage of Liquid and Solid Oxidizing Materials.* NFPA no 43A. Quincy, Mass, National Fire Protection Association, 1980.

86. New WJ: Pulse oximetry versus measurement of transcutaneous oxygen. *J Clin Monit* 1985; 1:126–129.

87. Nunn JF: *Applied Respiratory Physiology,* ed 2. Stoneham, Mass, Butterworth, 1977, p 409.

88. Pauling L, Wood RF, Sturdivant JH: An instrument for determining the partial pressure of oxygen in a gas. *J Am Chem Soc* 1946; 68:795–796.

89. Perkins JF: Historical development of respiratory physiology, in Fenn WO, Rahn H (eds): *Handbook of Physiological Society,* vol 3. *Respiration.* Washington, DC, American Physiological Society, 1964, pp 1–60.

90. Petty TL: Definitive criteria for prescribing home oxygen systems. *Respir Therapy* 1985; 15:13–21.

91. Redding JS, McAfee DD, Parham AM: Oxygen concentrations received from commonly used delivery systems. *South Med J* 1978; 71:169.

92. Richards CC: Oxygen-history, physics and chemistry. *Inhal Ther* 1968; 13:77–83.

93. Scacci R: Air entrainment masks: Jet mixing is how they work; the Bernoulli and Venturi principles are how they don't. *Respir Care* 1979; 24:928–931.

94. Schacter EN, Littner MR, Luddy P, et al: Monitoring of oxygen delivery systems in clinical practice. *Crit Care Med* 1980; 8:405–409.

95. Seager SL, Stoker HS: *Chemistry a Science for Today.* Glenview, Ill, Scott Foresman and Co, 1973, p 51.

96. Shapiro AR, Peters RM: A nomogram for planning respiratory therapy. *Chest* 1977; 72:197–201.

97. Sheffield PJ, Davis JC, Bell GC, et al: Hyperbaric chamber clinical support: Multiplace, in Davis JC, Hunt TK (eds): *Hyperbaric Oxygen Therapy.* Bethesda, Md, Undersea Medical Society, 1977, pp 25–39.

98. Shigeoka JW, Bonekat HW: The current status of oxygen-conserving devices [editorial]. *Respir Care* 1985; 30:833–836.

99. Slack WK, Thomas DA, DeJode LR: Hyperbaric oxygen in treatment of trauma, ischemic disease of the limbus and varicose ulceration, in *Proceedings of the Third International Conference on Hyperbaric Medicine,* Durham, NC. Washington, DC, National Academy of Sciences, 1965, pp 621–624.

100. Spearman CB, et al: Effects of changing jet flows on O_2 concentrations in adjustable air entrainment masks [abstract]. *Respir Care* 1980; 25:1266.

101. Swidwa DM, Montenegro HD, Goldman MD, et al: Helium-oxygen breathing in severe chronic obstructive pulmonary disease. *Chest* 1985; 87:790–795.

102. Tiep BL, Belman M, Mittman C, et al: A new pendant storage oxygen-conserving nasal cannula. *Chest* 1985; 87:381–383.

103. Tiep BL, Nicotra B, Carter R, et al: Evaluation of low flow oxygen-conserving nasal cannula. *Am Rev Respir Dis* 1984; 130:500–502.

104. Tobin MJ, Chadha TS, Jenouri G, et al: Breathing patterns: 2. Disease subjects. *Chest* 1983; 84:286–294.

105. Vital signs: *Product information.* Totwana, NJ, Vital Signs, 1983.

106. Ward JJ, Gracey DR: Arterial oxygen values achieved by COPD patients breathing oxygen alternately via nasal mask and nasal cannula. *Respir Care* 1985; 30:250–255.

107. Woodbury DM, Rollins LT, Gardner MD: Effect of carbon dioxide on brain excitability and electrolytes. *Am J Physiol* 1958; 192:79–90.

108. Woolner DF, Lanicin J: An analysis of the performance of a variable venturi-type mask. *Anesth Intensive Care* 1980; 8:44.

109. Yost LC, Barnhard WN, Kaiman A, et al: Oxygen air blending nomogram for medium and high flow rates. *Respir Care* 1977; 22:607–609.

110. Ziment I: *Respiratory Pharmacology and Therapeutics.* Philadelphia, WB Sanders Co, 1978, pp 442–478.

Aerosol Generators and Humidifiers

Timothy Op't Holt, M.H.P.E., R.R.T.

This chapter describes and illustrates equipment used for humidity and aerosol therapy. The assembly procedure for each piece of equipment as well as its operational capabilities, limitations, and applications will be covered. The procedures for administering aerosol and humidity therapy, its indications, contraindications, and hazards can be found in Chapter 6.

AEROSOL NEBULIZERS

A nebulizer is a device that produces an aerosol, the most common being the jet nebulizer. The jet nebulizer consists of a reservoir for solution, a jet, a capillary tube, and a baffle. The reservoir varies in capacity from 5 to 2,500 ml depending on the intended use of the nebulizer. The jet nebulizer operates using Bernoulli's principle of lowering the lateral pressure of gas around the jet to draw solution up the capillary tube where it is blasted into particles by the gas jet. A device that employs the jet and capillary tube without a baffle is called an *atomizer.* Atomizers produce larger particles than are deposited in the lung periphery and may be used to administer topical antibiotics or decongestants in the pharynx or nasal cavity.

Large aerosol particles are decreased in size by their impaction against the baffle. The baffle can be nearly any surface adjacent to the jet, such as a sphere, the sides of the container, or a bead. Following impaction, these smaller, therapeutically sized particles flow into the gas stream for delivery to the patient's airways.

Small Medication Nebulizers

The earliest medication nebulizers were operated by the patient by squeezing a bulb that powered the jet (Fig 13–1). A capillary tube was positioned adjacent to the jet, and following nebulization the particles were baffled by the sides of the container. The patient then inhaled the particles from the nebulizer. This type of nebulizer is currently in use to deliver small numbers of inhalations of bronchodilators in pulmonary function departments.

Pneumatic nebulizers are classified as either *mainstream* or *sidestream.* They are connected to the gas source at either a flowmeter or indirectly by a plastic tubing. The gas source is then directed into a jet to produce aerosol.

With a mainstream nebulizer, the main gas flow passes through the nebulizer, picking up the aerosol particles en route to the patient (Fig 13–2,A). The *Bird Micronebulizer* is used as a mainstream nebulizer since aerosol is produced in the "mainstream" of gas going to the patient (Fig 13–2,B and C). A slight modification of the nebulizer allows a portion of the mainstream gas to go through the nebulizer. The remainder of the flow passes over the nebulizer elements to the patient. The sidestream nebulizer is attached adjacent to the main gas flow (Fig 13–3). Gas powering the jet carries the aerosol particles into the main flow of gas going to the patient. The *Bennett Twin* is an example of a sidestream nebulizer (Fig 13–3,B and C).

The nebulizers just discussed are all nondisposable medication nebulizers. Currently, the majority of medicated aerosol treatments are being adminis-

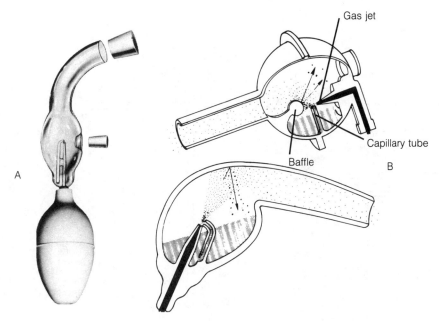

FIG 13–1.
A, early medication nebulizers. **B,** compression of the hand bulb supplies sufficient pressure to power jet. Lateral negative pressure at jet causes liquid entrainment from capillary tube. (Courtesy of Puritan-Bennett Corporation, Overland Park, Kansas.)

tered with disposable nebulizers. There are numerous brands of disposable nebulizers, but they all have basically the same features:

1. A medication cup with a capacity of 5 to 30 ml, which is threaded to fit or snap onto the top of the nebulizer or is molded into the nebulizer as a one-piece unit.
2. A jet, capillary tube, and baffle.
3. Appropriate attachments for a mouthpiece and gas delivery tube.

They may also include the following design features:

1. A gasket incorporated into the nebulizer top to prevent spilling and provide a seal within the device when in use.
2. The incorporation of an antispill barrier to prevent loss of solution if the nebulizer is tipped or inverted during therapy.
3. A slippery or treated interior to prevent solution droplets from accumulating within the nebulizer to assure optimal aerosol output.

Because the patient often holds onto these nebulizers during therapy, they have been referred to as *hand-held nebulizers* (Fig 13–4). Most of the disposable hand-held nebulizers are of the sidestream classification.

Assembly
Nondisposable Nebulizers.—The *Bennett Slip/stream nebulizer* is used as an example of nebulizer assembly (Fig 13–5). Following disinfection, the equipment should be aseptically assembled and packaged in a clean, dry area (see Fig 13–5):

1. Attach the capillary tube *(1)* to the jet *(2)*.
2. Connect a gas source to the jet, and assure that there is gas flow through the jet.
3. If there is no gas flow through the jet, use the probe provided to clear the jet orifice.
4. Assure the presence of the gaskets *(3* and *4)*.
5. Push the jet assembly into the nebulizer body *(5)*.
6. Secure the nut *(6)*.
7. Screw on the medication cup or vial *(7)*.
8. Package and store until use.

As with all jet nebulizers, the patency of the jet and capillary tube must be assured. If they are not patent, the nebulizer will not produce an adequate mist.

Nebulizer-Reservoir Combination.—The *Hudson Cloud Chamber* is a medication delivery device that incorporates a nebulizer and aerosol chamber (Fig 13–6). The aerosol flows into the aerosol chamber. When the patient inhales, the mist from the chamber

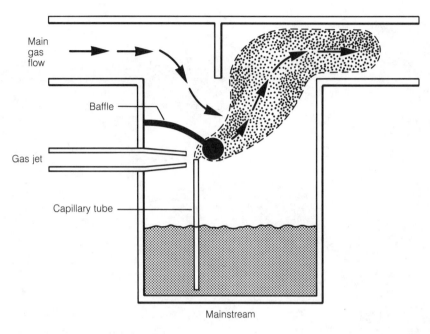

A

Main gas flow

Baffle

Gas jet

Capillary tube

Mainstream

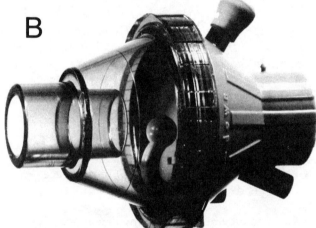

B

FIG 13–2.
A, schematic of a mainstream nebulizer. **B,** Bird Micronebulizer.
C, cutaway of Bird Micronebulizer. (Courtesy of Bird Products
Corporation, Palm Springs, Calif.)

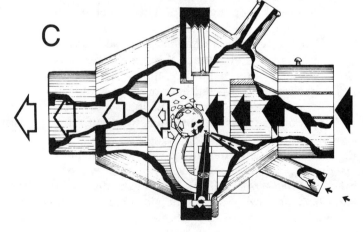

C

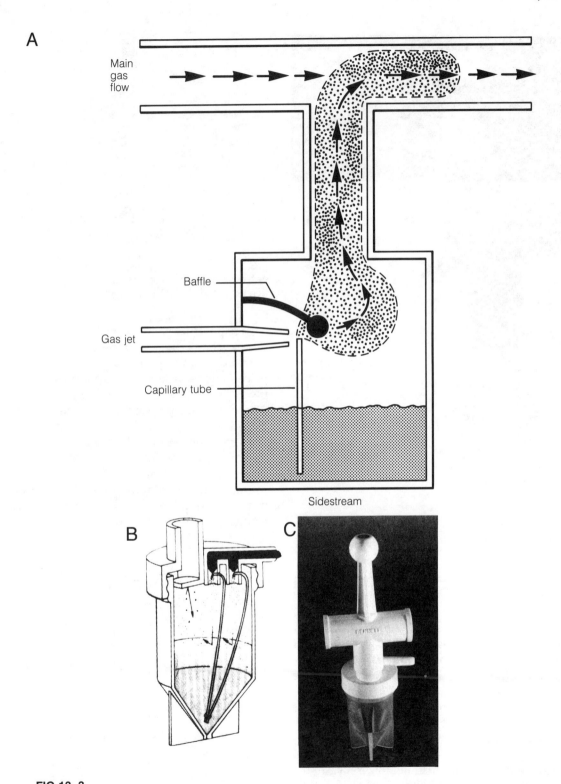

A, Main gas flow

Baffle

Gas jet

Capillary tube

Sidestream

B

C

FIG 13–3.
A, schematic of sidestream nebulizer. **B,** cutaway of sidestream nebulizer (Bennett Twin). **C,** Bennett Twin sidestream nebulizer. (Courtesy of Puritan-Bennett Corporation, Overland Park, Kansas.)

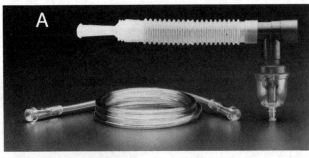

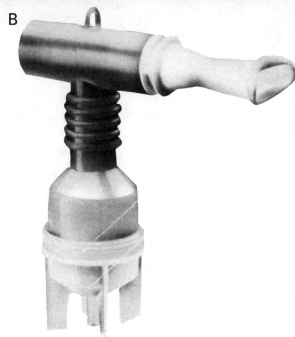

FIG 13–4.
Disposable sidestream medication nebulizers. **A,** Acorn nebulizer. (Courtesy of Marquest Medical Products, Inc., Englewood, Colo.) **B,** Inspiron nebulizer. (Courtesy of Inspiron, Division of C.R. Bard, Inc., Rancho Coucamonga, Calif.)

enters the lungs. On exhalation, exhaled gas exits the unit through an exhalation port. These exhaled gases do not enter the aerosol chamber because they hug the top of the device due to the fluidic principle of wall attachment (see Chapter 10).

The Hudson Cloud Chamber is a nondisposable device that uses disposable mouthpieces. The advantage of this unit is its ability to store aerosol particles, creating a dense mist in preparation for inhalation. Conventional hand-held nebulizers waste the medication nebulized during the expiratory phase because there normally is not any reservoir mechanism to trap newly generated or exhaled particles during expiration.

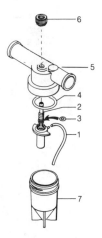

FIG 13–5.
Assembly of Bennett Slip/stream nebulizer. (Courtesy of Puritan-Bennett Corporation, Overland Park, Kansas.)

Disposable Nebulizers.—Most disposable nebulizers come preassembled from the factory. The only assembly required is placement of the mouthpiece, aerosol reservoir (if applicable), and gas supply tubing. Gas supply lines are generally 6 to 7 ft in length and are the same as the gas supply line for oxygen therapy equipment. The line may feature a universal connector, which eliminates the need for an adapter on the flowmeter used to power the nebulizer. Some gas supply lines may incorporate a thumb or finger control, which the patient occludes during inspiration and opens during expiration. It causes the nebulization of solution during only the

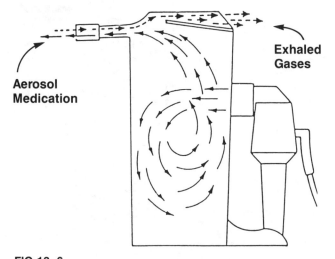

FIG 13–6.
Schematic diagram of the Hudson Cloud Chamber and its gas flow. (Courtesy of Hudson Oxygen, Temecula, Calif.)

inspiratory phase. Such a feature may alternatively be part of the nebulizer itself.

The most common patient attachment is the mouthpiece, which may connect directly to the nebulizer or can be spaced from it by a piece of reservoir tubing 3 to 6 in. long. A reservoir tubing may be placed distal to the nebulizer for enhanced aerosol particle availability at beginning inspiration. For patients with an artificial airway, a ventilator elbow or T piece may be used. During mechanical ventilation, the nebulizer can be placed into the inspiratory tubing without loss of tidal volume. An aerosol mask may also be used; however, it may promote nasal breathing and particle retention or deposition in the nasopharynx.

Performance Characteristics

These devices are designed to nebulize 3 to 5 ml of solution in 5 to 10 minutes with a source gas flow of 5 to 10 L/min. The F_{IO_2} at the patient's airway depends on the pattern of breathing and the F_{IO_2} of the source of gas. Although a given F_{IO_2} is generated by the device, the patient's F_{IO_2} will vary with different breathing patterns. Since these nebulizers are considered low-flow devices with a fixed output, patient breathing characteristics will cause the F_{IO_2} to vary as air mixes with inspired gas. Particle size and output varies among the nebulizers available (Table 13–1).

Limitations

Small medication nebulizers may be limited by any flaw in manufacturing or design that results in poor aerosol output, spilling of medications on tipping or inversion, entrapment of droplets within the nebulizer (effectively decreasing total output), and production of particles outside the therapeutic range. Particles of 1.0 to 10.0 μ have the greatest chance of depositing in the respiratory tract. Once particles reach 0.25 to 1.0 μ, there is deposition in

small airways and alveoli.[18] Often, patients who recline will tip the nebulizer from side to side. Manufacturers are now aware of this tendency and are constructing nebulizers that continue to nebulize when not in an upright position. Some claim to nebulize in a 90-degree-from-upright position.

Application

A medicated aerosol treatment may be administered using the following protocol:

1. The physician's order is checked for drug, dosage, and frequency of treatment.
2. The patient is assessed.
3. The necessary equipment is gathered: nebulizer and delivery device, flowmeter/compressor and adapter, if necessary, medication, and diluent.
4. The patient is instructed and informed of the indications and therapeutic procedure.
5. The equipment is assembled via the following procedure: hand washing, nebulizer assembly, placement of medication and diluent in reservoir, adjustment of flow to produce adequate mist, administration of treatment until medication is spent, and proper cleaning and storage of the nebulizer until the next treatment.
6. The patient responses are recorded.
7. Paperwork is completed (charge slip, records).

Large Mainstream Nebulizers

The component parts of the large mainstream nebulizers are equivalent to those of small medication nebulizers with several exceptions. Exceptions include a larger reservoir (250–2,500 ml), provisions for air entrainment (to allow high-flow aerosol-enriched oxygen therapy), and provisions for heating the liquid to be nebulized.

Nondisposable Large Mainstream Nebulizers

Ohmeda Ohio Deluxe Nebulizer.—The Ohmeda Ohio Deluxe nebulizer has been available in several models since its introduction (Fig 13–7). Two models, one with and one without an oxygen diluter control, have been available for use with Ohmeda Ohio-Armstrong incubators. The other two models differ in capacity and type of heater used. One of the therapy models comes with an 850-ml reservoir, an oxygen dilutor control for 40%, 60%, and 100% ox-

TABLE 13–1.

Reported Particle Sizes and Output of Small Medication Nebulizers*

COMPANY	MODEL	PARTICLE SIZE, μ	OUTPUT, (ML/MIN)†
Respiratory Care Inc.	—	1.5–4.0	0.35–0.85
Puritan-Bennett Corp.	Slip/stream 002200	—	0.15–0.45
Inspiron		3.5–7.0	—

*Manufacturers' data.
†Dependent on source gas flow.

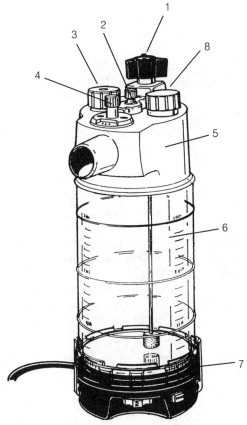

FIG 13–7.
Ohmeda Ohio Deluxe nebulizer (*outer view*): (*1*) nut for flowmeter attachment, (*2*) jet, (*3*) release valve, (*4*) diluter dial, (*5*) jar top, (*6*) reservoir, (*7*) clip-on heater, and (*8*) immersion heater port plug. (Courtesy of Ohmeda, Madison, Wis.)

ygen, and provision for a thermostatically controlled immersion heater. The other therapy model comes with an 800-ml reservoir, the same oxygen diluter control, and a steel base constructed to accommodate a thermostatically controlled clip-on heater. A 2 pounds per inch (psi) release valve is supplied with all models, although this device is functional only when the Ohmeda Ohio Deluxe is used in a closed system, as with an intermittent positive pressure breathing (IPPB) device.

Assembly.—Following disinfection, the equipment should be aseptically assembled and packaged in a clean, dry area (Fig 13–8):

1. Replace blank cap (*1*) and 2-psi pressure release assembly (*2*).
2. Replace jet (*3*).
3. Replace cleaning plug (*4*).

4. Turn the jar top over, and install the plate/baffle (*5*).
5. Screw in the capillary tube with the filter (*6*).
6. Screw jar top onto reservoir. Package and store.

If the clamp-on heater model reservoir is in use, the base plate is pushed into the base of the reservoir, and the retaining ring is screwed on securely. The jar top is replaced, followed by packaging and storage.

Ohmeda Ohio High Output Nebulizer.—The Ohmeda Ohio High Output nebulizer is used primarily in conjunction with the Ohio Pediatric Mist tent. It is designed to work at pressures ranging from 35 to 50 psi. The reservoir capacity is 2,500 ml. A damper control functions to vary the F_{IO_2} when the nebulizer is oxygen powered. The F_{IO_2} of the unit varies greatly depending on the configuration of the tent. Some tents are open at the top, whereas others are closed. Generally it is possible to achieve F_{IO_2} in the range of 0.25 to 0.40 using the damper control. The manufacturer claims the maximum flow is 250 L/min when it is operating at 50 psi without an air inlet filter.

Assembly.—Following disinfection, the equipment should be aseptically assembled and packaged in a clean, dry area (Fig 13–9):

1. Assure patency of the nebulizer tip (*1*) and insert it and the O ring into the nebulizer body (*2*).
2. Attach the capillary tube and filter (*3*) to the nebulizer body.
3. Screw the nebulizer body onto the threaded connection inside the nebulizer tube assembly (*4*).
4. Align the baffle duct (*5*) with the top cover (*6*).
5. Thread the filter on the end of the capillary tube through the hole in the baffle duct, and screw the nebulizer tube assembly into the top cover.
6. Screw the supply tube (*7*) into the top cap.
7. Secure the top cap onto the reservoir (*8*) with the clips (*9*).
8. Replace the fill plug (*10*).

Application.—The pediatric mist tent assembly is put in place at the bedside. The nebulizer is con-

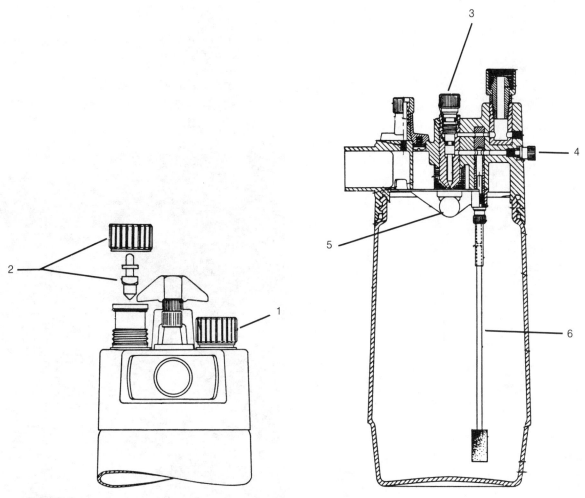

FIG 13–8.
Cutaway view of the Ohio Deluxe nebulizer. (See text for description of parts.) (Courtesy of Ohmeda, Madison, Wis.)

nected to the tent with 2.5-in. hoses. From the gas source, a high-pressure hose is connected to the threaded fitting on the nebulizer tube assembly. The reservoir is filled with 2.5 L of sterile water. The mist tent refrigeration unit is set as ordered, and the gas flow is set to 15 L/min. The $F_{I_{O_2}}$ is adjusted with the damper control as well as with supplemental oxygen sources or by opening the top of the tent canopy. The child should not be placed into the tent until proper operation is assured.

Bennett Nebulizer.—The Bennett nebulizer produced by Puritan-Bennett Corporation is similar in most respects to the Ohmeda Ohio Deluxe nebulizer. The unit has a 375-ml capacity, a 2-psi or 40 mm Hg release valve, and a removable plug for insertion of a nonthermostatically controlled immersion heater. Although the reservoir capacity is 375

ml, the usable volume is 200 ml, which necessitates frequent refilling. A dilution control is provided to allow adjustment of $F_{I_{O_2}}$. A cleaning button is provided to clear the capillary tube orifice at the jet (Fig 13–10).

Assembly.—Following disinfection, the equipment should be aseptically assembled and packaged in a clean, dry area (Fig 13–11):

1. Rebuild and replace the high pressure release (*1*) into the jar top (*2*).
2. Replace the immersion heater port plug (*3*) into the jar top (*2*).
3. Replace the filter and filter cap (*4*) onto the siphon tube (*5*).
4. Screw the jar top (*2*) onto the reservoir (*8*). Package and store.

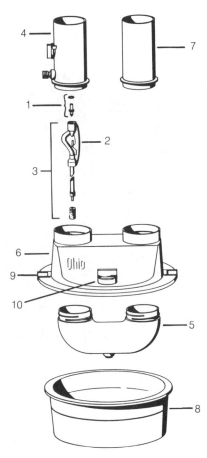

FIG 13–9.
Assembly of the Ohmeda Ohio High Output nebulizer. (See text for description of parts.) (Courtesy of Ohmeda, Madison, Wis.)

Puritan Bubble-Jet Humidifier.—The Puritan Bubble-Jet humidifier (Puritan-Bennett Corporation) doubles as either a bubble humidifier or jet nebulizer (Fig 13–12). A switch on the device that indicates bubble and jet is user selectable for the desired function. The device has a 375-ml reservoir that must be refilled at the 200-ml level, necessitating frequent refilling for continuous use. It does not have an air dilution feature; therefore, it delivers 100% source gas and flows up to approximately 17 L/min. Consequently, it may be used only for low-flow oxygen therapy. There is a 2-psi pressure release for use in closed-system applications.

Assembly.—Following disinfection, the equipment should be aseptically assembled and packaged in a clean, dry area (Fig 13–13):

1. Assemble and install the pressure release (*1*).
2. Assemble and install the switch assembly (*2*). A screwdriver is needed for this step.

3. Assemble the diffuser (*3*) and diffuser housing (*4*).
4. Set the cap (*5*) on the reservoir (*6*), and tighten the ring (*7*) to secure the cap to the reservoir.
5. Do not install the small-tube adapter (*8*) when using this device as an aerosol nebulizer.

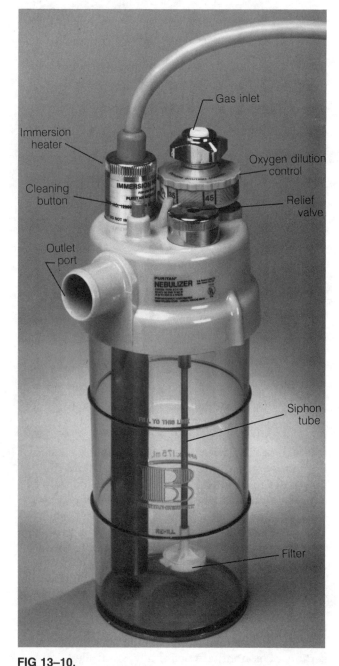

FIG 13–10.
Bennett nebulizer. (Courtesy of Puritan-Bennett Corporation, Overland Park, Kansas.)

sure release. If the release does not function, recheck the seal between the cap and reservoir, assuring correct position of the gasket. Attach the aerosol tubing, a water trap, and patient interface. Then adjust the flowmeter to the desired flow, and attach the patient interface.

For use as a bubble humidifier, the unit is assembled in the same manner except that the switch is placed in the bubble position, and the small-tube adapter is fitted into the aerosol outlet. The small-tube adapter is appropriate for low-flow oxygen delivery devices such as cannulas and masks.

Bird 500-cc Inline Micronebulizer.—The Bird 500-cc Inline Micronebulizer is available in two mod-

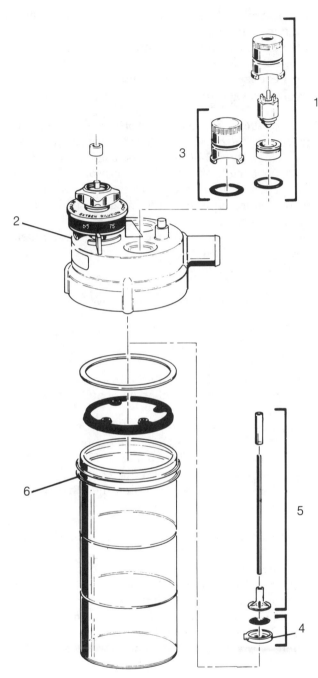

FIG 13–11.
Interior view of the Bennett nebulizer for assembly. (See text for description of parts.) (Courtesy of Puritan-Bennett Corporation, Overland Park, Kansas.)

Application as a Jet Nebulizer.—Attach the wing nut on the gas inlet connection to the flow source (flowmeter, hose connection, regulator). Detach the reservoir and fill it with 375 ml of the desired solution. Replace the jar. Select jet with the switch. Turn on the flow and obstruct the outlet to test the pres-

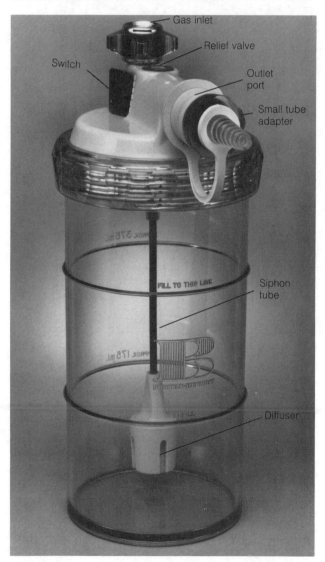

FIG 13–12.
Puritan Bubble-Jet humidifier. (Courtesy of Puritan-Bennett Corporation, Overland Park, Kansas.)

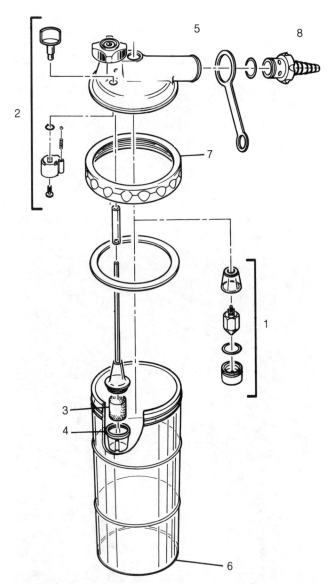

FIG 13–13.
Assembly of Bennett Bubble-Jet humidifier. (See text for description of parts.) (Courtesy of Puritan-Bennett Corporation, Overland Park, Kansas.)

els, differentiated by the ability to place one or two capillary tube-jet-baffle assemblies (Fig 13–14). This nebulizer is primarily for use with Bird ventilators. A gas supply from the ventilator supplies the pressure jet for the nebulizer. As gas passes through the nebulizer from the ventilator, it picks up the nebulized particles for delivery to the patient. This system holds the F_{IO_2} delivered by the nebulizer constant since the F_{IO_2} of the mainstream airway and pressure jet are equal and there is no outside air entrainment. When the accessory extension assembly is used, the mainstream airway opening is plugged

by the mantle. This system delivers a maximum of 15 L/min of 100% source gas. The nebulizer is similar to the Puritan Bubble-Jet humidifier because there is no provision for air dilution, which limits the use of this nebulizer to Bird ventilator applications and low-flow oxygen therapy.

Assembly.—The assembly of the two models of the Bird nebulizer is basically identical. Differences occur when the nebulizer is to be used as part of the ventilator circuit, as a low-flow aerosol delivery device, or with one or two jet assemblies. The following procedure is used to assemble the nebulizer to function as a mainstream low-flow aerosol delivery device. Following disinfection, the equipment should be aseptically assembled and packaged in a clean, dry area (Fig 13–15):

1. Connect the capillary tubing (*1*) to the crown (*2*).
2. Insert the pendant (*3*) into the crown (*2*).
3. Thread the capillary tube (*1*) through the dome (*4*), seating the crown on the dome.
4. Screw the dome onto the reservoir (*5*).
5. Screw the extension assembly (*6*) onto the dome.
6. Push the mantle (*7*) over the larger opening of the dome to occlude the opening.
7. Push the nebulizer connector (*8*) into the tallest tower in the crown.
8. Replace the stoppers (*9*) on the other two towers on the crown.

Mistogen High-Volume Pneumatic Nebulizer.—The Mistogen HV-12 pneumatic nebulizer is primarily intended for use with *CAM-2* and *CAM-3* pediatric mist tents (Fig 13–16,A). The nebulizer operates at 7–15 L/min and 50 psi. The reservoir capacity is 2 L with an output of up to 5 ml/min. An air dilution control allows an F_{IO_2} range of 0.35 to 0.70, although the F_{IO_2} will depend on the amount of room air allowed into the tent.

Assembly.—Following disinfection, the equipment should be aseptically assembled and packaged in a clean, dry area (Fig 13–16,B):

1. Assemble the oxygen dilute cap (*1*) and insert it into the cover (*2*).
2. Assure that the jet in the jet assembly (*3*) is clear.
3. Attach the jet assembly to the supply elbow (*4*).

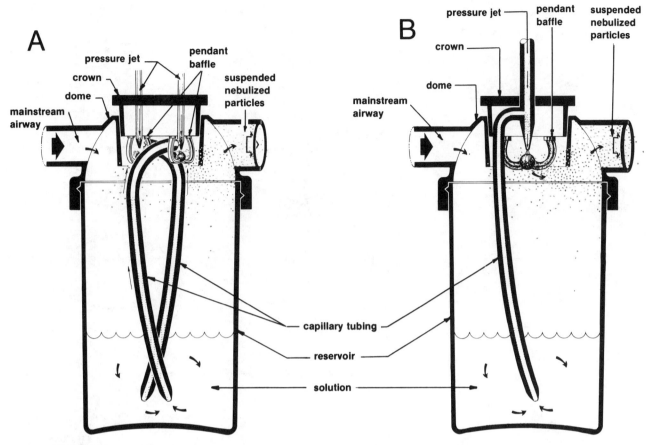

FIG 13–14.
A, single-jet Bird Micronebulizer. **B,** twin-jet Bird Micronebulizer. (Courtesy of Bird Corporation, Palm Springs, Calif.)

4. Attach the tube (5) and filter (6) to the jet assembly from the inside of the cover.
5. Seat the cover on the reservoir basin (7), and secure it with the clips (8).

Application.—The mist tent assembly is placed at the bedside. The reservoir basin of the nebulizer is filled with 2 L of sterile water. Once the proper function of the mist tent is assured, the child may be placed in the tent. Further discussion of mist tents is found in the section on pediatric mist tents.

Disposable Large Mainstream Nebulizers

There are numerous disposable large mainstream nebulizers. The variety of Fi_{O_2} settings, solution reservoir sizes, and types of solutions have been limited only by the customers' preference (Table 13–2). Common to all of these devices are a jet nebulizer, a fluid reservoir, and a variable air-entrainment port for changing the Fi_{O_2}. Table 13–3 lists set and actual Fi_{O_2} for these devices. Actual Fi_{O_2} is slightly higher than indicated on the nebulizer[8] due to back pressure on the venturi caused by the resistance of the aerosol tubing. Therefore, it is important to keep the tubing as straight as possible while in use. A water trap is also recommended because a fluid bolus will increase resistance and, therefore, Fi_{O_2}. If a precise Fi_{O_2} is desired during therapy, the therapist should analyze the Fi_{O_2} and make the appropriate change with the diluter ring. Because of the fixed nature of air/oxygen entrainment ratios, the Fi_{O_2} should not change when source gas flow is changed. Table 13–4 lists the actual and predicted flows at various Fi_{O_2} values. The predicted flows were calculated using the following formula:

$$\text{Predicted flow} = \frac{\text{Oxygen flow (L/min)} \times 0.8}{Fi_{O_2} - 0.2}.$$

Most flows are less than predicted due to back pressure on the venturi from the aerosol tubing. As was the case with Fi_{O_2}, the aerosol tubing must be kept as straight as possible. A water trap should be used because a fluid bolus will decrease delivered flow. This is a consideration in high-flow oxygen

A   INLINE nebulizer 890   B   INLINE nebulizer 4144

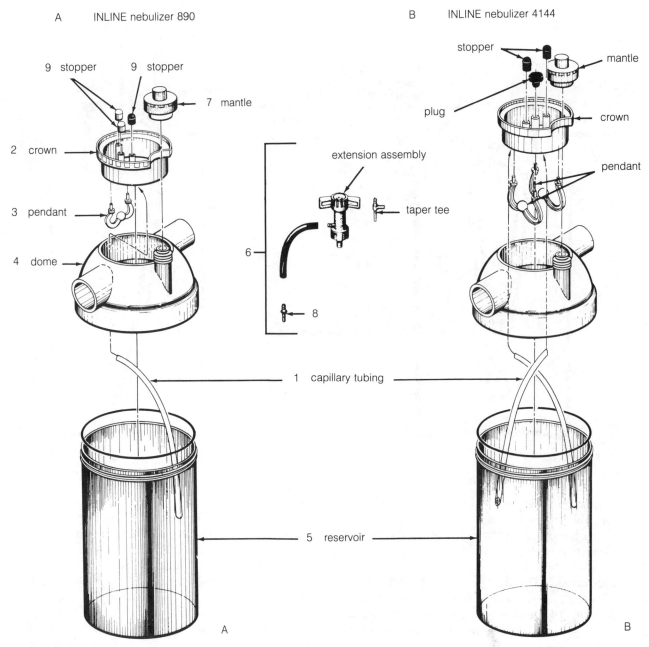

FIG 13–15.
Assembly of the Bird 500-cc Inline Micronebulizer. **A,** single-jet model (890). **B,** double-jet model (4144). (Courtesy of Bird Corporation, Palm Springs, Calif.)

therapy because total flow should be greater than or equal to three times the patient's minute volume to maintain the desired FI_{O_2}. At a high FI_{O_2}, it may necessitate using two or more nebulizers in a parallel circuit to obtain an adequate flow.

Table 13–5 lists humidity, output, and particle size data. For those units tested, relative humidity at room temperature ranged from 55% to 72%.[8] The relative humidity of the aerosol from the heated

Ohmeda Ohio Deluxe nebulizer was 135%. The U-Mid heated nebulizer produced 80% to 100% relative humidity at room temperature. The output of unheated nebulizers ranged from 0.5 to 5.0 ml/min. The output of heated nebulizers ranged fom 1.3 to 3.1 ml/min. Comparisons are difficult to make because the temperature of the heated aerosol varies, as does the source of the data. All reported particle sizes are within the 1.0 to 10.0-µ range. These par-

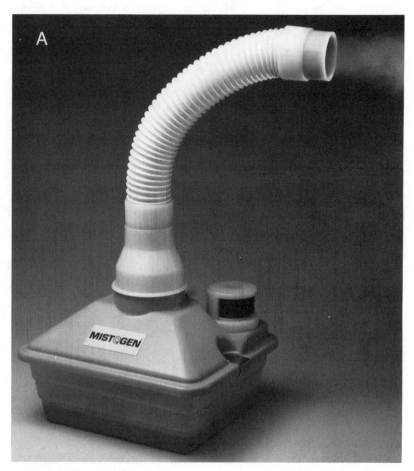
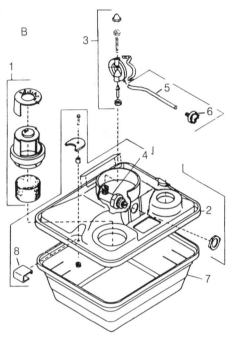

FIG 13–16.
A, Mistogen pneumatic nebulizer. **B,** assembly of the Mistogen HV-12 pneumatic nebulizers. (Courtesy of Mistogen/Timeter Products, Lancaster, Penn.)

ticle sizes were measured using a laser hologram method (a three-dimensional picture made without a camera on photographic film). Therefore, if the patient's pattern of breathing is optimal, there is the potential for small airways deposition and penetration when the patient is inhaling aerosol from these nebulizers.

Application.—The application of all of the large mainstream nebulizers is basically the same. Once the physician's order for aerosol and an F_{IO_2} are confirmed, the therapist can proceed with equipment assembly. After hand washing, the flowmeter is installed. The nebulizer is assembled. Usually, this step involves only the attachment of the nebulizer jet assembly to the reservoir bottle in a one- or two-step operation. If a non-prefilled nebulizer is used, the reservoir is filled at this point. If a heater is being used, it is put in place at this time. Heaters are generally used for patients with an artificial airway or if a greater volume of aerosol is indicated. The nebu-

lizer is firmly attached to the flowmeter. An aerosol hose of appropriate length with a water trap inline is attached to the nebulizer. An appropriate patient interface (mask, T piece) is attached to the patient end of the aerosol tubing. The ordered F_{IO_2} is set and the flowmeter turned on to deliver an adequate mist. Generally 8 to 10 L/min is sufficient. However, if a high F_{IO_2} is ordered, a total output of three times the patient's minute volume may be needed to assure the ordered F_{IO_2}. This may necessitate additional nebulizers in parallel. The delivery device is attached to the patient, and a no smoking sign is posted. Applicable notes are made in the patient's chart concerning date, time, device, F_{IO_2}, arterial blood gases, and breath sounds. Monitoring the system consists of assuring aerosol tube patency, adequate solution volume, and overall system cleanliness. Usually the entire system is replaced every 24 to 48 hours.

One must be aware of the possibility of electric shock if a heater should malfunction or if a saline

TABLE 13–2.

Nebulizers, Companies, Available Sizes, F$_{IO_2}$ Settings, Tested Heated, and Disposables

BRAND	COMPANY	AVAILABLE SIZES*	INDICATED F$_{IO_2}$ SETTINGS*	HEATER(S) AVAILABLE*	SOLUTIONS AVAILABLE*
Aquapak	Respiratory Care, Inc. Arlington Heights, IL 60004	440 ml 760 ml 1,070 ml 2,200 ml	0.28, 0.35, 0.40, 0.60, 0.80, and 0.98	One thermostatically controlled, one nonthermostatically controlled, nonimmersion	Sterile water, ½ normal saline, normal saline
Corpak	Corpak, Inc. Wheeling, IL 60090	465 ml 765 ml	0.28, 0.30, 0.40, 0.60, 0.80, and 0.96	Thermostatically controlled, nonimmersion	Sterile water, ½ normal saline, normal saline
Mistyox	Medical Molding Corp. of America Costa Mesa, CA 92626	400 ml 800 ml	0.28, 0.35, 0.40, 0.60, 0.80, 1.00	N/A	Sterile water
Travenol	Travenol Laboratories, Inc., Deerfield, IL 60015	1,000 ml	0.28, 0.30, 0.35, 0.40, 0.50, 0.70, and 1.00	Nonthermostatically controlled, nonimmersion	Sterile water, ½ normal saline, normal saline
U-Mid	Seamless Hospital Products Wallingford, CT 06492	500 ml	0.35, 0.40, 0.60, 0.70, 1.00	Nonthermostatically controlled, wrap-around	Sterile water, ½ normal saline, normal saline
Inspiron	Inspiron, Division of C.R. Bard, Inc. Upland, CA 91786	500 ml	0.35, 0.40, 0.50, 0.70, 1.00	Immersion, thermostatically controlled	Non-prefilled
Ohio Deluxe (Ohmeda)	Ohmeda Madison, WI 53707	800 ml (nondisposable)	0.40, 0.60, 1.00	Thermostatically controlled, clamp-on	Non-prefilled
Puritan-Bennett	Puritan-Bennett Corp. Lexana, KS 66211	375 ml (nondisposable)	0.40, 0.70, 1.00	Nonthermostatically controlled, immersion	Non-prefilled
Conchapak	Respiratory Care Inc. Arlington Heights, IL 60004	1,650 ml	Flush, 0.35, 0.40, 0.60, 0.80, 0.98	Thermostatically controlled, sleeve	Sterile water
High Output	Ohmeda Madison, WI 53707	2,500 ml (nondisposable)	No indicated values	N/A	Non-prefilled
Mistogen HV-12	Mistogen/Timeter Lancaster, PA 17601	2,000 ml (nondisposable)	0.35–0.70	N/A	Non-prefilled
Airlife	American Hospital Supply Evanston, IL 60201	500, 750, and 1,000 ml	0.28, 0.35, 0.40, 0.60, 0.98	Thermostatically controlled, nonimmersion	Sterile water, ½ normal saline, normal saline

*Manufacturer's data.

TABLE 13–3.

Set and Actual F$_{IO_2}$ of Large Mainstream Nebulizers*,†

NEBULIZER‡	SET F$_{IO_2}$										
	0.28	0.30	0.35	0.40	0.50	0.60	0.70	0.80	0.96	0.98	1.00
	ACTUAL F$_{IO_2}$										
Aquapak	0.31	N/A	0.38	0.44	N/A	0.62	N/A	0.82	N/A	0.94	N/A
Corpak	0.31	0.33	N/A	0.47	N/A	0.66	N/A	0.80	0.98	N/A	N/A
Mistyox	0.32	N/A	0.37	0.40	N/A	0.62	N/A	0.79	N/A	N/A	0.72
Ohmeda Ohio Deluxe	N/A	N/A	N/A	0.40	N/A	0.63	N/A	N/A	N/A	N/A	0.98
Bennett	N/A	N/A	N/A	0.42	N/A	N/A	0.70	N/A	N/A	N/A	100.0
Travenol	0.29	0.30	0.36	0.45	0.50	N/A	0.70	N/A	N/A	N/A	0.97
U-Mid	N/A	N/A	0.33	0.40	N/A	0.58	0.69	N/A	N/A	N/A	0.94
Inspiron§	N/A	N/A	0.37	0.42	N/A	N/A	0.72	N/A	N/A	N/A	0.96

*Unless otherwise indicated, data from Grose BY: Personal communication, 1985.
†N/A = data not available, not an indicated setting.
‡At 10 L/min of source oxygen flow at 50 psi.
§Manufacturers' data.

TABLE 13–4.

Actual and Predicted Flows at Indicated F_{IO_2}*

	PREDICTED FLOW, L/MIN										
	100	80	53.3	40	26.6	20	16	13.3	10.6	10.2	10
	SET F_{IO_2}										
	0.28	0.30	0.35	0.40	0.50	0.60	0.70	0.80	0.95	0.98	1.00
NEBULIZER†	ACTUAL FLOW,‡ L/MIN										
Aquapak Flow at 6 ft	53.5	N/A	37.9	33.6	N/A	19.7	N/A	13.8	N/A	10.9	N/A
Corpak Flow at 6 ft	41.9	37.8	N/A	21.5	N/A	14.4	N/A	12.3	10.9	N/A	N/A
Mistyox Flow at 6 ft	59.0	N/A	49.0	38.5	N/A	20.5	N/A	13.8	N/A	N/A	10.4
Travenol 28% Flow at 6 ft	67.1	66.3	55.6	32.6	28.6	N/A	17.0	N/A	N/A	N/A	10.6
U-Med Flow at 6 ft	N/A	N/A	51.9	40.9	N/A	20.8	16.6	N/A	N/A	N/A	11.8
Inspiron§ Flow at 5 ft	N/A	N/A	88	41.6	27.3	20.3	16.1	13.4	N/A	N/A	10
Ohmeda Ohio Deluxe Flow at 6 ft	N/A	N/A	N/A	35.1	N/A	19.0	N/A	N/A	N/A	N/A	10.7
Bennett Flow at 6 ft	N/A	N/A	N/A	35.4	N/A	N/A	14.9	N/A	N/A	N/A	10.2

*Unless otherwise indicated, data from Grose BY: Personal communication, 1985.
†At 10 L/min of source oxygen.
‡N/A = Data not available, not an indicated setting.
§Manufacturer's data.

TABLE 13–5.

Humidity, Output, and Particle Size Data for Large-Volume Mainstream Nebulizers*

BRAND	OXYGEN FLOW, L/MIN	F_{IO_2}	UNHEATED % RELATIVE HUMIDITY AT 37°C	HEATED % RELATIVE HUMIDITY AT 37°C	OUTLET TEMPERATURE °F	HEATED TOTAL OUTPUT, ML/MIN	NONHEATED TOTAL OUTPUT ML/MIN	PARTICLE SIZE†
Bennett	8	0.40	55		104.0	3.1	0.50	
Ohmeda Ohio Deluxe	8	0.40			96.8	2.6	1.0	
		1.00	72	135‡,§				
					95.0	2.2	0.47	96°F Mist 96°F 0.3–8µ Cold: 97°F 0.3–8µ
Aquapak	8	0.35	100‖		95.0	1.5	0.47	
Conchapak	8	0.35		157†,§	98.6	2.5		
Travenol	8	0.35			88.0	1.9	0.90	
Corpak	8	0.40			95.0	1.6	0.63	
U-Mid	8	1.00	60‡					
	8	0.40		80–100†,§	80.0	1.3†		70°F 0.3–6.0µ 100°F 0.3–10µ
Inspiron	8	0.50					0.90†	1–2.5µ
	8	0.35					1.40†	
Mistyox	8	0.35	76.2 at 70.5°F†				0.72	1–5µ
Ohmeda Ohio High Output	15						5.0†	
Airlife		0.40					2.2†	

*Unless otherwise indicated, data from Grose BY: Personal communication, 1985.
†Manufacturer's data.
‡Data from Klein EF, Shah DA, Shah NJ, et al: Performance characteristics of conventional and prototype humidifiers and nebulizers. *Chest* 1973; 64:690–696.
§Mean of all available F_{IO_2}.
‖Data from Giordano SP, Holland EL: A performance comparision of disposable humidifiers. *Respir Therapy*, July/Aug 1973.

solution is used and a current path provided. Some of the manufacturers warn not to use their heaters (particularly immersion heaters) when the solution level is below a recommended level. Otherwise, newer heaters have automatic shutoff features to protect the patient against tracheal burns.

Attachments for Aerosol Delivery.—Corrugated tubing is used to deliver aerosol from nebulizers and heated humidifiers to the patient. The tubing is flexible for its length and has 22-mm adapters at each end for attachment to the nebulizer and delivery device. The diameter of this tubing is ¾ in.

Smooth-bore sections that can be cut are often placed every 6 in. to allow installation of accessories or an adapter for attachment of another length of tubing. When cut, the loose ends have a 22-mm diameter. The internal surface of the tube may or may not be corrugated. A smooth-bore tube offers the advantages of decreased resistance and a more laminar flow than a corrugated surface. It may enhance aerosol delivery due to less internal surface area for impaction.

An effusion bag or water trap (Fig 13–17) is placed into the corrugated tubing wherever there is a dip where condensed solution may accumulate. Without a water trap, this solution bolus may cause one or more of the following problems:

1. Increased F_{IO_2} because of decreased air entrainment
2. Decreased total flow because of decreased air entrainment
3. Decreased or absent aerosol delivery because of the absorption of the aerosol particles
4. Patient discomfort if the tube is lifted and the bolus drains to the patient
5. Possible drowning or gagging if the bolus is drained into an artificial airway

Delivery of aerosol to the patient is made with several different devices depending on the type of airway available. The face mask (Fig 13–18) is made of vinyl and has a 22-mm connector for aerosol tubing. There are two holes in the mask for exhalation and escape of excess flow. A metal band over the nose bridge facilitates the mask-face seal. An elastic band that fits around the patient's head holds the mask in place. The face mask may be used for all spontaneously breathing patients who do not have artificial airways. The hazards of this device are pressure sores at contact points and the possibility of aspiration of vomitus if the mask is worn by a lethargic or comatose patient.

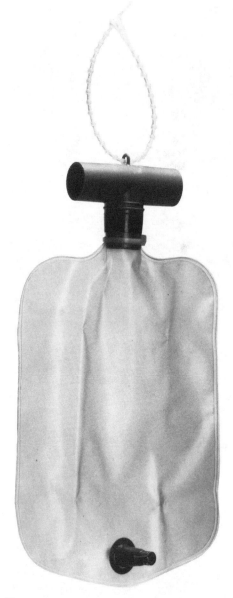

FIG 13–17.
Disposable effusion bag. (Courtesy of Hudson Oxygen, Temecula, Calif.)

For those patients who may be uncomfortable with a face mask on, the face tent is available. The face tent is a vinyl face enclosure that fits under the chin and is open above the nose (Fig 13–19). It too has a 22-mm adapter for aerosol tubing. Other than becoming easily dislodged and the possibility of pressure sores at contact points, there are no apparent hazards.

Oxygen concentration at the distal end of the aerosol tubing is easily obtained with an oxygen analyzer. However, the determination of the actual F_{IO_2} is more difficult, usually requiring a hypopha-

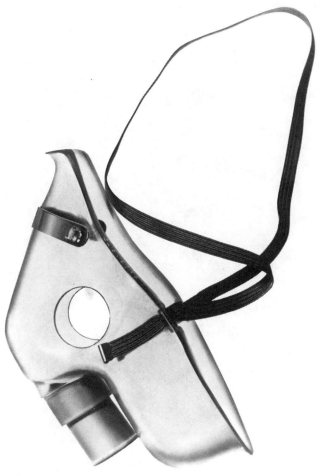

FIG 13–18.
Aerosol face mask. (Courtesy of Hudson Oxygen, Temecula, Calif.)

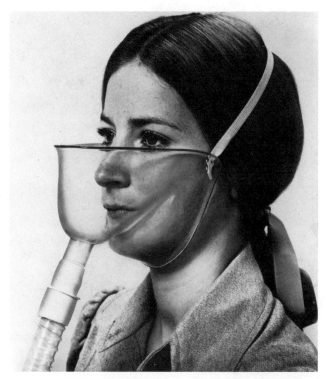

FIG 13–19.
The face tent. (Courtesy of Hudson Oxygen, Temecula, Calif.)

ryngeal oxygen sampler. It has been shown that when face masks and tents are used as described, the actual amount of oxygen delivered to the hypopharnyx ($F_{H_{O_2}}$) is far lower than the oxygen concentration at the end of the aerosol tube.[5, 7, 13, 16] These studies demonstrated that the $F_{H_{O_2}}$ decreases as inspiratory flow and tidal volume increase or nebulizer flow decreases. For example, in the Monast study, the $F_{H_{O_2}}$ had a range of 0.23 to 0.38 with the nebulizer $F_{I_{O_2}}$ set at 0.40.[13] This study was performed using a face tent and nebulizer with 12 to 14 L/min of 100% O_2 source gas. With the nebulizer set at $F_{I_{O_2}}$ of 1.0, the $F_{H_{O_2}}$ had a range of 0.33 to 0.66. In studies where the $F_{H_{O_2}}$ was measured with the aerosol face mask in use, the $F_{H_{O_2}}$ was closer to set $F_{I_{O_2}}$.[7, 16] However, as set $F_{I_{O_2}}$, tidal volume, and respiratory rate increased, the $F_{H_{O_2}}$ decreased. The $F_{H_{O_2}}$ remained less than 0.7 in all trials when set $F_{I_{O_2}}$ was 1.0. Thus, although the face mask and tent may deliver aerosol, the patient may *not* receive the fraction of oxygen indicated on the nebulizer diluter control.

The only way to assure a particular $F_{I_{O_2}}$ (without tracheal intubation) is with a tight-fitting mask with one-way valves and a reservoir bag in a nonrebreathing system. Otherwise, any change in the patient's pattern of breathing will affect the actual $F_{I_{O_2}}$.

The T piece with reservoir tubing is commonly used to deliver aerosol to a patient with an oral or nasal endotracheal tube. The T piece has a 22-mm adapter for the aerosol hose and a 15-mm inside-diameter (I.D.) adapter for the artificial airway (Fig 13–20). The reservoir tube may vary from 6 to 18 in. and is used to hold aerosol and oxygen. Provided that total flow is adequate, rebreathing and carbon dioxide retention should not be significant. If carbon dioxide retention does occur as a result of the reservoir, it can be shortened or removed. If a continuous stream of aerosol is observed exiting the reservoir during inspiration, it is reasonable to assume that the patient is receiving the entire inhaled volume from the nebulizer. If this flow is not evident, the total flow of source gas should be increased. The T piece may also be used with the tracheostomy tube; however, if the patient moves about excessively, the T piece will pull on the tracheostomy tube. This pulling may result in decannulation or damage to the tracheostomy site.

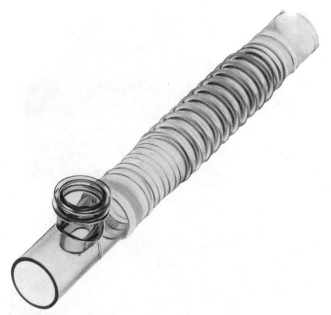

FIG 13–20.
T piece with reservoir. (Courtesy of Hudson Oxygen, Temecula, Calif.)

A less traumatic device for the tracheotomized patient is the tracheostomy mask (Fig 13–21). The tracheostomy mask is made of vinyl and has a swiveled 22-mm adapter for aerosol tubing. The mask fits over the tracheostomy tube but does not necessarily come in contact with it. The mask is held in place by an elastic band that fits around the neck. Because the mask does not attach to the tracheostomy tube, patient movement does not cause pulling on the tube as could occur with the T piece.

Accumulations of solution in the tubing should be drained periodically to assure aerosol flow. Patient attachments should be cleaned or replaced if they are fouled with secretions or are otherwise contaminated. The entire system must be checked periodically to assure proper function and patient attachment.

Ultrasonic Nebulizers

In an ultrasonic nebulizer, an electric current is used to produce sound waves that, when directed at the surface of a fluid reservoir, produce an aerosol (Fig 13–22). The electric current is a frequency-modulated signal of variable amplitude. The usual frequency is 1.35 MHz. This frequency is applied to a piezoelectric crystal, which is a substance that changes shape as a charge is applied. The piezoelec-

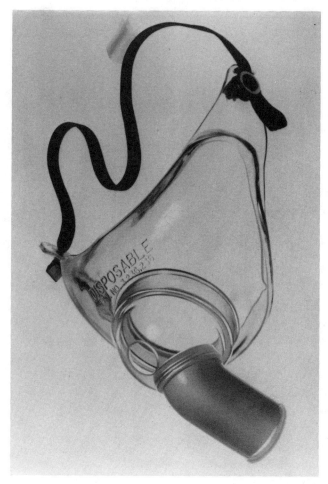

FIG 13–21.
Tracheostomy mask. (Courtesy of Hudson Oxygen, Temecula, Calif.)

tric crystal is the transducer in the ultrasonic nebulizer that changes the electrical energy into sound energy. This sound energy is focused on the surface of a fluid reservoir, where a geyser is generated. Aerosol particles then emanate from the geyser. In the geyser, surface tension and cohesive forces are overcome, causing continuous disintegration of the liquid into a fine aerosol. The typical ultrasonic nebulizer employs a couplant chamber, in the base of which is the transducer. This couplant chamber is filled with water. The couplant chamber helps absorb mechanical heat and acts as a transfer medium for the sound waves to the solution cup. The solution cup is immersed in the couplant, and it is in the solution cup that the geyser forms. A blower unit or external gas supply carries the aerosol from the solution cup through large-bore tubing to the patient. Aerosol output, that is, the density or amount of

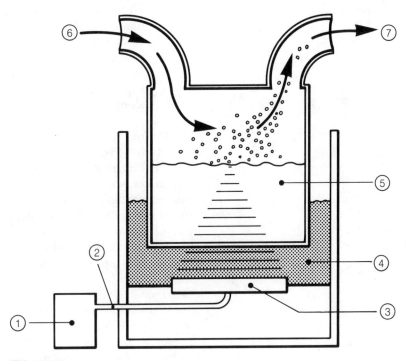

FIG 13–22.
Functional diagram of the ultrasonic nebulizer: *(1)* electric current generator, *(2)* cable, *(3)* piezoelectric crystal, *(4)* couplant chamber, *(5)* solution cup, *(6)* carrier gas inlet, and *(7)* aerosol outlet.

aerosol, is determined by the amplitude or strength of the frequency signal. The frequency is fixed; however, the amplitude is varied by a control on the ultrasonic nebulizer. Output ranges from 0 to 6 ml/min depending on the model in use.

Bennett US-1 Ultrasonic Nebulizer

The Bennett US-1 ultrasonic nebulizer (model 7301) is typical of the description just given, nebulizing solution at a frequency of 1.35 MHz. A blower with a flow of 0 to 60 L/min carries the aerosol to the patient and cools the power unit. A bacteria filter may be placed between the blower and the solution cup. The output control is adjustable to provide 0 to 3 ml/min of solution. The solution cup may be filled to 200 ml or kept continuously at that level by a float-feed system for continuous nebulization. If the nebulizer is inadvertently operated without water in the couplant chamber or solution cup, a protective circuit will turn off the power to the piezoelectric crystal, and the pilot lamp will flash. If the cooling blower inlet is blocked, another sensing device turns off the nebulizer circuit. If one of these events occurs, the unit is turned off for 30 seconds to allow the circuit to reset. The equipment should be checked for proper fluid levels and the blower inlet checked for obstruction.

Assembly.—Following disinfection, the equipment should be aseptically assembled and packaged in a clean, dry area (Fig 13–23):

1. Fit the crystal holder *(1)* into the coupling chamber *(2)* with a twisting motion, assuring a firm seat.
2. Lay the crystal cable in the slot at the rear of the unit. Push the clamp *(3)* with tooth forward onto two teeth inside the slot, as shown.
3. Fit the coupling chamber into the unit using the clamp to hold it in place.
4. Fill the coupling chamber with distilled water to a level between the minimum and maximum lines.
5. Fit the seal *(4)* into the groove around the solution cup *(5)*. Fill the cup with a maximum 200 ml of solution.
6. Place the discriminator *(6)* onto the cup, positioning it to accept the feeder tubes (for continuous feed).
7. Push the cover *(7)* over the solution cup.
8. Slide the edge of the cover under the two forward latches on the couplant chamber, pressing the ridge of the clamp *(3)* over the edge of the cover.

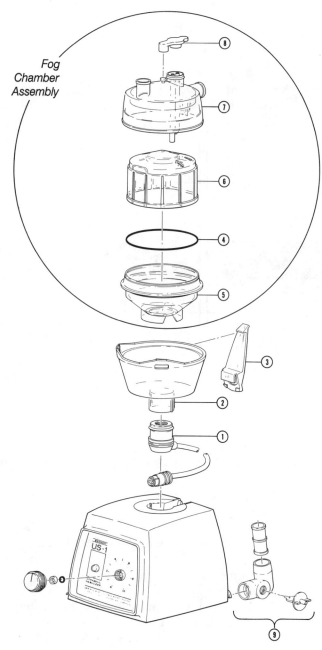

Fog Chamber Assembly

FIG 13–23.
Assembly of the Bennett US-1 ultrasonic nebulizer. (See text for description of parts.) (Courtesy of Puritan-Bennett Corporation. Overland Park, Kan.)

9. Secure the cap (*8*) on the feed port over the cover tubes.
10. Assemble the damper/flow control assembly, and push it onto the blower outlet (*9*).
11. Connect 8 in. of tubing between the flow control assembly and the cover inlet (port on the rear of the cover).

12. The unit is now prepared for single treatment use. A continuous feed system may be attached to the feeder port, allowing continuous nebulization. A jet-entrainment adapter can be adapted to the cover inlet to supply an increased $F_{I_{O_2}}$ to the patient along with the aerosol.

DeVilbiss Ultrasonic Nebulizers

Model 35B.—The DeVilbiss model 35B ultrasonic nebulizer is a pole-mounted nebulizer, producing an aerosol output of 0 to 3.0 ml/min with a particle size range of 1 to 10 μ. The particle size mode (most frequent size) is 3.0 μ. Relative humidity output of the model 35 varies with amplitude.[10] The maximum relative humidity at 37°C and a power setting of 1 is approximately 65% at a 6 L/min flow from the blower. At the highest power setting 5, approximately 190% relative humidity at 37°C is delivered with a blower flow of 8 L/min. As the flow from the blower is increased, the relative humidity at any power setting decreases. A blower module is attached to the nebulizer to deliver aerosol to the patient. The couplant chamber and transducer crystal on all DeVilbiss ultrasonic nebulizers is built into the unit. The only removable parts are the solution cup and the two-part plate that holds the cup in place. Solution cups are available for single-treatment use (up to 180 ml) and continuous use with a float-feed system and 2-L reservoir bottle. Only the output volume separates model 35B from model 65.

Model 65.—The DeVilbiss model 65 ultrasonic nebulizer is pole mounted and produces an aerosol output of 0 to 6.0 ml/min (Fig 13–24). Particle size is the same as that for the model 35B. The built-in blower incorporates an air control valve to vary the amount of air used to deliver aerosol to the patient. The nebulizer unit incorporates a lead zircon transducer. The power section develops a frequency of 1.35 MHz. The solution cup holds a maximum of 180 ml of solution, or a 3-L reservoir system may be attached to a continuous float-feed solution cup. Once assembled, the solution cup is filled for single use or by a reservoir system. The power toggle switch is placed in the on position, and the output control knob is set to deliver the desired amount of mist.

Assembly.—Following disinfection of the solution cup:

1. Place the drain tube into the drain tube clip (Fig 13–25).

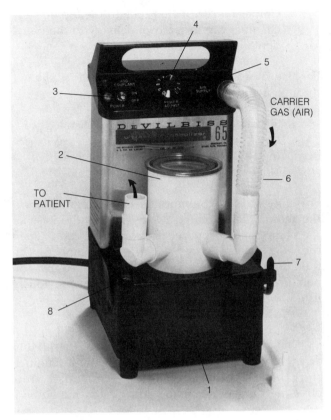

FIG 13–24.
The DeVilbiss model 65 ultrasonic nebulizer: *(1)* base containing transducer and couplant chamber, *(2)* solution cup, *(3)* power switch, *(4)* power adjust, *(5)* air control valve, *(6)* carrier gas tubing, *(7)* couplant drain hose, and *(8)* couplant indicator window. (Courtesy of DeVilbiss Health Care Division, Somerset, Penn.)

2. Fill the couplant chamber with distilled water until it reaches the fill line indicator. The float should now be up against the retaining clip.
3. Clip the solution cup between the two halves of the chamber cover (Fig 13–26). Place this assembly into the couplant chamber so that the hold-down tabs hold the couplant chamber cover in place. The indicator window will show black when there is sufficient water in the couplant chamber.
4. Connect a corrugated tubing between the blower outlet and the solution cup. An additional corrugated tubing goes to the patient (see Fig 13–24). At this point, any other carrier gas may alternately be connected to the solution cup inlet.
5. Fill the solution cup from the solution bottle or reservoir for patient use (Fig 13–27).

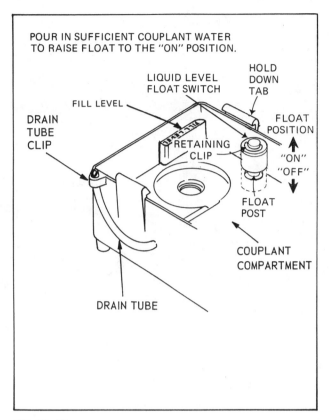

FIG 13–25.
Filling the couplant chamber of a DeVilbiss model 65 ultrasonic nebulizer. (Courtesy of DeVilbiss Health Care Division, Somerset, Penn.)

Pulmosonic Nebulizer

The Pulmosonic is a personal home-use ultrasonic nebulizer that comes in a carrying case. It is specifically designed and built for nebulization of a small amount of medication and diluent (no more than 10 ml). It functions the same as other ultrasonic nebulizers in that it generates a frequency of 1.35 MHz. Output of the Pulmosonic is 0.5 ml/min. When it is in use, the patient uncoils the cable and plugs in the power cord. The medication is put into the medication chamber. The nebulizer chamber, baffle, check valve, and mouthpiece are assembled (Fig 13–28). The unit is turned on and remains on until the medication is depleted. One-way valves prevent rebreathing of exhaled gas.

Mistogen MP-500 Ultrasonic Nebulizer

The Mistogen MP-500 ultrasonic nebulizer (Fig 13–29) has similar performance characteristics to the DeVilbiss 65 unit. It is usually mounted on a stand and has a built-in blower unit. The transducer is molded into the couplant chamber as a unit, which

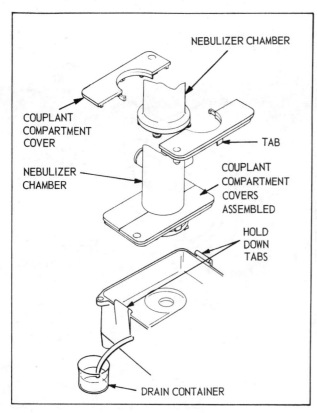

FIG 13–26.
Solution cup placement. (Courtesy of DeVilbiss Health Care Division, Somerset, Penn.)

is detachable for cleaning. The transducer/couplant chamber may double as the solution cup, or an additional solution cup may be immersed in the couplant chamber, depending on user preference.

Assembly.—Following disinfection (Fig 13–30):

1. Place the transducer/couplant chamber *(1)* in its socket at the right rear of the power unit.
2. Plug the hole in the base of the transducer/couplant chamber with the cap *(2)*.
3. Connect the cable *(3)* to its plug on the transducer/couplant chamber.
4. For a single treatment, fill the chamber with solution to a level no more than ¼ in. above the water inlet float *(4)* (float with retainer clip). It will provide an aerosol for approximately 15 minutes, until the switch float *(5)* shuts the unit off.
5. Place a clean filter *(6)* in the blower assembly *(7)*.
6. Screw the chamber cap *(8)* on.
7. Connect a corrugated tube *(9)* from the blower to the side of the chamber cap.

8. Connect a corrugated tube to the top of the chamber cap for aerosol delivery to the patient.

For use of a separate solution cup, follow steps 1 through 3 and then:

4. Fill the chamber with 200 ml of distilled water.
5. Install the solution cup, and attach the blower and patient corrugated tubing.

For use with a continuous-feed system, connect the feed system tubing to the hole in the base of the chamber (as opposed to using the cap). Open the feed system clamp to fill the chamber. The fluid level will adjust as it is consumed by the nebulizer. Follow steps 5 through 8 as previously listed.

Mistogen Electronic Humidilizer EH 147B

The Mistogen Electronic Humidilizer EH 147B is designed for two purposes: (1) as a room humidifier and (2) as an air-mist humidifier with mask-mouthpiece and large-bore tubing. As a room humidifier,

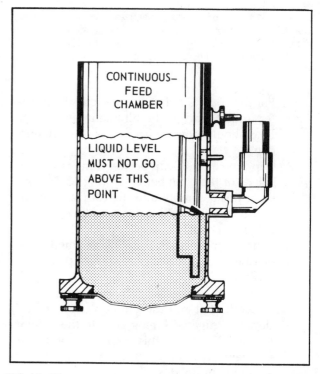

FIG 13–27.
Proper fill level of solution cup for DeVilbiss model 65 ultrasonic nebulizer. (Courtesy of DeVilbiss Health Care Division, Somerset, Penn.)

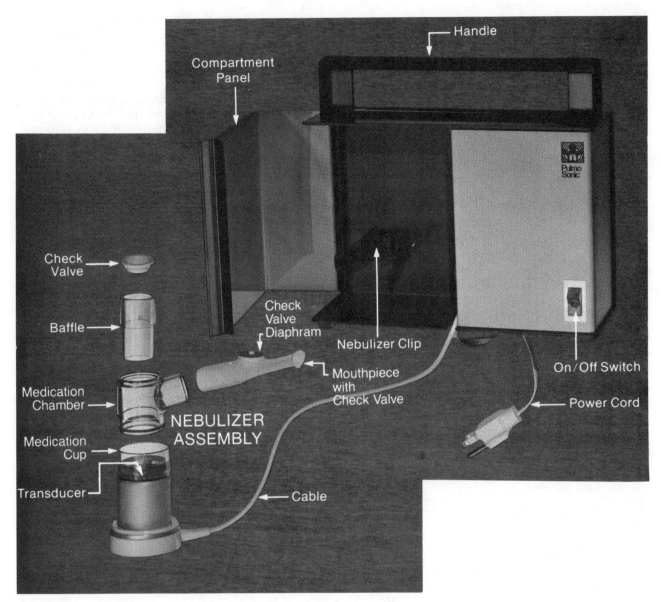

FIG 13–28.
The Pulmosonic ultrasonic nebulizer. (Courtesy of DeVilbiss Health Care Division, Somerset, Penn.)

it has a 6 ml/min output, operates continuously, and shuts off automatically when the 4.7-L reservoir becomes low.

Assembly.—Following disinfection (Fig 13–31):

1. Place the float assembly *(1)* into the oscillator chamber slots.
2. Place the blower stack *(2)* in position over the oscillator and float assembly.
3. Position the cover and nozzle *(3)* over the blower stack.

4. If preparing for patient use, fill the reservoir *(4)* with tap water and replace its lid *(5)*.
5. Invert the reservoir, and fit it in place adjacent to the cover.
6. Plug in the power cord, and turn on the unit.

The air-mist humidifier unit is optional. It is a one-piece unit that fits onto the oscillator chamber, having its own solution reservoir. This unit is used as other ultrasonic nebulizers. The output is approximately 3 ml/min.

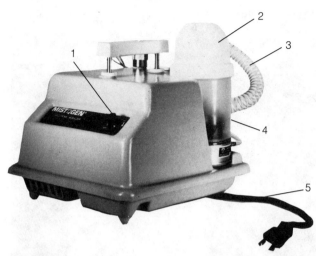

FIG 13–29.
Exterior and function control of the Mistogen EN-145 ultrasonic nebulizer: *(1)* on/off switch and output control, *(2)* solution cup cover, *(3)* corrugated hose from blower to solution cup cover, *(4)* transducer/couplant chamber/solution cup, and *(5)* power cord. (Courtesy of Mistogen/Timeter Products, Lancaster, Penn.)

Applications

Although the output of the nebulizer itself may be relatively constant, a number of variables will cause a decreased amount of aerosol actually delivered to the patient. These variables include baffling and condensation in the tubing, an increase in the gas flow carrying the aerosol, the temperature of the liquid in the solution cup, and high-viscosity solutions. The residue from soaps or plastics entering the solution cup may also decrease aerosol output.

Medications such as bronchodilators and chemical mucolytics should not be added to large-capacity ultrasonic nebulizer solution cups due to the possibility of drug reconcentration.[6] This occurs because different fluids nebulize at different rates. Water and saline nebulize faster than do other medications because of their lower molecular weights.

The ultrasonic nebulizer has been applied therapeutically in many ways, often without documented worth or scientific basis. Among these uses have been mist tent therapy, intermittent therapy with and without IPPB, and continuous therapy to patients with artificial airways. Particles produced by the ultrasonic nebulizer have a typical size of 3 μ, suitable for small airways deposition. Accordingly, the ultrasonic nebulizer could be used for aerosol therapy where solution particles are supposed to deposit in small airways (<2 mm in diameter). Since croup is an upper airway disorder, the ultrasonic nebulizer is not recommended and may be contraindicated in any case for small children and infants due to the possibility of fluid overload.[17] Care must be taken to assure that too much solution is not delivered. The ultrasonic nebulizer has been used to provide sterile water or hypertonic saline (10%) to

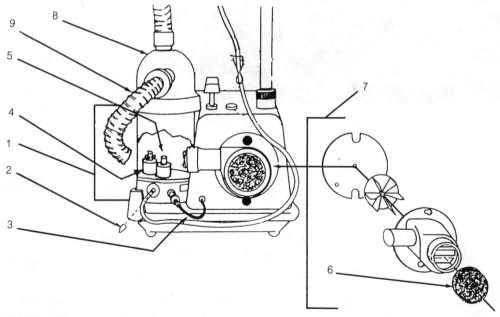

FIG 13–30.
Assembly of the Mistogen EN-145 ultrasonic nebulizer. (See text for description of parts.) (Courtesy of Mistogen/Timeter Products, Lancaster, Penn.)

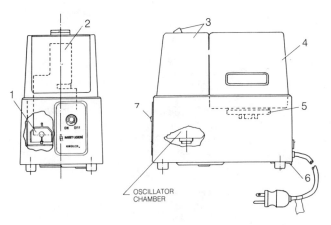

FIG 13–31.
The Mistogen Electronic Humidilizer EH 147B: *(1)* float assembly, *(2)* blower stack, *(3)* cover and nozzle, *(4)* reservoir, *(5)* reservoir lid, *(6)* filter, and *(7)* power knob. (Courtesy of Mistogen/Timeter Products,Lancaster, Penn.)

the airways to induce sputum for cytologic or bacterial studies (see Chapter 6).

Following assembly and filling, the operator should assure that all solutions spilled are wiped up. Solutions on the floor or on the nebulizer provide a current path and may contribute to an electric shock if improper contact is made with the operator or patient. The other hazard is contamination of the solution cup which may occur if one solution cup is used for several days. Daily replacement or use of a disposable solution cup should help to decrease the incidence of nosocomial infection.

Patient connection is made with the appropriate interface. For treatments, the mouthpiece should be used to assure mouth breathing. A port of exhalation, such as a T piece adjacent to the mouthpiece, should be provided to prevent rebreathing. The tracheostomy mask or T piece is used for patients with artificial airways. Large-bore aerosol tubing is always used to deliver ultrasonic mist. For continuous use, a water trap should be placed in the loop of the tubing. A water bolus in the tubing will drastically reduce the amount of mist delivered. Troubleshooting the ultrasonic nebulizer is basically the same for all units (Table 13–6).

Hydrosphere Nebulizers

The hydrosphere or Babington nebulizer differs from the jet nebulizer in that it has a glass sphere (1, Fig 13–32) over which a thin film of solution constantly flows. There is a hole in the sphere through which source gas exits at supersonic velocity. This blast of gas ruptures the film of solution into parti-

cles that are then impacted against a baffle. The resultant particle size is 3 to 5 μ. The solution in the reservoir is lifted up a capillary tube (2, Fig 13–32) by bubbles created as a result of splitting the source gas flow. Source gas flows into the nebulizer and splits, some of it going to the sphere, the rest to a tube that extends beneath the surface of the solution reservoir (3, Fig 13–32). The distal end of the tube is constructed such that solution is trapped above each bubble. Each bubble then lifts a small amount of solution through another tube to a reservoir above the sphere. The reservoir drains via gravity over the sphere.

Solo-Sphere Nebulizer

The Solo-Sphere nebulizer operates according to the previous description. It has an operating range

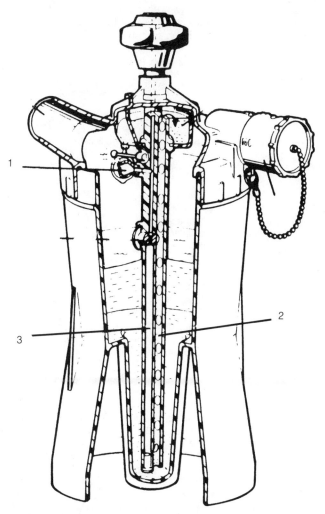

FIG 13–32.
The Solo-Sphere nebulizer and its component parts illustrate the Babington principle. (See text for description of parts.) (Courtesy of Airlife/American Pharmaseal Company, Montclair, Calif.)

TABLE 13–6.

Ultrasonic Nebulizer Troubleshooting*

SYMPTOM	POSSIBLE PROBLEM	SUGGESTED CHECK
1. Unit installed and connected as specified, but pilot light does not turn on when switch is turned to the "on" position.	Electrical outlet defective. Circuit breaker tripped. Fuse blown.	Check outlet with lamp or other appliance. Reset the circuit breaker or change fuse on the power switch. If the circuit breaker continues to trip or fuse blows again, service is needed.
2. Unit installed and connected as specified. Power pilot light turns on, and normal ultrasonic activity visible in nebulizer chamber, but no aerosol output.	Nebulizer chamber contaminated.	Wash nebulizer chamber, decontaminate.
3. Unit installed and connected as specified. Power pilot light turns on, but there is little ultrasonic activity visible in the nebulizer chamber, and aerosol output is low (even when on the no 10 power setting).	Couplant water excessively aerated. Nebulizer module and couplant water too cold. Diaphragm distorted, permitting air bubbles to interfere with proper transmission of vibrational energy into the nebulizer chamber. Couplant contaminated.	Wait for deaeration. Use warmer couplant water. Check to see that diaphragm is properly shaped and installed. Be sure the concave (recessed) side faces the interior of the chamber. Clean couplant compartment and replace couplant water.
4. Same as symptom no 3 but at a lower power setting.	Power setting too low to start and establish nebulization.	Turn output control knob to maximum power setting, then reduce to desired setting.
5. Unit installed and connected as specified. Power pilot light turns on. "Add couplant" light is on, and there is no ultrasonic activity visible in the nebulizer chamber.	Insufficient couplant water.	Add water to the couplant compartment.
6. Unit installed and connected as specified. Power pilot light turns on. "Add couplant" light is off, but there is no ultrasonic activity visible in the nebulizer chamber.	Power supply overheated and its thermostatic control opened.	The cooling air has been restricted or cooling fins need cleaning. The switch will reset when the equipment returns to room temperature.
7. Liquid reservoir filled and properly connected to nebulizer chamber, but chamber does not fill (for *continuous-feed system only*).	Foreign material or air bubbles in feed tubes. Liquid level control in nebulizer chamber plugged with foreign material. Air leaks at tube connections or reservoir cap.	Flush the system. Clean or flush the system. Tighten all connections by pushing tubes into fittings.

*Courtesy of DeVilbiss Health Care Division, Somerset, Penn.

of 10 to 50 psi and will deliver approximately 15 L/min undiluted source gas with the air-entrainment port blocked. The air-entrainment port is marked to deliver FI_{O_2}, of 0.40, 0.50, 0.60, 0.80, and 1.00. Table 13–7 lists manufacturer's air-entrainment ratios for these FI_{O_2} levels. Since the maximum source gas flow is 15 L/min, the maximum minutes output of a Solo-Sphere is 63 L/min of gas at an FI_{O_2} of 0.4. The aerosol output capacity is approximately 2 ml/min.

Assembly.—Following disinfection, the equipment should be aseptically assembled and packaged in a clean, dry area (Fig 13–33):

1. Replace the bottom diverting plug *(1)* into the base of the lift tube *(2)*.
2. Replace the bubble pump plug *(3)* with the flat side facing the sphere *(4)*.
3. Seat the large O ring *(5)* into the jar top *(6)*.
4. Align and insert the manifold *(7)* into the jar top (right and left sides are indicated.)
5. Secure the manifold with the thumb screws *(8)*.
6. Attach the reservoir *(9)* to the jar top. Package and store.

Application.—The Solo-Sphere is used in the same manner as the large-capacity jet nebulizer. Once an order for aerosol is confirmed, the nebulizer, aerosol tube, and patient attachment are taken to the patient's room. The nebulizer is attached to the flowmeter, and the reservoir is filled with solution to the fill line and replaced. The FI_{O_2} is set as prescribed. The aerosol tubing is connected to the nebulizer, and a water trap is placed. The patient attachment is connected to the aerosol tube. The gas flow is started, and patient attachment is made.

A heater that clips onto its base is available for the Solo-Sphere. The heater does not come in contact with the solution. The heater will warm the solution in a full nebulizer to 50°C in 20 minutes at the maximum temperature setting. The heater is de-

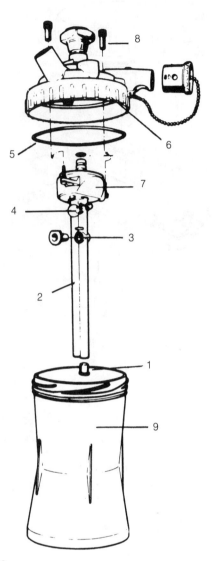

FIG 13–33.
Assembly of the Solo-Sphere nebulizer. (See text for description of parts.) (Courtesy of Airlife/American Pharmaseal Company, Montclair, Calif.)

signed to deliver a maximum aerosol temperature of 35°C at the high heat setting and low total flow. As always, when a heater is used, the temperature at the airway must be monitored.

Maxi-Cool Nebulizer

The Maxi-Cool hydrosphere nebulizer is intended for use with mist tents. It can be used interchangeably with the Ohmeda Ohio or Mistogen high-output nebulizers previously described. Mist tent assembly follows that of those described in the section on mist tents. The Maxi-Cool is pneumatically powered at 50 psi. A multiposition air-entrainment device attaches to the nebulizer. This device

TABLE 13–7.

Air-Entrainment Ratios for the Solo-Sphere Nebulizer FI_{O_2} Levels

FI_{O_2}	AIR/OXYGEN
0.40	4.20:1
0.50	2.70:1
0.60	2.00:1
0.80	1.25:1
1.00	1.00:1

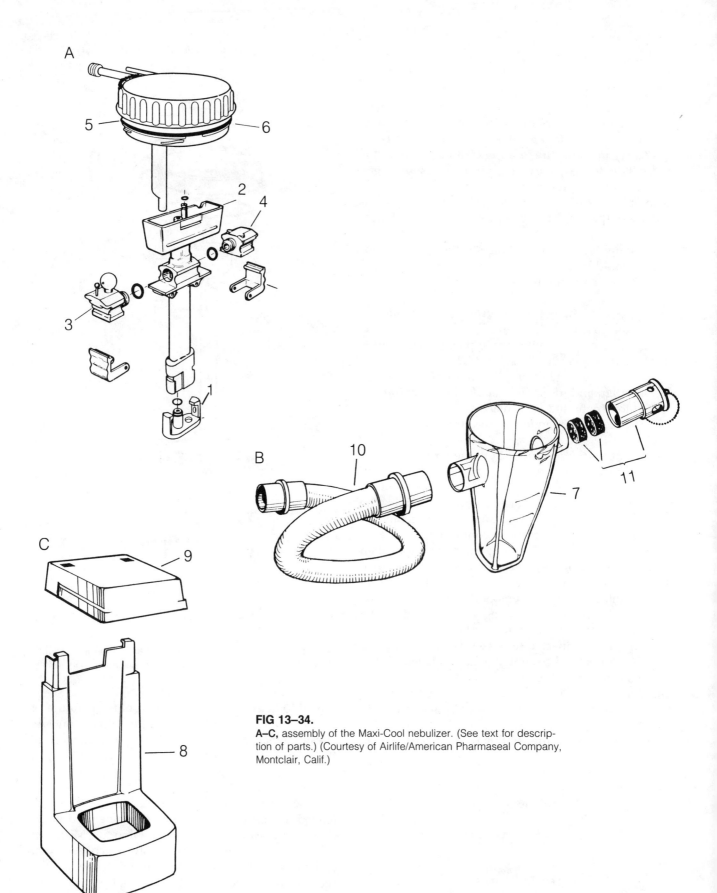

FIG 13–34.
A–C, assembly of the Maxi-Cool nebulizer. (See text for description of parts.) (Courtesy of Airlife/American Pharmaseal Company, Montclair, Calif.)

permits the FI_{O_2} to be adjusted to 0.28, 0.35, 0.40, 0.46, 0.67, or 0.98. Total flow may be varied from 30 to 285 L/min depending on entrainment setting and source gas flow. Aerosol output ranges from 1.5 to 7.7 ml/min, proportional to total flow.

Assembly.—Following disinfection, the equipment should be aseptically assembled and packaged in a clean, dry area (Fig 13–34,A–C):

1. Replace the pump plug *(1)* into the base of the manifold *(2)*.
2. Replace the sphere assembly *(3)* and low-flow adapter *(4)* into the manifold, and secure with catch-lock mechanisms.
3. Replace the large O ring *(5)* onto the jar top *(6)*.
4. Align the jar top and manifold, and press them together, assuring that the lid latches snap into the grooves on the manifold.
5. Place the vessel *(7)* into the housing base *(8)*.
6. Insert the manifold assembly into the vessel, and turn it clockwise to lock.
7. Attach the housing cover *(9)*.
8. Connect a high-pressure hose to the threaded outlet at the rear of the nebulizer.
9. Connect a large-bore aerosol hose *(10)* to the nebulizer outlet adjacent to the sphere.
10. Attach the air-entrainment device and filters *(11)* to the nebulizer adjacent to the low-flow adapter on the manifold.

Application.—The mist tent canopy is prepared at the bedside according to the manufacturer's instructions. The nebulizer is prepared by attaching the solution feed tubing to the ports adjacent to the high-pressure hose at the rear of the nebulizer. Water level in the nebulizer adjusts as it is consumed. The large-bore aerosol hose is attached to the tent canopy. The high-pressure hose is attached to a flowmeter, which is plugged in and turned on to 15 L/min. The desired FI_{O_2} is set and analyzed.

BUBBLE HUMIDIFIERS FOR OXYGEN THERAPY DEVICES

This discussion will concern bubble humidifiers used to humidify dry oxygen at flow rates more than 4 L/min.[1, 4, 11] The typical bubble humidifier consists of several components (Fig 13–35). Gas from the flowmeter enters the humidifier via a Diameter In-

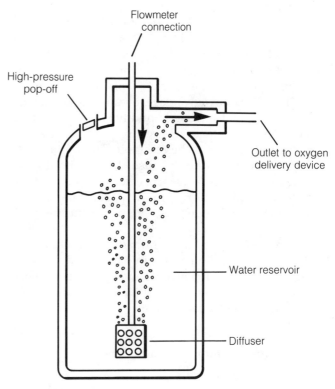

FIG 13–35.
Schematic of a nondisposable bubble humidifier.

dex Safety System (DISS) oxygen connector (see Chapter 12). The gas proceeds down a tube submerged in sterile water and is delivered to a diffuser. The diffuser, made of metal, plastic, porous rock, or other porous material, causes the gas to be broken into numerous very small bubbles. This action tends to increase relative humidity. The gas bubbles travel to the water surface, and gas escapes through a nipple designed to accommodate oxygen therapy small-bore tubing. A high-pressure release, which is usually audible, is incorporated into the humidifier. Usually, these devices sound if pressure meets a 2-psi limit. There are both nondisposable and disposable bubble humidifiers. They vary in respect to reservoir size and efficiency of the diffuser.

A second type of humidifier in use for oxygen therapy equipment is the jet humidifier. The jet humidifier is actually an atomizer, creating an aerosol. However, because of the presence of a sponge baffle, all particles are removed from the gas going to the therapy device. Because this device increases the gas-water interface, the relative humidity at a given flow is higher than that of a simple bubble humidifier.

A third type of humidifier used for oxygen therapy is the underwater jet humidifier. This humidifier incorporates the jet and bubble concepts. Gas blows through a jet below the water surface, creating aerosol particle-filled bubbles. When the gas bubbles reach the reservoir surface, they break, releasing humidified gas for delivery to the patient. The Ohio Jet humidifier is an example of this classification.

The apparent advantage of underwater jet humidifiers is that relative humidity is independent of the reservoir water level because the aerosol is produced at the base of the reservoir. There is a potential for contamination because these units do produce aerosols. If these particles are not baffled, bacteria could be carried to the patient. Careful disinfection on a 24-hour basis may prevent this problem.

The disposable bubble humidifiers in use are designed to deliver a high relative humidity at operating temperature. Relative humidity in these devices will decrease as water level drops because of decreased gas-water contact time.

Nondisposable Bubble Humidifiers

Chemetron Humidifier

The Chemetron humidifier is typical of bubble humidifiers. The humidifier consists of plastic reservoir and lid that incorporates a 2-psi pressure release (Fig 13–36). Following disinfection, the lid parts are reassembled and the reservoir attached. The unit is stored aseptically until use.

Ohmeda Ohio Jet Humidifier

The Ohmeda Ohio Jet humidifier is an example of a device that mixes water with oxygen through a jet system (Fig 13–37). The water-oxygen mix is forced through a sintered metallic diffuser to disperse the moisture-laden oxygen. The humidified oxygen bubbles to the surface of the reservoir and exits through the nipple in the cap into the therapy device. Assembly consists of replacing the diffuser following disinfection and replacing the reservoir onto the cap. The usable reservoir volume of this humidifier is 200 ml. Water consumption is 6.25 ml/hour when operated at 10 L/min.

Puritan Bubble-Jet Humidifier

The Puritan Bubble-Jet humidifier was also covered in the section on large mainstream nebulizers. Assembly and use are basically the same with two differences. The switch is put in the "bubble" position, and the small-tube adapter is fitted onto the aerosol outlet (see Fig 13–12). The 200-ml reservoir may last 2 to 3 days at a liter flow of 2 to 3 L/min.

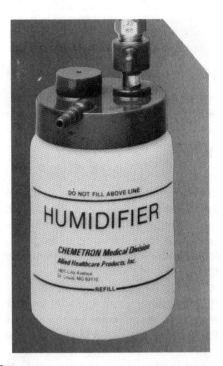

FIG 13–36.
The Chemetron bubble humidifier. (Courtesy of Chemetron/Allied Healthcare Products, St. Louis, Mo.)

The relative humidity (at 37°C) of this device ranges from 43% to 2.5 L/min to 29% at 10 L/min in a linear pattern.

Disposable Bubble Humidifiers

Most of the bubble humidifiers in use are disposable. They all have the same basic components described earlier. The major differences are the capacity of the reservoir and configuration of the diffuser. Those humidifiers that create smaller, more numerous bubbles are more efficient. A number of disposable bubble humidifiers with different performance characteristics are available (Table 13–8).

Assembly.—Most disposable units are in one or two pieces (Fig 13–38). Prefilled units include a sealed reservoir and a module that contains the DISS oxygen connector, the pressure release, and the nipple adapter. This module is in some way connected to the reservoir. Non-prefilled units come as a lid with the DISS connector, the pressure release, and the nipple adapter. The reservoir is filled to the indicated level, and the lid is screwed on.

Application.—Once the physician's order for oxygen therapy is confirmed, the flowmeter, humid-

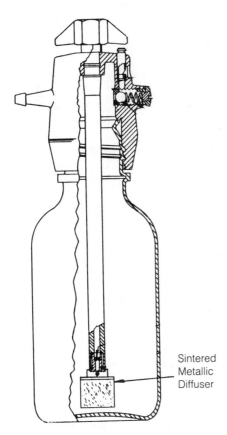

FIG 13–37.
The Ohmeda Ohio Jet humidifier. (Courtesy of Ohmeda, Madison, Wis.)

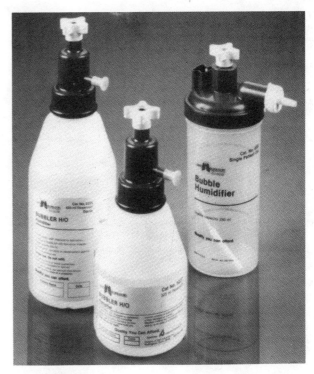

FIG 13–38.
Disposable bubble humidifiers. (Courtesy of Seamless/Dart Respiratory, Wallingford, Conn.)

ifier, and oxygen delivery device are taken to the patient's room. The patient is informed of the nature of the therapy and the device used. The flowmeter is installed. The humidifier is assembled and connected to the flowmeter. The oxygen delivery device (e.g., partial rebreathing mask) is connected to the nipple on the humidifier. The flowmeter is set to the prescribed flow, and the delivery tubing is kinked to check the pressure release. If the system is sealed and the release is working properly, there will be a hissing, rattling, or whistling, depending on the design of the release. The oxygen delivery device is then placed on the patient, and a no smoking sign is posted. Monitored parameters may include date and time, delivery device, oxygen flow rate, arterial blood gas analyses, and spontaneous ventilatory parameters. Monitoring the system consists of assuring cleanliness of the oxygen delivery device and the proper oxygen flow rate. Disposable prefilled humidifiers should be replaced when the water level reaches the specified level. Non-prefilled humidifiers are refilled until hospital policy dictates replacement. Disposable humidifiers are usually changed between patients.

HEATED MAINSTREAM HUMIDIFIERS

Heated humidifiers are used to heat and humidify the gas going through ventilator circuits and high-flow oxygen therapy devices such as masks and oxygen hoods. The American National Standard for Humidifiers and Nebulizers for Medical Use (ANSI Z-79.9, 1979) requires that the gas have a water content reaching the patient of at least 30 mg/L, which corresponds to 100% relative humidity at 86° F. The Emergency Care Research Institute (ECRI) recommends an output of at least 37 mg/L, which corresponds to 85% relative humidity at 93°F.[14] Saturated gas at 90°F is equivalent to approximately 70% relative humidity at body temperature (Fig 13–39). Additional components of these devices should include a temperature monitor, alarm or controller to limit maximum temperature at the airway to 104°F, a mechanism to sense if the temperature probe has become dislodged, and a low-temperature alarm set point above room temperature.[2]

There are four basic types of heated humidifiers in use. First is the heated pass-over type. Second are heated bubble humidifiers that employ a grid to decrease the size and increase the number of bubbles.

TABLE 13–8.

Performance Characteristics of Disposable Bubble Humidifiers*

HUMIDIFIER	MANUFACTURER	CAPACITY ML	DURATION	OUTPUT, ML/HR	% RELATIVE HUMIDITY AT ROOM TEMPERATURE	% RELATIVE HUMIDITY AT BODY TEMPERATURE	TYPE
Aquapak ("Quiet Humidifier")	Respiratory Care, Inc. Arlington Heights, IL 60004	340	64 hr at 5 L/min	4.61 at 5 L/min	71.1 at 5 L/min	35.0 at 5 L/min	Bubble
		650	138 hr at 5 L/min	4.55 at 5 L/min	70.2 at 5 L/min	34.4 at 5 L/min	
Aquapak ("Silent Humidifier")	Respiratory Care, Inc. Arlington Heights, IL 60004	440	91 hr at 5 L/min	4.40 at 5 L/min	67.4 at 5 L/min	33.1 at 5 L/min	Bubble
		760	156 hr at 5 L/min	4.62 at 5 L/min	71.1 at 5 L/min	34.8 at 5 L/min	
U-Mid	Seamless Hospital Products Wallingford, CT 06492	300	66 hr at 5 L/min	4.5 at 5 L/min	75 at 5 L/min	33 at 5 L/min	Jet
		500	111 hr at 5 L/min				
Inspiron	Inspiron Corp., Subsidiary of Omnicare, Inc. Rancho Coucamonga, CA 91730	300	79 hr at 4 L/min	3.8 at 4 L/min	95 at 4 L/min		Bubble
Corpak	Corpak, Inc. Wheeling, IL 60090	345	69.6 hr at 5 L/min	4.56 at 5 L/min	77 at 5 L/min	34 at 5 L/min	Bubble
		645	134 hr at 5 L/min	4.56 at 5 L/min			
OEM	OEM Medical Corp. Richmond, VA 23261	300 (non-prefilled)	9.6 hr to refill† at 5 L/min	4.15 at 5 L/min	62 at 5 L/min†		Bubble
IPI	Inhalation Plastics Niles, IL 60648	350, 550	Pending				Bubble
Airlife	American Hospital Supply Evanston, IL 60201	500	120 hr at 5 L/min	4.16 at 5 L/min	76 at 5 L/min		Bubble
Travenol	Travenol Laboratories, Inc. Deerfield, IL 60015	500					Bubble

*All data based on manufacturer's data unless otherwise noted.
†From Giordano SP, Holland EL: A performance comparison of disposable humidifiers. *Respir Therapy*, July/Aug 1973.

Third are heated wick humidifiers. These devices have a paper wick that is partially submerged in water. Surrounding the wick is a heating element. Fourth is the vapor-phase humidifier, which employs a hydrophobic filter. Water vapor is created below the filter, and only the water vapor created can diffuse through the filter en route to the patient. The most basic heated humidifier is the heated pass-over. This unit is found on the Emerson 3-PV Post-Operative volume ventilator and 3-MV intermittent mandatory ventilation (IMV) ventilator and has been known as the *hot pot*. Water is heated in the reservoir, and gas passes over it en route to the patient circuit. By itself, it is not as efficient as the other humidifiers discussed here.[14] The efficiency of the heated pass-over humidifier is enhanced in the Emerson IMV ventilator by passing the humidified gas through copper mesh that holds water and a heated inspiratory tube. If the tower is removed from a Cascade humidifier, it too becomes a heated pass-over type of humidifier. The tower has been removed to relieve inspiratory resistance when a Cascade humidifier is used in an IMV circuit without continuous flow.

Heated Bubble Humidifiers

In these devices, gas flows down a tube submerged in the water reservoir. The gas passes through a grid, which creates a large mass of bubbles. A heating element is either immersed in the reservoir or is beneath the reservoir, the base of

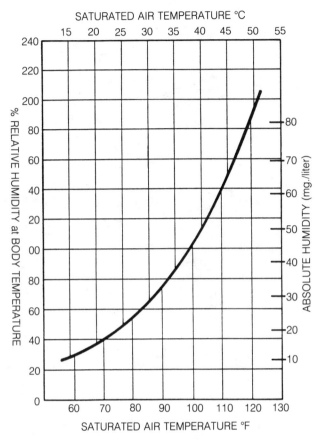

FIG 13–39.
Percent relative humidity at body temperature given saturated gas at different temperatures. (Courtesy of Ohmeda, Madison, Wis.)

which is metal. Water evaporates into the bubbles, which break at the reservoir's surface. The gas then proceeds to the patient.

Bennett Cascade Humidifiers

The Bennett Cascade I humidifier has been in use since the 1960s, often in conjunction with the Bennett MA-1 ventilator (Fig 13–40). the Cascade I is also useful for heated high-flow oxygen delivery. Gas enters the humidifier at the inlet and blows through a one-way valve, bubbling up through the grid. The sensing port is a hole in the tower. When the patient makes an inspiratory effort, this negative pressure is reflected through the sensing port so that an assisted breath may be delivered. Without the sensing port, the patient would have to exert an inspiratory effort equal to the depth of water in the reservoir in addition to the set assist effort. Heater temperature is controlled by the water temperature control. The numbers on this control indicate a range of temperatures (Table 13–9).

Since the Cascade I is not servo controlled, the water temperature control should be manipulated according to a thermometer placed at the airway. The heated, humidified gas exits the unit through the outlet.

Assembly.—Following disinfection, the equipment should be aseptically assembled and packaged in a clean, dry area (Fig 13–41):

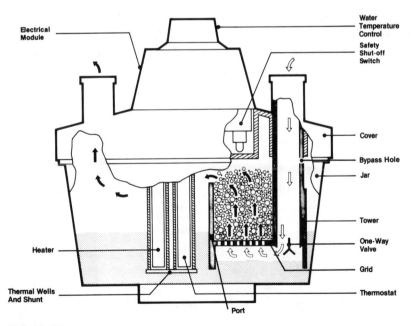

FIG 13–40.
Functional components of the Cascade I humidifier. (Courtesy of Puritan-Bennett Corporation, Overland Park, Kansas.)

TABLE 13–9.

Temperature Ranges for Particular
Control Numbers on the Cascade I

CONTROL NO.	RANGE OF TEMPERATURE, °C
1–5	20–35
5–6	35–37
6–7	> 37

1. Attach the heating element well *(1)* to the jar top *(2)* with the thumb screws *(3)*. Assure that the heating element well is firmly seated with the O rings *(4)*, because a loose connection here is a frequent source of leaks.

2. Assure that the seal *(5)* is in place in the jar top. If the seal is missing or torn, the jar will leak.

3. Insert the tower *(6)* into the jar top inlet and secure it with the screw *(7)*. Assure that the leaf valve *(8)* is in place in the tower.

4. Attach the reservoir *(9)*.

5. When the Cascade I is in use, it is attached to the heater control *(10)* with the locking tabs *(11)*.

Application.—The Cascade I reservoir is filled with sterile water and attached to the heater control. Once the unit is powered, it requires 20 minutes to warm up. The heater control should be adjusted to deliver gas at the desired temperature to the patient according to the thermometer proximal to the airway. Water consumption is proportional to gas temperature and flow. At any given heater setting, the gas temperature will decrease as the water level decreases and the gas flow decreases due to the increased time the gas is in the inspiratory tubing.[2] A float-feed system is available to maintain a constant water level. At flows of 8 to 14 L/min, the Cascade I produces a relative humidity at body temperature of 80%. A safety shutoff switch is incorporated into the heater control. When the jar is properly attached, the switch closes the power circuit of the heater.

Very similar to the Cascade I is the Ohmeda Ohio Heated Humidifier. The main difference between the two is in construction. The Ohmeda Ohio Heated Humidifier has a steel base that sits on a heater plate controlled by a thermostat. It is designed to deliver up to 100% relative humidity at body temperature at minute volumes up to 10 L/min.

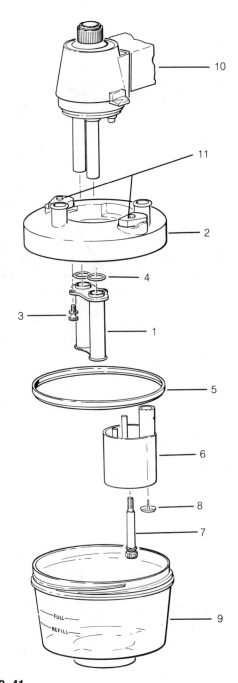

FIG 13–41.
Assembly of the Bennett Cascade I. (See text for description of parts.) (Courtesy of Puritan-Bennett Corporation, Overland Park, Kansas.)

Cascade II Humidifier

The Cascade II humidifier was introduced with the Bennett MA-2 ventilator. It is servo controlled by means of a thermistor at the proximal airway. Therefore, the operator sets the desired proximal airway temperature with a calibrated knob. An illuminated thermometer displays the proximal airway tempera-

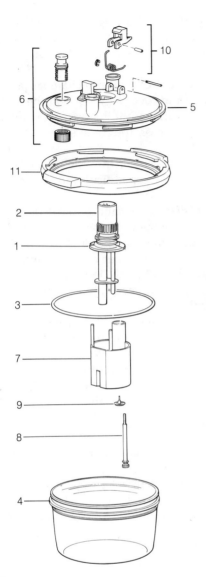

FIG 13–42.
Assembly of the Cascade II. (See text for description of parts.) (Courtesy of Puritan-Bennett Corporation, Overland Park, Kansas.)

ture. The temperature may be set in the range of 20° C to 42° C. The high temperature alarm can be set in the same range. If the water temperature should drop below 13° C, the humidifier recognizes a heater sensor failure condition, resulting in shutting off the humidifier power. A low water level condition is an additional alarm function.

Assembly.—Following disinfection, the equipment should be aseptically assembled and packaged in a clean, dry area (Fig 13–42):

1. Replace the O ring *(1)* on the heater core *(2)*.
2. Replace the jar seal *(3)* on the jar *(4)*.

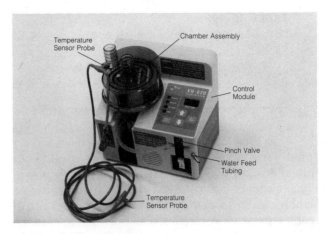

FIG 13–43.
BEAR VH-820 heated humidifier. (Courtesy of Bear Medical Systems, Inc., Riverside, Calif.)

3. Install the heater core into the jar top *(5)* from the inside, twisting the collar on the core to fix its position.
4. Replace the plug *(6)*.
5. Insert the tower *(7)* into the jar top inlet and secure it with the screw *(8)*. Assure that the leaf valve *(9)* is in place in the tower.
6. The latch assemblies *(10)*, used to hold the jar in place on the heater, are not disassembled for cleaning.
7. The locking ring *(11)* is affixed to the jar and is not removed for cleaning. When the jar top is latched to the heater, the locking ring is rotated to lock or loosen the jar.

The reservoir is filled with sterile water and latched to the heater control. The temperature probe is positioned in a socket at the patient wye. Warm-up time is 15 to 20 minutes. Temperature is maintained by the thermostat providing the water level is maintained between the full and refill levels. The humidifier can deliver gas at body temperature in the minute volume range of 3 to 25 L/min; however, the relative humidity of the delivered gas is not specified by the manufacturer.

BEAR VH-820 Heated Humidifier

The BEAR VH-820 humidifier (Bear Medical Systems, Inc,) can be mounted on a ventilator, column, or table and used with adults or infants (Fig 13–43). It is servo-controlled and has an alarm package to monitor proximal temperature, water level, and heater malfunction. A single, low-compliance and -resistance chamber serves both adult and infant applications (Table 13–10). The chamber assembly has

TABLE 13–10.

Compliance and Resistance of BEAR VH-820 Humidifier

RESERVOIR CAPACITY, ML	COMPLIANCE, ML/CM H$_2$O	RESISTANCE AT 60 L/MIN, CM H$_2$O/L/SEC
5–10	0.25	1.0

spiral vanes that provide a large surface area for humidification (Fig 13–44). The humidifier's operational systems include a rod heater, tube heater assembly, water level maintenance system, and proximal temperature controller. The operational systems are microprocessor-controlled by a closed-loop feedback servo-mechanism consisting of three thermistors and three controlled devices. The thermistors are located at the proximal airway, humidifier outlet, and within the rod heater. The controlled devices are the rod heater, the tube heater, and the solenoid-controlled pinch valve.

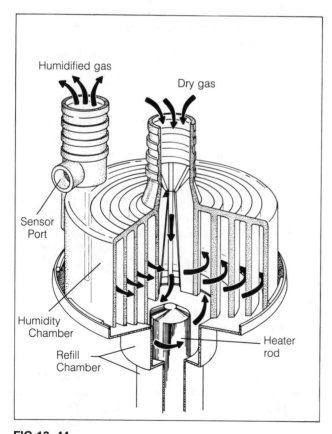

FIG 13–44.
Chamber assembly for BEAR VH-820 humidifier. (Courtesy of Bear Medical Systems, Inc., Riverside, Calif.)

Assembly.—Following disinfection, the equipment should be aseptically assembled and packaged in a clean, dry area (see Figs 13–43 and 13–44):

1. Install the O ring into chamber jar groove.
2. Place the cover assembly on the jar and turn it clockwise until it stops. The outlet port should be on the same side as the water feed port.
3. Insert the heater into the jar so that the flat surface is perpendicular to water feed tubing.
4. For infant application, install a 3/8-in. O.D. step-down adapter on the inlet and outlet ports of the chamber lid.
5. Install the chamber assembly into the control module and push down to secure.
6. Install water feed tubing in pinch valve assembly.
7. Connect tubing heater assembly to circuit and attach tube to the chamber outlet port.
8. Install probe jack into the receptacle on the left front of the control module.
9. Install probe sensors into the chamber outlet port and into the patient wye.

Application.—The humidifier is filled automatically by the pinch valve assembly, when the water level within the chamber assembly drops below the ⅛ level (approximately 1 ml). The humidifier normally operates at the ¼ to ½ level and has a normal water level of 5 to 10 ml. The humidifier takes 5 to 15 minutes to warm up. Once it is warm, the proximal temperature is displayed and servo-controlled at the desired level.

Heated Wick Humidifiers

Bird Wick Humidifier

The Bird wick humidifier has a cylindrical wick of blotter-type paper that is partially immersed in water (Fig 13–45). The wick soaks up the water, then it is warmed by the heating element that surrounds it. This humidifier is servo controlled by the thermistor readings at the airway. A float feed system holds the water level constant until the reservoir bag empties (Fig 13–46). Internal compliance is 0.23 ml/cm H$_2$O, and resistance is 0.3 cm H$_2$O at 60 L/min flow. One of the unique features of this humidifier is the ability to maintain 100% relative

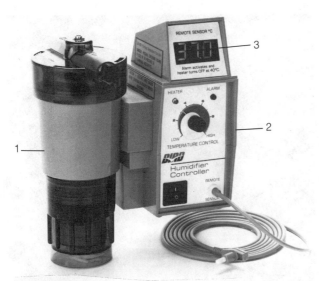

FIG 13–45.
Bird humidifier: *(1)* humidifier module, *(2)* humidifier controller, and *(3)* digital temperature readout. (Courtesy of Bird Corporation, Palm Springs, Calif.)

humidity at body temperature at continuous flows of up to 60 L/min. This is an important feature when continuous-flow IMV or continuous positive airway pressure (CPAP) ventilation is used. Alarms on this humidifier consist of an overheat audiovisual alarm, probe disconnect, and humidifier module disconnect.

Assembly.—Following disinfection, the equipment should be aseptically assembled and packaged in a clean, dry area (Fig 13–47):

1. Open and insert a wick *(1)* into the humidifier module *(2)*.
2. Place the float pad *(3)* into the lower float assembly *(4)*, and screw this assembly onto the bottom of the humidifier module, assuring correct placement of the bottom cap O rings *(5)*.
3. Twist the top cap *(6)* onto the humidifier module, assuring correct placement of the top cap O ring *(7)*.

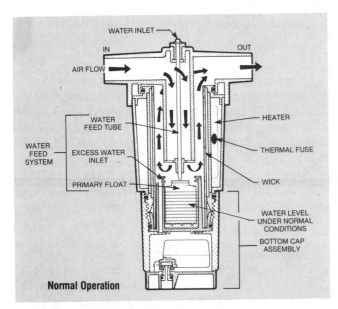

FIG 13–46.
Internal components of the Bird humidifier. (Courtesy of Bird Corporation, Palm Springs, Calif.)

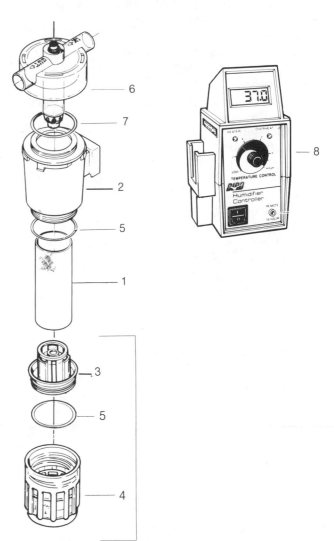

FIG 13–47.
Assembly of the Bird humidifier. (See text for description of parts.) (Courtesy of Bird Corporation, Palm Springs, Calif.)

4. The humidifier module may then be packaged and stored or installed onto the temperature controller (8) for use.

Application.—The humidifier module is installed on the temperature controller. A bag of sterile water is prepared with a *fill set*. The fill-set tubing adapts to the inlet on the top cap. The fill-set tube is left unclamped, and the water bag must be kept higher than the humidifier because it fills by gravity. The temperature sensor is plugged into the ventilator-patient circuit at the airway and into the temperature controller. Gas flow is started, and the humidifier is powered. The desired temperature is set by manipulating the temperature knob. The temperature should stay within ±1.0°C.

Fisher and Paykel Dual Servo MR450

The Fisher and Paykel Dual Servo MR450 is a servo-controlled heated wick humidifier that utilizes either disposable or reusable humidifier modules (Fig 13–48). The temperature control module features a temperature control knob, digital readout, power switch, probe plug, and alarm indicators for high temperatures (>38°C), low temperature (<30°C), and probe unplug. There are three humidifier modules: (1) disposable adult, (2) disposable infant, and (3) reusable adult. The reusable adult module has a wire, which when threaded into the patient circuit and heated, reduces condensation. Assembly consists of sliding a sterile humidifier module onto the temperature control module. The humidifier module is held in place by a spring and plastic tab.

Application.—The bag of sterile water is prepared with a fill set. The fill set is attached to the outlet (center pole) of the humidifier module. Ventilator-patient circuit tubing is placed appropriately. The humidifier module is filled to the indicated level. The probe is placed at the proximal airway and control module. After gas flow starts, the control module is powered and the temperature adjusted.

Respiratory Care Conchapak

The Respiratory Care Conchapak is similar to the Bird humidifier. The humidifier module, however, is disposable so there are no disinfection needs. The reservoir sits adjacent to the humidifier module (Fig 13–49). The humidifier is filled by gravity. As the water in the system is consumed, the surface area of the paper wick that is exposed to gas flow increases. Therefore, the relative humidity at a

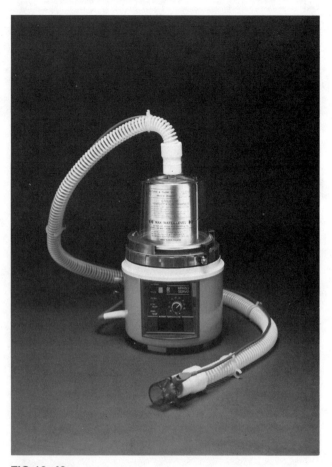

FIG 13–48.
Fisher and Paykel Dual Servo MR450 humidifier. (Courtesy of Fisher and Paykel/American Pharmaseal, Valencia, Calif.)

set gas flow may actually increase over the course of the consumption of the use of water in the reservoir bottle. The heater module consists of a power switch and heater control knob. This unit is not servo controlled, so a thermometer must be placed at the airway. Assembly consists of sliding a disposable humidifier module cylinder into the heater module, clamping the water reservoir in place, and attaching the two short tubes from the humidifier module to the reservoir.

Application.—The tubing clamps are opened to allow filling of the humidifier module. The unit is powered, and a 10-minute warm-up period should be allowed before temperature manipulation with gas flowing through the unit. A recent upgrade of the Conchapak is the Chonchatherm III, which incorporates a temperature probe and servo control. A

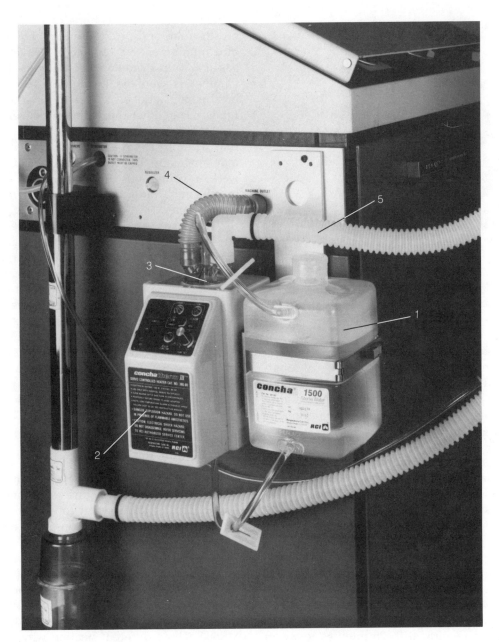

FIG 13–49.
Respiratory Care Conchapak: *(1)* reservoir, *(2)* heater module, *(3)* humidifier module, *(4)* tube from ventilator to humidifier, and *(5)* tube from humidifier to patient. (Courtesy of Respiratory Care Corporation, Arlington Heights, Ill.)

similar unit is the Travenol HLC 37, which is servo controlled, controls its water feed system, and has an alarm package.

Vapor Phase Humidifier

The Vapor Phase humidifier (Inspiron) is a servo-controlled unit incorporating a hydrophobic filter in its humidifier module (Fig 13–50). The disposable humidifier module sits on the heater unit in the same fashion as in the Fisher and Paykel humidifier. A reservoir of water adjacent to the humidifier supplies 10 ml of water at all times to the heated surface. The water is vaporized, and only water vapor passes through the hydrophobic filter. Because of this mechanism, sterile water is not required.

The heater module contains controls for power, a digital proximal airway temperature readout, alarm indicators, and a temperature set knob. Resistance

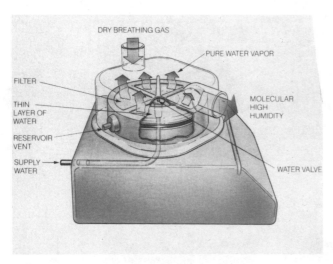

FIG 13–50.
Schematic diagram of the Vapor Phase humidifier. (Courtesy of Inspiron Corporation, Division of C.R. Bard, Inc., Rancho Coucamonga, Calif.)

and compliance are both very low because there is no liquid water for the patient to breathe through and the humidifier module is small. Relative humidity is reported to be adequate to eliminate humidity deficit. The Vapor Phase humidifier is also available in a non-servo-controlled model.

Application.—Heated humidifiers on ventilators are an essential part of the circuit unless a hygroscopic condenser humidifier is used. Typically, a flexible tube is placed between the mainstream bacteria filter and inlet of the humidifier. Then the inspiratory tube of the ventilator circuit is connected to the outlet side of the humidifier. The electric power for the humidifier is drawn from the ventilator. During ventilator setup, the humidifier's water reservoir is monitored, and the circuit is allowed to warm prior to patient application. Presently available humidifiers require 20 to 25 minutes to warm up to 30°C at the patient connection. Since it has been stated that relative humidity should be 100% at 86°F to prevent the pulmonary complications related to a dry mucosa, this should be taken into consideration in patient application.[14] The Cascade I, the Conchatherm, and the Bird humidifiers exceeded this specification at continuous flows of up to 30 L/min.[14] The Cascade humidifier exceeded this specification with flow rates up to 40 L/min, and the Bird humidifier exceeded the standard until flow rates reached 60 L/min. Each of these humidifiers delivered saturated gas at 37°C in simulated mechanical

ventilation at a tidal volume of 1,000 ml, rate of 12 breaths/min, and peak flow of 60 L/min.[14] Only the Bird humidifier was capable of delivering saturated gas at 37°C in a simulated continuous-flow IMV trial. Parameters were tidal volume 1,000 ml, rate of 7 breaths/min, and peak and continuous flows of 60 L/min. The other humidifiers delivered saturated gas at 28°C to 30°C in the IMV and continuous-flow trial. The BEAR VH-820 humidifier with tube heater may maintain 90% humidity at 35°C. Parameters were a continuous flow of up to 60 L/min, 14 breaths/min, and a peak flow of 40 L/min (manufacturer's data).

There are variables that will cause either a proportional increase or decrease in the amount of water vapor delivered to the patient. Variables that increase water vapor delivery are water reservoir temperature, ambient temperature, and heated inspiratory tubing. Variables that decrease water vapor delivery are water reservoir dead space and gas flow in the patient circuit. Therefore, the ideal humidifier is one that would deliver saturated gas at 32°C to 34°C, possess the ability to maintain a sufficient water reservoir temperature, heat the inspiratory tubing, and minimize or hold reservoir dead space constant.

Heated Ventilator Breathing Circuits

The inspiratory limb of a ventilator circuit, when heated, offers several distinct advantages over nonheated circuits: lower water consumption, little or no condensation, and elimination of the need for water traps. Two configurations are available.

First, a flexible wire is threaded into the inspiratory limb of the circuit. The fitting at the origin of the wire is joined to the cuff at the origin of the inspiratory tube, and this assembly is fitted to the humidifier output of the Fisher and Paykel Dual Servo MR500. Three different heating wires are available, depending on the length of the inspiratory tube. Temperature is sensed both at the humidifier and at the patient airway. The servo control unit and heated wire maintain an even temperature from the humidifier to the patient. This mechanism permits a lower water temperature in the humidifier module.

The control module houses alarms for circuit plug disconnection, high and low temperatures, a digital display of proximal airway temperature, and a temperature control knob. The performance characteristics of the Fisher and Paykel Dual Servo MR500 are similar to those of the MR450.

The only drawbacks of this system are the additional connections and the procedure involved in threading the heating wire into the ventilator circuit. These disadvantages emphasize the need for careful circuit integrity monitoring and infection control.

The other configuration for heated ventilator circuit is the wire-wrapped tubing. In the Emerson heated circuit, a wire is wrapped around the length of its permanent-type tubing. At each end of the wire there is a plug that fits a socket in the front panel of the Emerson IMV ventilator. There are no additional circuit connections in this system. However, it is not servo controlled, nor are there any alarms. Circuit temperature is regulated by a control knob on the control panel and monitored by a thermometer proximal to the airway.

Heat and Moisture Exchangers

These devices are the newest technology for airway humidification. They are known synonymously by several names: the heat and moisture exchanger, the hygroscopic condenser humidifier, and the artificial nose. The basic unit is the heat and moisture exchanger. The newer devices add a hygroscopic material. Therefore, even though they are referred to synonymously, there is a difference, primarily that the hygroscopic condenser humidifier is more efficient than the humidity and moisture exchanger. The principle behind the humidity and moisture exchanger and hygroscopic condenser humidifier is simply that the heat and humidity in exhaled gas is trapped and then released to dry inspired air, returning the heat and humidity to the patient's airways. The primary concern in the use of the hygroscopic condenser humidifier is efficiency. Research has been done to determine what humidity needs to be delivered to the lower airways to prevent the complications of pulmonary arteriovenous shunting, arterial desaturation, and decreased compliance, surfactant, and ciliary transport.[12, 16, 20] A study by Weeks and Ramsey found that a minimal level of 23 mg/L (100% relative humidity at 25°C) is acceptable.[20] Mebius reports a water content of 25 to 30 mg/L (57%–68% relative humidity at 37°C) and a temperature around 32°C at the upper part of the trachea to be adequate to preserve mucociliary and lung function.[12] The ECRI concluded that a hygroscopic condenser humidifier should have an output of 21 to 25 mg/L at 27°C to 30°C to properly condition inhaled gas.[16] These studies present a range in absolute humidity of 21 to 30 mg/L, which represents a range of approximately 43% to 65% relative humidity at 37°C. The ECRI also found that an artificial airway itself serves as a heat and moisture exchanger, adding 5 to 8 mg/L and 3°C to 5°C to inspired gas. It could therefore be concluded that the minimum output of a hygroscopic condenser humidifier should be 21 mg/L at 37°C, although more humidity and a higher temperature would be more acceptable.

Additional considerations that are important in the design and use of the hygroscopic condenser humidifier are low dead space, compliance and resistance, no water reservoir, no water source or electrical power required, and lightweight or easily supported so as not to pull on the artificial airway. There should be little or no gas leakage (<30 ml/min at 30 cm H_2O), and they should be able to withstand an internal pressure of 100 cm H_2O.[3]

Product Descriptions

The Dameca heat and moisture exchanger is a reusable device with a corrugated aluminum roll core. All of the devices have conventional 22- and 15-mm tapered connectors except the Dameca which has an 11-mm connector. The aluminum insert should be changed daily and between patients. One unique feature of this unit is an oxygen inlet port for low-flow oxygen administration. A smaller unit is available for low tidal volume and pediatric use. The Engström Edith hygroscopic condenser humidifier is a disposable device with a woven fiber core coated with lithium salts. The lithium salts are the hygroscopic agents. The unique feature of the Edith is that it incorporates a molded plastic flex tube for connection between the patient wye and swivel adapter (Fig 13–51,A). A further developed model, the Edith 1000, has a dead space of only 28 ml (Fig 13–51,B). The Portex Humid-Vent is a disposable hygroscopic condenser humidifier with a hygroscopic material coated paper roll core (Fig 13–51,C). The Siemens-Elema Servo 150 and 151 hygroscopic condenser humidifier units have reusable housings with a disposable hygroscopically coated cellulose and felt core. Newer models (152 and 153) are completely disposable and contain a flex tube (Fig 13–51,D). The Terumo Brethaid heat and moisture exchanger is a disposable unit with an aluminum and fabric disk core (Fig 13–51,E). The *Vitalograph* heat and moisture exchanger is a reusable unit with a stainless steel core (Fig 13–51,F). Comparative data on all of these heat and moisture exchangers and hygroscopic condenser humidifiers are found in Table 13–11.

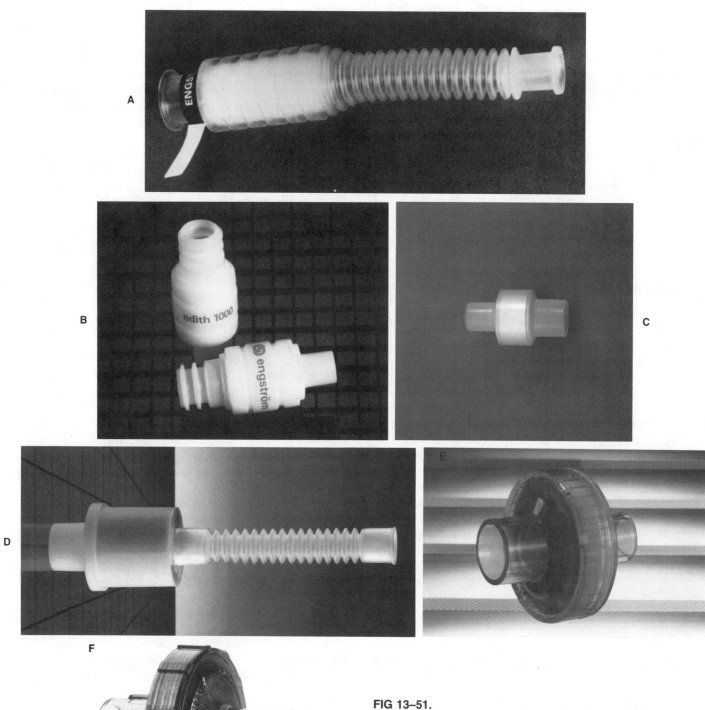

FIG 13–51.
Comparative sizes and shapes of available heat and moisture exchangers and hygroscopic condenser humidifiers. **A,** Engstrom Edith (Engstrom, Division of Gambro, Barrington, Ill.). **B,** Engstrom Edith 1000. **C,** Humid-Vent (Portex, Wilmington, Mass.). **D,** Servo 152 and 153 (Siemens-Elema, Schaumberg, Ill.). **E,** Brethaid (Terumo, Piscataway, N.J.). **F,** Vitalograph (Leaxana, Kansas).

TABLE 13–11.

Comparative Data on Heat and Moisture Exchangers and Hygroscopic Condenser Humidifiers*

MANUFACTURER	DAMECA	ENGSTROM†	PORTEX	SIEMENS-ELEMA		TERUMO	VITALOGRAPH
Model	Heat and Moisture Exchanger	Edith	Humid-Vent	Servo 150	Servo 151†	Brethaid	Vapor condenser
Dry weight, gm (oz)	44 (1.6)	25 (0.9)	9 (0.3)	41 (1.4)	25 (0.9)	14 (0.5)	67 (2.4)
Moisture output, mg/L (V_T = 666 ml; $\dot{V}$ = 40 L/min)	16	29 at V_T = 500 cc	21	25	27 at V_T = 500	14	16
Output gas temperature, °C	24	29	27	30	28.5	22	25
Compliance, ml/cm H_2O	0.062‡		0.01	0.09	0.03	0.01	0.03‡
Dead space, ml	62	90	10	90	30	10	30
Gas leakage at 30 cm H_2O, ml/min	0.800	0	0	0	0	0	50–500

*Unless otherwise noted data from Emergency Care Research Institute: Heat and moisture exchangers. *Health Devices* 1983;12:155–168.
†Data from Mebius C: A comparative evaluation of disposable humidifiers. *Acta Anaesthesiol Scand* 1983; 27:403–409, and manufacturer's literature.
‡Calculated from dead space due to excessive gas leakage.

Both the Siemens-Elema Servo and Engström hygroscopic condenser humidifier units have been studied for their properties as microbial filters. Following patient application, Stange and Bygdeman found no bacterial contamination in the expiratory limb of ventilator circuits when the Siemens-Elema Servo hygroscopic condenser humidifier was used.[19] In each case, bacteria were colonized in the patient's trachea and compared with cultures of the expiratory limb of ventilator circuits humidified by a heated water humidifier, where bacterial contamination was found in 2 of 15 cases. It has been reported that the growth of both bacteria and fungi were markedly reduced distal to the outlet of the Engström hygroscopic condenser humidifier.[9]

Application.—Heat and moisture exchangers are coming into wide use due to their low cost, ease of use, and elimination of need for water. However, there are a number of precautions the user must take. Since the heat and moisture exchanger is an attachment to the circuit, it provides two joints for possible airway disconnection. As a result, the airway disconnect pressure sensing line should be placed between the heat and moisture exchanger and the endotracheal tube. If this is not possible, the sensitivity pressure of the disconnect alarm should be set as close as possible to peak airway pressure. Heat and moisture exchangers should not be used in conjunction with heated humidifiers or placed downstream from nebulizers.

The use of multiple hygroscopic condenser humidifiers in series has been studied. The only successful application was when two and three Portex units were attached in series. This modification resulted in a moisture output of 22 and 23 mg/L at 30° C and 31° C, respectively. Other heat and moisture exchangers in series either did not provide adequate humidity or had too much dead space.[9]

Other than continuous use in mechanical ventilator circuits, a number of other uses have been suggested. In anesthesia, gas-tight heat and moisture exchangers can be used to humidify and decrease the amount of heat and moisture lost by the patient. Heat and moisture exchangers may also be used to humidify the airways of a spontaneously breathing patient with an artificial airway. The user would want to assure that the increased dead space the heat and moisture exchangers add does not interfere with ventilation. Patients who are being transported to special procedures or surgery and require ventilation may benefit from a heat and moisture exchanger since during transport it is not practical to use a heated humidifier.

It has been stressed that the use of heat and moisture exchangers and hygroscopic condenser humidifiers should be based on the requirements of the individual patient.[9] Patients with excessive secretions, damaged trachea, or impaired mucociliary clearance are not candidates for hygroscopic condenser humidifier use. During hygroscopic condenser humidifier use, more frequent tracheal suctioning and lavage may be necessary than when a conventional heated humidifier is used. If one or more of these problems develops during use of a hygroscopic condenser humidifier, it should be replaced by a conventional humidifier.

MIST TENTS

Croupette Cool Mist and Oxygen Tents

Croupette tents were introduced before the refrigerated tent units more commonly used now. Ice is used to cool the mist before delivery to the patient. In these units, a cooling chamber is secured to the base of an ice bath container so that the ice water does not enter the chamber. The nebulizer unit and distilled water reservoir are attached beneath the chamber. When gas is provided to the nebulizer, the aerosol particles flow into the chamber and out of the hose into the tent.

The Air-Shields Croupette Model D for infants has an output of 0.8 to 1.3 ml/min when supplied with oxygen at 8 to 10 L/min. The maximum F_{IO_2} supplied is 0.45 to 0.55. Using ice in the chamber will reduce the temperature of the tent environment 7°F to 10°F below room temperature. The larger Air-Shields Universal Croupette model for children has an output of 1.3 ml/min. With a 10 to 12 L/min source oxygen supply, the F_{IO_2} in the tent may reach 0.45 to 0.55. Use of ice in the chamber will reduce the temperature of the tent environment to 4°F to 5°F below room temperature.

Assembly

The Croupette Model D unit is a one-piece frame attached to a back panel that holds the nebulizer and ice chamber. The frame is unfolded, and the clear plastic tent is snapped in place. Ice is placed in the chamber, and distilled water is put in the nebulizer reservoir. Once adequate mist is assured, the infant can be placed in the tent. The Universal Croupette model has an over-bed frame from which the canopy is suspended. The nebulizer unit and ice chamber are attached to the head of the bed. Ice is placed in the chamber, and distilled water is put in the nebulizer reservoir.

Ohmeda Ohio Pediatric Aerosol Tent

The Ohmeda Ohio Pediatric Aerosol tent unit incorporates a refrigeration unit to cool the patient's environment, eliminating the need for ice. When in use, the unit is installed at the head of the bed with the canopy tucked under the mattress. The Ohmeda Ohio High Output nebulizer is used as previously described to provide aerosol. The refrigeration unit has two control settings. The cool setting causes cooling of the tent environment by 6°F to 16°F below room temperature. The circulate setting causes air to move within the canopy but will not provide cooling.

Assemble (Fig 13–52)

1. Assemble the condensate bottle (1) and bottle cap (2) through the condensate bottle bracket (3). The condensate tube (4) connects to the top of the condensate bottle.
2. Align the radial finned plate (5) on the evaporator (6), and secure it using the T-handle wrench (7) and four screws (8).
3. Attach the blower wheel (9) in place with the nut (10), and attach the condensate hose (4).
4. Push the evaporator shroud (12) over the evaporator, and rotate it counterclockwise into position.
5. Set the high-output nebulizer into the bracket (13). At this point, the tent may be stored until ready for use.
6. At the bedside, raise the canopy support rod (14) into position and secure.
7. Hang the canopy (15) from the canopy support arms (16), assuring that the three holes in the canopy are at the head of the bed. Smooth out the canopy wrinkles as much as possible.
8. Stretch the large round hole in the canopy around the evaporator shroud, assuring its fit in the shroud groove.
9. Attach the large white supply and return tubes to the canopy and towers of the high-output nebulizer.
10. Align the tent assembly with the head of the bed, and tuck the canopy under the mattress.
11. Attach a high-pressure hose to the high-output nebulizer. Attach the other end to a flowmeter, and plug it into the wall outlet.
12. Pour 2.5 L of sterile water into the reservoir.
13. Plug in the refrigeration unit.
14. Set the flowmeter for at least 10 L/min to avoid carbon dioxide accumulation and to provide adequate flow.
15. Set the refrigeration unit to cool or circulate as ordered.
16. Assure adequate mist and proper F_{IO_2} before placing the child in the tent.

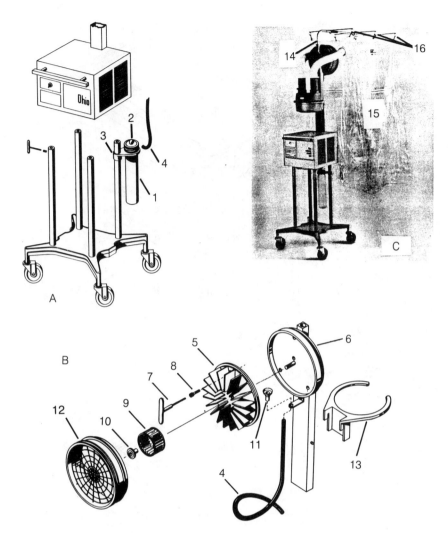

FIG 13–52.
A, assembly of the Ohio Pediatric Aerosol tent condensate trap. **B,** assembly of the cooling fan unit. **C,** bedside assembly of the canopy. (See text for description of parts.) (Courtesy of Ohmeda, Madison, Wis.)

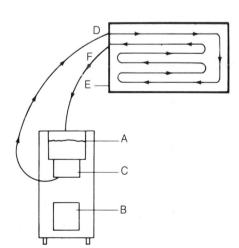

FIG 13–53.
Mechanism of atmospheric cooling in the Mistogen CAM-2 tent. How CAM operates: To start operation, first fill tank *(A)* with approximately 1 gal of distilled water. Refrigeration unit *(B)* chills this water. Pump *(C)* circulates chilled water first through line *D* through the channels of the Cool X Changer *(E)* and returns the water through line *F* back to tank *(A)* for rechilling. This is a continuous operation. (Courtesy of Mistogen/Timeter, Lancaster, Penn.)

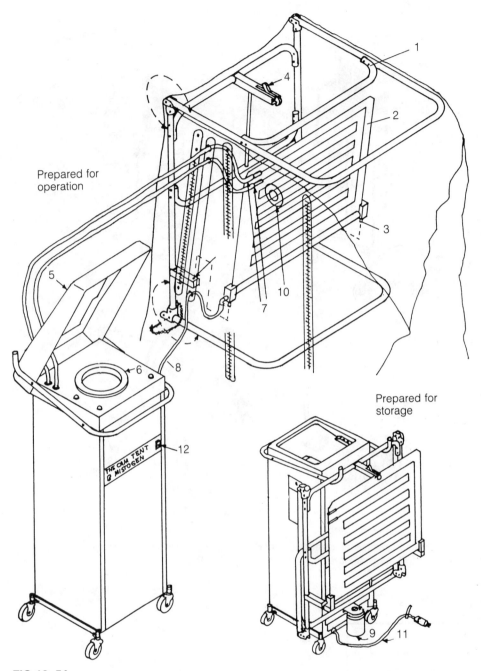

Prepared for operation

Prepared for storage

FIG 13–54.
Assembly of the Mistogen CAM-2 tent. (Courtesy of Mistogen/Timeter Products, Lancaster, Penn.)

Mistogen Child/Adult Mist (CAM) Tents 2 and 3

Both the CAM-2 and CAM-3 tents use the Mistogen HV-12 nebulizer previously described. The CAM-2 utilizes the refrigeration technique by chilling and circulating water through a panel inside the tent canopy (Fig 13–53). This mechanism does not circulate the air inside the tent as the Ohio tent does.

Assembly and Application

Following disinfection, aseptically (Fig 13–54):

1. Unfold the tent frame *(1)*, and slide the lower rail between the mattress and bedspring.
2. Install the cooling panel *(2)* in support block

holes *(3)* and hold in place with the latch *(4)*.

3. Attach the canopy to the frame as shown with the service holes adjacent to the control unit.

4. Do not allow the control unit to be less than 6 in. from the wall because heat is dissipated to the rear of the unit.

5. Lift the cover of the control unit *(5)*, and pour in approximately 1 gal of distilled water (to the lower lip of the circular collar *(6)*.

6. Connect the color-coded service tubes *(7)* to the fittings on the cooling panel and control unit. A click will be heard upon connection.

7. Connect the red color code tube *(8)* between the cooling panel and condensate drain assembly *(9)* (see folded storage diagram). Assure that there are no dips or loops in the condensate drain tube.

8. Assemble and place the nebulizer on the cover of the power unit. Connect the large white tube to the nebulizer and tent at *10*.

9. Attach a high-pressure gas hose to the nebulizer and a flowmeter, plugging it into the appropriate outlet.

10. Plug in the electrical cord *(11)*.

11. Turn on the power unit *(12)* and the gas flowmeter to 10 L/min.

12. Assure proper cooling, mist, and F_{IO_2} before placing the child in the tent.

CAM-3 Tent

The Cam-3 tent utilizes the *Peltier effect* for thermoelectric cooling. Peltier discovered that an electric current flowing across a semiconductor junction of dissimilar metals causes heat to be absorbed or released. If heat is removed from the hot side of the junction, the opposite side of the junction will cool. In the CAM-3, air from the tent environment flows over the cool air exchanger aided by a small fan. The patient environment heat is absorbed and transferred to the opposite side of the heat exchanger, where it is diffused by four small fans. In this process the air on the patient side of the thermoelectric cooling module is cooled and returned to the tent (Fig 13–55).

Use of the Peltier effect is the outstanding feature of the CAM-3 tent. Otherwise, its function, use, and assembly is similar to the Ohmeda Ohio tent. The unit is mounted on a frame with casters, supplies aerosol through a Mistogen HV-12 nebulizer, and has an optional float feed system. There are two operating modes, circulate and cool. In the circulate mode, heat is not exchanged in the thermoelectric mode.

Application

Several concerns are important in the management of mist tents. The F_{IO_2} may vary widely, depending on the amount of room air allowed into the tent. Most tents have zippers, holes, and an open front facing the foot of the bed. If a precise F_{IO_2} is

A

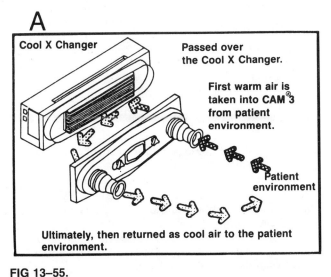

B

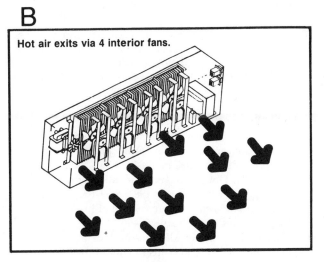

FIG 13–55.
Application of the Pelter effect in the Mistogen CAM-3 tent. **A,** front exploded view of module as it cools air. **B,** back interior view of module as it vents hot air. (Courtesy of Mistogen/Timeter Products, Lancaster, Penn.)

desired, these openings should be kept constant or closed altogether. The amount of aerosol needed has never been specified. However, there should never be so much that it is difficult to examine the patient. Ultrasonic nebulizers at high output should not be used with mist tents due to the possibility of fluid overload. Due to the property of oxygen to support combustion, every effort must be made to eliminate sources of sparks and flame. Nurse call buttons and bed controls must be certified as safe in oxygen environment. Toys should be checked to assure that they do not produce sparks. Smoking should be prohibited in rooms where mist tents are in use.

REFERENCES

1. Derry R: The evolution of heat and moisture for the respiratory tract during anesthesia with a nonrebreathing system. *Can Anaesth Soc J* 1973; 20:296–309.
2. Emergency Care Research Institute: Heated humidifiers. *Health Devices* 1980; 9:167–180.
3. Emergency Care Research Institute: Heat and moisture exchangers. *Health Devices* 1983; 12:155–168.
4. Esty W: Subjective effects of dry vs. humidified low flow oxygen. *Respir Care* 1980; 23:1143–1144.
5. Gibson RL, Comer PB, Beckham RW, et al: Actual tracheal oxygen concentrations with commonly used oxygen equipment. *Anesthesiology* 1976; 44:71–73.
6. Glick RV: Drug reconcentration in aerosol generators. *Inhal Ther* 1970; 15:179.
7. Goldstein RS, Young JH, R'buck AS: Effect of breathing pattern on oxygen concentration received from standard face masks. *Lancet* 1982; 2:1188–1190.
8. Grose BY: Personal communication, 1985.
9. *Independent Test on Filter Material Used in the Engstrom Edith: Report 08590.* Bromma, Sweden, Sylwan B, 1981.
10. Klein EF, Shah DA, Shah NJ, et al: Performance characteristics of conventional and prototype humidifiers and nebulizers. *Chest* 1973; 64:690–696.
11. Lasky MS: Bubble humidifiers are useful: Fact or myth? *Respir Care* 1982; 27:735–737.
12. Mebius C: A comparative evaluation of disposable humidifiers. *Acta Anaesthesiol Scand* 1983; 27:403–409.
13. Monast RL, Kaye W: Problems in delivering desired oxygen concentration from jet nebulizers to patients via face tents. *Respir Care* 1984; 29:994–1000.
14. Poulton TJ, Downs JB: Humidification of rapidly flowing gas. *Crit Care Med* 1981; 9:59–63.
15. Satewen WS: Temperature control of heated humidifiers. *Med Instrum* 1982; 16:55–56.
16. Schacter EN, Littner MR, Luddy P, et al: Monitoring of oxygen delivery systems in clinical practice. *Crit Care Med* 1980; 8:405–409.
17. Shapiro, BA, Harrison RA, Kacmarek RM et al: *Clinical Application of Respiratory Care*, ed 3. Chicago, Year Book Medical Publishers, 1985, p 108.
18. Spearman CV, Sheldon RL, Egan DF: *Egan's Fundamentals of Respiratory Therapy*, ed 4. St Louis, CV Mosby Co, 1982, p 348.
19. Stange K, Bygdeman S: Do moisture exchangers prevent patient contamination of ventilator? *Acta Anaesthesiol Scand* 1980; 24:487–490.
20. Weeks BD, Ramsey FM: Laboratory investigation of six artificial noses for use during endotracheal anesthesia. *Anesth Analg* 1983; 62:758–763.

LIST OF MANUFACTURER'S LITERATURE

Airlife, publication 2198. Airlife, Inc. Montclair, Calif, 1980.

Air-Shields Croupette cool mist and oxygen tents, detail aid 0131. Narco Air-Shields, Hatboro, Penn.

Aquapak humidification systems, form PL-0098. Respiratory Care, Inc, Arlington Heights, Ill, October 1984.

Aquapak nebulization systems, form PL-0097. Respiratory Care, Inc, Arlington, Heights, Ill, November 1983.

Bennett MA-2 ventilator, operating instructions, form 11040B. Puritan-Bennett Corp, Overland Park, Kan, January 1979.

Bennett nebulizer, operating and maintenance instructions, form 433044. Puritan-Bennett Corp, Overland Park, Kan, July 10, 1976.

Bennett Slip/stream nebulizer, instructions, form 3061F. Puritan-Bennett Corp, Overland Park, Kan, April 30, 1976.

Bennett US-1 ultrasonic nebulizer, operating instructions. Puritan-Bennett Corp, Overland Park, Kan, October 1982.

Bird heated humidifier, instructional manual, PNL 1001. Bird Corp, Palm Springs, Calif, 1985.

Bird Micronebulizer, specifications and instructions, form L746–8–76R2. Bird Corp, Palm Springs, Calif, August 1976.

Conchopak, publication PF–0071. Respiratory Care, Inc, Arlington Heights, Ill, March 1979.

Corpak nebulizer, output study. Corpak Respiratory Therapy, Wheeling, Ill, August 1982, pp 10–13.

Corpak prefilled humidifiers, performance study CP0330. Corpak Respiratory Therapy, Wheeling, Ill, August 1982, pp 1–2.

DeVilbiss 38B ultrasonic nebulizer, manual of instructions. DeVilbiss Co, Somerset, Penn, 1975.

DeVilbiss ultrasonic nebulizer 65 series, manual of instructions. DeVilbiss Co, Somerset, Penn, 1975.

Engstrom Edith, publication 55–10930–32. Gambro Engstrom AB, Bromma, Sweden, May 1984.

Fisher and Paykel MR450 and MR500 humidifiers, publications 5M/983A450 and 2.4M/385C500. Fisher and Paykel Medical Corp, Glen Falls, NY.

Humidification of respiratory gases, basic manual, publication 9034505E323E. Siemens-Elema, Elk Grove Village, Ill, October 1983.

Humidifier VH-820, instruction manual, publication 50000–10820. Bear Medical Systems, Inc, Riverside, Calif.

Humidifiers/nebulizers, publication 5300–S. Mistogen/Timeter, Lancaster, Penn, November 1979.

Inspiron disposable nebulizer with immersion heater adapter. Inspiron, Division of CR Bard, Inc, Upland, Calif, 1976, pp 2–13, 2–14.

Inspiron nebulizer, humidifier, and immersion heater kit. Inspiron, Division of CR Bard, Inc, Upland, Calif, 1976, pp 2–19, 2–20.

Maxi-Cool nebulizer, operations/technical manual, form R71–120, revision B. Airlife, Inc, Montclair, Calif, September 1978.

Mistogen CAM-2 refrigerated aerosol unit, operating instructions. Mistogen/Timeter, Lancaster, Penn.

Mistogen CAM-3 thermoelectric CAM tent, publication. Mistogen/Timeter, Lancaster, Penn.

Mistogen Electronic Humidilizer EH 147B, operation and maintenance manual. Mistogen/Timeter, Lancaster, Penn.

Mistogen EN-145 electronic nebulizer, operating instructions. Mistogen/Timeter, Lancaster, Penn, January 1980.

Mistogen HV-12 pneumatic nebulizer, operation manual. Mistogen/Timeter, Lancaster, Penn.

Mistogen oygen/aerosol mist tents, publication 4200–2. Mistogen/Timeter, Lancaster, Penn, November 1979.

Ohmeda Ohio Deluxe nebulizer, operation and maintenance manual, form 1774, 3/75–15M. Madison, Wis.

Ohmeda Ohio Heated Humidifier, operation and maintenance manual, stock no 178–1685–000. Madison, Wis, 1971.

Ohmeda Ohio High Output pneumatic nebulizer, operation and maintenance manual. Madison, Wis, 1983.

Ohmeda Ohio Jet and Bubble humidifiers, operation and maintenance manual, form 9794. Madison, Wis, 1980.

Ohmeda Ohio Non-Immersion nebulizer heater, temporary manual, publication 178–3028–000. Madison, Wis, 1984.

Ohmeda Ohio Pediatric Aerosol Tent, operation and maintenance manual. Madison, Wis, 1985.

Puritan Bubble-Jet humidifier, operation and maintenance instructions, form 944015. Puritan-Bennett Corp, Overland Park, Kan, July 15, 1977.

Solo-Sphere nebulizer, operations/technical manual, catalog no H2500/H2501. Airlife, Inc, Montclair, Calif, June 1980.

U-Mid/Prefil System, fact sheet, form 326. Bard-Parker, Lincoln Park, NJ, February 1980.

Vapor Phase humidifier, publication. Inspiron, Division of CR Bard, Inc, Rancho Coucamonga, Calif.

Intermittent Positive-Pressure Breathing Devices

Robert R. Fluck, Jr., M.S., R.R.T.

There are many brands and types of intermittent positive-pressure breathing (IPPB) machines. This chapter will concentrate only on those in common use today, both in the hospital as well as in the home. When many similar machines are made by a manufacturer, the most common model will be described in detail with only the differences between this model and the other discussed. Although some machines may also be able to function as ventilators for continuous mechanical ventilation, only their function as IPPB machines will be discussed here. Therefore, the operation of some controls or features may be omitted from the description. All values are taken from the respective manufacturer's literature unless specified otherwise.

BENNETT INTERMITTENT POSITIVE-PRESSURE BREATHING MACHINES

Puritan-Bennett Corporation makes two types of IPPB machines: electrically powered and gas powered. The prototype of this series is the AP-5 (AP denotes air powered) (Fig 14–1).

AP Series

We will discuss the electrically powered machines first. It is an electrically powered portable unit suitable for use in the hospital or the home. A compressor provides filtered air at a pressure adjustable from 0 to 35 cm H_2O and a maximum flow of 75 to 90 L/min at 20 cm H_2O pressure. A slipstream nebulizer, which operates continuously, has its output controlled by a needle valve.

The compressor draws in room air through a 10-μ filter, which then passes through a submicronic filter (Fig 14–2). At this point the gas flow splits, one path leading to the needle valve that controls flow to the nebulizer and the other leading to the pressure control mechanism. There is a venturi at the entrance to the pressure control mechanism that serves to augment flow. The pressure control mechanism consists of a spring-loaded disc that vents excess pressure to atmosphere. The gas next passes through the Bennett valve, the "valve that breathes with the patient." When the patient creates a subatmospheric pressure against the single vane on the drum, it rotates in a counterclockwise fashion, beginning inspiration; with increasing proximal airway pressure, the Bennett valve rotates partially clockwise, thus decreasing the flow rate. When the flow of gas through the Bennett valve drops to a terminal flow of 1 L/min, the counterweight in the valve closes it, thus beginning exhalation.

Many different manufacturers make disposable circuits for these machines. There is a single 22-mm large-bore tube that connects to a manifold. The manifold contains a slipstream nebulizer (part of the gas flow is diverted through the nebulizer) and an exhalation valve. For all Bennett equipment, there are separate accessory lines for the exhalation valve (smaller) and nebulizer (larger). In operation, the three tubes are attached to the appropriate connections on the machine. It is virtually impossible to

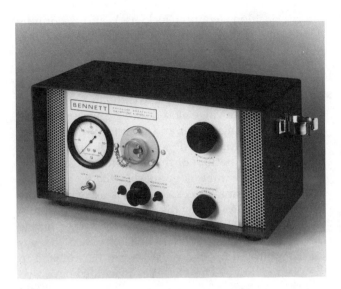

FIG 14–1.
Bennett AP-5. (Courtesy of Puritan-Bennett Corporation, Overland Park, Kansas.)

connect the accessory lines to the wrong nipples, because the smaller line (for the exhalation valve) will not fit the larger nipple, and the larger line (for the nebulizer) will fall off the smaller nipple. After the accessory lines are connected, the machine can be turned on. The pressure control is turned clockwise to increase the pressure to the desired starting value (usually 15–20 cm H_2O). The actual pressure is determined by lifting up the small handle on the Bennett valve, starting flow from the machine. The end of the 22-mm large-bore tube is then occluded, and the maximum pressure that registers on the manometer is noted. The nebulizer control should be turned counterclockwise to increase the flow until there is a visible aerosol being produced. Since there is continuous flow to the nebulizer as long as the compressor is on, it does not matter whether the machine is in the inspiratory or expiratory phase when this control is adjusted. Adjusting the nebulizer control has relatively little effect on the pressure or on available flow.

The Bennett AP-4 is identical to the AP-5 except for having a built-in support arm and covered storage compartment in the back. The Bennett AP-5B is an AP-5 with the capability of being operated from either 120 or 240 V alternating current (AC) at 60 Hz.

TA-1

The Bennett TA-1 is an electrically powered, manually controlled unit that falls somewhere between an IPPB machine and a simple aerosol generator (Fig 14–3). The compressor supplies a gas flow

of 16.5 to 18 L/min, which is increased by at least three volumes of entrained air for each volume generated by the compressor, giving a total gas flow to the patient of approximately 66 to 72 L/min. The unit can generate a maximum pressure of 7 to 34 cm H_2O. A handpiece contains a control valve, a medication nebulizer, and provision for flow augmentation by entraining room air. Approximate F_{IO_2} available with supplemental O_2 flow is 0.25 to 0.35 at 5 L/min of O_2, 0.28 to 0.38 at 7 L/min of O_2, and 0.3 to 0.4 at 9 L/min of O_2.

When the compressor is turned on, gas flows to the handpiece and out the control opening. If the control valve is held shut, gas flows to the lungs. The patient releases the control valve when ready to exhale through the mouthpiece.

The TA-1 is prepared for use by plugging in the electrical power cord and attaching a single gas line to a nipple on the front panel. The medication vial is unscrewed and the medication added. Then the pressure is set by turning the pressure control on the front panel until the dial indicates the desired peak inspiratory pressure. The machine is turned on and the treatment is begun under the control of the patient.

The TA-1, although out of production, seems ideally suited for home care. (Production was halted December 31, 1984, but Puritan-Bennett will continue to make parts available for 5 years.) It delivers a relatively safe pressure under complete control of the patient and has relatively few parts to clean and maintain.

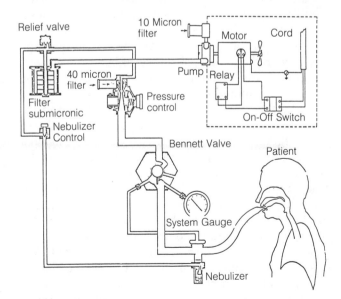

FIG 14–2.
Bennett AP-5 circuit diagram. (Courtesy of Puritan-Bennett Corporation, Overland Park, Kansas.)

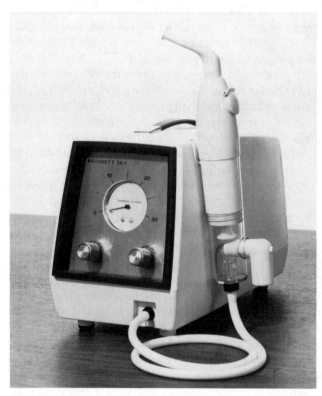

FIG 14–3.
Bennett TA-1. (Courtesy of Puritan-Bennett Corporation, Overland Park, Kansas.)

PR Series

The prototype of this series is the PR-2 (PR stands for pedestal respirator, Fig 14–4). Although these models can be used for mechanically assisted ventilation, their principal use now is for IPPB treatments. A detailed working knowledge of the internal circuit of the machine is unnecessary. Since they are powered by a 50-psi source of compressed gas, neither of the PR series IPPB machines would be suitable for home use.

The PR-2 operates off a gas source with a range of 40 to 70 psi, which first goes to a diluter regulator. This regulator contains a spring-loaded disc against which the gas presses. If the pressure falls below the set value, the disc flexes and a poppet valve opens, allowing more gas to enter the circuit. Integral with the pressure control is the provision for air dilution of the source gas. When the PR-1 or PR-2 is used for IPPB, the air dilution control should be in, or on (more about this under the discussion on controls). Gas then travels to the Bennett valve, which is slightly more complex in the PR series than in the AP series. When the patient creates subatmospheric pressure in the circuit, it draws against the lower vane on the Bennett valve, rotating it into the inspi-

ratory position (counterclockwise) and beginning flow to the circuit (maximum flow available is 80 L/min). The valve begins to rotate in a clockwise fashion as proximal airway pressure rises, decreasing flow. When the flow in the circuit reaches the terminal value of 1 L/min, the weight in the Bennett valve rotates the valve closed and expiration begins.

The breathing circuit and tubing nipples are the same as those for the AP series except that the nipples are on the bottom of the machine instead of the front. A 22-mm tube is connected to the main gas flow outlet, a small accessory line is attached to the smaller nipple to power the exhalation valve, and a large accessory line is attached to the larger nipple to power the medication nebulizer. Once the gas source is turned on, the pressure can be adjusted to the desired value. The PR series machines have two

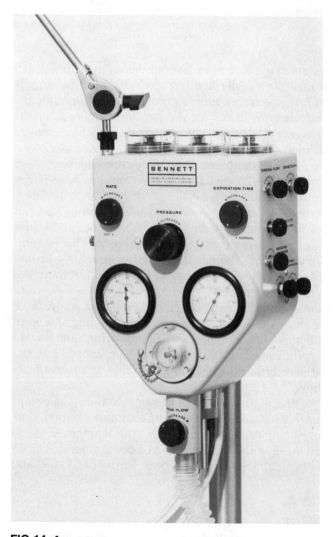

FIG 14–4.
Bennett PR-2. (Courtesy of Puritan-Bennett Corporation, Overland Park, Kansas.)

manometers on the front. The right-hand one is labeled control pressure and reads the pressure in the diluter regulator. This is the pressure that the PR-2 will achieve before beginning expiration. The left-hand manometer is labeled system pressure and reads the pressure in the patient circuit. The control pressure is increased by turning the large control in the middle clockwise until the desired pressure is indicated. The pressure available on the PR-2 is 0 to 50 cm H_2O. Once the desired pressure is set, attention should be turned to adjustment of nebulizer flow. On the right side of the machine, at the lower right corner as it is viewed from the side, are two nebulizer controls, inspiration and expiration. With the handle on the Bennett valve pushed up (to initiate inspiration), the inspiration nebulizer control is adjusted to provide a visible aerosol. Then with the Bennett valve rotated to the off position, the expiration nebulizer control is cracked. The purpose is to allow the accessory line and nebulizer to be pressurized so that the first portion of the inspired gas (presumably the part that will achieve the deepest penetration into the airways) will contain some aerosol. The nebulizer is powered by 100% source gas and will increase the delivered F_{IO_2} when the machine is operated in the air dilution mode and powered by 100% oxygen.

For use of the PR-2 as an IPPB machine, the remainder of the controls should be adjusted as follows. There are three smaller controls on the front (see Fig 14–4). In the upper left is the rate control; in the upper right, the expiratory time control; and below the Bennett valve in the center, the peak flow control. All three of these controls should be turned fully counterclockwise (off position). On the right side of the machine are four controls in addition to the nebulizer controls. The sensitivity control, located on the upper right, should be turned fully clockwise (off position). It will require the patient to exert a negative pressure of only 0.5 cm H_2O to trigger the machine. On the upper left is the terminal flow control, which should be cracked slightly. The purpose of the terminal flow control is to provide flow to the circuit distal to the Bennett valve, therefore allowing the Bennett valve to function properly even in the presence of a leak. Recall that the flow in the circuit must drop to 1 L/min for the Bennett valve to be able to terminate inspiration. The terminal flow control serves to compensate for leaks in the system up to 15 L/min. Directly below the terminal flow control is the air dilution control. It should be pushed all the way in (on position). When the air dilution control is on, unrestricted flow provides 3 L of room air for each liter of source gas, thus giving an F_{IO_2} of 0.40 if the machine is powered by 100% oxygen. However, as proximal airway pressure rises, so will the delivered F_{IO_2}. The delivered F_{IO_2}, with the air dilution control in the full on position, may be variable within a range of 0.40 to 0.60. Directly under the air dilution control is the negative pressure control. This control should be turned off (fully clockwise). The negative pressure control generates subatmospheric pressure via a venturi at the bottom of the machine to evacuate gas from the circuit during expiration (the negative pressure has a limited application, namely, only when the the PR-2 is used to ventilate infants).

Before beginning an IPPB treatment, one should double-check that the machine will cycle off at the preset pressure. The handle on the Bennett valve should be flipped up to begin inspiration, and the end of the circuit should be occluded. When the circuit is occluded, the system pressure manometer should be observed for the peak pressure. If the machine fails to cycle into expiration, the terminal flow control should be opened slightly until the inspiration ceases. If more than one-half turn is required to end inspiration, the circuit should be carefully inspected for leaks. There should be no interaction among the controls of either machine in the PR series when it is used for IPPB treatments.

The PR-1 is very similar to the PR-2 but has fewer controls (Fig 14–5). When viewed from the front, it has neither peak flow nor expiratory time controls. Viewed from the right, it does not have a negative pressure or terminal flow control. The only difference of importance for IPPB is in the controls for nebulization. Instead of inspiration and expiration, it has inspiration and continuous controls. Adjustment of the nebulizer is the same as with the PR-2. With the Bennett valve rotated into the on position (counterclockwise), the inspiration control is turned counterclockwise until there is a visible aerosol. The continuous control is just cracked. The only actual difference is that the flow from the continuous control is added to the flow from the inspiration control during inspiration; it will result in a slightly higher flow to the nebulizer during inspiration, which will probably not even be noticeable.

BIRD IPPB MACHINES

The Bird IPPB machines consist of a number of modifications of a basic unit, the Mark 7 (Fig 14–6). Continuing with the previous scheme, the Mark 7

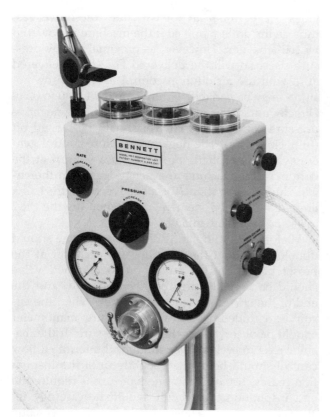

FIG 14–5.
Bennett PR-1. (Couresty of Puritan-Bennett Corporation, Overland Park, Kansas.)

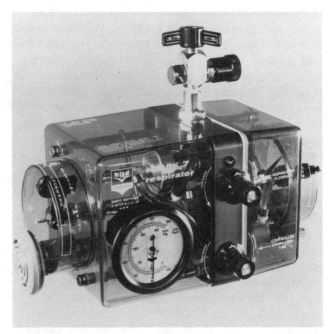

FIG 14–6.
Bird Mark 7 respirator. (Courtesy of Bird Corporation, Palm Springs, Calif.)

will be described and diagrammed in detail; the other machines will be mentioned only insofar as they differ from the basic model. The reader should be aware that the only Bird Mark series models presently being manufactured are the Mark 7, Mark 7A, Mark 8A, and the Bird ventilator (which will not be discussed here because it is intended primarily for mechanical ventilation).

All Bird machines with a Mark model designation are divided into essentially three parts:

1. The center body (also known as the control body) is made of metal, contains the major components of the machine, and is where it is attached to the gas supply.
2. The ambient compartment (chamber on the left) is where entrained air enters and where some control components are housed.
3. The pressure compartment (chamber on the right) is route for gas flow to the patient circuit.

Source gas is delivered to the inlet stem atop the center body at 50 psi (±5 psi). From there it flows through a filter to the sequencing switch (also known as a ceramic switch because of the material

of which it is made). The ceramic switch consists of a spool with inlet and outlet rings. Flow between the inlet and outlet rings is controlled by a movable spindle. With the spindle in the far right or on position, there is communication between the inlet and outlet of the switch and gas flows to the patient circuit. With the spindle in the far left (off position), no flow is allowed. The ceramic switch functions in either the on or off position (i.e., it cannot control flow). A central shaft holds the spindle in the spool. The left end of the shaft connects the spindle to the master diaphragm; it also has a manual timer rod, which enables the machine to be placed either in inspiration or expiration by the operator. There are also metal clutch discs at each end of the central shaft that allow for sensitivity adjustments and pressure control.

There is a threaded socket on the end of both the ambient and the pressure compartments. A lever moves a permanent magnet closer to or farther away from the metal clutch discs on the end of the central shaft. On the left side, this magnet-disc mechanism controls the amount of force needed to move the ceramic switch to the right (on) and thus serves as the sensitivity control. On the right side, the magnet-disc mechanism controls the amount of force needed to move the spindle to the left (off) and thus serves as the pressure limit control. The master diaphragm allows a subambient pressure exerted by the patient to move the ceramic switch to the right and thus initiate inspiration. It also allows the termination of inspiration when the force exerted on the diaphragm exceeds the force of attraction between the magnet and metal clutch disc in the pressure chamber.

When the Bird is first turned on, gas flows through the expiratory termination cartridge to the servoing/sensing Venturi, which generates subambient pressure on the pressure side and moves the ceramic switch into the on position. Gas now flows through the inlet of (1) inspiratory flow rate valve and (2) nebulizer pressure rise orifice. The inspiratory flow rate valve allows adjustment of flow delivered to the inlet of the master venturi. The master venturi entrains room air from the ambient compartment; this air is pulled in through the sintered brass filter (newer Bird models use an easily replaceable plastic filter). The gas stream passes through the venturi gate into the pressure compartment and then into the breathing circuit. Gas that passes through the nebulizer pressure rise orifice is metered to the inspiratory service circuit. This circuit powers both the exhalation valve and the Bird micronebulizer.

Pressure is monitored by a manometer that is mounted in the ambient chamber and connected to the pressure chamber through a restricting orifice; this orifice serves to dampen the movement of the manometer needle. The normal pressure limit is more than 60 cm H_2O. There can be a pressure pop-off installed in an opening in the pressure compartment, which limits pressure to 65 cm H_2O for therapy and 110 cm H_2O for mechanical ventilation.

There is no control for nebulizer flow rate. The only significant interaction among the controls is among inspiratory flow rate and air mix. With the air mix control in the out, or on, position, the maximum flow rate is 65 L/min against 15 cm H_2O back pressure. If the air mix control is in the in, or off position, the peak flow is limited to 40 L/min (personal measurement). When a higher peak inspiratory flow rate is needed, the Bird IPPB machines should always be operated with the air mix control in the on position.

In preparing the machine for use, one should first attach it to the gas source, preferably compressed air. Then an IPPB circuit should be attached. Assure that the circuit has provision for using one accessory line to power both the nebulizer and the exhalation valve, which usually involves a jumper tube that goes from the nebulizer to the exhalation valve (Fig 14–7). If the circuit is a Bird permanent circuit, there is no problem. If the circuit is a disposable one, however, be sure that there is a bleed hole

in the connection on top of the nebulizer. This bleed hole vents some of the flow being supplied to the inspiratory service line (remember that the inspiratory service line is fed at source gas pressure through a restricting orifice). If there is no bleed hole at the nebulizer, the first time the patient cycles the machine into the inspiratory mode, the exhalation valve line will be blown off.

Once the proper circuit has been attached, the gas supply to the machine should be turned on. It will result in the machine's cycling into the inspiratory phase. The flow rate control should be set around 20. Numbers next to the controls are for reference only and do not represent calibrated values. The flow rate should be adjusted to provide a smooth rise of the manometer once the patient begins the treatment. The pressure control should be set to 15 cm H_2O to start with and the outlet of the machine then occluded by the hand (this number may have no resemblance to the actual peak pressure unless the unit has been recently calibrated). The machine should be cycled into the inspiratory phase by pushing in on the control rod on the left (ambient) side of the machine, and the pressure control should be suitably adjusted until the indicated peak pressure is 15 cm H_2O. This value will be adjusted during the treatment to deliver the desired tidal volume. The inspiratory sensitivity should be set somewhere around the reference number 0. The range of inspiratory effort needed to trigger inspiration is 0 to -10 cm H_2O.

There are many variants on the basic Bird Mark 7 that may be found in respiratory therapy departments, even though only the Mark 7A, Mark 8A, and Bird respirator are presently being made. The

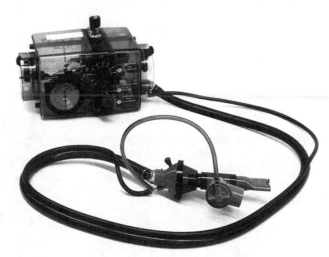

FIG 14–7.
Close-up of nebulizer of permanent circuit for Bird. (Courtesy of Bird Corporation, Palm Springs, Calif.)

special features of those models that are out of production will be described first, followed by the current machines.

Bird Mark 8

The Bird Mark 8 is a Mark 7 with an expiratory flow module added (Fig 14–8). This module was intended primarily for the Q and J circles used in ventilating infants. It can be distinguished from the Mark 7 by the fact that its center body is red, whereas the center body of the Mark 7 is green. There is also an additional flow control located on the center body behind the gas inlet stem. Finally, there is an additional small nipple for an accessory line located on the upper rear of the right (pressure) compartment.

Bird Mark 9

The Bird Mark 9 is identical to the Mark 8 with two exceptions (Fig 14–9). It has a larger pressure magnet, which allows it to deliver pressures to 200 mm Hg (approximately 270 cm H_2O). It also has a double venturi system to allow it to deliver higher flow rates.

Bird Mark 10

The Bird Mark 10 is a Mark 7 without the air mix control (Fig 14–10). It also has an inspiratory flow accelerator, which, if inspiration has not ended by a specified time, causes a sudden increase in flow resulting in a rapid rise in pressure that will terminate inspiration. There is a control on top of the center body behind the inlet stem that adjusts the delay before the extra flow is supplied to the master venturi.

Bird Mark 14

The Bird Mark 14 is essentially a Mark 10 with a larger pressure magnet to allow it to deliver pressures of about 140 mm Hg or 190 cm H_2O (Fig 14–11). It also features a vernier sensitivity control to allow finer adjustments of sensitivity.

Bird Mark 7A and Mark 8A

The Bird Mark 7A and Mark 8A are the Mark 7 and Mark 8 without an air dilution control (they are always on air mix) and with the addition of an apneustic flow rate module to the center body (Fig 14–12). Maximum inspiratory flow rate is specified as 80 L/min, and sensitivity is −0.5 to −5.0 cm H_2O. With the time/pressure cycled control pulled out, the machine is in the normal pressure-cycled mode. With this control pushed in, the machine is in the time-cycled mode. The Bird literature describes it as a ''dynamic inspiratory hold'' whose purpose is to optimize the distribution of inspired gas. In this mode, inspiration is actually split into two parts, pressure cycled and time cycled. Total inspiratory time is the sum of the time it takes to achieve the desired pressure plus the set apneustic time. This apneustic (inspiratory pause) feature is controlled by an apneustic hold timing circuit that is pressurized during the pressure-cycled phase. Following the termination of the pressure-cycled portion of inspira-

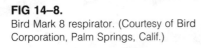

FIG 14–8.
Bird Mark 8 respirator. (Courtesy of Bird Corporation, Palm Springs, Calif.)

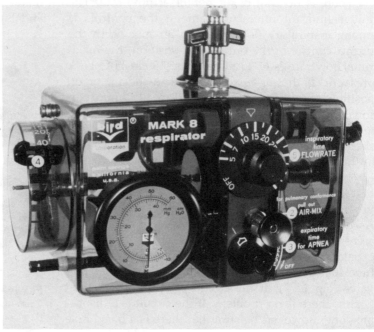

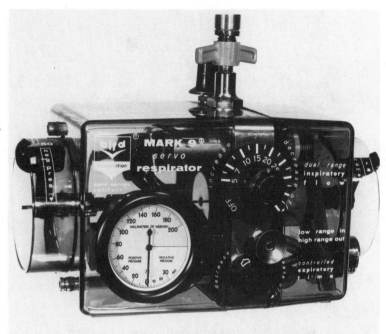

FIG 14–9.
Bird Mark 9 servo respirator. (Courtesy of Bird Corporation, Palm Springs, Calif.)

tion, this circuit continues to feed flow (150–200 ml/sec) through the inspiratory service line to the nebulizer, which also maintains the exhalation valve closed. As gas bleeds out of the apneustic hold timing cartridge, it feeds two auxiliary jets on the master venturi and thus provides some additional flow to the patient circuit from that source as well. The rate at which the gas bleeds out of the timing cartridge is controlled by a knob on top of the center body in front of the inlet stem. The range for this apneustic flow time is 0.3 to 3.0 seconds.

Minibird II

The Minibird II is a simple therapy unit with only pressure and flow controls (Fig 14–13). It is the same as the Portabird II, which is described in detail in the next section, with two exceptions: (1) it has no compressor and therefore requires a 50 pounds per square inch (psi) gas source; and (2) it has the apneustic flow feature, which functions in the same manner and has the same parts as in a Mark 7A or Mark 8A.

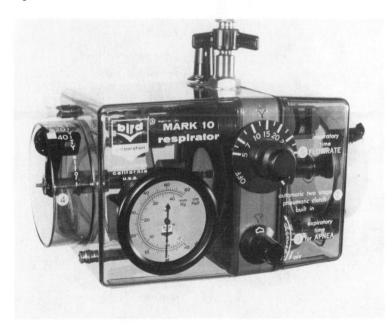

FIG 14–10.
Bird Mark 10 respirator. (Courtesy of Bird Corporation, Palm Springs, Calif.)

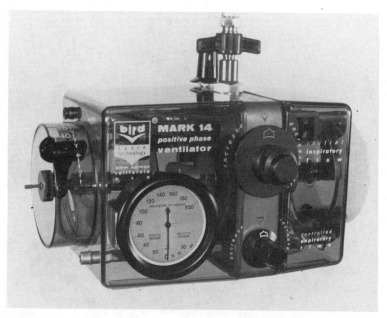

FIG 14–11.
Bird Mark 14 positive phase ventilator. (Courtesy of
Bird Corporation, Palm Springs, Calif.)

Portabird II

The Bird units previously described are restricted to hospital use because of their requirement of a 50-psi gas source for operation. Bird also makes an electrically powered unit, the Portabird II, which is suitable for home use. The Portabird II is a Minibird II with a compressor that frees it from external gas supplies (Fig 14–14). It is controlled by the Mark 1 sequencing servo (Fig 14–15), which is a modification of the ceramic switch found in the other Mark units. It has a single magnet with a metal clutch disc on either side for sensitivity and pressure regulation.

When gas is first supplied to the servo, it moves into the inspiratory position opening the ball valve (toward the right on Fig 14–15). Opening the ball valve allows gas to pass through the flow control valve. The gas flow then splits. One stream goes to the venturi jet to provide the main flow of gas for the patient; the other gas stream goes to the inspiratory service circuit to power the exhalation valve and the nebulizer. When the pressure in the circuit has reached the set level, the exhalation clutch disc is attracted to the magnet, and the valve moves to the left, closing the ball valve and beginning expiration.

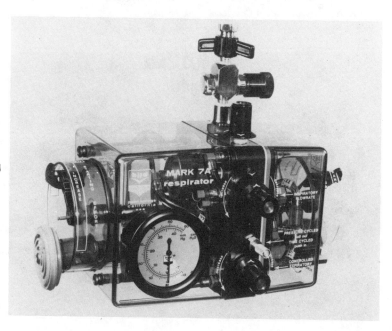

FIG 14–12.
Bird Mark 7A respirator. (Courtesy of Bird
Corporation, Palm Springs, Calif.)

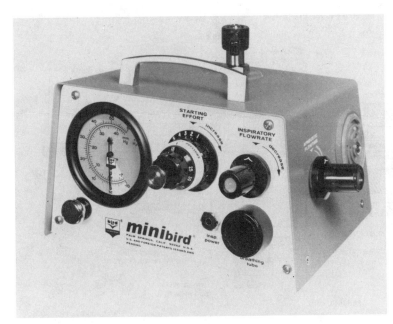

FIG 14–13.
Minibird II. (Courtesy of Bird Corporation, Palm Springs, Calif.)

The Portabird II has a maximum pressure of 45 cm H_2O and a maximum inspiratory flow rate of 45 to 50 L/min. Sensitivity is preset (nonadjustable) at -2 cm H_2O.

When using the machine, one first connects the patient circuit and inspiratory service line. Then medication is added to the nebulizer. The flow rate control is adjusted to "start" (about the middle of the flow range), and the pressure control is adjusted to 15 to 20 cm H_2O. The machine is turned on and the nebulizer inspected for proper aerosolization. Once the patient begins the treatment, the flow can be adjusted to provide a smooth rise of the manometer and the pressure adjusted to achieve the desired tidal volume. The machine can be cycled manually into either phase by use of the manual timer rod, which is found in the middle of the pressure control.

MONAGHAN 515

The Monaghan 515 is an electrically powered IPPB machine that provides a flow of 25 to 70 L/min with a maximum pressure of 30 cm H_2O (Fig 14–16).

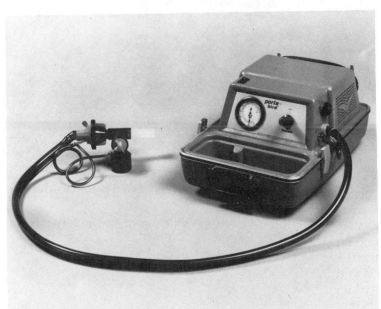

FIG 14–14.
Portabird II. (Courtesy of Bird Corporation, Palm Springs, Calif.)

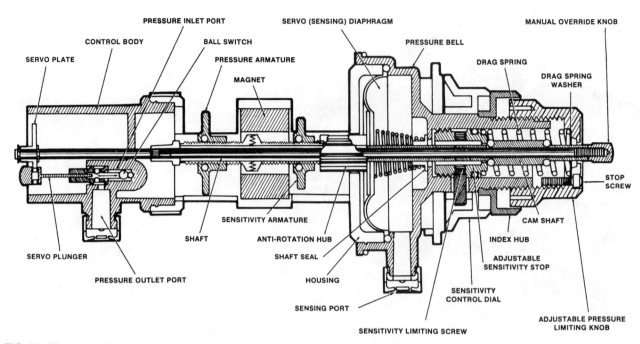

FIG 14–15
Circuit diagram of the Mark 1 sequencing servo. (Courtesy of Bird Corporation, Palm Springs, Calif.)

Sensitivity is fixed at less than 0.5 cm H_2O. The nebulizer operates continuously and has adjustable flow. The maximum flow is restricted by an orifice to 5 to 11 L/min. A companion model, the *Monaghan 517*, is identical to the Monaghan 515 with two exceptions: it is powered by 12 V DC instead of 120 V AC, and the maximum flow rate available is 55 L/min.

When the machine is turned on, flow from the compressor passes through a dump valve so that the compressor, a diaphragm type, will continue to run. (With no outlet for the compressed gas, the compressor would quickly stall.) When the patient generates a negative pressure in the circuit, this moves a disk off its seat. Attached to this disk is a rod that actuates the finger valve, (Fig 14–17). Gas now closes the dump valve, causing the compressor output to be supplied to the circuit. Part of the output goes to the needle valve, which controls flow to the nebulizer. The rest proceeds through the finger valve to a Venturi, which augments inspiratory flow. A small line goes from the main body to power the exhalation valve, thus maintaining the same pressure in the patient circuit and the exhalation valve. The maximum pressure is set by turning a knob on the front of the machine. This generates tension on a spring. When the pressure on the patient circuit side of the disk equals the pressure being exerted on the disk by the spring, the disk is returned to its seat and the machine cycles into expiration.

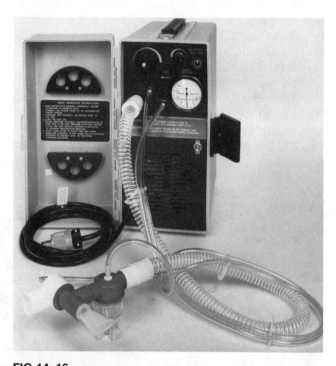

FIG 14–16.
Monaghan 515. (Courtesy of Monaghan Medical Division of Sandoz-Wander Corporation, Plattsburgh, N.Y.)

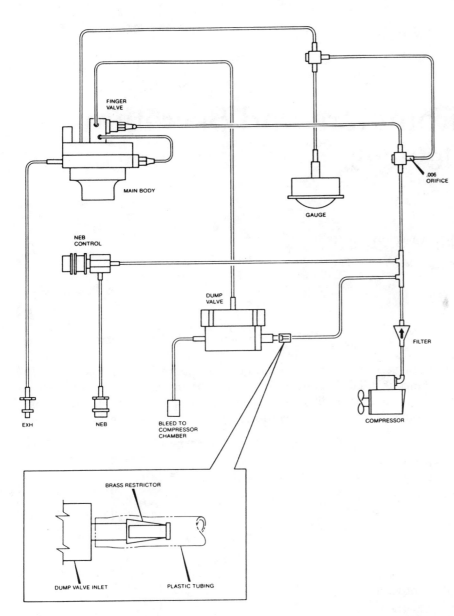

FIG 14–17.
Monaghan 515 circuit diagram
(Courtesy of Monaghan Medical
Division of Sandoz-Wander
Corporation, Plattsburgh, N.Y.)

To use the Monaghan 515, attach the circuit (Fig 14–16), which uses two accessory lines like the Bennett products, to the appropriate ports on the front of the machine. Add medication to the nebulizer, and adjust the flow and pressure controls to the middle of their ranges. Adjust the nebulizer to deliver a visible aerosol. Once the treatment has begun, adjust the flow to deliver the desired tidal volume.

SUGGESTED READINGS

1. Burton GG, Hodgkin JE (eds): *Respiratory Care*, ed, 2. Philadelphia, JB Lippincott, 1984.
2. McPherson SP: *Respiratory Therapy Equipment*, ed 3. St Louis, CV Mosby, 1985.
3. Spearman CB, Sheldon RL, Egan DF: *Egan's Fundamentals of Respiratory Therapy*, ed 4. St Louis, CV Mosby, 1982.

Incentive Spirometers and Secretion Evacuation Devices

William V. Wojciechowski, M.S., R.R.T.

INCENTIVE SPIROMETERS

Incentive spirometers are breathing devices designed to increase the patient's spontaneous tidal volume and assist in preventing atelectasis. Patients who undergo thoracotomies or laparotomies commonly develop postsurgical pulmonary complications ranging from atelectasis to acute ventilatory failure.[1, 7, 10] Clinical research has revealed that incentive spirometry may be a useful therapeutic adjunct that lessens the occurrence of postsurgical pulmonary complications.[3, 5, 8]

Voldyne Volumetric Exerciser

The Voldyne volumetric exerciser, manufactured by Chesebrough-Pond's, Inc., is an incentive deep-breathing exerciser capable of measuring large inspiratory volumes (Fig 15–1). Tidal volumes up to 4,000 ml can be measured. A slide pointer is used to indicate the inspiratory volume desired. The device contains a flow rate guide (indicator window) that helps the patient maintain a slow sustained maximal inspiration (SMI). According to the manufacturer, the function of this flow rate guide is to promote uniform distribution of the inspired gas throughout the tracheobronchial tree.[2] Assembly involves attaching one end of the patient tube to the exerciser and the other end to the mouthpiece (Fig 15–2).

When in use, the Voldyne should be held or placed in an upright position near the patient. The slide pointer (located on the left-hand side) should be elevated to the prescribed tidal volume level (Fig

15–3). The patient should be instructed by the respiratory care practitioner to exhale normally to the normal end-tidal expiratory level or FRC level. The patient should also be instructed to tightly seal his lips around the mouthpiece and slowly inspire, causing the piston to rise to the level of the slide

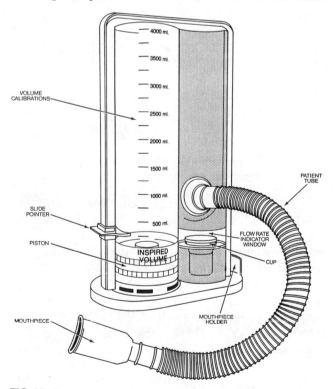

FIG 15–1.
Voldyne volumetric deep-breathing exerciser. (Courtesy of Chesebrough-Pond's Inc., Greenwich, Conn.)

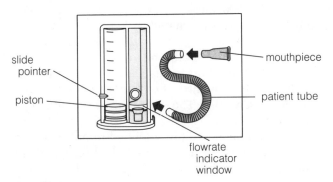

FIG 15–2.
Assembly of Voldyne breathing exerciser. (Courtesy of Chesebrough-Pond's, Inc., Greenwich, Conn.)

pointer. When the uppermost portion of the piston aligns with the slide pointer, the prescribed tidal volume has been achieved (Fig 15–4).

When the prescribed tidal volume has been achieved, the patient should be instructed to remove the mouthpiece from his lips and to exhale normally. Once the patient's inspiratory effort terminates, the piston returns to its resting level (Fig 15–5). The patient should repeat the inspiratory and expiratory maneuvers as frequently as recommended by the physician or the respiratory care practitioner. When the patient consistently achieves the preset tidal volume, a higher tidal volume should be set.

TRIFLO II Incentive Breathing Exerciser

The Triflo II is also manufactured by Cheseborough-Pond's, Inc. and consists of three individual chambers connected in series (Fig 15–6). Each chamber contains a ball that rises within the chamber when the patient's inspiratory effort generates a

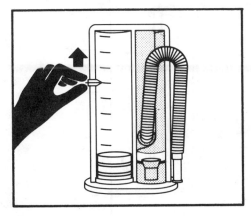

FIG 15–3.
Elevating slide pointer to desired tidal volume. (Courtesy of Chesebrough-Pond's, Inc., Greenwich, Conn.)

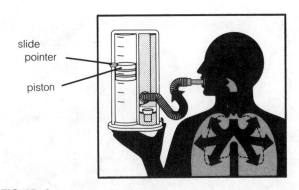

FIG 15–4.
Procedure: patient (1) exhales normally to function residual capacity (FRC) level, (2) creates a tight seal at mouthpiece, (3) inspires slowly, and (4) achieves preset tidal volume. (Courtesy of Chesebrough-Pond's, Inc., Greenwich, Conn.)

subatmospheric pressure above the ball. Assembly of the device is simple (Fig 15–7). One end of the patient tube is connected to the incentive spirometer, and the other end is attached to the mouthpiece.

When preparing to use the Triflo II, the patient should be instructed to maintain the unit in an upright position (Fig 15–8). The patient should hold the device and exhale to the normal end-tidal expiratory level. The patient should then create a tight seal around the unit's mouthpiece and commence inhaling.

With the Triflo II, the magnitude of inspiratory effort exerted will determine the number of balls that ascend within the entire device. For example, when a low inspiratory flow rate is prescribed, the patient's effort should be sufficient to raise only the ball in the first chamber on the right (Fig 15–9). An inspiratory flow rate of 600 ml/sec is needed for the ball in that chamber to rise to the top. When higher inspiratory flow rates are preferred, the patient is instructed to inhale faster, thereby causing two balls (middle and right) to rise (Fig 15–10). An inspiratory

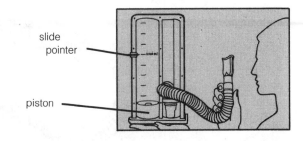

FIG 15–5.
Termination of maneuver: (1) patient exhales normally to FRC level, (2) patient removes mouthpiece from lips, and (3) piston returns to resting level. (Courtesy of Chesebrough-Ponds, Inc., Greenwich, Conn.)

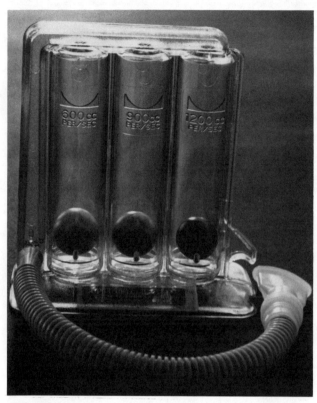

FIG 15–6.
Triflo II incentive breathing exerciser.

flow rate of 900 ml/sec is required to elevate both balls to the top of the chamber.

Regardless of the inspiratory flow rates prescribed, the patient should be told to sustain the desired inspiratory effort to suspend the ball or balls at the top of the chamber or chambers for approximately 3 seconds. The manufacturer's literature states that inspiratory flow rates of 600 and 900 ml/sec are acceptable and are intended to enhance uniform distribution of the inspired air throughout the lungs. However, inspiratory flow rates that achieve or exceed 1,200 ml/sec will cause the ball in the remaining chamber to rise to the top. Such inspiratory flow rates are considered by the manufacturer too rapid to promote uniform distribution of the inspired gas.[6] The patient should be instructed to keep the third ball at the bottom of its chamber.

When the patient's inspiratory effort is terminated, he or she should discontinue the tight seal around the mouthpiece and exhale normally. Termination of the patient's inspiratory effort causes the ball or balls to fall to the bottom of the chamber or chambers (Fig 15–11).

Tru-Vol Incentive Breathing Exerciser

The Tru-Vol incentive breathing exerciser, manufactured by Argyle (Fig 15–12), is a large-capacity incentive spirometer (capable of measuring up to 4,000 ml of lung volume). It was designed for promoting sustained maximum inspiration. The Argyle Tru-Vol incentive exerciser features (1) direct volume measurement, (2) low-resistance bellows, (3) single-

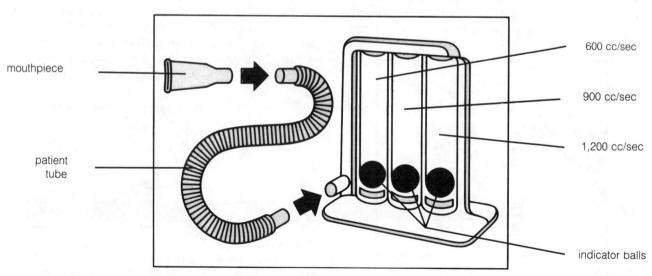

FIG 15–7.
Assembly of the Triflo II incentive breathing exerciser. (Courtesy of Chesebrough-Pond's, Inc., Greenwich, Conn.)

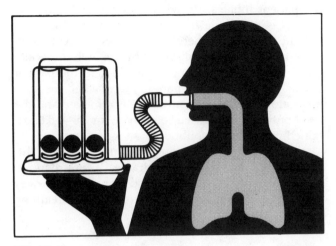

FIG 15–8.
The Triflo II incentive breather exerciser should be held upright during use. (Courtesy of Chesebrough-Pond's, Inc., Greenwich, Conn.)

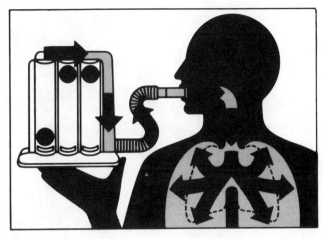

FIG 15–10.
Triflo II incentive breathing exerciser. High inspiratory flow rates are causing elevation of two chamber balls. (Courtesy of Chesebrough-Pond's, Inc., Greenwich, Conn.)

patient use, and (4) compactness. The unit requires assembly prior to use. To assemble the Tru-Vol, one has to comply with the following instructions (Fig 15–13):

1. Remove the unit from the bag with the top facing up. The corrugated hose and mouthpiece should be showing (Fig 15–13,A).
2. Lift and rotate the supporting arms of the spirometer to the vertical position. It is imperative that the graduated scale (tidal volume) be right-side up (Fig 15–13,B).
3. Place the unit on a flat surface, and push down the top and base housing (Fig 15–13,C).

4. Lay the unit on one arm support and separate the top housing from the base housing (Fig 15–13,D).
5. Place your fingers on the sides of the base housing, and push the arm of the spirometer with your thumbs until both sides of the arm click into place (Fig 15–13,E).
6. Place the unit on its opposite arm support and repeat step 5.
7. Repeat steps 4, 5, and 6 with the top housing.
8. Attach patient hose and mouthpiece (Fig 15–13,F).

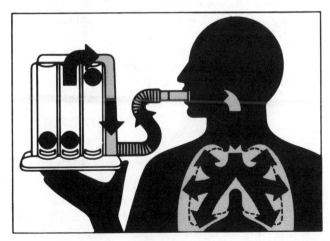

FIG 15–9.
Triflo incentive breathing exerciser. Low inspiratory flow rate is causing elevation of only one chamber ball. (Courtesy of Chesebrough-Pond's, Inc., Greenwich, Conn.)

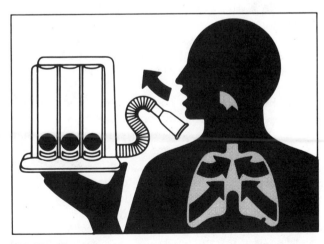

FIG 15–11.
Triflo II incentive breathing exerciser. Termination of maneuver: (1) patient exhales normally to functional residual capacity, (2) patient removes mouthpiece from lips, and (3) balls return to bottom of chamber. (Courtesy of Chesebrough-Pond's, Inc., Greenwich, Conn.)

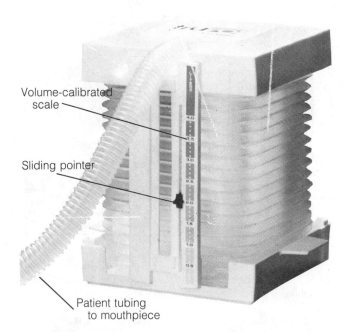

Volume-calibrated scale

Sliding pointer

Patient tubing to mouthpiece

FIG 15–12.
Argyle Tru-vol incentive breathing spirometer. (Courtesy of Sherwood Medical, St. Louis.)

Volurex Incentive Spirometer

The Volurex incentive spirometer is a volume displacement device with a 4,000-ml capacity and is calibrated in 200-ml increments (Fig 15–14). Since the Volurex is a volume displacement incentive spirometer, the accuracy of the device is not influenced by the inspiratory flow rate. The volume registered on the scale is the actual volume inspired by the patient.

The unit arrives in a collapsed position (Fig 15–15) and requires assembly according to the following procedure:

1. Separate the top portion (mouthpiece and reset button) from the bottom portion.
2. Align the vertical supports, making sure that the calibrated volume scale on the two portions match.
3. Secure the two portions together by snapping the male aspect (bottom portion) into the female aspect (top portion).

To use the Volurex, depress the reset button located atop the unit. The vinyl bellows will descend to the bottom of the unit. The patient should be instructed to create a tight seal around the mouthpiece and inhale slowly through the corrugated tubing. As the patient inhales, the vinyl bellows will rise. The bottom edge of the bellows serves as the inspired volume indicator. Therefore, wherever the bottom edge of the bellows aligns with the volume scale, that indicates the volume in millimeters the patient has inspired. When the patient has reached the end-inspiratory level, the mouthpiece is removed and the reset button is depressed to prepare for the next sustained maximum inspiration.

The vinyl bellows are thin and lightweight, thereby minimizing the inspiratory effort required by the patient. The Volurex also features a one-way valve that prevents the patient from rebreathing from the device.

Expand-A-Lung

The Dart Respiratory Expand-A-Lung incentive spirometer, manufactured by Seamless (Fig 15–16), is a single-use, flow-dependent incentive spirometer designed to provide SMI. The device comes in a re-sealable package and assembly involves connecting an 18-in. tube with preattached mouthpiece to a stem on the face of the unit. The goal can be set by a six-position variable-flow controller. The difficulty level can be adjusted from 1 (easiest: 150 ml/sec) to 6 (hardest: 1,000 ml/sec). The patient is instructed to hold the unit level, exhale, and then place lips around mouthpiece and inhale to raise the ball to the top of the viewing window. The ball should be kept elevated for 2 to 3 seconds for maximum inspiratory effect.

When the patient has completed the inspiratory effort or removes the mouthpiece from his mouth, the ball falls to the bottom of the viewing window. The Expand-A-Lung is then ready for another inspiratory effort.

The wide range of flow rates allows use with patients from pediatric to geriatric. The unit has a patient nameplate for personal identification, thereby minimizing the accidental use of the unit by another patient.

Spirocare Incentive Breathing Exercisers

The Spirocare (model 108B) incentive breathing exerciser, manufactured by Monaghan Medical, is a volume-oriented, battery-powered device that has the following volume ranges: 250–1,375, 500–2,750, and 1,000–5,500 ml (Fig 15–17). The volume range should be set according to physician or respiratory care practitioner recommendations.

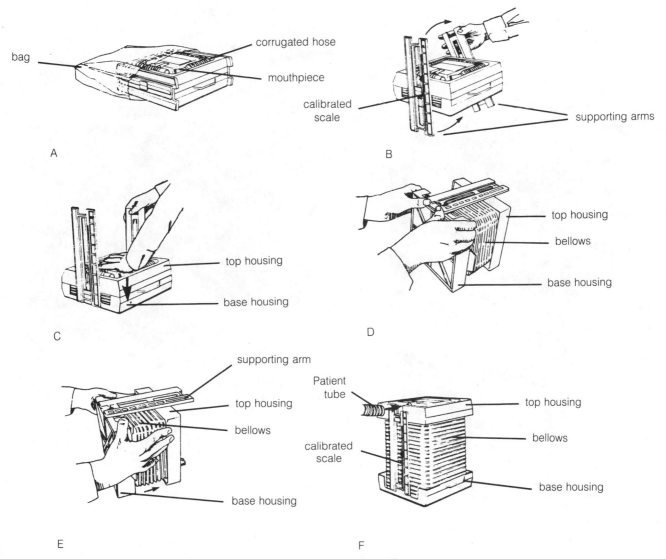

FIG 15–13.
Argyle Tru-vol. **A,** remove from bag. **B,** lift and rotate the supporting arm. **C,** push down the top. **D,** separate the top from the base.

E, push both sides of arm into place. **F,** attach patient hose and mouthpiece. (Courtesy of Sherwood Medical, St. Louis.)

The power switch must be placed in the on position for the unit to become operable. The spirometer is powered by four 1.5-V D-size alkaline batteries. Patient progress is indicated by goal lights on a multicolored display panel indicating a range of 1 to 10, with 10 representing the highest volume on the scale. A hold light is activated and remains lit for 2.5 seconds when the patient achieves the inspiratory goal. After each inspiratory effort, a reset button prepares the unit for another inspiratory maneuver. When the patient is finished with the spirometer, the power switch should be placed in the off position.

The Spirocare model 108M incentive breathing exerciser functions similarly to the Spirocare model 108B. However, the 108M model (Fig 15–18) allows the goal to be set on the unit in advance of the patient's performance of the inspiratory maneuver. Also, the 108M model is powered by 110-V alternating current (AC) instead of alkaline batteries.

CHEST PERCUSSORS

A variety of mechanical chest percussors are commercially available.[9] Models manufactured by

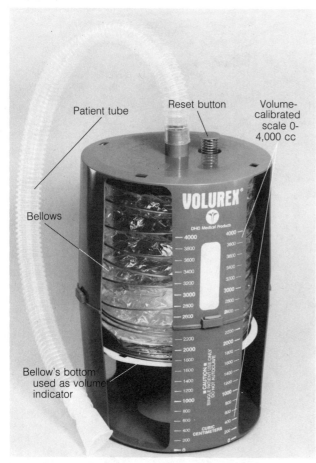

FIG 15–14.
Volurex incentive spirometer. (Courtesy of DHD Medical Products, Division of Diemolding Corporation, Canastota, N.Y.)

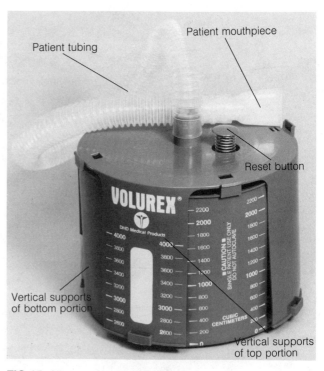

FIG 15–15.
Volurex incentive spirometer in a collapsed position before assembly. (Courtesy of DHD Medical Products, Division of Diemolding Corporation, Canastota, N.Y.)

General Physiotherapy, Inc. and Puritan-Bennett Corporation will be discussed here. A pediatric unit manufactured by Hudson will also be presented. Three models available through General Physiotherapy, Inc. include the *Vibramatic*, the *Multimatic*, and the *Flimm Fighter*.

The Vibramatic (Fig 15–19) features percussive directional stroking and is characterized by two force components (Fig 15–20). One component is directed perpendicular to the patient's body, and the other is directed parallel to the patient's body. The perpendicular component is intended to loosen tracheobronchial secretions, whereas the parallel component is designed to assist the movement of secretions in the direction deemed appropriate by the practitioner.[4]

The Vibramatic also features a variable percussion speed that is dial controlled, a speed indicator gauge, a timer with an automatic shutoff, and a stor-

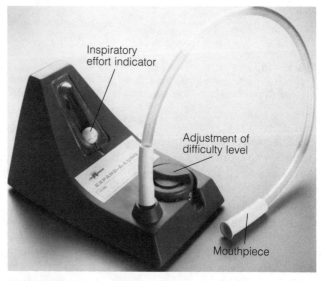

FIG 15–16.
Dart Respiratory Expand-A-Lung incentive spirometer. (Courtesy of Seamless/Dart Respiratory, Wallingford, Conn.)

tion on the patient for only 30 to 60 seconds. After 60 seconds or less, the applicator should be lifted from the patient's thorax and moved to another position.

3. The respiratory care practitioner should loosely hold the handle using the fingers only (Fig 15–22). The weight of the applicator and its assembly is sufficient to maintain contact with the patient's thorax. Additionally, less mechanical energy (vibrations) will be lost through the practitioner's hand and arm.

4. For average-sized patients, the variable-speed output control should be set at 20 to 30 cycles/sec. However, lower frequencies should be used on larger patients and higher frequencies should be used on smaller patients because effective drainage and vibratory action is inversely related to the body mass of the patient.

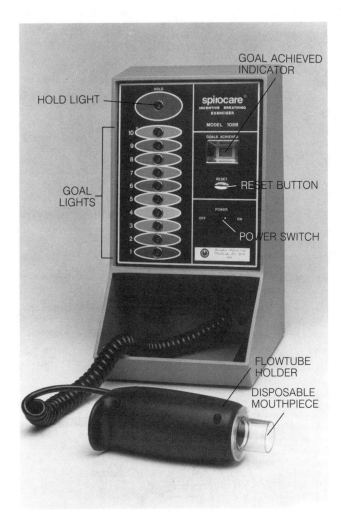

FIG 15–17.
Spirocare Model 108B incentive breathing exerciser. (Courtesy of Monaghan Medical Corp., Plattsburgh, N.Y.)

age compartment for the applicator. The Multimatic chest percussor has most of the features contained in the Vibramatic. Since the Multimatic is intended for use in clinics and offices, it does not include a timer, a speed indicator gauge, or a hospital-grade power cord and plug.

The manufacturer has a number of specific recommendations for using chest percussors featuring directional stroking activity. These recommendations include:

1. The applicator must always be attached to the percussor via the right-angle percussor adapter (Fig 15–21). The right-angle percussor adapter is responsible for producing the directional-stroking motion.

2. The applicator should be held in one loca-

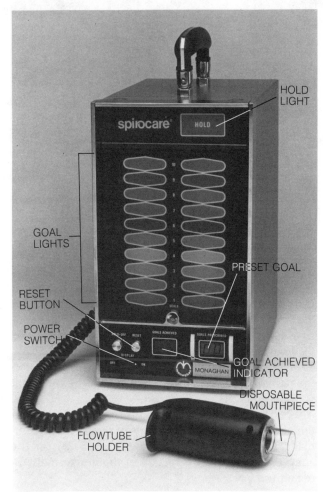

FIG 15–18.
Spirocare Model 108M incentive breathing exerciser. (Courtesy of Monaghan Medical Corp., Plattsburgh, N.Y.)

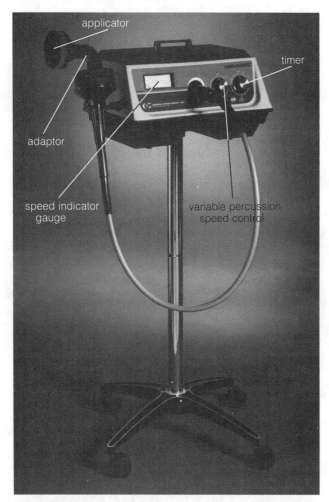

FIG 15–19.
Vibramatic chest percussor. (Courtesy of General Physiotherapy Inc., St. Louis, Mo.)

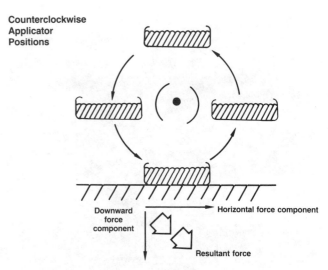

FIG 15–20.
Horizontal and perpendicular force components of applicator for Vibramatic chest percussor. (Courtesy of General Physiotherapy, Inc., St. Louis, Mo.)

sive directional stroking action, is secured to the patient's thorax in the following manner (Fig 15–25):

1. The applicator is placed within a depression located in a foam pad (Fig 15–25,A).

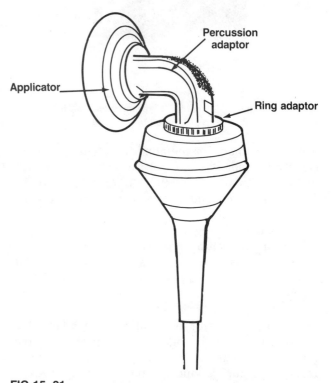

FIG 15–21.
Right-angle adapter for percussor of Vibramatic chest percussor. (Courtesy of General Physiotherapy, Inc., St. Louis, Mo.)

5. The practitioner's free hand should be placed lightly on the patient's thorax near the location of the applicator to monitor the percussive force. Increases or decreases in the frequency can then be made accordingly.

6. It is incumbent on the practitioner to position the patient according to the segment of the lung that is to be drained.

7. The practitioner should also utilize the directional stroking feature of the Vibramatic and Multimatic percussors. A red arrow (Fig 15–23) on the adapter indicates the direction of the horizontally directed force.

The Flimm Fighter is designed mainly for home care patients to allow them the opportunity to self-administer postural drainage and chest percussion (Fig 15–24). The applicator, which features percus-

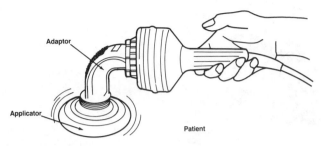

FIG 15–22.
Technique for holding the handle of the Vibramatic chest percussor. (Courtesy of General Physiotherapy, Inc., St. Louis, Mo.)

2. A Velcro positioning belt is attached to the foam pad (Fig 15–25,B).
3. The Velcro positioning belt is wrapped around the patient's thorax, positioning the applicator in its desired location (Fig 15–25,C).
4. The patient then assumes the appropriate position for the postural drainage and percussion of the desired segment (Fig 15–25,D).

The Puritan-Bennett Corporation manufactures an electrically powered, portable vibrator/percussor (Fig 15–26). The Puritan-Bennett model features a magnetically induced stroke that prevents excess vibration and pressure from being applied to the patient. The practitioner can control stroke intensity and frequency independently of each other. Stroke intensity and frequency should both be adjusted ac-

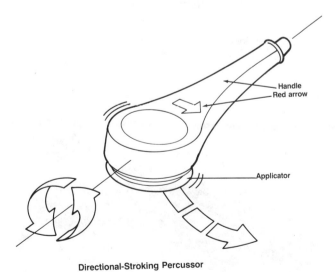

Directional-Stroking Percussor

FIG 15–23.
Directional stroking percussor for the Vibramatic and Multimatic chest percussors. (Courtesy of General Physiotherapy, Inc., St. Louis, Mo.)

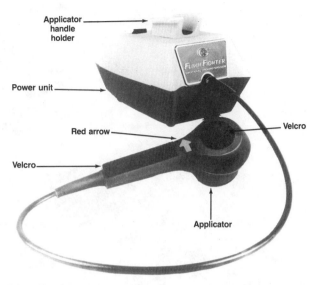

FIG 15–24.
The Flimm Fighter for self-application of postural drainage and chest percussion. (Courtesy of General Physiotherapy, Inc., St. Louis, Mo.)

cording to the patient's size, weight, and clinical condition.

A warning light on the unit alerts the practitioner that the motor is approaching overheating. The unit should then be turned off to allow the motor to cool. If the warning light is ignored, a thermal fuse inside the device safeguards the motor from overheating by causing the percussor to shut off automatically. The practitioner cannot reset the thermal fuse. The unit then needs to be sent to the manufacturer. Therefore, it is important for the operator to heed the red warning light (i.e., to manually turn off the unit and allow it to cool).

Hudson manufactures a pediatric percussor that is pneumatically powered (Fig 15–27). It is designed for clinical use on neonates, infants, and children. The unit features controls for percussion force and frequency. Both of these parameters can be adjusted accordingly to meet clinical needs.

The percussor can be powered by any medical-grade compressed air source. Required pressure ranges from 45 to 55 pounds per square inch (psi). The device includes the following equipment: (1) power unit, (2) remote head assembly, (3) high-pressure hose (6 ft long), (4) transmission hose (4 ft long), and (5) silicone diaphragms (five).

SUCTION CATHETER KITS

A number of manufacturers (e.g., Argyle, Portex, Inc., and Travenol Laboratories, Inc.) have suc-

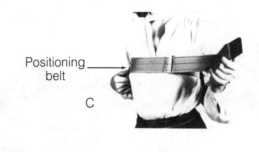

Positioning belt

C

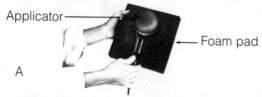

Applicator

Foam pad

A

A Velcro hook-and-loop secure the applicator handle.

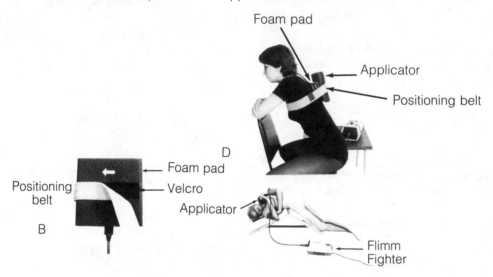

Foam pad

Applicator

Positioning belt

D

Foam pad

Positioning belt

Velcro

Applicator

B

Flimm Fighter

FIG 15–25.

Attaching the Flimm Fighter applicator. **A,** a Velcro hook and loop secure the applicator handle. **B,** the arrow in the foam pad indicates the direction of the horizontally directed force. **C,** the belt is then tightened and secured via a metal cinch. **D,** Flimm Fighter models can be obtained with a variable speed or with a single speed. (Courtesy of General Physiotherapy, Inc., St. Louis, Mo.)

FIG 15–26.

Puritan-Bennett vibrator/percussor. (Courtesy of Puritan-Bennett Corporation, Overland Park, Kansas.)

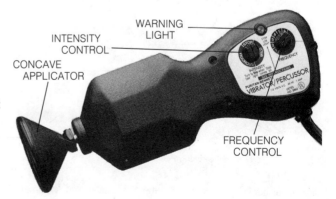

WARNING LIGHT

INTENSITY CONTROL

CONCAVE APPLICATOR

VIBRATOR/PERCUSSOR

FREQUENCY CONTROL

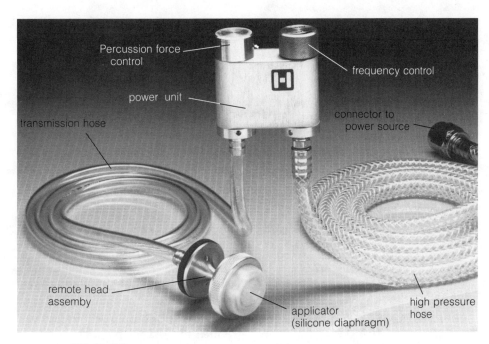

FIG 15–27.
Hudson pediatric percussor. (Courtesy of Hudson Oxygen, Temecula, Calif.)

tion catheter kits commercially available. The kits produced by these manufacturers do not vary considerably in their contents. Commonly, each provides sterile vinyl gloves, a sterile suction catheter, and a catheter rinse cup or rinse basin (Fig 15–28).

Argyle provides a number of choices for suction catheter kit selections. One of their kits contains (1) a rigid plastic basin; (2) a single-use, 120-ml sterile saline cup; (3) two vinyl gloves; (4) a drape; (5) and a suction catheter. The type of catheter chosen can be either the *Aero-Flo suction catheter* or the *DeLee tip*

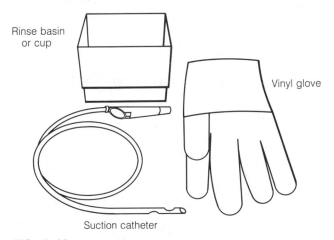

FIG 15–28.
Common components of suction catheter kits: suction catheter, rinse cup, and vinyl glove.

suction catheter (see later discussion). Other kits from Argyle can be stocked with one or two gloves, a pop-up basin and sterile field, or a rigid plastic basin and drape, and either Aero-Flo, DeLee tip, *whistle tip*, or *Safe-T-mark suction catheter*.

Portex provides the choice of suction catheter to include either the *Portex whistle tip* or the *Portex angled Coude*. The suction catheter available with the Travenol kit is the whistle tip type, which has dual opposing eyelets.

SUCTION CATHETERS

Suction catheters are manufactured according to a minimum of eight configurations that are intended to meet certain clinical needs (Fig 15–29). For example, the open-end suction catheter has a single orifice available for the aspiration of tracheobronchial secretions (Fig 15–29,A). When suction is applied to this catheter, the flow, produced by the negative (subatmospheric) pressure occurs through the suction catheter and the suction jar at the wall. Aspirated material moves into the open-end tip, travels through the entire length of the catheter, and deposits in the suction jar.

Caution must be exercised with open-ended suction catheters. If the open end impinges on the respiratory mucosal wall anywhere in the tracheobron-

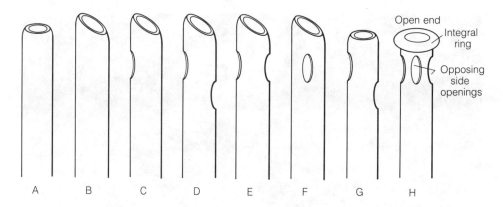

FIG 15–29.
A, open-end suction catheter with orifice perpendicular to long axis of catheter. **B,** open-end suction catheter with angular cut. **C,** Argyle whistle-tip catheter angular end and single side opening. **D,** Argyle whistle-tip catheter with angular end and two staggered side openings. **E,** Travenol whistle-tip catheter with angular end and two side openings. **F,** Portex whistle-tip suction catheter with angular end and single side opening. **G,** Argyle DeLee tip catheter with open end perpendicular to long axis of catheter , with two staggered side openings. **H,** Argyle Aero-Flo tip catheter with integral wing situated below four opposed eyes.

chial tree, the entire negative pressure will be exerted on that surface. In such instances, suction should be terminated by removing one's thumb from the suction control (Y or T). Continued negative pressure against the wall surfaces can damage or tear the mucosal layer. No attempts must be made in such a situation to maintain suction while withdrawing the catheter from the patient.

Another open-end suction catheter has an angular configuration of the tip (Fig 15–29,B). The slanted cut has been made obliquely to the long axis of the suction catheter. This design increases the area exposed to negative pressure. The same precautions apply to the open-end angular tip as pertain to the perpendicular cut. The open-end suction catheters are particularly useful for removing thick, tenacious secretions from the oral cavity.

The whistle-tip suction catheter is designed to reduce the risk of respiratory mucosal damage. Inspection of the whistle tip reveals that two openings are present (Fig 15–29,C). One is the angular cut made obliquely to the long axis of the catheter, and the other appears on the side wall of the catheter. The intention of this configuration is to prevent or, at least, minimize the chances of occluding the end of the catheter against the mucosal wall. If the whistle-tip catheter attaches to the mucosal wall, negative pressure would be directed through the other opening. Mucosal wall damage would thereby be reduced. Argyle manufactures a whistle-tip catheter that has a slanted open end and two opposed, but staggered, side openings, or eyes (Fig 15–29,D).

Travenol makes a suction catheter similar to the Argyle whistle tip previously described. It differs

FIG 15–30.
Argyle Aero-Flo tip catheter alongside mucosal wall. Integral ring reduces open-end or side-vent adherence to mucosal wall.

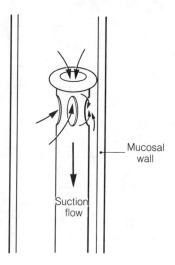

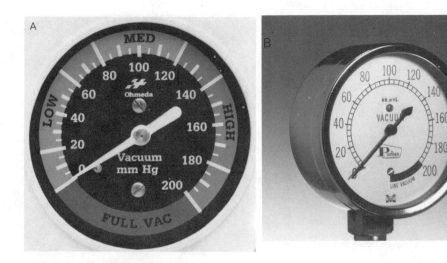

Ohmeda

FIG 15–31.
Suction regulators: Ohmeda **(A)** (Courtesy of Ohmeda, Madison, Wis.) and Puritan-Bennett **(B).** (Courtesy of Puritan-Bennet Corporation, Overland Park, Kansas.)

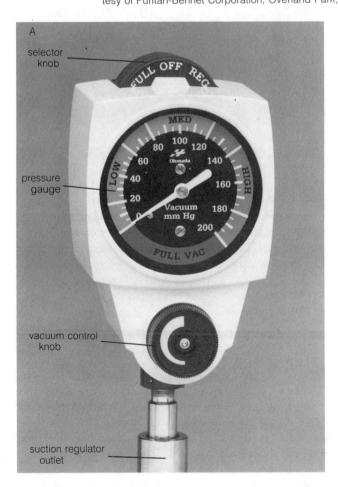

OHIO VACUUM REGULATOR

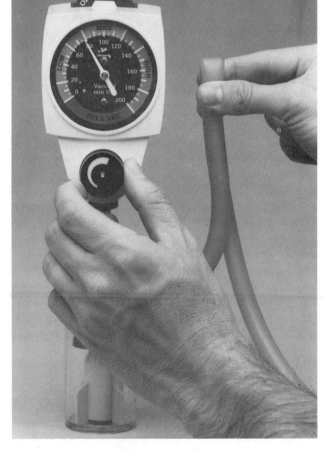

FIG 15–32.
A, Ohmeda vacuum regulator with three-position selector knob. **B,** establishing desired vacuum level by occluding suction regulator outlet and rotating vacuum control knob (Ohmeda vacuum regulator). (Courtesy of Ohmeda, Madison, Wis.)

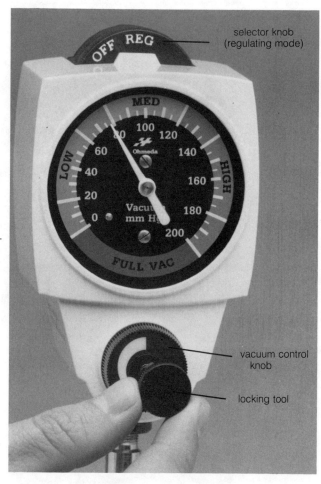

FIG 15–33.
Locking desired suction level in place (Ohmeda vacuum regulator). (Courtesy of Ohmeda, Madison, Wis.)

from the Argyle in that opposing side openings are not staggered (Fig 15–29,E). The Portex whistle-tip suction catheter has one port and a slanted open end (Fig 15–29,F).

Argyle produces two other suction catheters with unique characteristics, the DeLee tip and the Aero-Flo tip. The DeLee tip has an open end perpendicular to the long axis of the catheter (Fig 15–29G). The Aero-Flo suction catheter is characterized by an integral ring at its tip (distal end), above which four opposed eyes are situated (Fig 15–29H). The integral ring reduces the chance that the suction catheter will adhere to the mucosal wall, the protruding tip allows for suction to be applied through the four adjacent openings for the removal of mucus (Fig 15–30).

SUCTION REGULATORS

Wall vacuum is ordinarily provided by a centrally located vacuum pump. This vacuum pump supplies the negative (subatmospheric) pressure used for suctioning procedures. Ordinarily, the negative pressure created by the central vacuum system is much greater than that which is needed for airway suctioning. The negative pressure generated by such a system is usually within the range of 19 to 25 in. Hg.

The conversion of inches of mercury to millimeters of mercury is as follows:

$$1 \text{ in. Hg} = 25.4 \text{ mm Hg}$$
$$19 \text{ in. Hg} \times 25.4 \text{ mm Hg/in. Hg} = 482.6 \text{ mm Hg}$$
$$25 \text{ in. Hg} \times 25.4 \text{ mm Hg/in. Hg} = 635.0 \text{ mm Hg}$$

Therefore, in terms of millimeters of mercury, the central vacuum system operates within a range of 482.6 to 635.0 mm Hg. This amount of negative pressure is much greater than that required for tracheobronchial suctioning. The amount of negative pressure used for airway suctioning is controlled by attaching a suction regulator to the wall outlet. Suction regulators utilize either Quick Connect wall outlet connections or Diameter Index Safety System

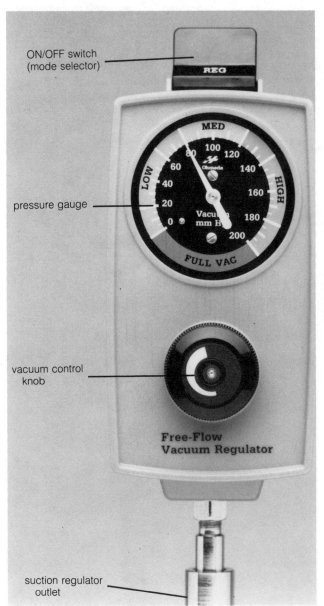

ON/OFF switch
(mode selector)

pressure gauge

vacuum control
knob

suction regulator
outlet

FIG 15–34.
Ohmeda Free-Flow regulator. (Courtesy of Ohmeda, Madison, Wis.)

(DISS) connections. The gauges or manometers on these regulators are generally calibrated in millimeters of mercury and can be adjusted to the desired negative pressure level (Fig 15–31).

The Ohmeda suction regulator has a selector knob that allows for the selection of any of three suction modes, that is, full suction, suction off, and regulated suction (Fig 15–32,A). When the selector knob is in the full-suction mode, full-line vacuum is provided. Full-line vacuum with this type of regulator can provide flow rates as high as 110 L/min. In the regulated suction mode, negative pressure can be set anywhere between 0 and 200 mm Hg. The desired vacuum level can be established by occlud-ing the suction regulator outlet and rotating the vacuum control knob located immediately beneath the pressure manometer (Fig 15–32,B). Once the vacuum level has been adjusted, it can be locked to prevent inadvertent alteration. A locking key located on the backside of the regulator can be removed and used to lock the vacuum control knob (Fig 15–33). In addition to being calibrated in millimeters of mercury, the pressure gauge on this regulator is color coded, indicating low, medium, high, and full vacuum.

Another type of suction regulator manufactured by Ohmeda is the *Ohmeda Free-Flow regulator* (Fig 15–34). The pressure manometer on this device is also color coded to indicate various levels of vacuum and

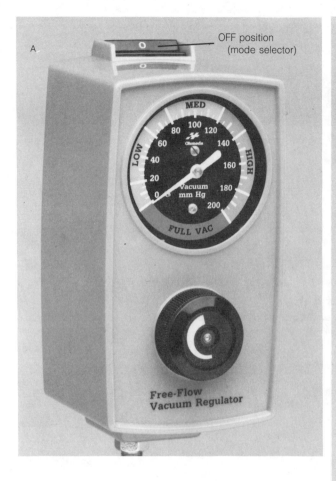

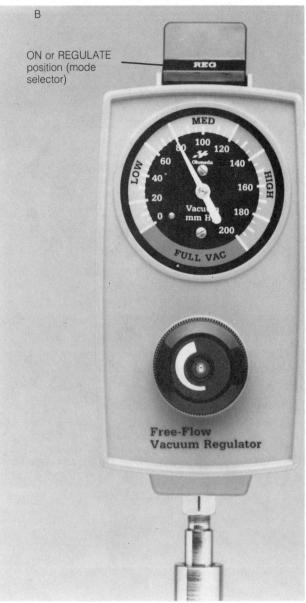

FIG 15–35.
Ohmeda Free Flow regulator in off position **(A)** and Ohmeda Free Flow regulator in on position **(B)**. (Courtesy of Ohmeda, Madison, Wis.)

displays a vacuum range of 0 to 200 mm Hg. Its flow rate capabilities range from 0 to 150 L/min. Having such high flow rate capabilities makes this regulator well suited for patient care facilities where central vacuum systems do not provide adequate vacuum levels.

A large on/off switch is located atop the regulator. In the off position the switch will lie flat across the top of the regulator (Fig 15–35,A). When the regulator is in the on position, the switch atop the reg-

ulator will be raised, indicating regulate (Fig 15–35,B). The vacuum control knob, located below the pressure gauge, can then be rotated to adjust the desired level of negative pressure. The locking tool can again be implemented to lock the vacuum control knob to prevent accidental pressure changes.

Once the vacuum control knob has been locked, the locking key can be returned to its housing located on the back side of the regulator (Fig 15–36,A). The ability of the Ohmeda Free-flow regulator to

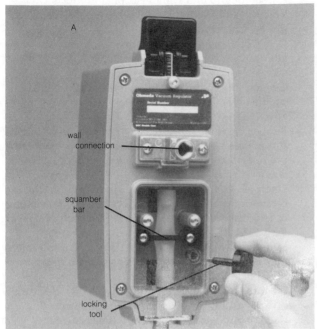
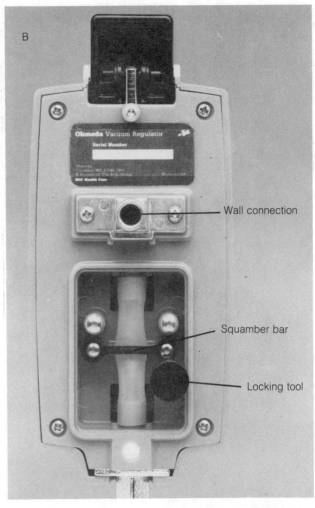

FIG 15–36.
Ohio Free Flow regulator. **A,** returning locking tool to its housing. **B,** locking tool secured on backside of regulator. (Courtesy of OHMEDA, Madison, Wis.)

maintain high flow rates even at low central vacuum levels exists because suction bypasses the regulator mechanism itself. Conventional suction regulators experience diminished capabilities under such conditions. Similarly, conventional suction regulators become less efficient as a result of contamination by foreign matter during use since suction is transmitted through the regulator mechanism. The Ohmeda Free-flow regulator eliminates much chance for foreign matter obstruction because suction bypasses the regulator mechanism.

Located on the Ohmeda Free-flow regulator's back side (Fig 15–36,B) is a small device called a *squamper bar.* The squamper bar controls the vacuum by compressing a flexible, clear, plastic tube in the suction circuit. The squamper bar alternately compresses and decompresses the tube as vacuum levels

change. Consequently, the vacuum control knob below the pressure gauge does not require repeated readjustments to maintain an adequate flow rate.

The Puritan-Bennett Corporation manufactures a general-purpose suction regulator (Fig 15–37). Its pressure gauge is calibrated in millimeters of mercury with a range of 0 to 200 mm Hg. To set a desired suction pressure setting, occlude the regulator, and rotate the vacuum pressure adjustment knob accordingly until the desired level is achieved. A safety lock is available to eliminate the chance of accidental pressure alteration.

Some regulators have a flag lever, located on the opposite side of the safety lock, that allows for an immediate switch to full-line vacuum if the need arises. If the flag is present, it should be in the regulated vacuum position when a preset suction level

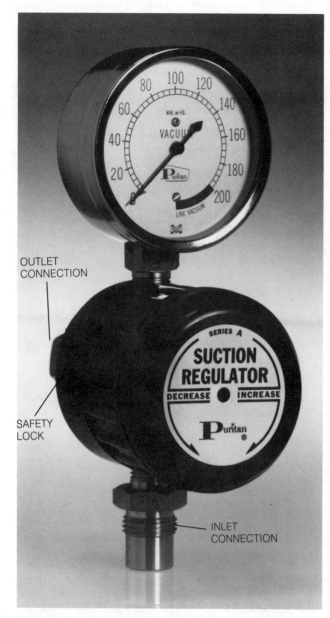

FIG 15–37.
Puritan-Bennett vacuum regulator. (Courtesy of Puritan-Bennett Corporation, Overland Park, Kansas.)

is being established. When the pressure manometer reading is adjusted beyond the 200 mm Hg level, full-line vacuum will be experienced at the regulator inlet.

REFERENCES

1. Bartlett RH, et al: Respiratory maneuvers to prevent postoperative pulmonary complications: A critical review. *JAMA* 1983; 224:1017–1021.

2. Chesebrough-Pond's, Inc, Hospital Products Division: Voldyne and Triflo II product literature. Greenwich, Conn., Chesebrough-Pond's, 1982.

3. Gale GD, Sanders DE: Incentive spirometry: Its value after cardiac surgery. *Can Anaesth Soc J* 1980; 27:475–480.

4. General Physiotherapy, Inc: Vibramatic/Multimatic product literature. St Louis, Mo, General Physiotherapy, 1984.

5. Indihar FJ, et al: A prospective comparison of three procedures used in attempts to prevent postoperative pulmonary complications. *Respir Care* 1982; 27:564–568.

6. Leigh IG, et al: A comparative study of IPPB, the incentive spirometer, and blow bottles: The prevention of atelectasis following cardiac surgery. *Ann Thorac Surg* 1978; 25:197–200.

7. Minschaert M, et al: Influence of incentive spirometry on pulmonary volumes after laparotomy. *Acta Anaesthesiol Belg* 1982; 33:203–209.

8. Pfenninger J, Roth F: Intermittent positive pressure breathing (IPPB) versus incentive spirometer (IS) therapy in postoperative period. *Intens Care Med* 1978; 3:279–281.

9. Radford R, et al: A rational basis for percussion—augmented mucociliary clearance. *Respir Care* 1982; 27:556–563.

10. Ros AM, et al: Incentive spirometry: Prevention of pulmonary complications after abdominal surgery. *Acta Anaesthesiol Belg* 1981; 32:167–174.

PRODUCT SOURCES

Airlife/American Pharmaseal Company
27200 N. Tourney Road
Valencia, CA 91355–8900

Argyle
Division of Sherwood Medical
Department AK
1831 Olive Street
St. Louis, MO 63103

Chesebrough-Pond's, Inc.
Division of Sherwood Medical
1831 Olive Street
St. Louis, MO 63103

Dart Respiratory
Seamless Hospital Products Company, Inc.
Barnes Industrial Park North
Wallingford, Ct 06492

DHD Medical Products
Division of Diemolding Corporation
125 Rasbach Street
Canastota, NY 13032

General Physiotherapy, Inc.
1520 Washington Avenue
St. Louis, MO 63103

Health Scan Products, Inc.
908 Pompton Avenue
Cedar Grove, NJ 07009

Hudson Oxygen
27711 Diaz Street
P.O. Box 66
Temecula, CA 92390–0066

Ohmeda
Division of Airco, Inc.
3030 Airco Drive
P.O. Box 7550
Madison, WI 53707

Portex, Inc.
42 Industrial Way
Wilmington, MA 01887

Puritan-Bennett Corporation
9401 Indian Creek Parkway
P.O. Box 25905
Overland Park, KS 66225–5905

Shiley, Inc.
17660 Gillette Avenue
Irvine, CA 92714

Travenol Laboratories, Inc.
Medical Products Division
One Baxter Parkway
Deerfield, IL 60015

16

Mechanical Ventilators

J. Douglas Vandine, R.R.T.

The responsibilities of the respiratory therapist in intensive care units include the monitoring and management of patients on mechanical ventilators. It is essential that respiratory therapists have a working knowledge of both the mechanisms and capabilities of the devices used to provide ventilatory support. To understand how mechanical ventilators work, we must identify the tasks we expect the machine to perform. The subsequent analysis of how a particular ventilator accomplishes these tasks will define its operational characteristics.

Five important independent variables associated with mechanical ventilation are:

1. The rate of breathing (breaths/min).
2. The size of each breath (tidal volume).
3. How fast the breath is given (inspiratory time, inspiratory flow rate).
4. The mixture of gas used ($F_{I_{O_2}}$).
5. The pressure in the system at end expiration (positive end-expiratory pressure, PEEP).

Also, there are several different modes of mechanical ventilation that may be available on a single ventilator (see Chapter 10). The operational characteristics of the machine will depend on the mode of ventilation selected.

This chapter will analyze several representative types of mechanical ventilators in terms of the modes of ventilation available and look at how the independent variables of ventilation are determined. The goal of this chapter is to teach the principles of ventilator operation with the expectation that the reader will be able to extend the application of this knowledge to devices not specifically discussed in this book.

PHYSICAL LAWS AND MECHANICAL VENTILATION

Before the various types of ventilators are classified and described, the gas laws involved in mechanical ventilation will be reviewed. Operation of mechanical ventilators requires a knowledge of pressure, volume, and flow relationships for gases. Interaction between ventilator controls is based on some of the principles described in the sections that follow.

Boyle's Law

Given a fixed mass (n) of gas during mechanical ventilation, bulk movement of gas (flow) occurs only in response to a pressure difference. As pressure changes in the ventilator circuit, the volume of gas delivered by the ventilator varies inversely with the pressure change, provided the gas temperature (T) is held constant (Boyle's law: PV = constant). The degree to which the delivered volume is affected by system pressure describes the internal compliance of a ventilator.

Example: A volume-preset ventilator has a bellows volume of 2,200 ml. The volume of the gas conduction system from the bellows to the patient is 800 ml.

1. What is the internal compliance of the system?
2. If the bellows delivers 1,000 ml to the conduction system and the pressure in the system reaches 50 cm H_2O, how much of that 1,000 ml will actually go to the patient?

Solution 1: Compliance (C) equals the change in volume (ΔV) divided by the change in pressure (ΔP).

$$C = \frac{\Delta V}{\Delta P}$$

$$\text{Compliance} = \frac{V_1 - V_2}{P_1 - P_2}$$

Using Boyle's law, we find that $V_2 = V_1 \times (P_2/P_1)$. Substituting V_2 into the compliance equation:

$$\text{Compliance} = \frac{V_1 (1 - P_2/P_1)}{(P_1 - P_2)}$$

If an arbitrary pressure (20 cm H_2O) is selected for P_2, and P_1 is set at atmospheric pressure (1,034 cm H_2O) the internal compliance can be calculated:

where

$$P_1 = 1,034 \text{ cm } H_2O$$
$$P_2 = 1,054 \text{ cm } H_2O$$
$$V_1 = 3,000 \text{ ml}$$

$$\text{Compliance} = \frac{3,000 \ (1 - 1,054/1,034)}{1,034 - 1,054}$$

$$= 3 \text{ ml/cm } H_2O$$

Solution 2: If the pressure in the system reaches 50 cm H_2O, the compressed volume will be 3 ml/cm $H_2O \times 50$ cm H_2O, or 150 ml. Actual delivered volume is $1,000 - 150$ or, 850 ml.

Poiseuille's Law

The physical law governing gas flow through conduction system is Poiseuille's law, which states, in its simple form:

Pressure difference (ΔP) = flow ($\dot{V}$) × resistance (R)

Rearranged to express flow:

$$\dot{V} = \frac{\Delta P}{R}$$

The application of this principle to mechanical ventilation is of key importance to understanding the principles of mechanical ventilation. Consider the following practical application:

The working pressure of a given ventilator is 3 pounds per square inch (psi) (approximately 210 cm H_2O). The resistance of the ventilator circuit and valve is fixed at 100 cm H_2O/L/sec. If during inspiration, the pressure in the patient circuit rises evenly from ambient pressure to 60 cm H_2O, how will the flow change during the course of inspiration?

Answer: Since the resistance is constant, the flow is proportional to the pressure difference driving the gas. The initial pressure in the patient circuit is atmospheric, and the driving pressure is 3 psi (210 cm H_2O). The initial flow, then, is:

$$\dot{V} = \frac{\Delta P}{R}$$

where
$\Delta P = 210 - 0 = 210$ cm H_2O (start of inspiration)

$R = 100$ cm H_2O/L/sec.

$$\text{Initial } \dot{V} = \frac{210 \text{ cm } H_2O}{100 \text{ cm } H_2O/L/sec}$$

$$= 2.1 \text{ L/sec, or } 126 \text{ L/min}$$

At the end of inspiration, the driving pressure is less by the pressure in the patient circuit. Under these conditions, the flow is reduced:

$$\Delta P = 210 - 60 = 150 \text{ cm } H_2O$$
(end of inspiration)

$$R = 100 \text{ cm } H_2O/L/sec$$

$$\text{Terminal } \dot{V} = \frac{150 \text{ cm } H_2O}{100 \text{ cm } H_2O/L/sec}$$

$$= 1.5 \text{ L/sec, or } 90 \text{ L/min}$$

This decrease represents about a 28% reduction in flow. As an exercise, calculate the initial and terminal flows using the data just given but applying it to a ventilator whose driving pressure is only 100 cm H_2O:

$$\Delta P = 100 - 0 = 100 \text{ cm } H_2O$$
(start of inspiration)
$$R = 100 \text{ cm } H_2O/L/sec$$

$$\text{Initial } \dot{V} = \frac{100 \text{ cm } H_2O}{100 \text{ cm } H_2O/L/sec}$$
$$= 1.0 \text{ L/sec, or } 60 \text{ L/min}$$
$$\Delta P = 100 - 60 = 40 \text{ cm } H_2O$$
(end of inspiration)
$$R = 100 \text{ cm } H_2O/L/sec$$

$$\text{Terminal } \dot{V} = \frac{40 \text{ cm } H_2O}{100 \text{ cm } H_2O/L/sec}$$
$$= 0.4 \text{ L/sec, or } 24 \text{ L/min}$$

These two concepts, Boyle's law and Poiseuille's law, are crucial to the understanding of the workings of pneumatic systems, and it is important to have a firm grasp of these principles before proceeding to the next section.

CLASSIFICATION OF MECHANICAL VENTILATORS

One accepted means of classifying ventilators involves specifying (1) the *cycling mechanism*, or how the start of inspiration is determined; (2) the *limit factor*, or how the end of inspiration is determined; and (3) the *motive force*, or how the device acts on the patient to deliver a breath. Using this system, one would classify the Emerson iron lung, for example, as a time-cycled, pressure-limited, negative-pressure ventilator.

However, as one deals with more sophisticated ventilators, it becomes difficult to classify them with these basic terms. Many state-of-the-art ventilators have several modes of operation that determine how the machine is cycled or limited.

A more practical way of describing late-generation mechanical ventilators is to identify (1) their *source of power*, (2) their *control mechanisms*, and (3) the *mode capabilities* of the machine being discussed. For example, the BEAR I ventilator (Bear Medical Systems, Inc.) is pneumatically powered and electronically controlled with assist, control, synchronized intermittent mandatory ventilation (SIMV), and continuous positive airway pressure (CPAP) capabilities. This method of classification will be used in this chapter, along with discussion of cycling and limiting mechanisms for particular modes.

The characteristics of ventilators belonging to four basic groups will be discussed: (1) the negative-pressure ventilators (Emerson iron lung), (2) the pressure-preset positive-pressure ventilators (Bird Mark 7), (3) the volume-preset positive-pressure ventilators (piston-driven, bellows-driven, flow-integrating, servo-controlled, and microprocessor-controlled ventilators), and (4) continuous flow–type neonatal ventilators (Bourns BP200 produced by Bear Medical Systems, Inc.). The discussion will include control interaction, monitor and alarm systems, and an operational description.

Negative-Pressure Ventilators

Iron Lung

Although not in common use today, the iron lung is of interest from both a historical and a physiologic standpoint. A body-enclosing respirator in which the patient sat upright was described in 1838 by John Dalziel, a Scottish physician.[1] The first iron lung used in the United States was built at the Harvard School of Public Health in 1929 by Philip and Cecil Drinker.[2] The most important improvement of the iron lung was made by John H. Emerson in 1932 when he added a transparent airtight dome over the patient's head so that positive-pressure ventilation could be given when nursing care was needed.[3] The Emerson iron lung was used extensively for 30 years in the treatment of polio victims.

The iron lung is an electrically powered and controlled, time-cycled, pressure-limited ventilator and can be used only in the control mode. It consists of a steel tank with openings in either side for patient access and at one end for the patient's head (Fig 16–1). The opposite end of the lung is closed by a diaphragm that is driven by a lever attached to an electric motor. The lever can be moved independently of the motor in the event of a loss of electrical power.

Control Mechanism.—The respiratory frequency is determined by varying the speed of the motor (see Fig 16–1)*(1)*. The depth of inspiration is determined by the excursion of the diaphragm. It can be adjusted by turning the control wheel at the base of the drive lever *(2)*. The inspiratory flow rate of delivery depends entirely on the inspiratory/expiratory (I/E) ratio and cannot be altered by the operator. The composition of the inspired gas is not controlled by an iron lung. All controls function independently. A Bourdon-type pressure gauge *(3)* is mounted on the top of the iron lung to allow attendants to monitor ventilation pressure. A pressure vent *(4)*, operated by a thumbscrew, protects the patient against excessive pressure.

Operation.—During inspiration, the motor moves the drive lever, displacing the diaphragm outward. The increase in tank volume causes the pressure to fall, which pulls outward on the patient's chest wall. As the patient's intrathoracic volume increases, air is drawn in through the upper airway and into the lungs. Then the motor moves the diaphragm back to the starting position, the pressure in the tank returns to atmospheric pressure, and passive exhalation occurs.

Pressure-Preset Ventilators

Bird Mark 7

The Bird Mark 7 is an example of a pneumatically powered and controlled, pressure-preset positive-pressure ventilator. It is capable of operating in either a control or an assist/control mode and has the advantage of small size, quiet operation, and independence from electrical power (Fig 16–2).

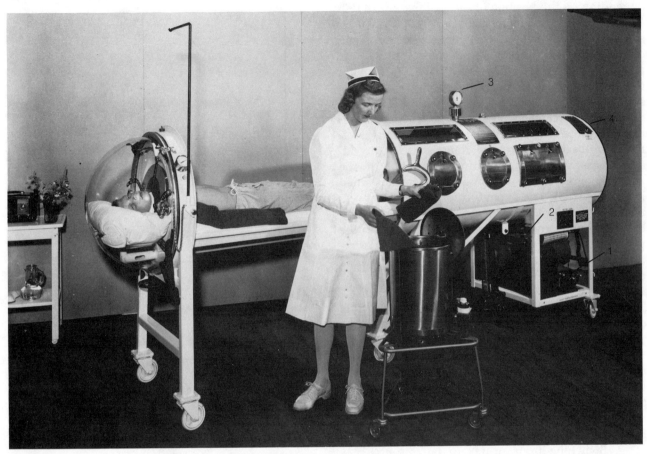

FIG 16–1.
Emerson iron lung. Respiratory frequency is determined by varying the speed of the motor (1). Depth of inspiration is determined by turning the control wheel at the base of the drive lever (2). Bour- don-type pressure gauge to minotor ventilation pressure (3). Pres- sure vent protects patient against excess pressure (4). (Courtesy of J.H. Emerson Company, Cambridge, Mass.)

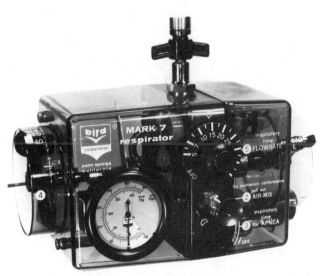

FIG 16–2.
Bird Mark 7. (Courtesy of Bird Corporation, Palm Springs, Calif.)

Control Mechanism.—In the control mode the rate is determined by the inspiratory time, which is a function of the flow rate, and the pressure limit, and apnea controls. The inspiratory time will in- crease if the flow rate decreases or the pressure limit increases. The expiratory time is shortened as the apnea control is turned clockwise. The apnea control is not calibrated, but for a given combination of flow rate and pressure limit, the rate can be varied by ad- justing the apnea control and timing the rate for a minute. The pressure limit control is the major de- terminant of the tidal volume. The tidal volume and the peak inspiratory pressure are dependent on the patient's total compliance (see Appendix B). The ac- tual tidal volume delivered should be monitored continuously during pressure preset ventilation. The flow rate control determines how quickly gas will flow into the lungs during inspiration. It may be var- ied from zero to approximately 80 L/min and will be either a square wave or flow-tapered wave pattern depending on the position of the air-mix control (Fig 16–3). The Bird ventilators are dependent on their source of gas (usually oxygen) for the composition of inspired gas. With the air-mix control in the "in" position, the patient will receive 100% O_2. Moving the air-mix control to the "out" position diverts the source gas through a venturi (see Chapter 12), which mixes the source gas with gas in the ambient chamber. Since the entrainment rate of the venturi is affected by back pressure, the composition of the inspired gas will change during inspiration if the machine is driven by oxygen and the gas entrained is air (Fig 16–4). End-expiratory pressure is not regulated by the Bird Mark 7, and it will return to ambient pressure unless modifications are made to the patient circuit. An airway pressure monitor is incorporated into the machine and allows attendants to observe fluctuations in airway pressure.

Control Interactions.—The following controls on the Bird Mark 7 interact with each other:

1. Changing the peak inspiratory pressure can affect the cycle rate since the inspiratory time will vary directly with the peak inspiratory pressure. In the air-mix configuration, increasing the peak inspiratory pressure will also result in a higher mean F_{IO_2}.

2. Switching from air-mix to 100% source gas will result in decreased inspiratory flow and a slowing of the respiratory rate due to a longer inspiratory time.

3. Changing the flow rate will affect the respiratory rate since the inspiratory time varies inversely with the flow rate. Marked increases in flow rate may also decrease the delivered volume due to more turbulence in the airway and a shorter inspiratory time.

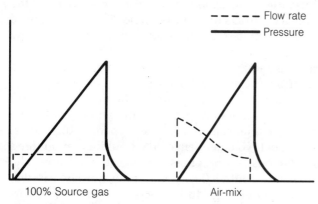

FIG 16–3.
The affect of the air-mix control on the inspiratory flow wave form.

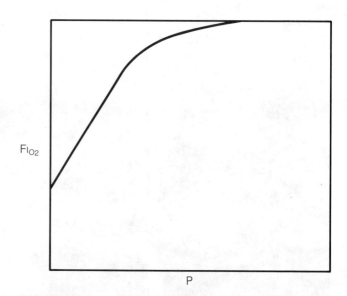

FIG 16–4.
The effect of the back pressure on the F_{IO_2} of a Bird Mark 7 when set on air dilution.

4. Large changes in the sensitivity control will effect changes in the peak inspiratory pressure. The interaction occurs because both controls are linked by the magnetic clutch system that cycles the ventilator (Fig 16–5).

Circuit Assembly and Testing.—The patient circuit consists of three tubes, a nebulizer, and an exhalation valve assembly (Fig 16–5). The main flow

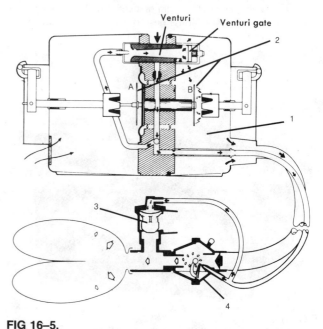

FIG 16–5.
Structure of Bird Mark 7. (Modified from McPherson SP: *Respiratory Therapy Equipment*, ed 3. St. Louis, CV Mosby, 1985, p 272.)

line fits a 22-mm inside-diameter (I.D.) outlet port from the pressurized chamber of the machine. The two smaller-bore (⅛-in. I.D.) pieces of tubing drive the nebulizer and activate the exhalation valve. After assembly, test the circuit by setting the flow rate control at 5, the pressure limit at 40, and the air-mix on "in." With the patient connector occluded, manually cycle the machine by pushing in the red control rod on the left-hand side of the ventilator. If the circuit is properly assembled, the pressure will rise steadily to the pressure limit, and the machine will cycle off.

Operation (see Fig 16–5).—Inspiration may be initiated in one of two ways. In the assist mode, a drop in pressure in the pressurized chamber *(1)* opens the magnetically balanced main flow valve (ceramic control). In the control mode, this valve is opened by a timer mechanism that is regulated by a bleed valve. As pressurized gas bleeds out of the chamber, the trip arm pushes against the steel disc *(2A)*, which is attached to the ceramic flow control. Once the control is opened, source gas, at 50 psi, enters the system at a rate determined by the flow control. After traversing the ceramic control, the source gas either passes directly into the pressurized chamber and on to the patient circuit, or, if the air-mix option is employed, the source gas is split so that part of the source flow is diverted to the air-mix venturi. In both cases part of the source gas is then diverted to pressurize the exhalation valve *(3)* and to operate the mainstream nebulizer *(4)*. Inspiration is terminated when the pressure on the patient side of the ventilator is great enough to overcome the magnetic force on the steel clutch plate *(2B)*. It forces the plate, along with the ceramic control, back into the closed position.

The problems associated with pressure-preset ventilation combined with the unwieldy assortment of accessories needed to adapt this machine to the demands of the intensive care unit have, in most hospitals, relegated these devices to the role of backup ventilators; however, the fact that they are small, lightweight, and pneumatically powered (as well as inexpensive) makes them attractive as critical care transport ventilators.

Volume-Preset Positive-Pressure Ventilators

Piston-Driven Ventilators
Emerson 3-PV Post-Operative Ventilator.—The Emerson 3-PV Post-Operative ventilator was selected for discussion because the simple pneumatic

mechanisms incorporated in its design make it easy to see how the principles of ventilator operation apply (Fig 16–6). It is an electronically powered and controlled, volume-preset, positive-pressure ventilator. The Emerson 3-PV ventilator can operate in the control or assist/control modes, although the responsiveness of the assistor is somewhat poor.

Control Mechanisms.—The cycle time of the Emerson 3-PV ventilator is determined by independently setting the inspiratory time and the expiratory time, which controls the speed of the driving motor during the respiratory cycle (see Fig 16–6,A). Since the controls are not calibrated, the cycle rate must be counted by the operator and adjusted as needed. During operation the easiest method of adjusting the cycle rate is to vary the expiratory time. Care must be exercised to avoid undesirable short expiratory times.

A hand-operated crank on the front of the ventilator adjusts the tidal volume by varying the stroke of the piston (see Fig 16–6,B). The window above the wheel displays the approximate volume being delivered. The flow wave form of the Emerson 3-PV ventilator is sinusoidal as a result of the circular motion of the driving cam (Fig 16–7,A). The flow starts low, peaks at midinspiration, then falls off to zero at end inspiration. The peak flow depends on the tidal volume and the inspiratory time. Room air is drawn into a reservoir during the recovery phase of the piston (Fig 16–7,B). Other gases (usually oxygen) may be introduced into the reservoir to displace all or part of the tidal volume (Fig 16–7,C). The flow of these gases must be titrated against the minute volume and analyzed to assure an accurate F_{IO_2}.

Positive end-expiratory pressure (PEEP) can be applied by adding the weight of a column of water to the exhalation valve (Fig 16–7,D). A calibrated tube is supplied for this purpose. A low inspiratory pressure alarm is available as an option. The airway pressure is measured by a Bourdon-type gauge mounted on the control panel. Exhaled tidal volume is measured and displayed on a top-mounted spirometer (see Fig 16–6). The patient is protected against high-system pressure by a manually adjustable, spring-loaded release valve mounted on the heater/humidifier (Fig 16–7,E). The pressure release valve triggers no audible or visible indicators when opened.

Circuit Assembly and Testing.—The external circuit for the Emerson 3-PV ventilator consists of an inspiratory water trap, an inspiratory arm, a Y con-

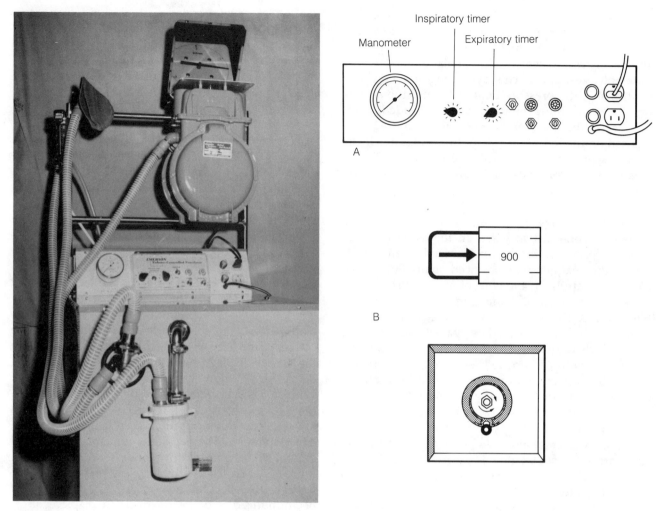

FIG. 16–6.
Emerson 3-PV Post-Operative volume ventilator. (See text for description of control mechanisms *A* and *B*.)

nector with 15-mm endotracheal tube connector, and an expiratory arm. Testing for leaks is done by capping the patient connector and occluding the outflow port of the exhalation valve. The ventilator is then allowed to cycle, pressurizing the circuit. If the circuit is intact, the pressure will drop no more than 5 cm H_2O in 10 seconds (expiratory time must be of adequate length to perform the test). Should the machine fail this test, the most likely sources of a leak are the water trap, the humidifier, and the exhalation valve.

Operation (see Fig 16–7).—At the beginning of inspiration, the drive cam (Fig 16–7,A) closes a microswitch (see Fig 16–7,F) that allows the motor speed during inspiration to be controlled by the inspiratory timer. As inspiration occurs, the piston (see Fig 16–7,G) forces the tidal volume out of the

cylinder (see Fig 16–7,H) and into the patient circuit. Backflow through the reservoir (see Fig 16–7,B) is prevented by a one-way valve at I. The pressure line to the exhalation valve originates at J just proximal to a second one-way valve (see Fig 16–7,K). This valve has two functions. It prevents the backflow of gas during the piston's downstroke, and its resistance assures that the pressure in the exhalation valve line will be greater than that in the patient circuit throughout inspiration. Without this pressure differential, at the exhalation valve, the ventilator could not function. Then the gas flows through a pass-over humidifier (see Fig 16–7,L) that incorporates an emergency pressure relief valve (see Fig 16–7,E). After passing up through a condensation tube, losing excess moisture, the gas passes the patient trigger sensor (see Fig 16–7,M), inactive during inspiration, and the pressure line port (see Fig 16–7,N)

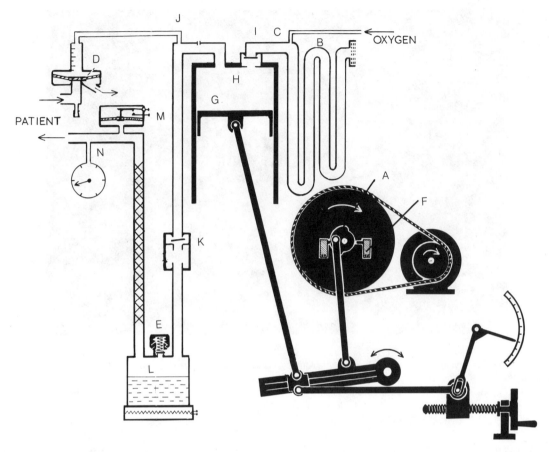

FIG 16–7.
Schematic diagram of the Emerson 3-PV Post-operative ventilator. *A,* driving cam. *B,* reservoir. *C,* oxygen inlet. *D,* exhalation valve. *E,* release valve. *F,* microswitch. *G,* piston. *H,* cylinder. *I,* one-way valve. *J,* pressure line to exhalation valve. *K,* one-way valve. *L,* blow-across heated humidifier. *M,* patient trigger sensor relief valve. *N,* pressure line point. (Modified from Mushin WW, Rendell-Baker L, Thompson PW, et al.: *Automatic Ventilation of the Lungs,* ed 3. Oxford, Blackwell Scientific Publications, 1980, p 557.)

before leaving the machine to be delivered to the patient. At the beginning of the expiratory phase, a microswitch (see Fig 16–7,F) is opened, allowing the motor speed during the expiratory phase to be controlled by the expiratory timer. The descent of the piston closes the one-way valve at K dropping the pressure on the machine side of the exhalation valve (see Fig 16–7,D). The positive pressure on the patient side forces the exhalation valve open, and the patient is allowed to exhale until the pressure in the circuit is no longer able to support the weight of water (if any) in the PEEP column. The descent of the piston opens the one-way valve at I and draws fresh gas from the reservoir into the cylinder. Should the patient trigger sensor be activated during expiration, the motor speeds up to complete the cycle, then starts the next inspiration. There is, however, a time lag while the machine runs through the accelerated expiratory phase.

Bellows-Driven Ventilators

Bennett MA-1 Ventilator.—The Bennett MA-1 ventilator (Puritan-Bennett Corporation) is an electrically powered and controlled, volume-preset ventilator. It can operate in either assist or assist/control mode.

Control Mechanism.—The ventilatory rate is determined by setting the cycle rate control (Fig 16–8,A). Since the position of this calibrated dial may drift with use, the actual cycle rate should be timed by the operator. The range of cycle rates is continuously adjustable from 0 to 60 breaths/min. The size of the delivered breath (tidal volume) is determined by the normal volume control (see Fig 16–8,B) and is adjustable between approximately 200 to 2,200 ml. The normal tidal volume can be periodically altered to deliver large inflation volumes, or sighs. The sigh volume control (see Fig 16–8,C) is used to set the size of the sigh breaths (typically $1.5 \times V_T$), and the

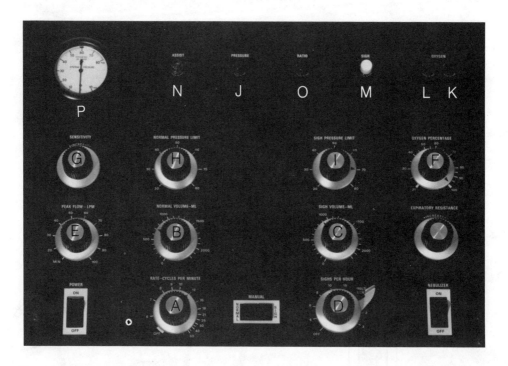

FIG 16–8.
Bennett MA-1 ventilator: *A*, cycle rate control. *B*, normal volume control. *C*, sign volume control. *D*, signs per hour control. *E*, peak flow control. *F*, FI$_{O_2}$ control. *G*, sensitivity setting. *H*, high-system pressure limit. *I*, high-system pressure limit for sighs. *J*, pressure limit lamp. *K*, loss of O$_2$ warning lamp. *L*, lamp indicat-ing O$_2$ supply is pressurized. *M*, sign indicator lamp. *N*, assist indicator lamp. *O*, reverse I/E ratio lamp. *P*, inline manometer. (Courtesy of Puritan-Bennett Corporation, Overland Park, Kansas.)

cycle rate of occurrence is determined by the sighs per hour control (Fig 16–8,D).

The peak flow control determines how rapidly the tidal volume is delivered (see Fig 16–8,E). The control is calibrated in liters per minute, and the flow wave form is essentially a square wave that is modified only slightly by downstream impedance. The wave form is not adjustable.

The FI$_{O_2}$ control enables the operator to select an appropriate mixture of air and oxygen (F). The mixing occurs within the machine and requires an oxygen source of 50 pounds per square inch (psi). The oxygen pressure is reduced inside the ventilator and stored in an accumulator. After each breath, a proportioning valve mixes oxygen from the accumulator with air drawn in through a filter while the bellows is refilling.

Positive end-expiratory pressure is applied by a valve inserted into the exhalation valve line (see Fig 16–9,H). The PEEP valve causes a residual pressure to be maintained in the exhalation valve during exhalation. As long as the pressure in the patient circuit is higher than the exhalation valve pressure, gas will flow through the valve. Once the pressures equalize, gas flow ceases, and an expiratory plateau

is maintained until the beginning of the next inspiration.

Control Interaction.—The most significant interaction is between the sensitivity and PEEP controls. The sensitivity setting (see Fig 16–8,G) determines the trigger level of the machine for patient efforts. Failure to adjust this parameter for high levels of PEEP could result in excessive work on the part of the patient to activate an assist breath. Care must also be taken to assure that the chosen peak flow is appropriate for the selected tidal volume. Too high a flow rate results in turbulence and increased airways resistance, whereas too low a flow rate could mean an inverse I/E ratio.

Monitor and Safety Systems.—The following monitor and alarm systems are available on the MA-1 ventilator (see Fig 16–8):

1. High-system pressure relief can be set independently for normal and high volumes (see Fig 16–8,H and I). Violation of the set relief pressure results in immediate termination of inspiration and activa-

tion of the red pressure limit lamp (see Fig 16–8,J) accompanied by an audible alarm.

2. Loss of oxygen supply while operating above 21% activates a red warning lamp (see Fig 16–8,K) and an audible alarm. During normal operation, a green indicator lamp (see Fig 16–8,L) signifies that the oxygen supply is pressurized and in use.

3. A white indicator lamp (see Fig 16–8,M) is activated each time a sigh breath is delivered, but it is not accompanied by an audible signal.

4. Each time the machine is triggered in the assist mode, a yellow indicator lamp (see Fig 16–8,N) is activated, but is not accompanied by an audible signal.

5. Should the combination of tidal volume, cycle rate, and peak flow settings result in a situation where the inspiratory phase is longer than the expiratory phase, a red warning lamp (see Fig 16–8,O) is activated.

6. Loss of power while the ventilator is turned on results in a battery-powered, audible alarm.

7. Inspiratory and expiratory pressures are monitored by an inline manometer (see Fig 16–8,P). The pressure line monitors pressure inside the machine proximal to the humidifier. Consequently, the manometer reading will always be slightly higher than the proximal airway pressure.

8. Tidal volume is monitored by a bellows-type spirometer mounted on a pole to the left side of the machine. An optional low-volume alarm can be added to the spirometer.

Circuit Assembly and Testing (Fig 16–9).—The external circuit connections are all on the left side of the ventilator. Inspiratory gas leaves the machine and passes through a humidifier (see Fig 16–9,A). The inspiratory limb of the circuit (see Fig 16–9,B) conducts the gas to a mainstream nebulizer (see Fig 16–9,C) and then on to a Y connector (see Fig 16–9,D). The expiratory limb (see Fig 16–9,E) runs from the Y connector to the exhalation manifold (see Fig 16–9,F). The exhaled gas is carried from the mani-

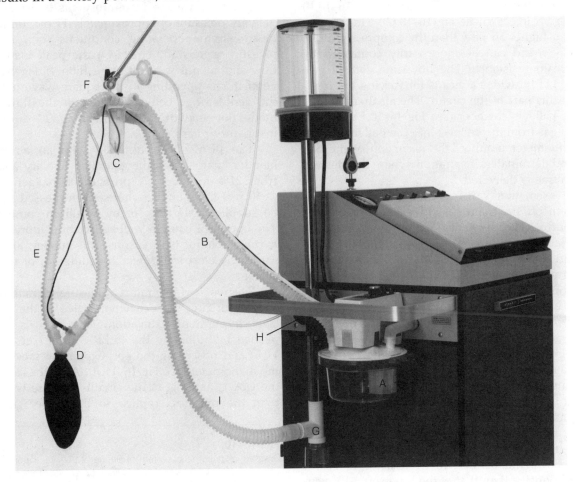

FIG 16–9.
Bennett MA-1 ventilator. *A,* humidifier. *B,* inspiratory limb. *C,* mainstream nebulizer. *D,* Y connector. *E,* expiratory limb. *F,* ex-halation manifold. *H,* PEEP valve. (Courtesy of Puritan-Bennett Corporation, Overland Park, Kansas.)

fold to a water trap (see Fig 16–9,G) by a wide-bore, corrugated tube (see Fig 16–9,I). The water trap is mounted at the base of the spirometer pole so that the volume of each exhaled breath is registered by the spirometer. Separate lines supply gas to the nebulizer and the exhalation valve. To test the circuit, set the cycle rate at 6/min, the tidal volume at 1,000 ml, and the peak flow at 30 L/min. Attach a test lung to the patient connector, and observe that the spirometer registers 1,000 ml ± 50 ml. To check for small leaks, crimp the exhalation valve tubing during inspiration. Check to see that the system pressure does not fall by more than 5 cm H_2O over 10 seconds. Should these tests indicate a leak, the more common problem points on this circuit are the exhalation diaphragm and seat, the nebulizer cup gasket, and the Cascade humidifier gasket.

Operation (Fig 16–10).—At the start of inspiration, a solenoid (see Fig 16–10,A) is activated, allowing air from the main compressor (see Fig 16–10,B) to power an injector (see Fig 16–10,C). The injector allows for higher air flow than the compressor alone can deliver and can be more easily controlled by downstream resistance. The flow rate control (see Fig 16–10,D) provides a means for varying the resistance in this part of the circuit. The air then passess into the bellows chamber (see Fig 16–10,E), driving inspired gas from the bellows into the patient circuit. A potentiometer monitors the excursion of the bellows and terminates inspiration when the desired tidal volume is delivered.

The exhalation valve is pressurized by a split line taken off the main gas drive just prior to the flow control. The resistance of the flow control assures that the pressure in the exhalation valve is always greater than the pressure in the inspiratory line during inspiration.

During the changeover to exhalation, the solenoid (see Fig 16–10,A) is returned by a spring to its resting position. It directs the output of the main compressor through a second injector (see Fig 16–10,F), closing the outlet valve of the bellows. A split line taken off prior to the injector drives a Venturi that simultaneously depressurizes the bellows chamber and the exhalation valve, allowing the patient to exhale and the bellows to refill with fresh gas. The refilling of the bellows is accomplished by gravity and augmented by a return spring. This rapid refilling allows the Bennett MA-1 assistor to be far more responsive than that of the Emerson 3-PV ventilator.

Flow-Integrating Ventilators

BEAR I.—The BEAR I (Bear Medical Systems, Inc.) is a pneumatically powered, electronically controlled volume-preset ventilator capable of performing in four modes: control, assist/control, SIMV, and CPAP (Fig 16–11).

Control Mechanism.—The cycle rate control (see Fig 16–11,A) determines the respiratory frequency. The range may be varied from 0.5 to 60 breaths/min by using a divide-by-10 control (see Fig 16–11,B). The size of each machine delivered breath is determined by the tidal volume control (see Fig 16–11,C) and may be set between 100 to 2,000 ml. The volumes delivered during spontaneous breathing in the SIMV and CPAP modes are dependent on the degree of patient effort. Sigh breaths may be selected at cycle rates and volumes independent of the normal machine delivered breaths.

The peak flow control (see Fig 16–11,D) is calibrated in liters per minute and has a range of 20 to 120 L/min. Since the inspiratory gas is driven by a delivery pressure of approximately 11 psi, under the most extreme operating conditions (i.e., systems pressure equals 100 cm H_2O) the peak inspiratory flow should not vary by more than 15% when the ventilator is operating in the square wave mode. If the ventilator is being operated in the flow taper mode, flow may drop by as much as 50% during the inspiratory phase.

The BEAR I is equipped with an air-oxygen blender that allows the operator to vary the F_{IO_2} from 21% to 100%. A pressurized oxygen source (>30 psi) is required, whereas compressed air may be supplied externally or by a built-in compressor. The option of using a wall source of compressed air is preferable for two reasons. It is quieter, and it reduces the electrical power consumption of the ventilator.

Positive end-expiratory pressure is maintained by pressurizing the exhalation valve to the desired level throughout exhalation. This task is accomplished by adjusting the PEEP control (see Fig 16–11,E) and observing the end-expiratory pressure on the manometer (see Fig 16–11,F). As is the case with the MA-1, as long as the circuit pressure is greater than the pressure applied to the valve, gas flow

FIG 16–10.
Diagram of pneumatic system of Bennett MA-1 ventilator. *A,* main solenoid. *B,* main compressor. *C,* injector. *D,* flow rate control. *E,* bellows chamber. *F,* injector for depressurizing bellows chamber. (Courtesy of Puritan-Bennett Corporation, Overland Park, Kansas.)

Model MA-1 Pneumatic System

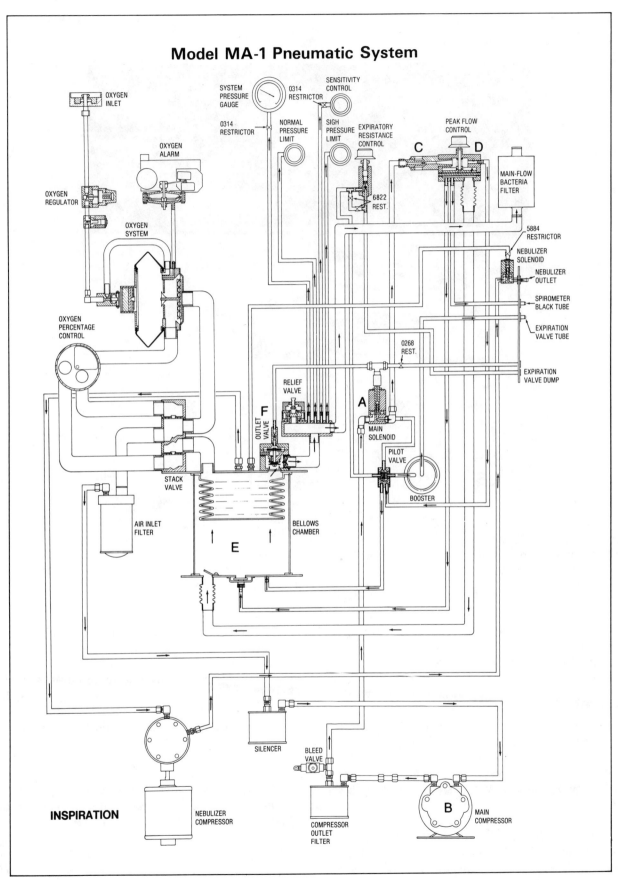

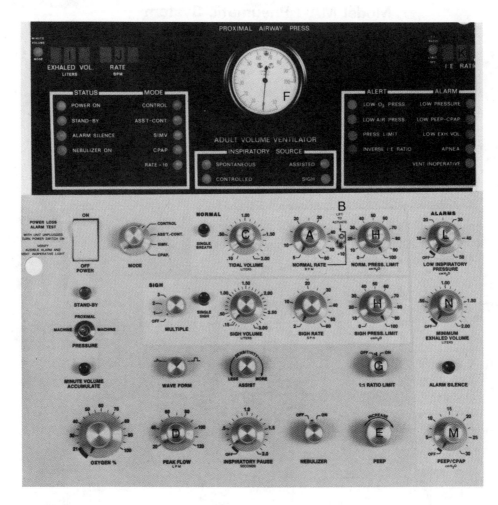

FIG 16–11.
BEAR I ventilator: *A,* cycle rate control. *B,* divide-by-10 control. *C,* tidal volume control. *D,* peak flow control. *E,* PEEP control. *F,* pressure manometer. *G,* I/E ratio limit control. *H,* high-system pressure control. *I,* exhaled volume display. *J,* cycle rate display. *K,* I/E ratio display. *L,* low-pressure alarm. *M,* low-PEEP alarm. *N,* minimal exhaled volume alarm. (Courtesy of Bear Medical Systems, Inc., Riverside, Calif.)

through the valve will continue. When circuit pressure equals the valve pressure, gas flow ceases, and an expiratory plateau is maintained at the equilibrium point. The BEAR I is also equipped with a compensator valve on the PEEP system that injects flow into the patient circuit if the PEEP level drops below its set level. This compensation is managed through the demand valve that provides flows up to 100 L/min for spontaneous breathing during SIMV. A patient disconnect will result in this valve opening all the way and a high flow of gas passing through the patient line.

Control Interaction.—The only significant control interaction is the relationship between peak flow, tidal volume, and inspiratory time. As the peak flow is decreased, the inspiratory time increases for any fixed tidal volume. The BEAR I allows the user to employ inverse I/E ratios, although a visual indicator will alert the operator to this condition. A limit control for inverse I/E ratios is located on the right side of the control panel (see Fig 16–11,G). When engaged, this control terminates inspiration and sounds an alarm when the time allotted for inspiration exceeds one half of the total cycle time.

Monitor and Safety Systems.—The following monitoring and safety systems are available on the BEAR 1 (see Fig 16–11):

1. High-system pressure controls that can be set independently for sigh and normal breaths (see Fig 16–11,H) are available. Should the machine pressure

exceed the set pressure limit, inspiratory flow is terminated.

2. An antisuffocation valve is incorporated into the inspiratory line. Should the air pressure fail during operation, this valve opens, allowing the patient to breath spontaneously through the ventilator. The resistance of this valve is quite high, however, and the patient should be removed from the ventilator and hand ventilated as soon as possible.

3. Digital monitors provide continuous display of the following parameters: exhaled volume (see Fig 16–11,I), cycle rate (see Fig 16–11,J), I/E ratio (see Fig 16–11,K).

4. Proximal airway pressure is displayed via a Bourdon-type manometer.

5. Indicator lights continuously display the following information: mode, power, minute-volume accumulator, rate/10 selected, alarm silence, or stand-by status.

6. Intermittent indicator lights display the inspiratory source of each breath (i.e., spontaneous, control, assist, or sigh).

7. There are five operator-selected alarm settings on the BEAR I that provide both audible and visual indicators when an alarm parameter is violated:

   a. *Low pressure (L)*. The operator selects a *minimum* peak airway pressure based on observation of the patient (usually 5 to 10 cm H_2O below the average peak inspiratory pressure).

   b. *Low PEEP* (M). If PEEP is ordered, a drop in expiratory pressure to more than 3 cm H_2O below the desired plateau level indicates excessive work on the part of the patient. This adjustable alarm monitors the PEEP level and sounds when the parameter is violated. The usual remedy for this situation is to increase the patient sensitivity.

   c. *Minimal exhaled volume* (N). This alarm should be set approximately 100 ml below the patient's exhaled tidal volume. If, on any breath, the exhaled volume is less than that designated by the operator, an alarm sounds, accompanied by a red indicator lamp. It is important to note that if the patient is breathing spontaneously in the IMV mode, the minimal exhaled volume setting must reflect the lowest expected spontaneous tidal volume. Failure to consider the size of the patient's spontaneous breaths will result in frequent, un-

necessary, annoying alarms. This alarm is automatically reset when the minimal exhaled volume parameter returns to an acceptable level.

   d. *Apnea*. Should the patient fail to make an inspiratory effort, or should the machine not cycle a control breath within 15 seconds of the previous breath, this alarm will sound, accompanied by a red indicator lamp.

   e. *Ventilator inoperative*. This alarm is most often triggered by a patient disconnect when the patient is on PEEP. Since the BEAR I has a built-in leak compensator, disconnect results in high (100 L/min) flow delivered to the patient circuit. If no resistance is encountered, the ventilator interprets it as a disconnect and responds with a ventilator inoperative signal.

In addition to the alarm package, there are four system alert indicators that will respond to any of the following conditions with audio and visual signals: (1) drop in O_2 pressure, (2) drop in air pressure, (3) inverse I/E ratio, and (4) high airway pressure limit. The one drawback of this comprehensive monitor package is that the audible signals are indistinguishable from one another. In the event of an alarm or an alert, the operator must examine the ventilator to determine the source of the problem.

Circuit Assembly and Testing (Fig 16–12).—The inspired gas mixture exits the machine via a white elbow connector. A universal rubber adapter must be mounted on the elbow to install the main-flow bacteria filter (see Fig 16–12,A). A 9-in. flex tube (see Fig 16–12,B) is used to conduct the gas from the bacteria filter to the humidifier (see Fig 16–12,C). From the humidifier, the gas is conducted to the nebulizer–exhalation valve manifold (see Fig 16–12,E) by a suitable length of large-bore tubing (see Fig 16–12,D). Similar tubing connects the out port of the nebulizer to the patient Y. An auxiliary port on the patient Y (see Fig 16–12,F) allows for proximal airway pressure monitoring via a ⅜-in. I.D. tubing (see Fig 16–12,G). This tubing is attached to a water trap/cooling coil that prevents water condensate from reaching the internal parts of the pressure monitoring system and causing a machine malfunction. A shorter length of ⅜-in. tubing is used to connect the cooling coil to the proximal pressure monitor port on the ventilator. The expired gas is carried to the exhalation valve by a length of wide-bore tubing. The

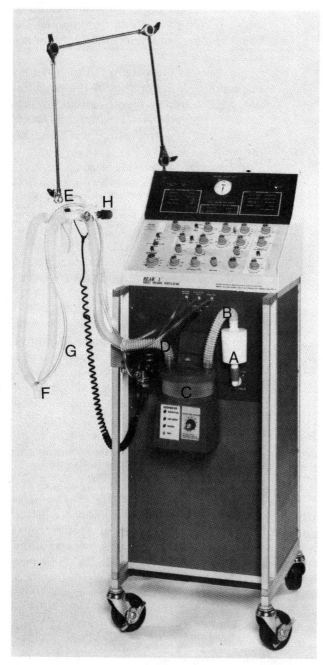

FIG 16–12.
Circuit assembly of the BEAR I ventilator *A*, bacteria filter. *B*, flex tube. *C*, humidifier. *D*, tubing to nebulizer. *F*, patient Y. *G*, 3/8-in. tubing for proximal airway pressure monitoring. *H*, flow sensor assembly. (Courtesy of Bear Medical Systems, Inc., Riverside, Calif.)

exhalation valve is pressurized through a 1/8-in. tubing that runs from the valve stem to the exhalation valve: port adjacent to the proximal pressure monitor port on the front of the machine. The flow sensor assembly (see Fig 16–12,H) is connected directly to the distal side of the exhalation valve, and the signal

it generates passes through a cable that connects to the pin-indexed, exhaled-flow sensor port.

To test the circuit for leaks, set the tidal volume and flow controls at their minimum position, and block the patient end of the Y connector. Allow the ventilator to cycle, and pinch off the exhalation valve line before the ventilator cycles into expiration. Since the exhalation valve remains pressurized, the pressure in the circuit should not fall by more than a few centimeters of water over a 10-second period. A drop of more than 10 cm H_2O indicates that a significant leak is present and should be located and corrected before the machine is put in service.

Operation (Fig 16–13).—The flow of gas to the patient is controlled by the main flow solenoid (see Fig 16–13,A). The operation of the solenoid is controlled by the main electronic control circuit. This circuit receives input from the cycle rate generator, the assist sensor, the mode selector control, the system pressure monitor, and the I/E ratio monitor circuits. The logic used to then operate the solenoid valve is dependent on the status of these input parameters. For the purpose of this discussion, we will stipulate that the ventilator is operating in the assist/control mode to limit the number of cases we might have to consider.

Oxygen and air are supplied to the ventilator through inlet ports on the back panel (see Fig 16–13,B). The supply pressures are monitored both by Bourdon gauges and electronic pressure controls that control the gas supply alarm circuits. The source gases are then reduced from 50 to 11 psi by a step-down regulator on the air line and a relay valve slaved to the regulator on the oxygen line. Each line is directed to the oxygen blender before the inspired gas mixture reaches the main flow solenoid. The main flow solenoid opens in response to either a patient effort (assist) or a signal from the cycle rate generator (control), and the inspiratory phase begins. Before exiting the machine, the inspiratory gas passes a vortex generator (see Fig 16–13,C), which creates a turbulent area between two sensor heads (see Fig 16–13,D). The degree of disturbance in this area is directly proportional to the flow and, as such, allows the sensors to monitor the flow and compute the delivered volume. When the sensor computes the delivered volume to be that dialed in on the control panel, inspiration is terminated. The exhalation valve is pressurized by a separate line that is a branch of the main air supply line (see Fig 16–13,E). This air is reduced in pressure to about 2 psi by a low-pressure regulator (see Fig 16–13,F). From the regulator the air supply is controlled by a three-way

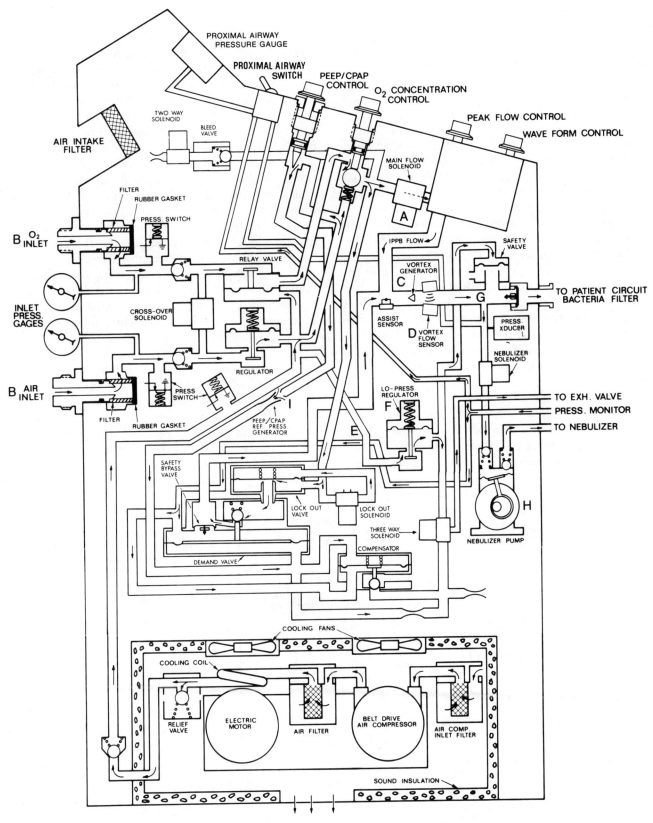

FIG 16–13.
Diagram of pneumatic system of BEAR 1 ventilator. *A*, main flow solenoid. *B*, air and oxygen inlet parts. *C*, vortex generator. *D*, sensor heads. *E*, line to exhalation valve. *F*, low-pressure regula-tor. *G*, line to nebulizer. *H*, compressor pump. *I*, main com-pressed air line. (Courtesy of Bear Medical Systems, Inc., River-side, Calif.)

solenoid valve that responds to commands from the main control circuit. The nebulizer is driven with gas taken from the main line flow distal to the flow sensors (see Fig 16–13,G) (the tidal volume is not affected by the use of the nebulizer). A compressor pump (see Fig 16–13,H) assures that the gas is delivered to the manifold at a sufficiently high pressure to drive the nebulizer. Positive end-expiratory pressure is provided by an injector system that operates off of the main compressed air line (see Fig 16–13,I). The air diverted to the PEEP control circuit is regulated by the same three-way solenoid that operates the exhalation valve. The purpose of this solenoid is to differentiate between the pressure seen by the exhalation valve during the inspiratory phase and the pressure used to deliver PEEP. It is of more than passing interest that all of the pneumatic controls operate off of the main air supply line. This design characteristic makes it possible to operate the ventilator in the absence of a compressed gas source by using the on board compressor and selecting an $F_{I_{O_2}}$ of 21%.

Servo-Controlled Ventilators

A servo controller is responsible for maintaining some critical parameter within a prescribed range. The mechanism a servo uses to accomplish this is a feedback loop. Assume that a task is initiated by the servo controller (see Fig 16–14), which monitors the task through sensors. These sensors provide input to the servo controller. This input is compared with the reference value supplied to the controller (this reference value may be either preprogrammed or may be in the form of alternate input). Any variance between the reference value and the input signal results in a change in the output from the servo unit, which will bring the task back on track. Servo controllers are most useful in situations where unpredictable changes in a system can affect task performance. Under these circumstances, the servo, via the feedback loop, can adapt the performance of the task to feedback loop to changes in the operating system that might otherwise cause the system to fail. The critical parameter being controlled in the Servo Ventilator 900C by Siemens-Elema, for example, is the inspiratory flow.

Siemens-Elema Servo Ventilator 900C.—The Servo 900C is a pneumatically powered, electronically controlled, volume- or pressure-preset (or both) ventilator. It is capable of operating in seven modes of ventilation, and its classification depends largely on the mode in which it is being used. The modes available on the 900C are (1) volume control (assist/

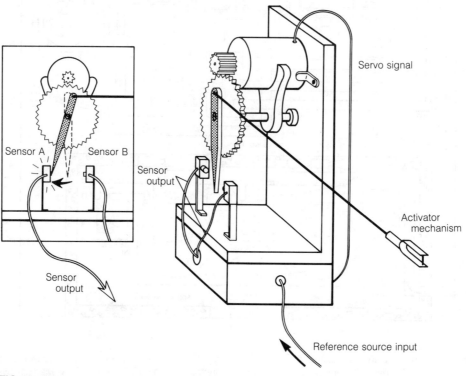

FIG 16–14.
Conceptual model of a servo controller.

control), (2) SIMV, (3) pressure support, (4) SIMV with pressure support, (5) CPAP, (6) pressure control, and (7) manual.

First the 900C ventilator will be described in the volume-control mode. The other modes will then be discussed to the extent that they differ in control settings and interaction from those in the volume-control mode.

Control Mechanism (Fig 16–15).—The respiratory rate is set by adjusting the breaths per minute control to the desired cycle rate. The tidal volume is determined by the relationship between the preset minute volume control (see Fig 16–15,A) and the breaths per minute control (see Fig 16–15,B). There is no flow rate control on the 900C. The flow rate can be calculated, however, from the relationship of the preset minute volume to the inspiratory time

percent (see Fig 16–15,C). The ventilator is set to provide X liters of gas to the circuit each minute. The inspiratory time percent control limits the actual duration of flow to a certain fraction of a minute, Y. The flow rate during inspiration, therefore, will be X liters divided by Y fractions of 1 minute.

Example: Consider a patient whose settings on the 900C are 12.0 L/min for minute volume, 10 breaths/min for cycle rate, and 33% for inspiratory time percent. What is the inspiratory flow rate?

Solution: There are, in fact, two ways to solve this problem. With each breath the patient receives 1.2 L in one third of the cycle time. For a cycle rate of 10/min, the cycle time is 60 sec/10 cycles, or 6 seconds. One third of that is 2 seconds, or $\frac{1}{30}$ of a minute. The flow rate, then, is calculated by division:

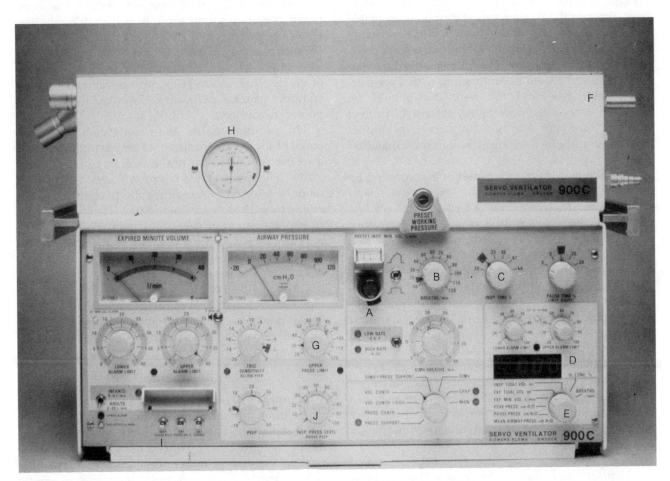

FIG 16–15.
Siemens-Elema Ventilator 900C. *A,* preset minute volume control. *B,* breaths per minute control. *C,* inspiratory time percent control. *D,* digital display. *E,* digital display selector control. *F,* low-pressure inlet. *G,* upper pressure limit control. *H,* working pressure manometer. *I,* inspiratory hold button. *J,* pressure level above PEEP control. (Courtesy of Siemens-Elema Corporation, Schaumburg, Ill.)

$$\dot{V} = \frac{1.2 \text{ L}}{1/30 \text{ min}}$$
$$= 36 \text{ L/min.}$$

A somewhat easier solution is to use the X liters/Y fraction method:

$$\dot{V} = \frac{12 \text{ L}}{0.33}$$
$$= 36 \text{ L/min.}$$

The second method eliminates the need to perform calculations based on the rate and limits the calculation to a single step.

The composition of the inspired gas delivered by the 900C is determined by the use of auxiliary blenders, vaporizers, or both that supply gas to either a high-pressure or a low-pressure inlet (Fig 16–15,F). This arrangement allows for tremendous versatility since several combinations of gases can be used to drive the ventilator. Some of the options available are air-oxygen blender, oxygen–nitrous oxide blender, halothane vaporizer, enflurane vaporizer, and isoflurane vaporizer. The volatile anesthetic vaporizers must be used in conjunction with a pressurized carrier gas, and the ventilator should be equipped with a gas-scavenging system to protect intensive care unit and operating room personnel from the anesthetic discharge through the exhalation port.

Positive end-expiratory pressure is controlled by the solenoid that operates the exhalation valve. (Since there are, in fact, no external valves on this ventilator, the flow controllers on the inspiratory and expiratory limbs are called *gates*.) There are two inputs to this solenoid. One simply controls its action during inspiration by closing the expiratory gate. The second input is referenced against the pressure measured in the expiratory limb and compared against the set PEEP level. In the expiratory phase, the expiratory gate is open until the pressure approaches the PEEP setting. At this point the solenoid is activated, and the expiratory gate is closed. Should the pressure fall below the PEEP reference level, the inspiratory gate will allow gas to leak into the system until equilibrium is restored between the reference level and the pressure measured in the expiratory limb.

Monitor and Safety Systems.—The monitor functions of the 900C include analog display of airway pressure and minute volume (see Fig 16–15). The minute volume display, however, fluctuates with the ventilatory cycle and should not be taken as an accurate measure of the patient's actual minute volume. More accurate readings of the status of the ventilator can be obtained from the digital display at the lower right corner of the machine (see Fig 16–15,D). A selector control (see Fig 16–15,E) changes the display to one of the following: the respiratory rate, FI_{O_2}, inspiratory tidal volume, expiratory tidal volume, peak inspiratory pressure, pause pressure, or mean airway pressure.

The functions of the 900C that are monitored by alarm circuits are minute volume (high and low), gas supply, apnea, high peak pressure, and high and low FI_{O_2}. When an alarm parameter is violated, a high-pitched, intermittent beep sounds from the side of the machine. The beep is accompanied by a flashing red indicator light that allows the operator to determine which parameter is out of range. Should an electrical disconnect occur, a slower-paced beep will sound for approximately 6 minutes. It is not accompanied by an indicator lamp. All of the alarm circuits need to be manually set except for gas supply (failure to maintain a working pressure of greater than 20 cm H_2O), apnea (failure of the inspiratory gate to open over a 15-second interval, and power disconnect).

In addition to the alarm indicators, the front panel of the ventilator has nine amber indicators that alert the operator to current mode, monitor, or alarm status. The mode status lamps will light whenever a mode is selected that requires the patient or the operator to initiate every inspiration. These modes are pressure support, CPAP, and manual. Two of the indicator lamps alert the operator to the status of the minute volume display (adult, 0–40 L/min; or infant, 0–4 L/min) and the status of the SIMV cycle rate control knob (4–40 breaths/min, or 0.4–4 breaths/min). One lamp, located next to the trig sensitivity control, lights whenever a patient-initiated breath occurs. The last two alert lamps indicate a failure on the part of the operator to establish alarm limits on the minute volume and FI_{O_2} alarms.

Control Interactions.—Control interaction is the single most difficult aspect of the 900C that must be faced when one is learning how to operate the ventilator. Since the 900C evolved from constant minute volume ventilators rather than from constant tidal volume machines, the control setup varies markedly from ventilators like the BEAR I and the Bennett MA-1. It is so important that the operator be aware of the potential control interactions of this ventilator that we will examine several of the controls independently and describe the effect changes will have on other ventilatory parameters.

Preset Inspiratory Minute Volume.—Changes in the preset minute volume control, when in a volume ventilation mode, directly affect both tidal volume and inspiratory flow rate. That is, when the minute volume setting is increased, the flow rate and the tidal volume both increase proportionately.

Breaths Per Minute.—The delivered tidal volume depends on the breaths per minute setting; changes in the position of this control will result in changes in the tidal volume. In a volume ventilation mode, if the minute volume is constant, the tidal volume will vary inversely with the breaths per minute setting. The same is also true in the SIMV modes.

Inspiratory Time Percent.—Because the flow rate is determined by this control in conjunction with the minute volume, changing the inspiratory time percent results in a change in the flow rate provided the minute volume setting is unchanged. The relationship between the inspiratory time percent control and the flow rate is inverse. That is, decreasing the inspiratory time increases the flow rate and vice versa.

Pause Time Percent.—The addition of an inspiratory pause will affect the I:E ratio to a greater or lesser degree. The important aspect of the pause control, however, is the imposed limitation that the combination of the inspiratory time percent and pause time percent cannot exceed 80% of the total cycle time as determined by the breaths per minute control.

SIMV Breaths Per Minute.—The significant interaction between this control and the normal breaths per minute control is that the SIMV cycle rate can never exceed the cycle rate set on the normal breaths per minute control.

Circuit Assembly and Testing.—Since the exhalation valve is incorporated into the machine itself, the external circuit need consist of only gas conduction tubing and a humidification system. A short length of large-bore tubing can be used to connect the inspired gas outlet to the humidifier. The inspiratory line carries the gas to the patient Y, and the expiratory tubing returns the expired gas to the ventilator. A hydroscopic, bacteria filter should be used to prevent contamination of the internal parts of the

ventilator and to protect the expiratory flow transducer from damage or erroneous readings that might result from water condensing on the transducer screen.

Testing the circuit for leaks is easily done by setting the upper pressure limit (see Fig 16–15,G) higher than the working pressure (see Fig 16–15,H) and occluding the patient Y. The airway pressure manometer should rise rapidly to the level of the working pressure and stay there for the duration of the inspiratory phase. Depressing the inspiratory pause hold button (see Fig 16–15,I) will then allow the system pressure to be observed under static conditions. The system pressure should not drop by more than 5 cm H_2O in 10 seconds.

Operation.—The operational description of the 900C must necessarily include descriptions of four different types of breaths. A constant-volume breath, a spontaneous breath, a pressure-controlled (time-limited) breath, and a pressure-support breath. Since all ventilatory modes consist of some combination of these, the descriptions should suffice to cover all of the ventilatory modes except the manual mode. Since the manual mode is used only in anesthesia (and only with specially designed accessories), it will not be discussed.

Volume-preset breaths may be initiated either by patient effort (assist mode) or by the ventilator (control mode). At the beginning of the breath, the servo controller opens the inspiratory gate (see Fig 16–16,B) to an intermediate position and closes the expiratory gate (see Fig 16–16,E). The flow through the gate results from the pressure difference between the bellows (see Fig 16–16,A) and the patient circuit. This flow is measured by the inspiratory flow transducer (see Fig 16–16,C) and monitored by the servo controller. The signal monitored by the controller is compared with inputs from the preset minute volume and breaths per minute controls. If there is a difference between the two signals, the servo controller increases or decreases the gate opening to either increase or decrease the flow until the signals balance. This process is repeated continually throughout inspiration and results in a good approximation of a square wave flow through the inspiratory gate. Inspiration is terminated when either the time limit is reached or circuit pressure at (see Fig 16–16,F) exceeds the upper pressure limit. If any inspiratory pause is selected, both gates (see Fig 16–16,B and E) will remain closed for the duration of the pause. At the start of exhalation, the expiratory

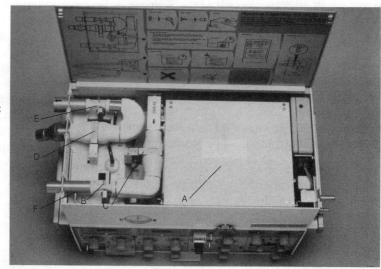

FIG 16–16.
Diagram of pneumatic system of the Servo 900C ventilator. *A,* bellows. *B,* inspiratory gate. *C,* inspiratory flow transducer. *D,* expiratory flow transducer. *E,* expiratory gate. *F,* inspiratory pressure point. (Courtesy of Siemens-Elema Corporation, Schaumburg, Ill.)

gate is opened to its maximum width, and expired gas is allowed to flow from the patient through the expiratory limb of the ventilator. The expiratory flow transducer (see Fig 16–16,D) measures the flow throughout exhalation, and its signal is integrated over time to monitor the exhaled tidal volume. These conditions hold for all breaths in the volume control mode and for the mandatory ventilation breaths in SIMV or SIMV and pressure support.

A spontaneous patient effort is measured as a drop in pressure distal to the inspiratory gate (see Fig 16–16,B). The response of the ventilator is to open the inspiratory gate and allow fresh gas to flow into the patient circuit. The amount of flow provided is directly related to the magnitude of the pressure drop (patient effort). The expiratory gate maintains its position until the pressure in the patient circuit exceeds the designated PEEP. If no PEEP is set, the expiratory gate closes during the time that the inspiratory gate is open. These conditions hold for all breaths in the CPAP mode and for all spontaneous patient breaths in SIMV.

In the pressure control mode, inspiration may be initiated by either time cycling or patient effort. In the time-cycled mode, the cycle rate is determined by the breaths per minute control (see Fig 16–15,B) and the duration of positive pressure by the inspiratory time percent setting (see Fig 16–15,C). If the breath is patient initiated, the duration of positive pressure will remain the same but the cycle rate will increase depending on how much the expiratory time is shortened. The size of the breath is determined by the pressure level above PEEP control (see Fig 16–15,J), and the preset minute volume is disabled.

All breaths in the pressure support mode must be initiated by the patient. Inspiration begins when the patient triggers the ventilator and ends when one of the following conditions is met:

1. The pressure in the patient circuit exceeds the preset pressure by 2 cm H_2O.
2. The flow rate drops to 25% of its peak value.
3. Inspiration is time cycled by exceeding the time designated by the breaths per minute control and the inspiratory time percent controls.

It is noteworthy that the flow pattern produced in pressure support is a sharply tapered one due to the relatively low working pressure of the ventilator and to the fact that as the pressure rises in the circuit, the machine interprets it as a lower patient demand for flow and allows the inspiratory flow gate to slowly close. These conditions hold for all breaths in the pressure support mode and for the nonmandatory breaths in SIMV and pressure support.

Microprocessor-Controlled Ventilators

Advances in solid-state electronics have made microprocessors (computer microchips) available that are capable of performing complex tasks, have the ability to perform data acquisition and storage, and are relatively inexpensive. Several ventilators utilize microprocessors to control pneumatic systems, monitor ventilator function, and store and analyze patient data.

Using what is essentially a small computer to run a ventilator has a number of advantages. First, since these chips have such tremendous capabilities, it is possible to program them with a wide variety of sophisticated options. Second, the computer can monitor the performance of individual components within the machine and either alter performance to meet changing needs or at least alert the operator to such a need. Third, the microprocessor-controlled ventilator is the ideal research tool since output from the microprocessor is easily handled by more sophisticated computers. This capability reduces the difficult task of data gathering for research. Perhaps the most significant advantage of the microprocessor-controlled ventilators is their adaptability. As new modalities of mechanical ventilation are developed, the microprocessor can be reprogrammed to give the ventilator the desired capabilities.

Hamilton Veolar.—The Hamilton Veolar ventilator (Fig 16–17) is a pneumatically powered, microprocessor-controlled ventilator capable of operating in five modes: (1) assist (AMV), (2) control (CMV), (3) SIMV, (4) mandatory-minute ventilation (MMV), and (5) CPAP. Pressure support is available not as a discrete mode but as a sort of extension of the PEEP function. Microprocessor ventilators are simply servo controllers that analyze input and regulate output. In this context, it is advisable to consider the microprocessor to be just a black box and to concentrate on understanding the pneumatics of a particular ventilator.

From a design standpoint, the Veolar has several excellent capabilities. One such point is that the manufacturer did not succumb to the temptation of high technology and substitute touch keys for more conventional controls. Although such control systems do reduce the potential for accidental parameter change, they also require an inordinate amount of training time, and since the function of any one key may not be self-evident, staff who work infrequently with a key pad control may periodically need additional training. Another nice feature of the control panel is its organization. The front panel (Fig 16–17) is divided into three, well-defined areas, each devoted to a different set of functions and each clearly labeled as to what those functions are. The first area to be discussed is the control panel.

The rate control (see Fig 16–17,A) is functional in the CMV and SIMV modes. The rate knob is actually a dual control with separate position indicators for the CMV rate and the SIMV rate. Special attention should be paid to the fact that the CMV control must always be set equal to or higher than the SIMV setting. The range of cycle rates for the Veolar ventilator is from 0.5 to 60 breaths/min.

The size of each mechanical breath is determined by the tidal volume control (see Fig 16–17,B). The range of this control is from 30 ml to 2 L, but it is of dubious accuracy at settings less than 100 ml. There is no flow rate control on the Veolar. The flow pattern control simply modifies the flow configuration seen during inspiration; it does not determine how rapidly the breath is delivered, though it may have an effect on peak flow. The mean flow rate is determined by the relationship between the tidal volume control, the CMV rate setting, and the percent of insufflation time (see Fig 16–17,C).

The $F_{I_{O_2}}$ control (see Fig 16–17,D) may be varied between 0.21 and 1.0. The Veolar is not equipped to handle gas mixtures other than air-oxygen. The PEEP/CPAP control (see Fig 16–17,E), like the rate control, has dual functions. The PEEP/CPAP control, the large, outer knob, is adjustable between 0 and 50 cm H_2O. The smaller, inner control determines what level (if any) of inspiratory pressure support should be given on any spontaneous breath.

Control Interaction.—All controls except those with dual action function independently. As previously mentioned, the flow rate depends on the relationship between several controls, and constitutes the only major interaction between the controls.

Patient Monitors.—Indicator lamps alert the operator to patient trigger conditions and inspiratory plateau. Digital display windows allow continuous monitoring of tidal volume, respiratory rate, peak, baseline, or mean airway pressure and minute volume. An analog LED display monitors airway pressure.

Alarms.—Audible alarms accompanied by a warning lamp alert the operator to failure of power or gas supply and ventilator dysfunction. Adjustable alarms will sound if the patient exceeds a user-defined maximum respiratory rate or airway pressure. Maximum and minimum alarms to alert operators to changes in minute volume or inspired oxygen concentration are also available. User-defined alarms may be silenced for 120 seconds.

Operational Description (Fig 16–18).—The gas supply of the Veolar ventilator consists of air and oxygen delivered separately at 50 psi. After the gas passes a check valve (see Fig 16–18,A), the inlet pressure of each gas is monitored by a pressure switch (see Fig 16–18,B). The inlet pressure of each gas is reduced to 20 psi by internal pressure regula-

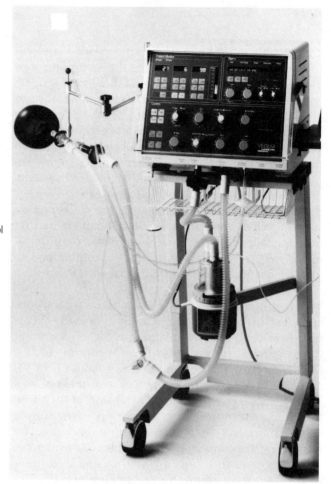

FIG 16–17.
Hamilton Veolar ventilator. Rate control *(A);*. tidal volume control *(B);* percent insufflation time *(C);* Fl$_{O_2}$ control *(D);* PEEP/CPAP control *(E);* Pmax control *(F).* (Courtesy of Hamilton Medical Corporation, Reno Nev.)

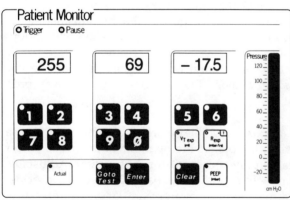

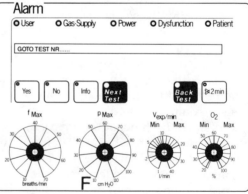

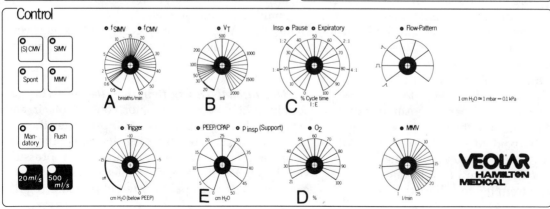

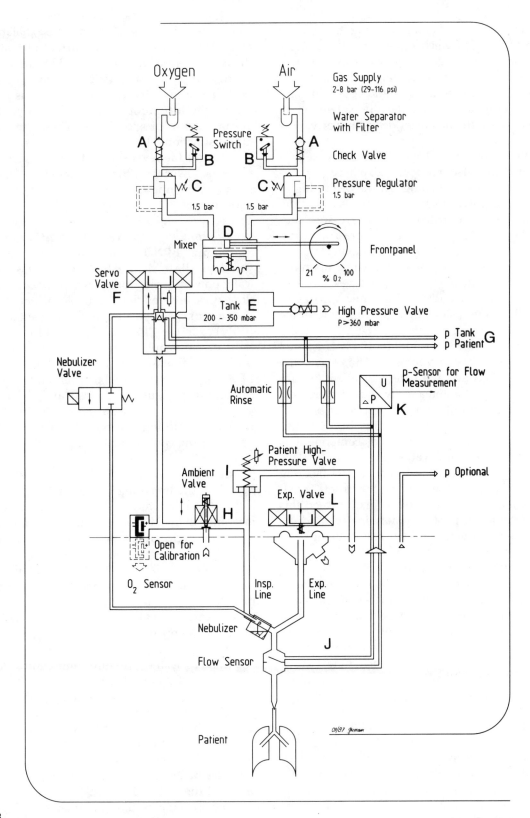

FIG 16–18.

Diagram of pneumatic system of the Hamilton Veolar ventilator. *A,* check valve. *B,* pressure switch. *C,* internal pressure regulators. *D,* mixing valve. *E,* reservoir tank. *F,* plunger valve. *G,* pressure sensors. *H,* ambient valve. *I,* patient high-pressure valve. *J,* low-compliance tubing. *K,* differential pressure transducer. *L,* exhalation valve. (Courtesy of Siemens-Elema Corporation, Schaumburg, Ill.)

tors (see Fig 16–18,C) before entering the mixing valve (see Fig 18,D), which determines the composition of the inspired gas. The gas mixture then passes into a reservoir tank (see Fig 16–18,E), which maintains a pressure between 3 and 5 psi. Inspiratory gas from this tank may enter the patient circuit either directly, via the nebulizer drive line, or via the main gas flow circuit.

The main flow controller consists of an electrodynamically controlled plunger valve (see Fig 16–18,F) with a triangular opening. At the beginning of inspiration, the valve opens, allowing gas to flow from the tank into the patient circuit. Pressure sensors (see Fig 16–18,G) measure the pressure drop across the valve, and a linear potentiometer accurately determines the height of the valve opening. Using preprogrammed values for the resistance of the valve in various positions, the microprocessor calculates the flow using the pressure differential across the valve.

The ambient valve (see Fig 16–18,H) is located on the inspiratory line just before the line leaves the ventilator and becomes the external patient circuit. This valve is opened automatically should there be a failure of the gas supply, power supply, or both. It is essentially a fail safe, much like the BEAR I anti-suffocation valve. The final internal component is the patient overpressure valve (Fig 16–18,I). This valve is set by adjusting the Pmax control (see Fig 16–17,F) in the alarm section of the front panel. Should the pressure in the patient circuit exceed this designated value, inspiration is terminated, and excess pressure is vented from the patient tubing.

At the proximal airway, inspired and expired volumes are monitored by a flow sensor. The flow sensor is connected by 4-mm I.D. low-compliance tubing (see Fig 16–18,J) to a differential pressure transducer (see Fig 16–18,K). These two components comprise a pneumotachometer of broad linearity. The signal from the transducer is then integrated by the micropressor to calculate volume. One advantage of this system is that the tidal volume reading is actually the volume being exhaled through the patient's airway, and the display reflects no component of volume lost due to pressurization of the patient circuit. The expiratory limb of the circuit carries the exhaled gas directly to the exhalation valve (see Fig 16–18,L). The exhalation valve is electronically activated and occludes the expiratory arm of the circuit during inspiration. Positive end-expiratory pressure is also maintained by this valve through a constant coil current to the valve motor. The force with

which the valve pushes against the exhalation membrane is proportional to the current in that coil, and the current, in turn, is controlled by the PEEP/CPAP control. If a pressure-assist option (pressure support) is selected, the desired pressure is maintained during the inspiratory phase by the identical mechanism used to provide PEEP. There are two important distinctions. Pressure assist occurs during inspiration, and the level selected for pressure assist can never be lower than the designated PEEP level. This constraint is inherent in the design of the dual pressure control.

Continuous-Flow Neonatal Ventilators

Bourns BP200 Ventilator.—The Bourns BP200 ventilator (Bear Medical Systems, Inc.) is a pneumatically powered, electronically controlled, continuous-flow pressure ventilator capable of operating in either intermittent positive pressure ventilation mode (IPPV) or in the CPAP mode. All of the control functions of the ventilator are incorporated into the face of the machine and are distinctly labeled. After the BP200 is connected to both air and oxygen lines (minimum pressure of 35 psi) and the machine is plugged into an electrical outlet, the machine is activated by turning the mode control in the upper corner of the control panel (Fig 16–19).

Control Mechanism.—The cycle rate is determined by the breathing rate control and is calibrated in breaths per minute. The original version of this machine allowed continuous adjustment of the breathing cycle rate from 0 to 60 breaths/min. More recently, however, clinicians have frequently had to use respiratory rates in the 60 to 120/min range to ventilate smaller, more unstable neonates. Most BP200 ventilators have now been retrofitted with cycle rate cards that allow the cycle rate to go to a maximum of 150 breaths/min.

The size of the breath delivered by the BP200 is determined by the pressure limit control located at the bottom of the machine (see Fig 16–19). Since this control is not calibrated, its setting must be compared against the reading of airway pressure as taken from the proximal airway pressure gauge during the inspiratory phase, with the patient connector blocked. The maximum pressure plateau attainable with the BP200 is approximately 80 cm H_2O and is preset at the factory.

The inspiratory time parameter is analogous to the cycle rate of delivery on an adult ventilator. The inspiratory time can be determined by the interac-

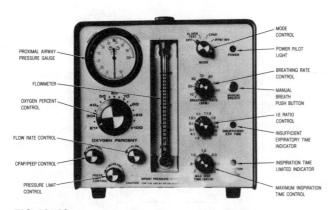

FIG 16–19.
Bourns BP200 ventilator. (Courtesy of Bear Medical Systems, Inc., Riverside, Calif.)

tion of the (1) cycle rate control and the (2) I:E ratio control.

Example: An infant's ventilator orders call for a cycle rate of 20 breaths/min and inspiratory time of 0.5 seconds. If the maximum inspiratory time is set at 1.0 seconds, what I:E ratio would you select to comply with the ordered inspiratory time?

Answer: The maximum inspiratory time control is, in this case, acting only as a default limit. The I:E ratio determines the inspiratory time. The cycle time is 60 sec/20 breaths/min, or 3 seconds:

$$\text{Expiratory time} = \text{cycle time} - \text{inspiratory time}$$
$$= 3.0 - 0.5$$
$$= 2.5 \text{ seconds}$$

The I:E ratio is most often represented with *I* equal to unity or 1.0. One way to calculate the *E* portion of the ratio, when I = 1.0, is to divide the expiratory time by the inspiratory time:

$$\text{I:E ratio} = 1 : E_t \div I_t$$
$$= 1 : 2.5 \div 0.5$$
$$= 1 : 5$$

The I:E ratio must be set at (3.0 minus 0.5) divided by 0.5 equals 1 to 5.0 to achieve the correct inspiratory time.

The F_{IO_2} can be continuously adjusted from 21% to 100% using the oxygen percent control located under the proximal airway pressure gauge. The CPAP/PEEP control can provide end-expiratory plateaus from 0 to 15 cm H_2O. On the BP200, PEEP is achieved by increasing or decreasing the resistance to flow through the exhalation valve. One potential problem with continuous-flow pressure ventilators is

that inadvertent PEEP is sometimes measured at the proximal airway. It occurs when the flow needed to ventilate the patient is so high that there is continuous positive pressure at the proximal airway even when the PEEP control is turned off. Later-generation ventilators have eliminated this problem by modifying the design of the exhalation valve.

The flow rate control is of far greater consequence in the neonate than it is in the adult, primarily because the newborn lung has an extraordinarily high specific airways resistance. The flow control on the BP200 can be adjusted to deliver flows from 0 to 20 L/min, which can be monitored by the Thorpe tube incorporated into the control panel. It is important to make sure that the flow used is sufficient to allow the patient to reach the desired peak airway pressure. The index for it is that the proximal airway pressure should be the same when the patient is on the machine as it is during the pressure check with the patient connector blocked. If these pressures are not within 1 to 2 cm H_2O of one another, either the flow is too low or there is too large a leak around the infant's endotracheal tube.

Control Interactions.—There are two major control interactions on the BP200. The first is the relationship between I:E ratio, cycle rate, and inspiratory time. Since the inspiratory time is dependent on the rate and the I:E ratio, a change in one of these

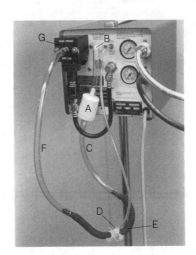

FIG 16–20.
Circuit assembly of the Bourns BP200 infant pressure ventilator. *A,* extenal bacteria filter. *B,* outflow port. *C,* inspiratory tubing connects to a humidifier (not shown) and O_2 sampling port (not shown). *D,* pressure-monitoring port. *E,* proximal temperature probe is inserted here (not shown). *F,* expiratory limb. *G,* exhalation block. (Courtesy of Bear Medical Systems, Inc, Riverside, Calif.)

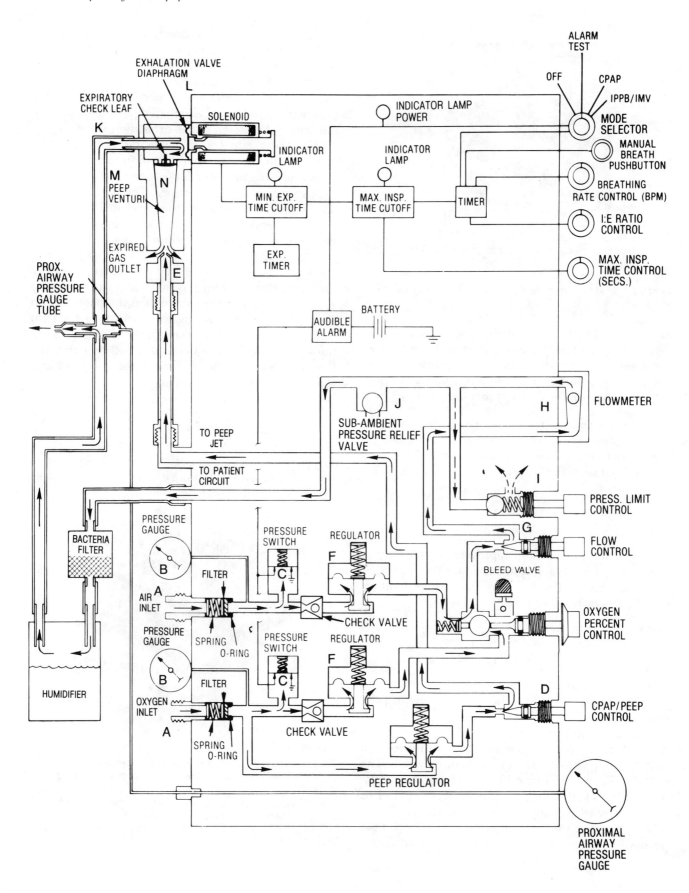

controls will result in a change in the inspiratory time. The second control interaction is the dependency of the peak pressure on flow. Low flow rates, especially when combined with short inspiratory times, might result in failure of the ventilator to reach the desired ventilating pressure.

Monitor and Safety Systems.—An audible alarm powered by an internal battery will sound if the mode control is turned on and either the power, air, or oxygen supply is interrupted. The only other monitor functions of the BP200 are two red indicator lamps that alert the operator to the presence of a time-limited inspiration or of an expiratory phase of less than 0.2 seconds. Supplementary breaths can be given by depressing the manual breath button while in the IPPV mode. The pressure limit and inspiratory time of these breaths are the same as those for machine-initiated breaths. This button is not functional in the CPAP mode.

Circuit Assembly and Testing (Fig 16–20).—An external bacteria filter (see Fig 16–20,A) is connected to the outflow port (see Fig 16–20,B) of the ventilator by a short length of latex tubing. A 24-in. length of low-compliance tubing, such as Tygon, connects the bacteria filter to an O_2 sampling port. Because of the premature newborn's sensitivity to fluctuating PaO_2, it is prudent to continuously monitor the FiO_2. The O_2 sampling port is attached directly to the inlet of the humidifier. From the humidifier, the inspiratory tubing (see Fig 16–20,C) carries the gas to the patient wye. At the proximal airway are ports for pressure monitoring (see Fig 16–20,D) and a proximal temperature probe (see Fig 16–20,E).

The expiratory limb of the circuit (see Fig 16–20,F) is connected directly to the exhalation block (see Fig 16–20,G) on the back of the machine. If some form of heated wire system is not used to prevent rainout of water in the patient circuit, water traps must be incorporated into both the inspiratory and expiratory limbs of the circuit.

To test the circuit prior to use, turn the pressure limit control fully clockwise. With a 1-second inspi-

ratory time and the flow set at 6 L/min, occlude the patient connector. The system pressure should rise to at least 80 cm H_2O. Failure to reach this pressure indicates a leak in the system. Commonly leaks are found in the humidifier, in the water traps, or around the temperature probe at the patient connector. The test flow of 6 L/min is recommended for patient circuits with a compliance of less than 1.5 ml/cm H_2O. Circuits with higher tubing compliance may require higher test flows.

Operation (Fig 16–21).—Air and oxygen enter the rear panel of the ventilator through their respective ports (see Fig 16–21,A). The delivery pressure of each is monitored by both a pressure gauge (see Fig 16–21,B) and a pressure control (see Fig 16–21,C), which activates the gas supply alarm if either delivery pressure falls below 35 psi. From the oxygen delivery line, a high-pressure conduit diverts a portion of the oxygen supply to the PEEP control valve (see Fig 16–21,D). This valve controls the oxygen flow to the PEEP venturi (see Fig 16–21,E), which, in turn, regulates the resistance of the exhalation valve.

Both the air and oxygen are next dropped to an operating pressure of 10 psi by independent pressure reduction valves (see Fig 16–21,F). This level allows the oxygen percent control to maintain reasonably constant FiO_2 even if the delivery pressure of one or both of the gases fluctuate. The mixed gases then traverse a needle valve assembly (see Fig 16–21,G), which is the main flow control. The flow is displayed by the Thorpe tube (see Fig 16–21,H), which is the next component in the gas conduction system. From the Thorpe tube, the inspired gas mix passes the pressure limit control (see Fig 16–21,I). This control is a simple, spring-loaded valve that allows gas to vent to the atmosphere when the pressure in the gas conduction system exceeds the tension placed on the valve spring. The tension on the valve spring is adjusted by turning the pressure limit control on the front panel. An antisuffocation valve (see Fig 16–21,J) provides for some measure of safety in the event of a gas supply failure. From here the inspired gas is delivered to the patient circuit.

The expiratory limb of the ventilator consists of the exhalation valve/PEEP assembly. Expired gas from the patient is carried to the exhalation valve, which is comprised of a block housing the exhalation channel (see Fig 16–21,K) and the exhalation valve diaphragm (see Fig 16–21,L). The diaphragm is activated by a solenoid, which, during inspiration, rapidly and completely occludes the expiratory channel, causing pressure to rise in the patient circuit and di-

---

FIG 16–21.
Rear view of Bourns BP200 infant pressure ventilator flow diagram. *A,* air and oxygen inlet ports. *B,* pressure gauge. *C,* pressure control. *D,* PEEP control valve. *E,* PEEP Venturi. *F,* pressure reduction valves. *G,* needle valve assembly. *H,* Thorpe tube. *I,* pressure limit control. *J,* antisuffocation valve. *K,* exhalation channel. *L,* exhalation valve diaphragm. *M,* Venturi throat. *N,* expiratory check leaf. (Courtesy of Bear Medical systems, Inc., Riverside Calif.)

verting flow to the endotracheal tube. This single-step closure of the exhalation valve is the major advantage the BP200 has over ventilators with later-generation exhalation valves. The insignificant amount of time that it takes to effect closure allows the operator to achieve an almost square inspiratory flow pattern, something that is difficult to accomplish with a differential pressure–type valve. The PEEP assembly is simply a Venturi throat (see Fig 16–21,M) that increases the flow resistance characteristics of the exhalation valve by retarding the movement of the expiratory check leaf (see Fig 16–21,N).

REFERENCES

1. Dalziel J: On sleep and an apparatus for promoting artificial respiration, in *British Association for Advancement of Science*. Report no 2. 1838, p 127.
2. Drinker P, McKhann CF: The use of a new apparatus for prolonged administration of artificial respiration. *JAMA* 1929; 92:1658.
3. Emerson JH: *The evolution of "Iron Lung."* JH Emerson Co, Cambridge, Mass, 1978.

SECTION IV

Strategies for Modifying Respiratory Care

Ongoing Patient Assessment

Glen G. J. Low, M.Ed., R.R.T.

The role of the respiratory care practitioner in health care delivery systems requires in-depth skills for evaluating patient care and physiologic effects. Although the traditional focus of evaluation has primarily been the cardiopulmonary system, the complexity of multiple system failure found in the patient population today requires an understanding of the relationship of the cardiopulmonary system to other organ systems. For prospective patient assessment and care, the respiratory care practitioner must have an understanding of the related functions and special problems of other physiologic systems.

This chapter will provide a basis for (1) understanding the rationale for continuous assessment, (2) developing a systematic physiologic approach to treatment, (3) evaluating respiratory modalities based on therapeutic objectives, and (4) evaluating the systems for processing and documenting the information obtained. The rationale for continuous assessment and monitoring is to:

1. Update physiologic assessments
2. Identify the therapeutic objective
3. Initiate and maintain therapy that has been prescribed
4. Evaluate the patient's response to the care provided
5. Suggest modifications in respiratory management
6. Provide a basis for documentation of care given
7. Assure patient safety

CONTINUOUS PHYSIOLOGIC ASSESSMENTS

Information utilized for continuous patient assessment share common evaluations with those used for initial assessment covered in Section I. However, this chapter will focus on applying this data to ongoing patient evaluation.

Patient evaluation should precede the first respiratory care treatment so that a data base can be established. Assessment can range from simple observations to more complex and technically oriented evaluations such as those performed in the intensive care units. The evaluation should be appropriate for the suspected pathologic condition. For example, when the heart rate is evaluated in a healthy patient, assessing the peripheral pulse fits the therapeutic objective better than performing a 12-lead ECG.

The initial assessment of the patient should provide the respiratory care practitioner with the physiologic basis for respiratory care to be administered. The level of initial assessment can vary with a given patient; however, a useful data base should include chief complaint, patient history consisting of: patient profile, family history, and past medical history, and review of respiratory system and other related areas. Laboratory data should be selected from those items useful for proposed therapeutic goals and typically includes: arterial blood analyses, chest x-ray, ECG, hemoglobin level, hematocrit, and electrolyte concentrations.

Cardiovascular Examination

Evaluation of the cardiovascular system, such as heart rate and rhythm and perfusion state, can provide important and easily accessible information. For ongoing patient assessment to yield the highest results, a baseline assessment is necessary. Frequently when respiratory care services are implemented, direct assessment of baseline information is not always possible. However, the data can generally be solicited from nursing and medical personnel.

Heart Rate and Rhythm

An assessment of heart rate, strength, and rhythm can be accomplished by evaluating the peripheral pulse by palpating the radial, brachial, femoral, pedal, tibial, or carotid artery (Fig 17–1). A normal adult heart rate is between 60 and 100 beats/min. The most common site for assessment is the radial artery. Caution should be exercised when palpating the carotid artery of cardiac patients since firm pressure applied to this site can result in vagal stimulation leading to bradycardia.

The examiner's fingers should be placed on top of the artery, parallel with it (Fig 17–2). The examiner's thumb should not be placed on the artery since the thumb's own pulse is strong enough to be mistaken for a patient's beat. The pulse should be counted for 1 minute. The strength (bounding, weak) and regularity should be noted. An irregular peripheral pulse should be compared with the apical pulse rate.

The strength of the pulse can provide valuable information about the cardiovascular system. A weak pulse may occur with cardiac failure, shock, decreased circulatory blood volume, or peripheral vasodilation. A bounding pulse may be indicative of hypoxemia, anemia, exercise, or hypermetabolic states such as fever and hyperthyroidism. Anxiety, peripheral arteriosclerotic disease, or medications may result in a bounding pulse. Irregular rhythm may indicate the presence of premature ventricular contractions connected with cigarettes, caffeine, anxiety, hypoxemia, and certain medication. Hypoxemia causes an increase in heart rate, stroke volume, and cardiac output as a compensation mechanism to deliver more available oxygen to the tissues. Evaluation of pulse is readily available, whereas the assessment of stroke volume and cardiac output requires more sophisticated and invasive procedures. Although heart rate is a sensitive indicator, it is not specific. Therefore, it must be considered as an im-

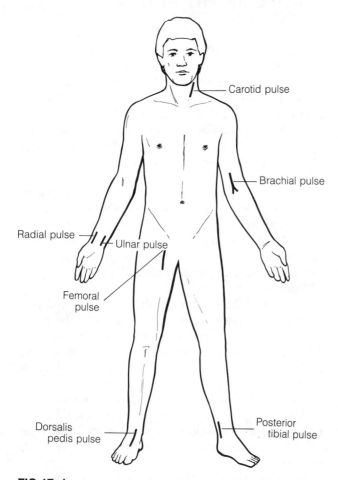

FIG 17–1.
Locations for assessing the radial, brachial, femoral, pedal, tibial, and carotid pulse.

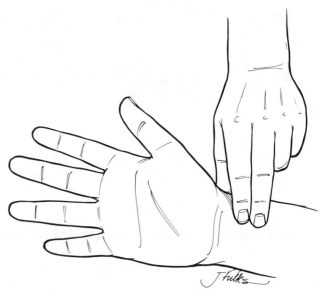

FIG 17–2.
Radial pulse being taken.

portant evaluation parameter that needs to be used in conjunction with other monitoring tools, such as clinical diagnosis and patient history.

The most common cardiac rhythm associated with hypoxia is sinus tachycardia. Evidence of premature ventricular contractions (PVCs) will occur as the level of hypoxia increases and the myocardium weakens. If left untreated, PVCs can lead to ventricular tachycardia and fibrillation. Successful treatment of hypoxemia can be documented by a return in the heart rate to baseline.

Perfusion State

Blood Pressure.—Arterial blood pressure is the result of the force of blood against the walls of the arteries. Systolic blood pressure is the peak force exerted during contractions of the left ventricle (normal range, 90 to 140 mm Hg). Diastolic pressure is the force exerted when the heart relaxes (normal range, 60 to 90 mm Hg). Pulse pressure represents the difference in systolic and diastolic pressures (normal range, 35 to 40 mm Hg).

Arterial hypertension is present when the blood pressure is greater than 140/90 mm Hg. Hypertension results when peripheral vascular resistance increases, increasing the force of ventricular contraction, or from fluid overload. Hypotension is present when the blood pressure is less than 90/60 mm Hg. Hypotension is the result of peripheral vasodilation, left ventricular failure, or low blood volume. Prolonged hypotension may result in an inadequate circulation and impaired oxygen delivery, resulting in tissue hypoxia.

Since blood pressure is a dynamic measurement directly affecting oxygen transport, it should be continually monitored. The measurement of blood pressure can readily be performed using a sphygmomanometer (blood pressure cuff) and a stethoscope, or an arterial line can be inserted for continuous assessment (Fig 17–3).

Neurologic Function.—Assessment of neurologic status can provide valuable information. The level of consciousness is a good indicator of the extent of hypoxemia, low cardiac output, compromised perfusion state, acid-base imbalance, accumulation of metabolic waste products, and low glucose level. Positive pressure ventilation can affect the neurologic system by increasing the intracranial pressure. Intracranial pressure can be increased if the venous pressure increases or the cerebral blood flow decreases. Neurologic acuity is a sensitive indicator; however, it is not specific. Therefore, it

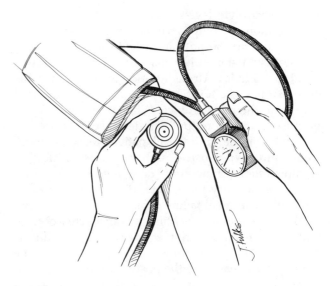

FIG 17–3.
Blood pressure being taken from the brachial artery.

must be considered as an important evaluation parameter that needs to be used in conjunction with other monitoring tools, clinical diagnosis, and patient history.

Several abnormal ventilatory patterns are associated with direct injury to or a lesion of the brain. Cheyne-Stokes respiration can result from central nervous system lesions or accumulation of metabolic waste products. Apneustic breathing, apnea, and Biot's breathing can occur from indirect injury to the respiratory control centers of the pons and medulla.

The practitioner should assess neurologic function by observing ventilatory patterns, airway reflexes (e.g., gag and swallow), response to pain, purposeful movement, and level of consciousness. The observation can aid in selecting the extent of artificial airway management of such patients. Patients who are confused, irritable, and agitated should be assumed to have an inadequate cerebral oxygenation until other causes can be eliminated.

Skin.—The patient integument is an important parameter used to evaluate perfusion state. Normally, the skin is warm and dry. Hypoxemia leads to peripheral shunting of blood from the skin to more central organs. When a patient's perfusion state is compromised, the skin appears pale, sweaty, and cold.

Renal Function.—An evaluation of renal function is performed by monitoring the fluid balance, intake and output, specific gravity, daily weights, serum electrolyte levels, urine and blood osmolarities, pulmonary compliance, and blood gases.

The urinary output can provide an indication of the perfusion status. Normal urine output in adults is 1.0 to 1.5 L/day. Urine filtration in the glomerulus of the kidney is a function of the blood pressure and volume in the renal arteries. When perfusion is compromised, urinary output will decrease. It is not uncommon for the critically ill patient to be hypovolemic and hypotensive. Other factors, including administration of nephrotoxic agents and existing renal disease, may make determination of the exact cause of acute renal failure difficult.

Positive pressure ventilation can decrease renal perfusion, resulting in the release of antidiuretic hormone (ADH) and aldosterone.[4, 5, 33] Antidiuretic hormone is released by the posterior pituitary gland. It acts on the kidney tubules, causing a reduction in urinary output and a retention of sodium and water.

Pulmonary problems can occur with renal failure, including excessive water imbalance, which results in an increased pulmonary extravascular water and pulmonary edema. To evaluate the effects of renal failure on respiratory function, one must monitor the peak inspiratory pressure, plateau pressure, effective static compliance, and PaO_2. Increased pressures, a decreased compliance, and falling PaO_2 can be early indications of pulmonary extracellular fluid. Cardiac output, arterial pressure, central venous pressure (CVP), and pulmonary artery wedge pressure (PAWP) can be observed and are useful indicators of fluid and electrolyte balance. Hypovolemia may also result in thickened and encrusted bronchial secretions.

Chest Assessment

Inspection

Visual examination of the chest is a technique used to assess the thoracic configuration, pattern, and effort of breathing. It can give the respiratory care practitioner valuable information on the mechanical ability to maintain ventilation. For adequate inspection to occur, the room must be well lighted and the patient must be sitting in an upright position. Male patients should be stripped to the waist, and female patients should be given some type of drape.

The chest should be inspected for dimensions. The anteroposterior dimension normally increases gradually with age; however, a premature increase occurs in patients with chronic obstructive lung disease. The abnormal increase in the anteroposterior

dimension is called *barrel chest*. Other abnormal deformities of the thorax include:

1. *Kyphosis.*—Spinal deformity in which the spine has an abnormal anteroposterior curvature.
2. *Scoliosis.*—Spinal deformity in which the spine has a lateral curvature.
3. *Kyphoscoliosis.*—Combination of kyphosis and scoliosis, which may produce a restrictive lung defect as a result of poor lung expansion.
4. *Pectus carinatum.*—Sternal protrusion anteriorly.
5. *Pectus excavatum.*—Depression of part or all of the sternum, which can produce a restrictive lung defect.

Assessment of respiratory rate and effort should be included. The counting of respiratory rate should be performed in an inconspicuous manner so as not to skew the patient's normal pattern. Evaluation of the use of the accessory muscles for ventilation can provide the practitioner with valuable information. When accessory muscles (scalene and sternomastoid) become active at rest, pulmonary conditions such as acute and chronic airway obstruction, acute upper airway obstruction, and reduced lung compliance may be present.

Palpation

Palpation involves touching the chest wall in an effort to evaluate underlying lung structure and function. Palpation is performed to (1) evaluate vocal fremitus, (2) estimate symmetry of thoracic expansion, (3) establish the position of the trachea, and (4) assess the skin and subcutaneous tissues of the chest.

Vocal fremitus is the term referring to the vibrations created by the vocal cords and transmitted to the chest wall. When these vibrations are felt on the chest wall, it is called *tactile fremitus*. During the assessment, the patient is asked to repeat the word 99 while the examiner's hands systematically palpates the thorax from superior to inferior. The anterior, lateral, and posterior chest walls should be evaluated. The normal lung structure is a combination of fluid- and air-filled tissue. Increased fremitus results from the transmission of the vibration through a more solid medium such as the consolidation typical of pneumonia. If the area of consolidation is not in connection with patent bronchus, fremitus will not be increased but will be absent or decreased. Patients who are obese or who have a large chest wall often have a reduced tactile fremitus. Also, when the pleural space lining the lungs become filled with air (pneumothorax), the vocal fremitus is reduced significantly or is absent. Patients with emphysema have hyperinflated lungs with a reduction in the density of lung tissue. In this situation, the vibrations transmit poorly through the lung tissue, resulting in bilateral reduction in tactile fremitus.

The passage of air through airways containing thick secretions may produce palpable vibrations referred to as *rhonchial fremitus*. Rhonchial fremitus are often audible during inhalation and exhalation and may clear if the patient produces an effective cough.

The practitioner should evaluate the characteristics and quality of the thoracic expansion. It should occur simultaneously and equally during a deep inhalation. This expansion can be evaluated on the anterior and posterior chest walls. Anteriorly, the practitioner's hands are placed over the anterolateral chest wall with the thumbs extended along the costal margin toward the xiphoid process (Fig 17–4). On the posterior side of the chest, the hands are positioned over the posterolateral chest wall with the thumbs meeting at approximately the eighth thoracic vertebra (Fig 17–5). The patient is instructed to exhale slowly and completely while the practitioner's hands are positioned on the chest. When the patient

has exhaled maximally, the tips of each thumb meet at the chest, and the thumbs are extended toward the midline until the tip of each meets at the midline. The patient then is instructed to take a full, deep breath. The distance each thumb moves from the midline should be noted. Normally, each thumb moves an equal distance of approximately 3 to 5 cm. Diseases that effect the expansion of the thorax include kyphosis, scoliosis, atelectasis, lobar pneumonia, pleural effusion, and pneumothorax.

The surface of the chest can be assessed for the presence of subcutaneous emphysema. When air leaks from the lungs into subcutaneous tissue, fine pockets of air travel underneath the skin, producing a crackling sound and sensation when palpated.

Percussion

Percussion is the technique of tapping on a surface to evaluate the underlying structure. Percussion of the chest wall produces sound and a palpable vibration useful in the evaluation of the underlying lung tissue. The technique requires the practitioner to place the middle finger of one hand firmly against the chest wall parallel to the ribs with the palm and other fingers off of the chest wall. The tip of the middle finger on the other hand strikes the middle finger on the chest wall with a quick, sharp blow (Fig 17–6). The practitioner should assess systemati-

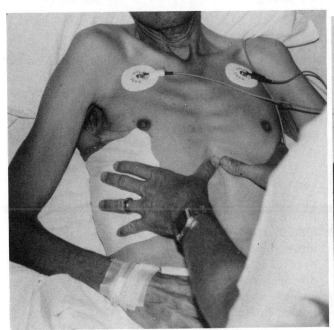

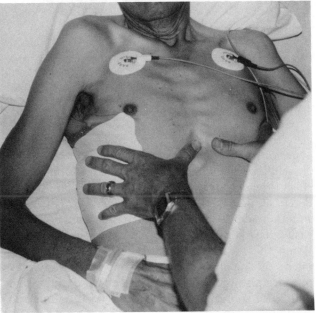

FIG 17–4.
Evaluation of chest expansion by placing hands anterolaterally over the chest with thumbs extended along the costal margin toward the xiphoid process. (From Frownfelter DL: *Chest Physical*

Therapy and Pulmonary Rehabilitation: An Interdisciplinary Approach, ed 2. Chicago, Year Book Medical Publishers, 1987, pp 166–167. Used with permission.)

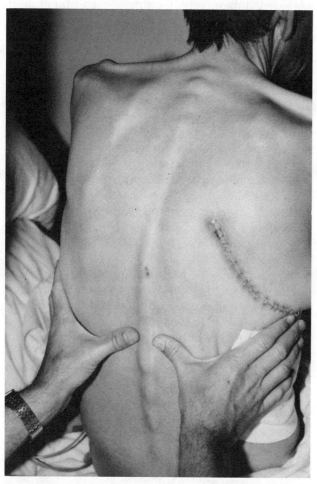

FIG 17–5.
Evaluation of chest expansion by placing hands posteriorly over the posterolateral chest wall with thumbs meeting at approximately the eighth thoracic vertebra. (From Frownfelter DL: *Chest Physical Therapy and Pulmonary Rehabilitation: An Interdisciplinary Approach*, ed 2. Chicago, Year Book Medical Publishers, 1987, p 168. Used with permission.)

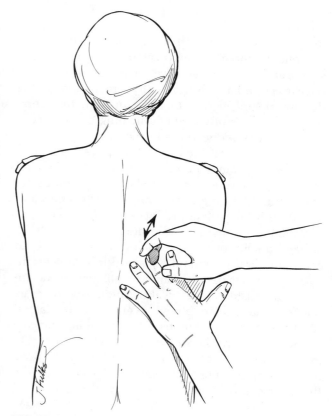

FIG 17–6.
Posterior side of the chest with the examiner's middle finger on it and the other hand striking with the opposite middle finger.

cally from one side to the other, working from the superior to the inferior aspect of the thorax.

The sound generated during percussion of the chest is evaluated for intensity (loudness) and pitch. Percussion over normal lung fields produces a sound moderately low in pitch that can be heard easily. The sound is referred to as *normal resonance.* When the percussion note is louder and lower in pitch, the resonance is increased. Percussion may produce a sound with characteristics of a dull or flat note. The sound is generally short in duration and not loud.

Percussion should be considered an assessment tool to be considered with other physical findings and history. Any abnormality that tends to increase the density of the lung tissue, such as consolidation of pneumonia, lung tumors, hemothorax, pleural effusion, or atelectasis, results in a loss of resonance and a dull percussion note over the affected area. An increase in resonance is detected in patients with hyperinflated lungs, as in asthma and chronic obstructive pulmonary disease (COPD), or when the pleural space is contained with air (pneumothorax).

Diaphragmatic excursion can be assessed by percussion done over the posterior chest wall. Diaphragmatic movement is estimated by instructing the patient to take a deep, full inspiration and to hold it. The respiratory care practitioner then determines the lowest margin of resonance by percussing over the lower portion of the lung fields and moving downward in small increments until a distinct change in the percussion note is detected. The patient is instructed to exhale fully, holding this position while the percussion note is assessed (Fig 17–7). The range of diaphram excursion during a deep breath is about 5 to 7 cm. Diaphragmatic movement is decreased in patients who have neuromusclar diseases and severe COPD.[47]

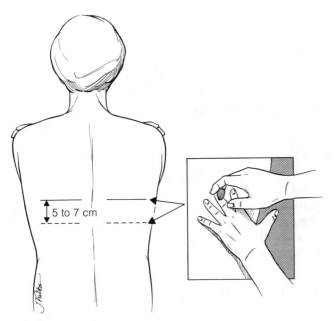

FIG 17–7.
Posterior side of the chest with diaphragm at the end of a deep exhalation and deep inhalation. Examiner's hands percuss as previously described at the two positions approximately 5 to 7 cm vertical distance apart.

Auscultation

Auscultation of the patient's chest can provide valuable information of airway patency and level of ventilation. It can provide useful information on a variety of diseases. Although subjective, the experienced respiratory care practitioner skilled in the technique can document and monitor a patient's progress through chest auscultation. When one is listening to breath sounds, the diaphragm of the stethoscope should be placed against the chest wall, since clothing may alter lung sounds or produce distorted sounds (Fig 17–8). The tubing should not be rubbing against any objects, since it may produce extraneous sounds.

In most of the conducting airways of the lungs, gas flow is described as laminar. This smooth flow is replaced by turbulent, unsteady flow in large airways. The vibration of the gas in the large airways is transmitted to the walls of the airways and hence to the surface of the chest. As sound travels toward the periphery and chest wall, it is progressively filtered and attenuated. The following are breath sounds the respiratory care practitioner will encounter:

1. *Normal, or vesicular breath sounds.*—In healthy individuals, lung sounds have a characteristic quality that varies with the area of the chest where they are heard. Over the large airways, a tubular quality

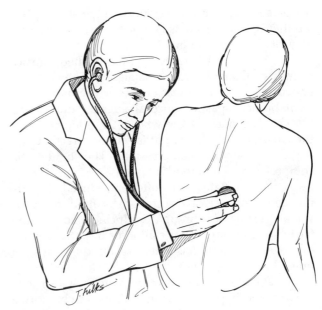

FIG 17–8.
Auscultation of the chest.

is normally present, such sounds are bronchial, or tubular, breath sounds (see 2). The sounds heard over the chest at a distance from the airways have a lower pitch and frequency. The vesicular sound is heard over all areas of the lungs except where large airways are close to the surface.

2. *Bronchiolar,* or *tubular breath sounds.*—As noted, bronchiolar or tubular breath sounds are normally heard over larger airways. Sounds heard over the large airways are relatively louder than the vesicular sound. The difference is particularly noticeable during expiration. In the normal person, the bronchial sound is heard over the trachea or in the midline of the upper anterior portion of the chest, both to the right and left of the sternum. It is also heard in the right upper anterior portion of the chest and on the back between the scapulas. Bronchial breath sounds heard over the base of the lung are abnormal. Often times the finding of bronchial breath sounds in this area is a result of the better transmission of them from centrally located areas to the periphery; however, it can result from lung consolidation such as pneumonia.[19]

3. *Bronchovesicular breath sounds.*—Areas of the chest intermediate between those where bronchial sounds are heard and those where vesicular sounds are heard, resulting in a mixture of the bronchial and vesicular qualities.

4. *Rhonchi.*—Rhonchi are generated by the vibrations of the wall of a narrowed airway. Low-pitched continuous sounds are often associated with

the presence of excessive sputum in the airways. Often they are described as low-pitched wheezes. They may clear with coughing.

5. *Wheezes.*—Wheezes are high-pitched, musical sounds generally heard on exhalation. They are generated when the diameter of the airway narrows, as from bronchospasm, mucosal edema, and foreign objects. The pitch of the wheeze is independent of the length of the airway but is related directly to the degree of airway compression. The tighter the compression, the higher the pitch.

6. *Rales.*—Rales are often produced by the movement of excessive secretions or fluid in the airways as air passes through producing a sound similar to soda fizzing. Rales can occur in patients without excessive secretions when collapsed airways pop open during inspiration.[18]

7. *Decreased* or *absent breath sounds.*—Obstructed airways and hyperinflated lung tissue inhibit normal transmission of sounds through the lung. Air or fluid in the pleural space and obesity reduce the transmission of breath sounds through the chest wall. Patients with chronic air flow obstruction often have a reduced transmission throughout all lung fields, resulting in decreased breath sounds. Shallow breathing patterns also contribute to reduced breath sound intensity in patients with chronic obstructive airway disease.

Cough Assessment

Coughing is the most common symptom in patients with pulmonary complications. Coughing is a mechanism for expulsion of foreign material and secretions. A cough is produced by mechanical, inflammation, or temperature stimulation of the cough receptors located in the conducting airways. Although sometimes annoying, the cough provides a protective mechanism for the airways.

Evaluation of the changes in the quality, characteristics, and frequency of the cough can provide valuable information about the patient's status. A cough may be acute (sudden onset, short course), chronic (daily for more than 8 weeks), or paroxysmal (periodic, prolonged, forceful episodes). Often a cough occurs in conjunction with other symptoms such as pain, headache, or fainting and can result in rib fractures for those patients on long-term steroid therapy.

A description of the cough should be noted as effective (strong enough to clear the airways) or inadequate (too weak to mobilize secretions) and as productive (mucus or other material is expelled) or dry (secretions not produced). Documentation is important since changes in its characteristics are common and generally follow a chronologic order of dry to a productive cough.

The quality and characteristics of the cough can also provide assessment information that may give clues to the underlying pathologic condition. A barking (seal-like bark) quality to the cough generally indicates croup. A brassy (harsh, dry) hoarse quality and an inspiratory stridor to the cough generally are associated with problems of the upper airway. Wheezy coughs suggest lower airway pathologic conditions, and chronic productive coughs are generally indicative of chronic bronchitis. Hacking (frequent periods of coughing or clearing the throat) may be the result of smoking, viral infections, or sinus infections.

Sputum Assessment

Ongoing evaluation and documentation of the patient's sputum for changes in color, volume, and consistency is essential in assessing the pulmonary flora. The normal healthy adult sputum is composed of 95% water, 2% lipoprotein, 1% carbohydrate, and trace amounts of lipids and DNA.[41] Sputum should be evaluated grossly and microscopically. The gross examination will yield information concerning its thickness. The normal sputum is watery, whereas tenacious mucus usually represents dehydration. Retained secretions have solid flecks of green or yellow, which may represent cast formations from the bronchioles.[8] Signs of pulmonary infection result in changes in the sputum color. Sputum is normally white and translucent. Yellow sputum denotes pus, since white blood cells seen microscopically have a yellow appearance. Green usually means old, retained secretions, since—when seen microscopically—the proteolysis of the mucopolysaccharide bonds that provide a bonding of mucus results in a green color. Sputum that is green and has a foul smell usually indicates a *Pseudomonas* infection. A brown color usually denotes old blood, whereas red denotes fresh blood.[15]

PULMONARY MECHANICS

Pulmonary mechanics are an important component of objective evaluation for ongoing assessment of pulmonary function. Utilization of information from pulmonary function testing usually fits in one of the following categories: (1) determines if an abnormality exists, (2) classifies the type of abnormality, (3) assesses the severity of the abnormality, (4) assesses therapy or follows the course of the disease.[3]

Ventilatory Rate

The normal range of ventilatory rate for an adult is 12 to 20 breaths/min. Ventilatory rate should be assessed for 1 minute and notations concerning any irregularities noted. Assessment of the ventilatory rate should be done in an inconspicuous manner so as not to make the patient aware, which may result in artificial changes.

The breathing rate is controlled by the respiratory centers in the pons and medulla. Increases in carbon dioxide tension, decreases in pH (acidosis), and decreases in blood oxygen tension result in increases in both rate and tidal volume. An increase in the metabolic rate, as in thyroid disease, exercise, stress, infections, fever, hypoglycemia, pulmonary edema, hepatic coma, and ketoacidosis results in an increased rate and depth of respiration. The rate and tidal volume are gross indicators of the mechanical work of breathing. Also, rapid shallow breathing is usually associated with a pulmonary or thoracic restriction, such as pleuritic chest pain. Depression of the respiratory center results in slowing of the respiratory rate. It can occur in the following situations: arterial pH greater than 7.45 (alkalosis), severe hypoxemia and hypercapnia, drug overdose, and administration of narcotics, sedatives, and anesthetic agents.

Tidal Volume

Tidal volume is the amount of gas exhaled during normal ventilation. Normal tidal volume (V_T) is 7 to 9 ml/kg (3 to 4 ml/lb) of ideal body weight. The depth of tidal volume is controlled by the respiratory centers in the pons and medulla. Tidal volume is composed of two components: alveolar ventilation ($\dot{V}_A$), the portion that effectively exchanges with alveolar capillary blood, and dead space ventilation ($\dot{V}_D$), the portion that primes the conducting airways but does not take place in alveolar gas exchange (Fig 17–9). The dead-space volume is normally about 1 ml/lb of ideal body weight, or about one third of the tidal volume. Evaluation of the subunits of tidal volume are equally important to determine, since the respiratory care practitioner needs to know effective alveolar ventilation ($\dot{V}_A$) as well as the amount of bulk gas movement.

An individual's tidal volume can vary greatly. Intermittent increases in tidal volume as much as three to four times normal occur 6 to 10/hour. The increase in tidal volume is known as a *sigh* and has a physiologic benefit of recruiting maldistributed

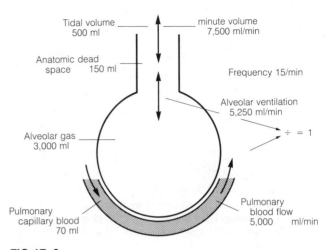

FIG 17–9.
Conducting airways and alveoli indicating dead-space volume and alveolar ventilation subsectioned as the portions of tidal volume.

ventilation. If shallow breathing without occasional sighing is maintained for prolonged periods of time, atelectasis and pneumonia may result.[2] Conditions that may cause tidal volume to be smaller than normal include pneumonia, atelectasis, postoperative thoracic and abdominal surgery, chest trauma, congestive heart failure, restrictive pulmonary disease, neuromuscular disease, and central nervous system depression of the respiratory centers. Abnormally large tidal volumes may indicate the presence of metabolic acidosis or severe neurologic injury.

Tidal volume measurements can be assessed with any number of commercially available bedside pulmonary function units. Equipment generally consists of a spirometer, mouthpiece/mask, one-way valves, and large-bore tubing (Fig 17–10).

Breathing Pattern

An evaluation of the patient's pattern of ventilation is an important parameter to document. The pattern of ventilation can give valuable information concerning pulmonary mechanics and neurologic lesions. *Eupnea* is referred to as a normal rhythmic respiratory pattern. *Bradypnea* implies a slow respiratory rate with slight increases in the depth of respiration. *Tachypnea* is a shallow rapid breathing pattern. *Hyperpnea* indicates an increased depth of breathing with some increase in respiratory rate. Tachypnea and hyperpnea are generally significant of midbrain upper pontine lesions. *Biot's respiration* is irregular with regular intervals of apnea, characterized by abrupt periods of hyperventilation. The pattern is seen with pontine lesions. *Cheyne-Stokes respiration* is a respiratory pattern characterized by cycles of increasing tidal volume, followed by de-

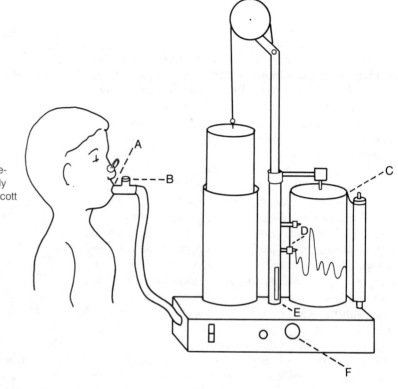

FIG 17–10.
Portable bedside spirometer, mouthpiece, one-way valve, and large-bore tubing. (From Grady D: *Laboratory Exercises.* New York, JB Lippincott Co, 1987, p 298. Used with permission.)

creasing tidal volume. Respirations may cease for 5 to 30 seconds. *Apnea* is a cessation of respiration in the resting expiratory position. *Apneustic respiratory pattern* is a cessation of breathing in the inspiratory position interrupted periodically by expiration. The pattern is seen with low pontine lesions. *Ataxia* is a respiratory pattern characterized by chaotic irregular breathing. The pattern is significant of lesions of the medulla. Patients with a restrictive pulmonary dysfunction will maintain their level of minute ventilation by increasing their tidal volume.

Vital Capacity

The vital capacity is the maximal amount of air that can be exhaled from the lungs after a maximal inspiration. The vital capacity is measured in liters or milliliters. There are many commercially available spirometers with varying degrees of portability that can be used at the patient's bedside. The technique of measurement requires the patient to inspire maximally and then exhale into a spirometer. Vital capacity can be measured from maximal inspiration to maximal expiration or vice versa. Actual patient values need to be compared with predicted normal values. A decreased vital capacity could be indicative of loss of functional or actual lung parenchyma characterized by such abnormalities as pulmonary edema, bronchogenic carcinoma, extrapulmonic ab-

normalities such as pneumothorax, pleural effusion, or cardiac enlargement. A decreased vital capacity could be the result of extrathoracic restrictions, such as ascites, obesity, pregnancy, kyphoscoliosis, or by the loss in integrity of the conducting airways to support the bulk movement of gas during the maneuver, as in bronchiolar obstruction, asthma, and COPD. A decrease could also result from neuromuscular diseases and depression of the respiratory center.

Airway Patency

Airway patency is fundamental to the effectiveness of spontaneous ventilatory support. The ability of the patient to voluntarily sustain comfortable ventilation is proportional to the extent of airway patency. In a patient with decreased patency, flow rate measurements will be decreased. Airway patency in various lung disorders is a dynamic process, as with asthma. The assessment of airway patency provides the practitioner with an evaluation of the therapeutic regimen for reversible airway disease treated with sympathomimetics. Bedside evaluation of airway patency can be documented with pulmonary function testing. Flow rate measurements commonly assessed at the bedside are:

1. The peak expiratory flow rate (PEFR)
2. Volume of gas exhaled in a given time inter-

val during the execution of a forced vital capacity (FEV_1, FEV_2, FEV_3),

3. Ratio of timed forced expiratory volume to forced vital capacity, expressed as a percentage (e.g., $FEV_1/FVC\%$),
4. Forced expiratory flow between 200 and 1,200 ml of the vital capacity ($FEF_{0.2-1.2\ L}$), and
5. Forced expiratory flow during the middle half of the forced vital capacity ($FEF_{25\%-75\%}$)

The validity of the test depends largely on patient effort and cooperation. Spirometry may fail to provide evidence of diffuse obstructive lung disease when it is of slight degree.[41] Only when lung disease progresses do lung capacities such as forced vital capacity (FVC) and inspiratory capacity (IC) decrease while residual volume (RV), functional residual capacity (FRC), and total lung capacity (TLC) increase.[10]

Prebronchodilator and Postbronchodilator Evaluations

Serial bedside pulmonary function testing is an important tool to chart the progress of the therapeutic regimen for lung disease. The effectiveness of bronchodilator therapy can be assessed by prebronchodilator and postbronchodilator studies. Bronchodilator administration is a substantial component of respiratory care, and its effects warrant continuous evaluation by the practitioner. Although bronchodilator therapy has been somewhat routinely prescribed in the management of obstructive airway disease, not all patients demonstrate a significant reversible component of their disease.[27] Optimum pharmacologic effect is best determined by objective measurement and evaluation of the patient's ventilatory state. In 1982, Kasik et al.[27] encouraged objective evaluation with specific reference to the measurement of forced expiratory flow.[10] Equipment for measuring expiratory flow is available and can provide practitioners with a rapid and simple means of obtaining more objective data for the assessment of bronchodilators.[16] A bronchodilator has a significant effect when there is a greater than 15% increase in flow rate measurement as determined by changes in the $FEF_{25\%-75\%}$ and $FEF_{0.2-1.2\ L}$. The criteria for using serial bedside pulmonary function testing would be the patient's cooperation and ability to perform the test successfully. In a patient with no significant increase in expiratory flow rates following bronchodilator therapy, evaluation of the patient's clinical findings should reveal a disease pattern characteristic of COPD.

Forced Expiratory Volume.—As previously noted, when the FVC is measured over a given time interval, it is referred to as the forced expiratory volume (FEV), with a subscript to indicate the time (FEV_t). The times generally used are 0.5 second, 1.0 second, 2.0 seconds, and 3.0 seconds. The FEV is determined once the FVC maneuver has been performed utilizing a mechanism to denote time on the horizontal axis (Fig 17–11). The significance of the test is that it allows the assessment of volume over a given period of time, thus providing the measurement of flow rate. The flow rate assessment can provide the practitioner with information relating to the level of airway obstruction. Nomograms are available to compare an individual patient's results with predicted normal values. The FEV and flow rate measurements can vary as much as 20% from the predicted value and still be considered normal. Postoperative cough effectiveness can be judged by the flow rate indicated by the FEV rate in 1 second (FEV_1). The average cough generates flow rates of 4 to 6 L/sec.

Forced Expiratory Volume/Forced Vital Capacity Ratio.—As defined earlier, the forced expiratory volume/forced vital capacity is a ratio that expresses a given timed volume to the vital capacity. It is a mathematical computation from the FEV_t and FVC. A normal individual should be able to exhale 60% of FVC in 0.5 second, 83% in 1 second, 94% in 2 seconds, 97% in 3 seconds. Nomograms are available to compare an individual patient's results with predicted normal values. The FEV can vary as much as 20% from the predicted value and still be considered normal. Patients with a reduced value will fall into a

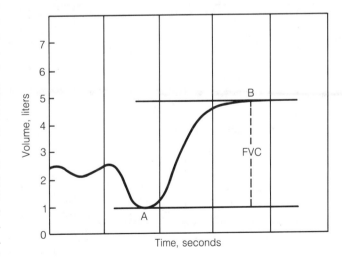

FIG 17–11.
Tracing of a forced vital capacity with time lines on the x axis denoting time.

category of obstructive airway disease; patients with restrictive disease often show a normal $FEV_t/FVC\%$ ratio.

Forced Expiratory Flow Between 200 and 1,200 ml.—The FEF between 200 and 1,200 ml is the flow rate measured during the first 200 to 1,200 ml of FVC maneuver (Fig 17–12). The $FEF_{0.2-1.2 L}$ is usually recorded in liters per second but is reported in liters per minute. The average flow rate measurement is 6 to 7 L/sec (400 L/min).

The $FEF_{0.2-1.2 L}$ is an indicator of air flow in the large airways. Decreased flow rate measurements are indicative of obstructive lung disease; restrictive lung disease patterns will generally be normal.

Peak Expiratory Flow Rate.—Peak flow is the maximum flow rate attainable at any time during a forced expiratory volume (PEF rate). It is recorded in liters per second. The value tends to vary and is markedly effort dependent. The average peak flow attainable in healthy young men is 10 L/sec (600 L/min). The procedure can be easily performed with a Wright peak flowmeter. The device is easily portable and requires no electrical power. However, a drawback of the device is the lack of hard copy. Flow rates are best measured by a pneumotachograph in which the flow signal can be integrated to a given volume. Maximum expiratory flow rate (MEFR) curves are obtained when flow is measured throughout the FVC. Maximum expiratory flow rate measurements can be useful in assessing the ability to generate a cough.[3]

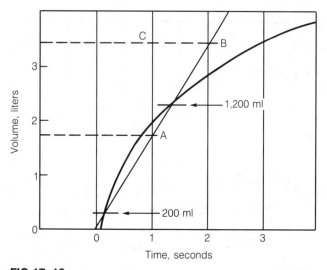

FIG 17–12.
Forced vital capacity showing $FEF_{200-1,200L}$ calculations.

ARTERIAL BLOOD GAS MEASUREMENTS

Arterial blood gas measurements are an important component of ongoing patient evaluation. It is an important part of the documentation of hypoxemia, ventilation, and acid-base balance. However, the information obtained from the blood gas measurement provides only a snapshot evaluation at that moment. The information must take into account the F_{IO2}, hemoglobin level, and acid-base status for the assessment of oxygenation and ventilation to be significant. Documentation of cardiopulmonary status at the moment the arterial gas was drawn is important. The relationship of the information from a blood gas must be related to the effects it has on the cardiopulmonary system. An in-depth discussion of arterial blood gas analysis can be found in Chapter 18. The intent of this section is to provide the respiratory care practitioner with a system to integrate and utilize the information as it clinically relates to the patient's oxygenation and ventilation status.

Assessment of Oxygenation

Tissue oxygenation is the end product of a number of complex steps. Initially, the amount of oxygen available at the alveolar level to cross the alveolar-capillary membrane depends on the inspired oxygen concentration and distribution of ventilation. Oxygen in the alveoli crosses the alveolar-capillary membrane into the blood. Factors influencing the ease with which this process occurs include the partial pressure, the pressure gradient, and the thickness of the alveolar-capillary membrane. Once oxygen is in the arterial blood, the ability of the blood to transport adequate volumes of oxygen to the tissues depends on the hemoglobin level, cardiac output, the vasomotor tone, and the integrity of the cardiovascular system. At the tissue level, oxygen movement into the tissue across the capillary membrane is dependent on the pressure gradient. Once oxygen is in the tissues, its utilization depends on the tissues metabolism. The clinical assessment of tissue oxygenation cannot be measured directly; therefore, the following indirect measurements can be used:

1. Measuring the effectiveness of matching ventilation with perfusion and by calculating the degree of shunt
2. Measuring the ability of oxygen to cross the alveolar capillary membrane by calculating the alveolar-arterial oxygen gradient

3. Measuring the PaO_2 and the oxyhemoglobin content, which allows the evaluation of the ability of the arterial blood to transport adequate amounts of oxygen
4. Measuring the arterial and venous oxygen contents and calculating the difference between these two values, which allows the amount of oxygen utilized by the tissues to be identified

Ventilation-Perfusion Relationships

The purpose of ventilation is to provide oxygen at the alveolar level where it will be matched with arterial blood flow and to remove carbon dioxide from alveoli and venous blood. The adequacy of alveolar ventilation is a dynamic process, dependent on the tissue oxygenation requirements, carbon dioxide level, and acid-base balance. The ideal relationship of ventilation and perfusion is one where they would be matched equally. However, equal matching does not occur, causing variations in this relationship, affecting the ability of tissues to receive adequate supplies of oxygen and remove carbon dioxide. Ventilation without perfusion results in a condition called *dead space,* and perfusion without ventilation results in a condition called *shunt.*[12]

Dead-Space Ventilation.—Dead-space ventilation is that portion of the inspired volume that does not reach the alveolar level to participate in gas exchange. Total or physiologic dead space normally is composed of anatomical and alveolar dead space. Anatomic dead space is the volume of gas in the conducting airways of the tracheobronchial tree.

Alveolar dead space is the volume of gas within the alveoli that are being ventilated but not perfused. Normally, 20% to 40% of tidal volume does not participate in gas exchange and is dead-space ventilation.

Dead space can be calculated by a technique that utilizes the Bohr equation, defining respiratory dead space as:

$$\dot{V}_D = \frac{(FA_{CO2} - FE_{CO2}) \times \dot{V}_E}{FA_{CO2}}$$

where:

$\dot{V}_E$ = expired volume (tidal volume)
FA_{CO2} = fraction of CO_2 in alveolar gas
FE_{CO2} = fraction of CO_2 in expired gas.

Modifications of this equation are necessary since measuring alveolar concentration of carbon dioxide is clinically difficult, requiring the partial pressures of the component gases to be substituted. The modified equation is:

$$\dot{V}_D = \frac{(Pa_{CO2} - P\bar{E}_{CO2}) \times \dot{V}_E}{Pa_{CO2}}.$$

The procedure requires the practitioner to collect exhaled gas over several respiratory cycles and to measure the volume and concentration of carbon dioxide while obtaining simultaneous carbon dioxide arterial blood gas measurement. Placing the variables into the equation will allow the practitioner to calculate a reasonably accurate measurement of physiologic dead space.

Because of the difficulty in measuring the anatomic dead space, for the purposes of clinical purposes, the anatomic dead space is sometimes equated with the subject's ideal weight in pounds (1 ml/1b). The measurement of respiratory dead space yields information regarding the status of functional lung tissue. The anatomic dead space is larger in men than in women and with larger tidal volumes caused by exercise or pulmonary disease.[10] The anatomic dead space increases in patients with large functional residual capacities and in diseases such as bronchiectasis.[10] It may decrease in asthma or in diseases characterized by bronchial obstruction.

Alveolar ventilation is the volume of gas that participates in rapid gas exchange in the lungs. It can be calculated by subtracting the dead-space ventilation from the total. The alveolar ventilation is normally about 4 to 5 L/min in the adult patient and is subject to wide variations. The adequacy of alveolar ventilation must be determined by arterial blood gas analysis.

Dead-space ventilation can be expressed in terms of the relationship to the volume of wasted ventilation on the conducting airways and nonfunctioning alveoli. It is usually expressed as a fraction of the tidal volume (V_D/V_T) and is considered normal if the derived value is less than 0.3. Mechanical ventilatory support may be required if the V_D/V_T ratio increases to more than 0.6.[22] For the V_D/V_T ratio measurement to be clinically useful, the ventilatory pattern, metabolic function, and cardiovascular function must be stable.

Intrapulmonary Shunting.—Shunting is the portion of the cardiac output that perfuses nonventilated alveoli and can be divided into two types (anatomical and physiologic). Anatomic shunt comprises the greater portion of the normal intrapulmonary shunt and is the normal blood flow through the pleural, bronchial, and thebesian veins. In the normal individual, approximately 2% to 5% of the cardiac output is returned to the left side of the heart without being oxygenated. Its effect is a lowered oxygen content when the blood returns to the left atrium. A small amount of physiologic shunt is normal; however, increased physiologic shunt is associated with atelectasis, pneumonia, pneumothorax, and pulmonary edema.

An equation for determining the shunt fraction relates the total cardiac output to that portion of cardiac output that has not been oxygenated. The mathematical derivation is based on Fick's equation. The proportion of shunt is determined by calculating the oxygen content of pulmonary end-capillary (Cc'_{O_2}), arterial (Ca_{O_2}) and mixed venous ($C\bar{v}_{O_2}$), blood. The Fick equation states that:

$$\frac{\dot{Q}_S}{\dot{Q}_T} = \frac{Cc'_{O_2} - Ca_{O_2}}{Cc'_{O_2} - C\bar{v}_{O_2}}$$

Where:

$\dot{Q}_S$ = shunted cardiac output
$\dot{Q}_T$ = total cardiac output
Cc'_{O_2} = pulmonary end-capillary oxygen content
$C\bar{v}_{O_2}$ = mixed venous oxygen content.

To use the shunt equation, calculate the oxygen contents of the pulmonary end-capillary, arterial, and mixed venous blood by the following equation:

O_2 content (vol%)

= (Hb con) (Hb %sat) (1.34) + (0.003) (P_{O_2})

where:

Hb con = hemoglobin content
Hb %sat = hemoglobin saturation percentage
P_{O_2} = partial pressure of oxygen.

The oxygen content is expressed in milliliters of oxygen per 100 ml of blood (vol%).

The arterial oxygen content Ca_{O_2} is calculated from arterial blood gas values, and mixed venous oxygen content ($C\bar{v}_{O_2}$) is calculated from pulmonary artery blood gas values. To calculate Cc'_{O_2}, one would have to obtain a pulmonary capillary blood gas sample from an ideally ventilated and perfused alveolus, which is not possible. Therefore, Cc'_{O_2} is calculated based on the assumption that pulmonary end-capillary gas tension is equal to the alveolar oxygen tension, thus requiring the alveolar-air equation (Fig 17-13).

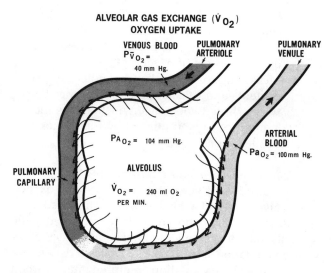

FIG 17–13.

Lung with enlargement at the alveolar-capillary level denoting PA_{O_2} approximately equivalent to capillary oxygen. (From Barnes T: *Brady's Programmed Introduction to Respiratory Therapy*, ed 2. (Bowie, Md, Brady Communications, 1980, p 72. Used with permission.)

As a result, shunt determination can be made utilizing the clinical shunt equation as follows:

$$\frac{\dot{Q}_S}{\dot{Q}_T} = \frac{(PA_{O_2} - Pa_{O_2})\,(0.003)}{Ca_{O_2} - C\bar{v}_{O_2} + (PA_{O_2} - Pa_{O_2})\,(0.003)}$$

where:

$\dot{Q}_S$ = shunted blood flow
$\dot{Q}_T$ = total blood flow
PA_{O_2} = pressure of oxygen in the alveoli
Pa_{O_2} = pressure of oxygen in arterial blood
Ca_{O_2} = oxygen content in arterial blood
$C\bar{v}_{O_2}$ = oxygen content in mixed venous blood.

The clinical shunt equation requires 100% saturation of hemoglobin with oxygen in arterial blood, and pulmonary artery sample is needed to determine $C\bar{v}_{O_2}$. When a pulmonary artery sample is not available, the modified shunt equation can be utilized as follows:

$$\frac{\dot{Q}_S}{\dot{Q}_T} = \frac{(PA_{O_2} - Pa_{O_2})\,(0.003)}{(4.5\ \text{vol\%}) + (PA_{O_2} - Pa_{O_2})\,(0.003)}$$

where:

$\dot{Q}_S$ = shunted blood flow
$\dot{Q}_T$ = total blood flow
PA_{O_2} = pressure of oxygen in the alveoli
Pa_{O_2} = pressure of oxygen in arterial blood.

This equation assumes a normal arterial-venous content difference of 4.5 vol%. Limitations to this equation are that the patient must have a stable cardiovascular status and metabolism.

The equipment required to collect the data for shunt determination includes a blood gas analyzer, a humidifier, an oxygen source connected to a reservoir system, and a one-way valve. The procedure requires the patient to be at rest in the semi-Fowler's position and connected to the system. Analyze the F_{IO_2}, and allow the patient to breathe from the system for 20 minutes to ensure that the nitrogen is washed out, which will minimize the effects of diffusion and ventilation and perfusion abnormalities. After 20 minutes, obtain arterial and mixed venous blood samples. The samples should be prepared properly and sent to the laboratory for analysis of Pa_{O_2}, Pa_{CO_2}, and $P\bar{v}_{O_2}$.

Complications from the procedure itself are minimal. However, if the patient is breathing from hypoxic drive, the administration of 100% oxygen may result in hypoventilation. Other complications from the administration of high concentration of oxygen include absorption atelectasis and pulmonary vasodilation, which increases intrapulmonary shunting. To overcome the effect of absorption atelectasis, one should perform routine shunt measurements on a F_{IO_2} of less than 0.6.[36]

The assessment of the degree of shunting can be a clinically useful tool to evaluate the effectiveness of oxygen therapy and the adequacy of spontaneous ventilation as well as to differentiate among shunt, ventilation and perfusion problems, and cardiac failure as a cause of hypoxemia.[14] Oxygen therapy will have a minimal effect when increased anatomic or physiologic shunt is present. A shunt of 0.30 indicates that mechanical ventilatory support will be required. This percentage correlates with an approximate alveolar-arterial oxygen pressure difference, $P(A-a)O_2$, of 300 to 350 mm Hg.

PA_{O_2}, Pa_{O_2}, and Pa_{CO_2} Relationships

The relationship between the alveolar and arterial oxygen tensions can be used to assess the ability of the lung as a gas transfer organ. The alveolar-arterial oxygen pressure difference, $P(A-a)O_2$, is calculated by subtracting the arterial oxygen tension from the alveolar oxygen tension ($PA_{O_2} - Pa_{O_2}$). The $P(A-a)O_2$ is a measurement of the pressure difference between alveolar and arterial blood tension; normal range is 10 to 15 mm Hg on room air. The partial pressure of alveolar oxygen can be calculated from the alveolar-air equation (see Fig 17–16). In normal lungs, the gas transfer occurs readily; with

pulmonary disease, oxygen gas exchange is hindered, and a large $P(A-a)O_2$ will exist. The predicted $P(A-a)O_2$ is dependent on the F_{IO_2} and the age of the patient. When the patient is breathing room air, the normal $P(A-a)O_2$ can be estimated by multiplying 0.4 times the patient's age. Gilbert and associates have demonstrated using adult subjects that the $P(A-a)O_2$ is affected not only by the severity of respiratory disease but also by acute changes in F_{IO_2}.[21] Because of the partial dependence of $P(A-a)O_2$, on F_{IO_2}, patients breathing differing oxygen concentrations and having the same $P(A-a)O_2$ may have differing severity of lung disease. An evaluation of the relationship between PA_{O_2}, Pa_{O_2}, and Pa_{CO_2} can provide the practitioner with the possible causes of the patient's hypoxemia. Hypoxemia occurring with a normal $P(A-a)O_2$ may be the result of a low ambient P_{O_2} or hypoventilation. If hypoxemia exists on an F_{IO_2} of 0.21 and the sum of the Pa_{O_2} and Pa_{CO_2} is 110 to 130 mm Hg, the cause of the hypoxemia is hypoventilation. If the sum is less than 110 mm Hg, the cause of the hypoxemia is related to defects in the lung's ability to oxygenate the blood. If the sum of the Pa_{O_2} and Pa_{CO_2} is more than 130 mm Hg, the patient is probably receiving supplemental oxygen or an analysis error has occurred.

Pa_{O_2}/PA_{O_2} Ratio

The arterial oxygen tension ratio (Pa_{O_2}/PA_{O_2}) has been suggested as an alternative index of gas exchange.[21] The normal ratio range is 0.75 to 0.90. In adult subjects breathing an F_{IO_2} of 0.40 to 1.00, Pa_{O_2}/PA_{O_2} has been shown to be less affected by F_{IO_2} changes than $P(A-a)O_2$, particularly when shunt is the primary derangement of gas exchange.[21] Pa_{O_2}/PA_{O_2} may provide misleading information in infants with respiratory distress syndrome (RDS) due to opened fetal anatomic shunts. Should right-to-left shunting occur at the ductus arteriosus, the value of Pa_{O_2} obtained from the umbilical artery will be lower than the value of Pa_{O_2} measured preductally. Therefore, the severity of disease, quantified with Pa_{O_2}/PA_{O_2}, using the umbilical artery Pa_{O_2}, may be overestimated.[9] Pulmonary fibrosis, pulmonary edema, interstitial edema, and adult respiratory distress syndrome (ARDS) are pulmonary abnormalities characterized by an increased $P(A-a)O_2$.

Pa_{O_2}

The assessment of arterial oxygenation provides information about the ability of oxygen to be transported. Oxygen is transported in two compartments: attached to hemoglobin and dissolved in plasma. The assessment of the oxygen-hemoglobin transport is dependent on the actual amount of hemoglobin and oxygen saturation; decreases in either will decrease the amount of oxygen being transported. The second compartment, the plasma component, is smaller and directly related to the partial pressure of oxygen ($PaO_2 \times 0.003$). The total oxygen-carrying capacity is a combination of both compartments.

The normal range of arterial PaO_2 is 80 to 100 mm Hg. The normal oxygen tension is directly related to age and can be estimated by:

Predicted PaO_2 (supine) =
$$103.5 - (0.42 \times age) \pm 4 \text{ mm Hg}.$$
Predicted PaO_2 (seated) =
$$104.2 - (0.27 \times age) \pm 4 \text{ mm Hg}.$$

Hypoxemia occurs when the respiratory system fails to oxygenate arterial blood, generally resulting in decreased PaO_2, SaO_2, and CaO_2. The practitioner needs to quantitate the severity of the abnormality by looking at the relationship between FI_{O_2}, PA_{O_2}, and Pa_{O_2}.

$P\bar{v}O_2$

A sample to determine the partial pressure of oxygen in mixed venous blood can be obtained from a Swan-Ganz catheter.[7] The normal value is 40 mm Hg. It can give the practitioner an indication of the level of oxygenation at the tissue level as blood is returning from there. However, only a decreased value has interpretative significance. It has been demonstrated that normal or supranormal values of $P\bar{v}O_2$ can coexist with severe tissue hypoxia caused primarily by arterial admixture.[24, 30] Some conditions that fall under this category are septicemia, hemorrhagic shock, congestive heart failure, and some febrile states.[20, 23] Therefore, only when circulatory function is intact and tissue oxygen is unimpaired can $P\bar{v}O_2$ in the normal ranges indicate adequate oxygenation, and evaluation of normal and high values must be made with caution in conjunction with other physiologic values.

Cyanosis

Cyanosis is not always a reliable indicator of hypoxemia; for example, the level of unsaturated hemoglobin and oxygen must reach 5 gm% before cyanosis can be observed. Since cyanosis is hemoglobin dependent, patients with anemia may not show visible signs of cyanosis until dangerous levels of hypoxemia exist.

When malfunction of the oxygen-hemoglobin mechanism is suspected, actual analysis of the hemoglobin using co-oximetry should be performed. Information obtained from such studies yields actual hemoglobin content, saturation, methemoglobin, carboxyhemoglobin, and oxygen content.

Transcutaneous Gas Monitoring

Noninvasive clinical transcutaneous gas monitoring employs a heated oxygen and carbon dioxide electrode placed on the skin. The oxygen electrode works on the same principle as that in the blood gas analyzer and is a development of the original type.[26] The O_2 and CO_2 electrode is housed in a heated plastic case, with the membrane making contact with the skin (Fig 17–14). The electrode, when connected to the monitor, performs three basic functions:

1. Measures the flow of current between the silver and platinum electrodes and digitally displays oxygen tension in millimeters of mercury
2. Measures the change in hydrogen ion concentration, thus measuring carbon dioxide tension, and digitally displays CO_2 tension in millimeters of mercury
3. Measures temperature by means of a thermistor (temperature-sensing electrode) located inside the electrode housing; heat energy in the electrode core is varied to maintain the temperature at the desired level
4. Monitors the level of heat energy being expended at any moment, measuring the rate of skin heating by capillary blood flow. The monitored value is referred to as the *relative heating power*.

The electrode is calibrated with gas (high and low concentrations) similar to the procedure used for arterial blood gas analysis equipment. After calibration, an adhesive disk is attached, a small drop of

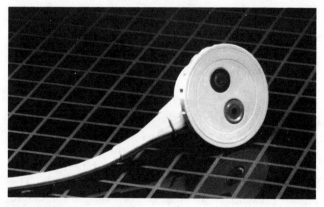

FIG 17–14.
Transcutaneous oxygen–carbon dioxide electrode head.

water is applied to the electrode to form a seal, and the disc is applied after the skin placement site is cleansed with alcohol. By heating the skin, it causes the capillary bed to arterialize, forcing oxygen and carbon dioxide to migrate to the corresponding electrode where it can be read. The relative heating power indicates the amount of energy needed to maintain the desired temperature, and it can be continuously recorded. This data can provide information relative to the underlying perfusion.[11] A change in blood flow or perfusion leads to changes in the energy required to maintain the desired electrode temperature. Assuming that the change in required energy varies with perfusion state, we can indirectly monitor continuous changes in blood pressure, cardiac output, and heart rate or when a vasodilating or vasoconstricting agent has been administered. The placement of the electrode is relatively noninvasive and allows for continuous assessment of oxygenation and ventilation. Comparison of transcutaneous oxygen tensions and arterial blood gases indicates a correlation coefficient of 0.97 TcP_{O_2}/Pa_{O_2} for healthy neonates and 0.94 for premature neonates; 0.94 for obstetric, gynecologic, and surgical patients have been reported.[25]

Although transcutaneous gas monitoring has been used extensively for several years with the neonatal population, it has had limited success in the adult population due to the thickness of the skin causing a barrier for gas diffusion resulting in erroneously low and high oxygen tensions. Once a correlation between the transcutaneous partial pressure of oxygen (TcP_{O_2}) and carbon dioxide (TcP_{CO_2}) have been established with arterial blood gas analysis, the data can be used for monitoring the respective values. This technique does not do away with arterial blood gas sampling but can decrease the frequency of them. The responsibility of maintenance and clinical application of transcutaneous gas monitoring is an appropriate function of the respiratory care practitioner. A practitioner must have total knowledge of its operation and factors influencing its application to make it a useful and reliable clinical ongoing evaluation tool.[17]

Pulse Oximetry

Pulse oximetry is a method of hemoglobin-oxygen saturation determination utilizing the spectrophotometry principle. The principle requires a light directed through the capillary bed and a mechanism to receive light on the other side (Fig 17–15). The color of the hemoglobin (saturated, unsaturated) effects the light wave frequency and intensity received. The pulse oximeter is able to isolate the pul-

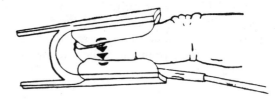

FIG 17–15.
Pulse oximeter probe.

sating bed and therefore is capable of discriminating toward the arterialized sample. The probe is noninvasive and can be used on the ear or finger of adults and on the wrist, ankle, or foot of neonates.

ASSESSMENT OF VENTILATION ADEQUACY

Arterial Carbon Dioxide Tension

Arterial carbon dioxide tension is an indication of the body's ability to sustain adequate alveolar ventilation. The amount of carbon dioxide produced by the body is determined by the metabolic rate. Under normal conditions, the amount of carbon dioxide excreted by the lungs is equal to the amount of carbon dioxide produced by the tissues. The normal production is about 200 ml/min.

Alterations in carbon dioxide production leads to changes in the depth and rate of ventilation. Alveolar ventilation is assumed to be adequate when the Pa_{CO_2} is maintained between 35 and 45 mm Hg. Under normal circumstances, a minute ventilation of 5 to 7 L/min is adequate to maintain a normal Pa_{CO_2}.

Although alveolar ventilation is regulated primarily by arterial carbon dioxide levels, hypoxemia may increase alveolar ventilation. Alterations in minute ventilation, respiratory rate, or physiologic dead space will change the amount of alveolar ventilation, thus affecting the arterial carbon dioxide level. A decreased respiratory rate can decrease alveolar ventilation because a smaller volume of air is available for gas exchange. If respiratory rates decrease, larger tidal volumes are required to maintain the same volume of alveolar ventilation.

An increase in physiologic dead space affects the relationship between minute ventilation and Pa_{CO_2}. To maintain the same Pa_{CO_2}, increased dead space may necessitate an increase in minute ventilation of two to three times the patient's normal value. Consequently, the work of breathing is increased.

The respiratory care practitioner can manipulate the Pa_{CO_2} of patients committed to mechanical ventilation by an appropriate increase or decrease in minute alveolar ventilation ($\dot{V}_A$). An equation can be used to calculate the $\dot{V}_A$ required to achieve a specific Pa_{CO_2}. The equation states that the desired $\dot{V}_A$ is equal to the production of CO_2 per minute times 0.8 (a constant taken from the equation for $\dot{V}_A/Q$) divided by Pa_{CO_2}:

$$\dot{V}_A = \frac{\dot{V}_{CO_2} \times 0.8}{Pa_{CO_2}}.$$

In clinical practice, $\dot{V}_{CO_2}$ can be calculated by using body weight in kilograms times 3.5, which is the milliliters of CO_2 production per kilogram per minute. Then the formula is:

$$\dot{V}_A = \frac{(\text{Body weight/kg} \times 3.5) \times 0.8}{Pa_{CO_2}}.$$

Since $\dot{V}_A$ is about 0.8 of $\dot{V}_E$, the Pa_{CO_2} can be estimated from measurement of $\dot{V}_E$. The formula is:

$$Pa_{CO_2} = \frac{(\text{Body weight/kg} \times 3.5) \times 0.8}{\dot{V}_E \times 0.8}$$
$$= \frac{(\text{Body weight/kg} \times 3.5)}{\dot{V}_E}.$$

End-Tidal Carbon Dioxide Monitoring

Continuous assessment of carbon dioxide excretion can be monitored by analysis of exhaled CO_2. The technique utilizes a mechanism for microsampling volumes of exhaled gas. Analysis of the gas can be performed by the infrared principle or mass spectrometry. Increased values may indicate hypoventilation or airway obstruction. Decreased values indicate hyperventilation such as those associated with head trauma and hypoxemia. Capnography can provide important ventilatory management information during weaning of patients.

Invasive Hemodynamic Monitoring

The continuous assessment of critically ill patients requires invasive monitoring to provide moment-to-moment evaluation of electromechanical physiologic functions.[28] Noninvasive methods, with the exception of ECG, usually cannot be read continuously and may not be obtainable in low-flow or shock states. Due to the nature of the population that the respiratory care practitioner cares for, a knowledge of noninvasive monitoring as a tool for continuous patient care is required.

Direct pressure measurements, in which the cardiovascular system is invaded, have been used in operating rooms and cardiac catheterization laboratories for some time. In recent years, the application of this technology has found its way into almost all intensive care units. With invasive monitoring, direct pressure measurements are obtained from catheters inserted into blood vessels. These catheters connect to transducers, which sense pressure changes. Changes in pressure causes an electronic signal to be emitted, displayed, and stored if necessary. Invasive monitoring includes the use of arterial, central venous, and pulmonary artery catheters.

There are several advantages to direct pressure monitoring. There is an immediate indication of the response of the vascular system to therapy, and long-term continuous monitoring permits the detection of subtle, trend-setting changes. Even when a patient is in shock, when other methods of evaluation fail, continuous, accurate measurement of peripheral or central vascular pressures can be made. Disadvantages include added risk to the patient, because invasion of the cardiovascular system carries with it the dangers of embolization, bleeding, vessel and tissue damage, and infection. Central arterial or venous catheters carry the added risk of stimulating cardiac arrhythmias.

Arterial Pressure Monitoring

Arterial pressure should be monitored continuously in the unstable patient. A pressure transducer system attached to an indwelling arterial line can provide a continuous pressure tracing. Situations indicating the need for an arterial line include hypotension, low cardiac output, administration of potent vasoactive drugs, and the need for frequent arterial blood gas determinations. Common sites for indwelling arterial catheters are the radial, brachial, axillary, and femoral arteries. The radial artery usually is the vessel of choice.

Once inserted, the catheter is connected to the oscilloscope, and a visual display can be monitored continuously. The wave form that is displayed consists of (1) the anacrotic limb, (2) the systolic peak, (3) the dicrotic notch, and (4) the diastolic pressure (Fig 17–16). The location of the dicrotic notch should be at least one third the height of the systolic peak. Normal arterial pressure range is 140/90–90/60 mm Hg.

Potential complications of an indwelling arterial catheter include infection, air embolism, thromboembolism, arrhythmia, catheter displacement, electromicroshock, hemorrhage, and impaired peripheral circulation.[35]

Blood Gas Sampling From an Arterial Line.— Arterial blood can be easily aspirated from an indwelling arterial catheter and sent to the laboratory for Pa_{O_2}, Pa_{CO_2}, and pH analysis. With patients who require frequent samples, an arterial line for such

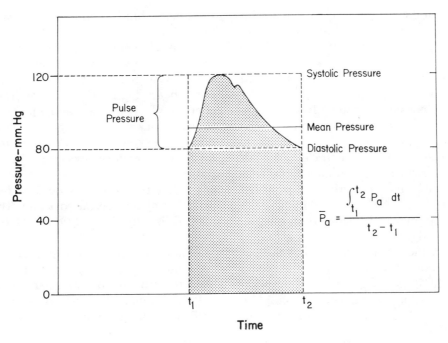

FIG 17–16.
Arterial pressure wave form showing anacrotic limb, systolic peak, dicrotic notch, and diastolic pressure. (From Berne RM, Levy MN: *Cardiovascular Physiology.* St Louis, CV Mosby, 1967, p 90. Used with permission.

purposes is more convenient, is more accessible, and minimizes patient discomfort.

The setup for an indwelling arterial catheter may vary slightly depending on the type of catheter and transducer used. Generally, the system consists of the line, a flush solution, a series of stopcocks, and a pressure transducer.[32] When the stopcock position is changed, blood is drawn from the catheter; the pressure tracing reading is visible on the oscilloscope, or the transducer-catheter system is flushed with solution from an intravenous bag via intraflow flush valve. The flush solution is heparinized to prevent clotting of blood in the line. Supplies for drawing the gas include a 10-ml sterile syringe to flush the line, a 5-ml heparinized syringe, a patient label, and a container in which to ice the blood.

The respiratory care practitioner should be proficient in the sampling technique. First, evaluate the pressure tracing to determine whether the line is patent and functioning. Sluggish tracings may indicate partial obstruction by a clot or displacement of the catheter. Prior to drawing the sample, aspirate the line until blood is obtained. Observe the blood color for homogeneity. It should not be diluted by the flush solution. Turn the stopcock off to the sample port, replace the aspirating syringe with a heparinized syringe, and obtain the blood sample (normally 3 ml). Eject any air bubbles from the sample, and ice it immediately. Pull on the tail of the intraflow system, and observe the blood returning into the patient. The line should be cleared with the flush solution. Care must be taken so that air bubbles or clots are not injected into the arterial line. Observe the arterial pressure tracing to determine whether the line is functioning properly. The sample can be sent to the laboratory for analysis.

Complications of this procedure are associated with the invasive aspect of the line. Observe the pressure wave form for resistance in line or obstruction. Care must be taken to prevent disconnection of the line. Also, improper positioning of the stopcock can result in blood loss. Infection and air embolism can result from improper aspiration techniques. The catheter can cause vessel irritation and spasm, resulting in impaired circulation and ischemia distal to the catheter. In addition, thromboemboli, electromicroshock, and hemorrhage are potential complications.[35]

Central Venous Pressure Monitoring

The purpose of CVP monitoring is to assess the hemodynamic status and the need for fluid replacement. In addition, certain medications can be administered and frequent blood samples can be obtained without causing the patient discomfort. Regulation of fluid replacement can be managed by using CVP monitoring as a guide. In patients with normal cardiac reserve and pulmonary vascular resistance, CVP reflects the ability of the myocardium to pump blood.

Usually CVP is measured from a catheter located in the superior vena cava or right atrium. When the catheter is properly positioned, the CVP reflects the pressure of the right atrium. Right atrial pressure, in turn, reflects right ventricular end-diastolic pressure and the performance of the right ventricle.[35] The adequacy of right ventricular function affects the ventilation-perfusion ratio and proportion of right-left shunting of blood.

The CVP catheter may be threaded from the jugular, subclavian, or right brachial vein. Insertion of a CVP line through the subclavian vein has the potential complication of a pneumothorax if the pleura is nicked during the insertion procedure. Complications of a CVP line include pulmonary emboli, phlebitis, pneumothorax, malposition of the catheter, arrhythmias, fluid overload, air emboli, and electromicroshock.[40]

Central venous pressure may be monitored continuously as a wave form on an oscilloscope or intermittently with a water manometer held at the level of the heart (Fig 17–17). Positive pressure ventilation alters CVP readings, and, if possible, readings should be taken with the patient off the ventilator or during the expiratory phase of respiration.[6, 13] If positive end-expiratory pressure (PEEP) or continuous positive airway pressure (CPAP) is used, the amount of positive pressure must be considered in the interpretation of the measured value. The normal value for CVP is 3 to 15 cm H_2O, or 1 to 6 mm Hg.

Pulmonary Artery Pressure Monitoring

Pulmonary artery pressure (PAP) monitoring is used to evaluate intravascular volume and cardiac output. Pulmonary artery pressure is preferred to CVP monitoring because the CVP is not always a

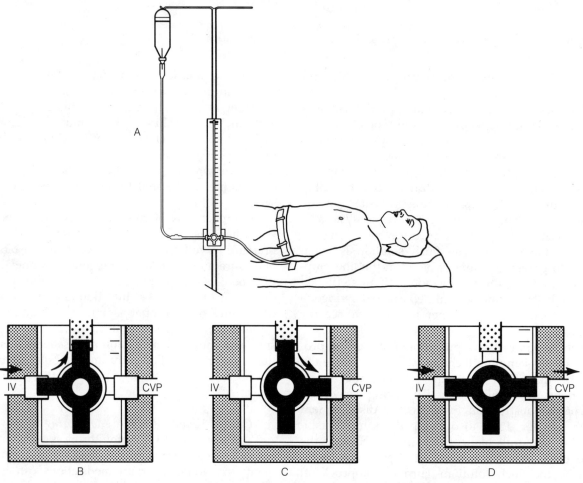

FIG 17–17.
Patient lying flat with a CVP catheter inserted, connected to a water manometer at the midchest level.

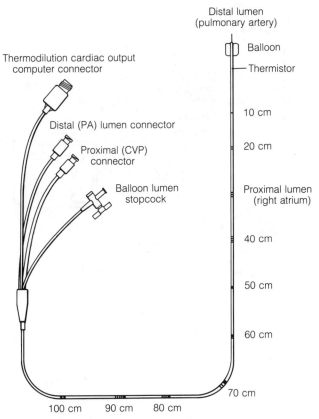

Distal lumen
(pulmonary artery)

Balloon

Thermodilution cardiac output
computer connector

Thermistor

10 cm

Distal (PA) lumen connector

20 cm

Proximal (CVP)
connector

Balloon lumen
stopcock

Proximal lumen
(right atrium)

40 cm

50 cm

60 cm

70 cm

100 cm   90 cm   80 cm

FIG 17–18.
Swan-Ganz catheter indicating all the ports.

reliable guide to left ventricular filling pressure or left atrial pressure, whereas PAP reflects atrial pressure and the adequacy of left ventricular function.

The Swan-Ganz catheter is a special balloon-tipped flow-directed catheter used for PAP and PAWP monitoring (Fig 17–18). The catheter is inserted through a cutdown in a brachial vein, usually in the antecubital space, and floated through the superior vena cava, right atrium, right ventricle, pulmonic valve, and into the pulmonary artery (Fig 17–19). The position of the catheter determines the pressure being measured. With the catheter tip in the pulmonary artery, measurement of the pulmonary artery pressure may be obtained. A tracing of the pressure wave may be visualized on an oscilloscope or a digital display.

When the balloon of the Swan-Ganz catheter is partially inflated, the catheter floats forward to lodge itself in a pulmonary capillary. When the balloon is fully inflated, blood flow behind the balloon (right side of the heart) is obstructed, and PAWP, reflecting left atrial pressure, is measured.[42] If pulmonary disease exists, which would increase resistance to blood flow through the pulmonary capillary bed,

PAWP will reflect the increased pressure created by the resistance.[42] Under normal circumstances, left atrial pressure indicates the effectiveness of the heart as a pump. The catheter may be used also for thermal dilution measurements of cardiac output and as a site for obtaining mixed venous blood samples.

Normal pulmonary artery pressures are systolic 20 to 30 mm Hg and diastolic 0 to 10 mm Hg, with a mean PAP of 20 mm Hg. An elevated PAP may indicate left-to-right shunt, left ventricular failure, mitral stenosis, or pulmonary hypertension. The normal mean PAWP is 4 to 12 mm Hg. An elevated PAWP may indicate left ventricular failure, mitral stenosis, or cardiac insufficiency.[43]

With a thermodilution Swan-Ganz catheter positioned in the pulmonary artery, it is possible to repeatedly and reliably determine cardiac output. The cardiac output can be measured by injecting an exact amount of solution into the circulation. The change in temperature allows the volume of blood to be calculated.

With the Swan-Ganz catheter, 10 ml of cooled 5% dextrose in water is introduced into the right atrium via the catheter. A thermistor located in the tip of the catheter measures the blood temperature in the pulmonary artery. The temperature of the patient, the injection solution, and the change in blood temperature are the variables to compute cardiac output. The procedure can be repeated without delay.

Mixed venous sampling is useful in evaluating tissue oxygenation and cardiac output. A mixed venous sample and an arterial sample may be sent for blood gas analysis. The oxygen content is determined for both samples, and the arterial-venous oxygen content difference is calculated. Increased oxygen content difference indicates an increased oxygen extraction at the cellular level. Tissues will extract a greater amount of oxygen if a hypermetabolic state exists or if cardiac output is reduced.

The information from the pressure readings (PAP, PAWP, CVP, cardiac output) of the Swan-Ganz catheter can be used to assess and guide the management of the patient's hemodynamic status. In left atrial failure, PAWP will be elevated, with CVP remaining normal. If the PAWP is greater than 20 to 25 mm Hg, it indicates left ventricular failure and can be treated with diuretic therapy and possible reduction of the afterload using a vasodilator or an intra-aortic balloon pump. Frank pulmonary edema is generally exhibited at a PAWP of 25 to 30 mm Hg.[34] All pressures will be elevated in concurrent right and left atrial failure. Primary right atrial

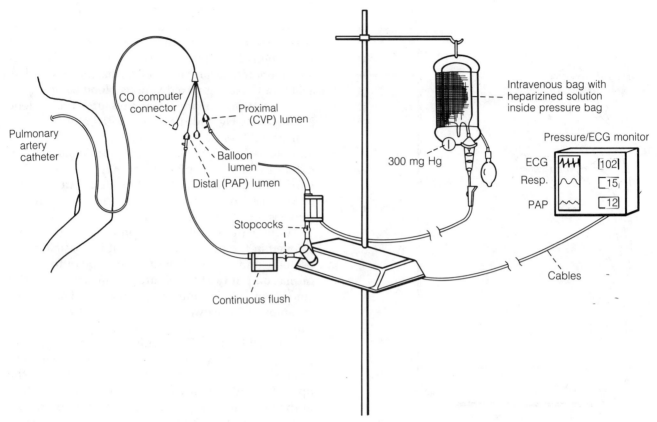

FIG 17–19.
Swan-Ganz catheter in a patient through a cutdown in the antecubital fossa. (Note tip of the catheter in the pulmonary artery.)

failure will be indicated by normal PAWP and elevated CVP. Hypovolemia is indicated by a decrease in CVP, PAWP, and cardiac output. Volume should be replaced to return PAWP to normal levels. A PAWP 18 mm Hg or greater may signal impending pulmonary edema. Pulmonary embolism results in a high PAP in the presence of a low or normal PAWP.

The Swan-Ganz catheter plays a very important role in the care of the critically ill patient in shock. Management of the fluid balance and vasopressor therapy is more precise when a pulmonary artery line is used to monitor PAP, PAWP, and cardiac output. Complications of pulmonary artery monitoring include arrhythmias, infection, catheter knotting, microembolism, balloon rupture, pulmonary artery rupture, air emboli, thromboembolism, lung ischemia, and pulmonary infection.

Therapeutic Objectives

Identification

It is important to have the therapeutic objective of respiratory care clearly understood by all members of the health care team participating in the clinical care of a patient. It is the function of the respiratory care practitioner to provide not only quality care but also therapy that clearly fits the therapeutic goals of a given patient's physiologic situation. To establish a clear therapeutic objective, the respiratory care practitioner must have a comprehensive understanding of the indications, expected outcomes, and potential side effects anticipated for every therapy and modality administered. Changing the therapeutic regimen without physiologic assessment should be avoided to reduce the risk of the therapy being potentially dangerous, costly, and unnecessary.

Establishing the therapeutic objective is the first step in documenting the need for intervention. The comprehensive plan should always involve (1) the expected outcome, (2) the means of evaluation, and (3) the modifications when the implementation phase is approached. Generally, the assessment includes observations, physical examinations, and clinical tests.

It should be noted that some life-threatening situations may not allow the practitioner the completeness of assessment before therapeutic intervention begins. In those cases, the level of assessment does require the practitioner to establish the nature of the condition present rather than the extent of the condition. An example is the finding of cyanosis as a sign of hypoxemia rather than the arterial oxygen partial pressure and hemoglobin saturation to establish the hypoxia level. In this example, the practitioner establishes cyanosis as the basis of hypoxia, administers appropriate therapeutic support, and later establishes the level of hypoxemia. With an appropriate oxygen delivery system in place, expected therapeutic outcomes such as a decrease in the patient's breathing rate and myocardial work should be seen. A follow-up evaluation should include an arterial blood gas study to document the effectiveness of the emergency treatment and a plan for reevaluation such as a periodic arterial blood gas analysis.

The practitioner should aim toward the goal of reducing the therapy as soon as possible. To initiate a responsible effort in this direction requires continual assessment of the patient's status so that suggestions can be made regarding the discontinuance of unneeded treatments.

Therapeutic Objectives for Respiratory Therapy Modalities

The practitioner should have an understanding of the physiologic basis for respiratory care. Continuous assessment of the patient requires the practitioner to periodically reference the changes in the patient's physiology to the expected therapeutic goals. To fulfill this function within the ongoing assessment model, a review of the goals of basic respiratory therapy is provided.

Clinical Goals for Oxygen Therapy.—The goals of oxygen therapy are to (1) treat hypoxemia, (2) decrease the work of breathing, and (3) decrease the myocardial work. The treatment of hypoxemia involves the application of oxygen. When arterial hypoxemia is the result of decreased alveolar oxygen tensions, hypoxemia may be dramatically improved by increasing the inspired oxygen tensions. Increased ventilatory work is a common response to hypoxemia. Enriched inspired oxygen may allow for more alveolar gas exchange to maintain adequate alveolar oxygen levels, resulting in a decreased need for total ventilation. The cardiovascular system is a primary mechanism for compensation of hypoxemia. Oxygen therapy can effectively support many disease states by decreasing or preventing the demand

for increased myocardial work. Effective oxygen therapy will decrease the myocardial work.[37]

Clinical Goals for Aerosol Therapy.—The goals of aerosol therapy are to (1) aid bronchial hygiene, (2) provide a means to humidify inspired gas, and (3) provide a means to deliver medication.[1, 31, 37] The application of aerosol therapy requires the respiratory care practitioner to have an understanding of its purpose. Its application as an aid to bronchial hygiene can be utilized to hydrate dried, retained secretions, restoring and maintaining the mucous blanket, promoting expectoration, and improving the effectiveness of the cough.[38] In addition, its application can be used for the administration of medical gases because of their anhydrous nature. To prevent mucosal drying of the patients with their upper airway bypassed as a result of artificial airway requires the application of aerosol therapy to ensure proper humidification of inspired gas. Aerosol therapy is a method of administration of medication via the inhalation route. The types of pharmacologic agents the respiratory care practitioner commonly administers are catecholamines, decongestants, mucokinetic agents, steroids, and antibiotics.

Clinical Goals for Intermittent Positive-Pressure Breathing Therapy.—The goals of intermittent positive-pressure breathing (IPPB) therapy are to (1) increase tidal volume (sometimes as much as three to four times), (2) provide mechanical bronchodilation, and (3) increase collateral ventilation.[29, 44, 48, 49] Intermittent positive pressure breathing can be used to increase a patient's tidal volume in those individuals who are unable to breathe deeply.[49] Its application should increase the patient's tidal volume between two and three times normal. Documentation of the increase in exhaled tidal volume can be accomplished with volume-measuring devices; bedside pulmonary function spirometers typically used for assessment of continuous mechanical ventilation can be used to determine tidal volume.

Clinical Goals for Chest Physical Therapy.—The goals for chest physical therapy are to (1) prevent the accumulation and improve the mobilization of bronchial secretions, (2) improve the efficiency and distribution of ventilation, and (3) improve cardiopulmonary reserve using exercise techniques to promote physical conditioning.

The techniques of chest physical therapy involve (1) bronchial hygiene, (2) breathing exercises, and (3) physical reconditioning. Bronchial hygiene involves the use of postural drainage, chest percussion, and vibration to aid the removal of secretions from the tracheobronchial tree. Breathing exercises encompass techniques that include coughing instructions and diaphragmatic breathing.

Clinical Goals for Incentive Spirometry.—The goals for incentive spirometry are to (1) optimize lung inflation, (2) optimize the cough mechanism, and (3) allow early detection of acute pulmonary disease.[39] Incentive spirometry is a cost-effective technique for the administration of prophylactic administration of bronchial hygiene therapy. The technique requires patient cooperation and motivation. The lungs should be without acute atelectasis, pneumonia, and retained secretions. Patients should have forced vital capacity of more than 15 ml/kg and a respiratory rate of less than 25/min. The respiratory care practitioner should provide the initial instructions and be assured that the patient is capable of self-administering the therapy. The patient should be instructed to perform incentive spirometry every waking hour. One deep breath should be performed every 30 seconds and repeated 8 to 10 times.

THERAPEUTIC PLAN

The therapeutic plan should always state the goal of therapy as well as the details of the way in which the drug or procedure is to be used. At least as important as the preceding is the plan for patient education in which detailed plans for instruction of the patient about his or her problem, its management, and the effect on the patient's life-style. The planning portion of patient care involves a team approach. Health care providers involved in chronic and long-term illness should develop a care team approach. Members from at least the following disciplines should be included: social work, dietary, psychiatry, physical therapy, nursing, respiratory therapy, and the primary physician.

DOCUMENTATION

Documentation of respiratory care is an essential component of comprehensive care to the patient. Documentation serves as a mechanism for continuity of care and provides for communication to co-workers on the health care team. It serves as a legal record for the protection of the respiratory care practitioner and the patient. The extent of the doc-

umentation should be consistent with the expected use of the information. It may range from a concise statement indicating the therapy performed, patient response, and findings to a more involved explanation and discussion often used in discharge planning summaries. The record of care placed in the patient's chart by the respiratory care practitioner must be specific, explicit, and accurate. Some methods of charting are too often random, routine, and mindless of documentation of patient care, with diagnosis and crucial observations buried among trivia. A problem-oriented medical record (POMR), developed by Lawrence Weed,[45] is a clearly defined thesis and a data base on which to build decisions about the care.[46] Each member of the team contributes to the gathering of data and the assessment of its significance.

A POMR is primarily a way for caretakers to communicate in clear statements the patient's medical problems and a plan for solution. The implementation of this type of record keeping is justified by the outcomes relating to health care delivery, not just a better record. Some of the potential benefits are:

1. Facilitates care of the whole patient by displaying all important problems
2. Improves communication among health care providers
3. Organizes the record to reduce needless duplication of data acquisition and recording
4. Displays medical logic and plans to facilitate record review and quality control
5. Facilitates data retrieval for teaching and research and for transfer of health care records
6. Facilitates preparation of insurance forms and other administrative documents
7. Facilitates preventive care and health maintenance

The POMR consists of four parts: (1) data base, (2) problem list, (3) initial plans, and (4) progress notes. The data base is the supporting structure of problem identification. It includes such items as medical history and physical examination, nursing and respiratory practitioners' assessment, laboratory reports, consultant assessments, previous medical record summaries, and pertinent communications. The problem list constitutes anything that has, does, or may require health care management and has or could significantly alter a person's physical or emotional well-being. The problem list should state the number and whether it is active, inactive, or re-

PROBLEM SHEET					
No.	Date	ACTIVE PROBLEM	Date End	No.	INACTIVE PROBLEM
1	5/23	Myocardial Infarction		1	Hernia
2	5/23	Heart Block	6/1		
3	5/27	Pulmonary Edema	5/28		
4	5/28	Pneumonia			
5	6/2	Anemia			

FIG 17–20.
Example of a problem list with active, inactive, and resolved clinical entities.

solved and a date its status developed (Fig 17–20). The problem list functions as a reference for coordination of all of the patient's health problems, provides a visual representation of past and present problems as well as pointing out possible problem interactions, and allows a reference of which problems are being managed. Generally the physician and nurse are responsible for documentation of the problem list. However, the respiratory care practitioner at some institutions may input into the record or have a separate problem list specific to the cardiopulmonary system. Examples of problems are previous diagnosis, symptoms or conditions reported in the patient interview, physical findings, abnormal laboratory findings, or emotional problems.

The systematic organization of data so that the information in it can easily be accessed and effectively utilized can be accomplished by the format that it is presented in. A four-section format called the S-O-A-P format—subjective data, objective data, assessment, and plan—is a record-keeping system that organizes data so that information can be clearly identified with a specific problem being addressed (Fig 17–21). The subjective data are patient input about complaints from the patient's point of view, feelings, reactions, and observations. For example, it can also include information from nonhealth personnel, including the patient's family and friends. A foundation of information can be developed during the patient interview. Documentation of dialogue

can be essential in evaluating changes in the levels of oxygenation and carbon dioxide removal influencing the patient's neurologic response.

The objective data include clinical signs, laboratory tests and x-rays, and observations by the health care team. A flow sheet can be used to organize the data. As the name denotes, the information recorded represents a summary of events over a given period of time (Fig 17–22). Additional examples of the type of information found in this section are parameters that practitioners can measure such as heart and respiratory rates.

The assessment section discusses the severity, diagnosis, prognosis, and other changes in patient status. The documentation is important for comparative evaluation of the course of the patient's pathophysiology. The assessment of the patient's problems should be summarized by relating the clinical findings to the patient's condition or disease entity. Examples are: "the patient is not responding to therapy," "the patient is improving rapidly," "the patient is in respiratory failure," or "the patient had an acute asthma attack."

The plan section describes what will be done for the patient, including the therapy to be administered, the type of additional information needed, and patient education requirements.

PATIENT NAME John Doe	COMPREHENSIVE EPISODIC CARE
DATE: 9/2/87	
Problem no.: 1 ___	Problem Title: Dyspnea

Subjective: Patient complains of shortness of breath while in bed.

Objective:

Physical Exam: Patient diaphoretic. RR: 28 breaths/ minute, Heart rate: 112 beats/minute. Moderate use of accessory muscles of respiration,

Laboratory: ABG's drawn; pH:7.36, $PaCO_2$:48 mm Hg, PaO_2: 42 mm Hg, HCO_3: 30 mEq/L

Assessment: Patient moderately hypoxic.

Plan: Administer O_2 at 4 L/min, observe closely, obtain ABG in 45 minutes.

_____
Signature

FIG 17–21.
Example of an S-O-A-P note.

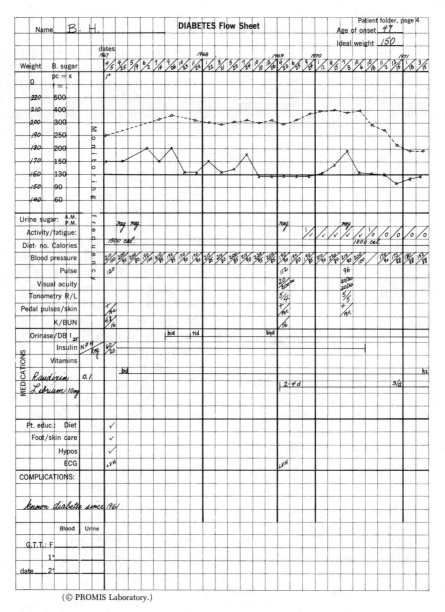

(© PROMIS Laboratory.)

FIG 17–22.

Example of a clinical flow sheet. (From Hurst JW, Walker HK: *The Problem-Oriented System.* New York, Medcom Press, 1972, p. 149. Used with permission.)

An important point to emphasize using the S-O-A-P method is to record only changes in progress and unusual events. The benefits of the S-O-A-P method include the economy of time for health care providers (e.g., easier and faster to read) and better patient care by setting goals for each specific problem. The S-O-A-P method of charting makes users conscious of logic and forces them to reason clearly.

The S-O-A-P method of documentation does have some drawbacks. It is only as good as the weakest entry. An assessment based on insufficient data is an inductive conclusion. The assessment becomes the major premise from which one deduces a plan of treatment, and if the information is incomplete or inaccurate, the plan on which it is based could be faulty or potentially harmful.

The respiratory care practitioner, as an intermediary in patient care, should carefully document information that will be potentially useful, recording unusual as well as routine events. A good practitioner, like a writer, is a good observer. One is more likely to think clearly if one commits the process to writing. It requires practitioners to take responsibility for their decisions and the care they provide.

Computer Application for the Medical Record

With the application of sophisticated computer systems, more health care professionals are turning toward their use for processing and storing medical, financial, and administrative information. For the most part, however, the recording of information in the medical record has undergone little metamorphosis. The clinical information utilized and inputted by the respiratory care practitioner and other health care professionals at most institutions follows a manual model. The manual input of information has stood the test of time. Although workable, it does have significant drawbacks. Perhaps a paramount barrier of the manual medical record is the lack of communication it sometimes presents as a result of poor handwriting, incomplete information, and inaccessibility. A foreseeable solution to this problem is the application of the computer for processing information and charting mechanisms.

The application of computer charting requires the institution to have an extensive networking of terminals for ease of access. From the standpoint of the respiratory care practitioner, a comprehensive system should have access to laboratory, blood gas and radiology results, physician orders, patient history and progress notes, and respiratory care notes. The computer system should be menu driven and user friendly. The respiratory care practitioner gains access to appropriate levels of information determined by his or her individual security code. The charting model for the respiratory care practitioner should follow a comprehensive template that standardizes the information recorded. An example of a charting template for routine respiratory therapy could be inclusive of (1) medications delivered, (2) the patient's condition (e.g., effects of therapy, adverse reactions), (3) changes in breath sounds, (4) heart rate before and after treatment, (5) sputum production and cough effort, and (6) the therapist's signature. In addition, the system can be cross-referenced for billing purposes, audits, quality control, monitor management, and medical errors.

Because of the volume of data generated in the medical environment, computers are quickly becoming valuable tools. The computer enhances the availability of information, automatically processes requests so that the derived information is available and chronologically organized, and presents the data in a form that aids the decision-making process.

It not only saves the health care practitioner time but also improves the quality of the decisions being made. The computer applications for critical care medicine will help cope with data overload until standards can be set to determine and answer questions concerning how much data, what types, and how often its accumulation is necessary. The final outcome of computer application should not stray away from the patient's bedside with an intrigue of the factual application but should help the practitioner more effectively utilize and document information about the patient's well-being.

Patient Safety

Ongoing patient assessment can provide a certain measure of patient safety. It is always important but especially with critically ill patients dependent on life support systems. Maintaining a correct interface between the patient and life support equipment is a high priority in the critical care area. The respiratory care practitioner can play a major role in this regard by providing a comprehensive physiologic and mechanical alarm system that is set and maintained appropriately. In addition, the practitioner needs to educate other health care professionals regarding the meaning and value of alarm systems.

REFERENCES

1. Abramson H: Proceedings of the second conference on clinical application of the ultrasonic nebulizer. *J Asthma* 1968; 5:213.
2. Askanazi J, et al: Patterns of ventilation in postoperative and acutely ill patients. *Crit Care Med* 1979; 7:41.
3. Bailey WC: Respiratory function evaluation. *Ala J Med Sci* 1977; 14:43–47.
4. Baratz R, et al: Urine output and plasma levels of antidiuretic hormone during intermittent positive-pressure breathing in the dog. *Anesthesiology* 1970; 32:17.
5. Baratz R, et al: Plasma antidiuretic hormone and urinary output during CPPB in dogs. *Anesthesiology* 1971; 34:510.
6. Cengiz M, Crapro RO, Gardner RM: The effects of ventilation on the accuracy of pulmonary artery and wedge pressure measurements. *Crit Care Med* 1983; 11:502.
7. Certelli R, Cruz JC, Farhi LE, et al: Determination of mixed venous O_2 and CO_2 tensions and cardiac output by rebreathing method. *Respir Physiol* 1966; 1:258–264.
8. Chodosh S: Examination of sputum cells. *N Engl J Med* 1970; 282:854.
9. Cohen A, Taeusch W, Stanton C: Usefulness of the

arterial/alveolar oxygen tension ratio in the care of infants with respiratory distress syndrome. *Respir Care* 1983; 28:169–173.

10. Comroe J, Forster R, Dubois A, et al: *The Lung*, ed 2. Chicago, Year Book Medical Publishers, 1979.

11. Conner E, Berkowitz G, Colvin E, et al: Transcutaneous oxygen tension measurements in necrotizing enterocolitis (NEC). *Clin Res* 1978; 26:825.

12. Dantzker DR, et al: Ventilation-perfusion distribution in the adult respiratory distress syndrome. *Am Rev Respir Dis* 1979; 120:1039.

13. Davidson R, Parker M, Harrison RA: The validity of determinations of pulmonary wedge pressure during mechanical ventilation. *Chest* 1978; 73:352.

14. Dimas S, Kacmarek RM: Intrapulmonary shunting, part II. *Curr Rev Respir Ther* 1978; 1:35–39.

15. Dulfano MJ: *Sputum, Fundamentals and Clinical Pathology*. Springfield, Ill, Charles C Thomas, Publishers, 1973.

16. Eichenhorn MS, Beauchamp RK, Harper PA, et al: An assessment of three portable peak flowmeters. *Chest* 1982; 82:306–309.

17. Emrico J: Transcutaneous oxygen monitoring in neonates. *Respir Care* 1979; 24:601–605.

18. Forgacs P: The functional basis of pulmonary sounds. *Chest* 1978; 73:399.

19. Forgacs P, Nathoo AR, Richardson HD: Breath sounds. *Thorax* 1974; 29:223–227.

20. Geunter C, Hinshaw L: Comparison of septic shock due to gram-negative and gram-positive organisms. *Proc Soc Exp Biol Med* 1970; 134:780–783.

21. Gilbert R, Auchincloss JH, Kuppinger M, et al: Stability of the arterial/alveolar oxygen partial pressure ratio. *Crit Care Med* 1979; 7:267–272.

22. Hedley-Whyte J, Burgess GE, Feeley TW, et al: *Applied Physiology of Respiratory Care*. Boston, Little, Brown & Co, 1976.

23. Hemreck A, Thal A: Mechanisms of high circulatory requirements in sepsis and septic shock. *Ann Surg* 1969; 170:677–695.

24. Hiller C, Bone R, Hill D, et al: Mixed venous oxygen tensions as a measure of oxygen delivery in endotoxin shock. *Clin Res* 1979; 27:399.

25. Huch A, Huch R: Transcutaneous noninvasive monitoring of PO_2. *Hosp Pract* 1976; 6:43–52.

26. Huch A, Huch R, Arner B, et al: Continuous oxygen tension measured with a heated electrode. *Scand J Clin Lab Invest* 1973; 31:269.

27. Kasik JE, Alexander MR: Reversing the irreversible [editorial]. *Chest* 1982; 82:517–518.

28. Loantiegne KC, Civetta JM: A system for maintaining invasive pressure monitoring. *Heart Lung* 1978; 7:610.

29. Menkes HA, Traystman FJ: Collateral ventilation: State of the art. *Am Rev Respir Dis* 1977; 116:287.

30. Miller M, Cook W, Mithoefer J: Limitations of the use of mixed venous PO_2 as an indicator of tissue hypoxia. *Clin Res* 1979; 27:401.

31. Miller W: Fundamentals of aerosol therapy. *Respir Care* 1972; 17:295.

32. Morton BC: Basic equipment requirements for hemodynamic monitoring. *Can Med Assoc J* 1979; 121:879.

33. Murdaugh WV, Sieker HO: Effect of altered intrathoracic pressure on renal hemodynamics, electrolyte excretion and water clearance. *J Clin Invest* 1959; 38:834–842.

34. Robin ED, Cross CE, Zelis R: Pulmonary Edema. *N Engl J Med* 1973; 288:239, 292.

35. Schroeder JP, Daily EK: *Techniques in Bedside Hemodynamic Monitoring*. St Louis, CV Mosby Co, 1981.

36. Shapiro BA, Cane RD, Harrison RA, et al: Changes in intrapulmonary shunting with administration of 100 percent oxygen. *Chest* 1980; 77:138–141.

37. Shapiro BA, Harrison RA, Kacmarek RM, et al: *Clinical Application of Respiratory Care*. ed 3. Chicago, Year Book Medical Publishers, 1985.

38. Shapiro BA, Harrison RA, Kacmarek RM, et al: *Clinical Application of Respiratory Care*, ed 3. Chicago, Year Book Medical Publishers, 1985, p 106.

39. Shapiro BA, Harrison RA, Kacmarek RM, et al: *Clinical Application of Respiratory Care*, ed 3. Chicago, Year Book Medical Publishers, 1985, p 146.

40. Shoemaker WC, Thompson WC, Holbrook PR: *Textbook of Critical Care*. Philadelphia, WB Saunders Co, 1984.

41. Slonim NB, et al: *Respiratory Physiology*, ed 5. St Louis, CV Mosby Co, 1987.

42. Spring CL: *The Pulmonary Artery Catheter: Methodology and Clinical Application*. Baltimore, University Park Press, 1983.

43. Tarnow J: Swan-Ganz catherization: Application, interpretation and complications. *Cardiovasc Surg* 1983; 30:130.

44. Terry PB, et al: Collateral ventilation in man. *N Engl J Med* 1978; 298:10.

45. Weed LL: *Medical Records, Medical Education and Patient Care: The Problem-oriented Record as a Basic Tool*. Cleveland, Case Western Reserve University Press, 1969.

46. Weilacher RR: Using the problem-oriented approach in respiratory therapy. *Respir Care* 1975; 20:272–275.

47. Williams TJ, Ahmand D, Morgan WK: A clinical and roentgenographic correlation of diaphragmatic movement. *Arch Intern Med* 1981; 141:878.

48. Wilson FHL, et al: IPPB: A clinical evaluation of its use in certain respiratory diseases. *Calif Med* 1957; 87:161.

49. Ziment I: Why are they saying bad things about IPPB? *Respir Care* 1973; 18:677.

Blood Gas Interpretation

Patrick F. Plunkett, Jr., Ed.D., R.R.T.

Blood gas analysis is the measurement of the partial pressures of oxygen (PO_2) and carbon dioxide (P_{CO_2}) in the blood, along with the determination of the plasma hydrogen ion concentration (pH). Blood gases are measured in a variety of clinical situations and are used to monitor the following physiologic parameters: (1) arterial oxygenation, (2) oxygen delivery to the tissue, (3) alveolar ventilation, and (4) acid-base balance.

Blood gas interpretation requires the systematic analysis of the PO_2, P_{CO_2} and pH taken in light of the patient's total clinical condition. A clinical diagnosis is not based entirely on blood gas results. Rather, clinical findings should be the prime determinant of a diagnosis. Laboratory data, such as blood gases, are used to either confirm the preliminary diagnosis, quantitate the severity of the disorder, or assess the effectiveness of therapy (Table 18–1).

Arterial blood is most often used in blood gas analysis. The reason arterial, as opposed to venous, blood is sampled is due to the fact that the arterial PO_2 and P_{CO_2} are determined by the function of the patient's cardiopulmonary system, whereas venous PO_2 and P_{CO_2} are determined primarily by the state of the tissue surrounding the capillary beds drained by the vein from which the blood was drawn. Therefore, arterial blood gas values reflect the patient's total cardiopulmonary performance, whereas venous blood gas values reflect only the condition of isolated tissue. An exception to this distinction is made with mixed venous blood samples. Mixed venous blood is found within the pulmonary artery and is used in the assessment of oxygen delivery. Mixed venous PO_2 is reflective of the state of total body be- cause it is composed of blood draining from all the organs, which is mixed together in the right atrium and ventricle before entering the pulmonary artery.

BLOOD GAS SAMPLE

Arterial blood can be drawn from the radial, femoral, and dorsalis pedis arteries. Arterial spasm, hematoma formation, and intraluminal clotting are all possible adverse consequences of arterial punctures.[8, 13] The radial artery is most often the site of choice for arterial punctures because of its easy accessibility and stability, plus the presence of good collateral circulation to the hand via the ulnar artery. The radial artery is considered the safest site for arterial punctures.[17]

TABLE 18–1.
Common Clinical Indications for Blood Gas Analysis

I. Arterial oxygenation and oxygen delivery
   Unexplained tachypnea, dyspnea, restlessness, tachycardia, and anxiety
   Decreased cardiac output
   Precardiothoracic and postcardiothoracic surgery
   Cardiopulmonary arrest
II. Alveolar ventilation
   Unexplained drowsiness, confusion, and tachycardia
   Bradypnea
   Cardiopulmonary arrest
III. Acid-base balance
   Tachypnea or abnormal breathing patterns such as Kussmaul's ventilation
   Renal failure
   Drug intoxications
   Cardiopulmonary arrest

Whenever the radial artery is chosen as the puncture site, the extent of collateral circulation to the hand is assessed by the modified Allen test.[2] The steps in the modified Allen test are as follows:

1. Palpate the radial artery in both wrists to identify the wrist with the strongest pulse. If both pulses are equal, choose the artery on the nondominate side. For example, if the patient is right handed, use the radial artery on the left.
2. Once the artery is chosen, have the patient extend his or her arm with the hand held open.
3. Instruct the patient to close his or her hand tightly, forming a fist, thereby forcing blood out of the hand.
4. Apply direct occluding pressure to both the radial and ulnar arteries using your index and middle fingers.
5. Instruct the patient to open his or her hand. Release the pressure from only the ulnar artery, and watch for the restoration of color to the hand.
6. If color is restored within 10 to 15 seconds, the test result is positive and a sign that the patient has adequate collateral circulation to his or her hand. A positive modified Allen's test signifies that an arterial puncture can be performed.
7. If color is not restored to the hand after the ulnar artery is released, the test result is negative and a sign that the patient does not have adequate collateral circulation. A negative modified Allen test signifies that it is unsafe to perform an arterial puncture on that wrist. The opposite wrist should then be tested as described in steps 2 through 7.

OVERVIEW OF BLOOD GAS THEORY

The survival of most animal and plant cells requires the maintenance of fairly constant levels of intracellular oxygen and carbon dioxide. Oxygen is used in the process of metabolism. Molecular oxygen is combined with electrons in the mitochondria of aerobic cells to form water. Carbon dioxide is produced in the process of carbohydrate metabolism and must be removed from the cell. Cells require a continuous supply of oxygen and the continuous removal of carbon dioxide to maintain their viability.

The process of meeting the oxygen and carbon dioxide needs of a *single-cell organism* is not complex (Fig 18–1). Oxygen from the atmosphere diffuses directly into the single-cell organism, whereas carbon dioxide produced by the cell diffuses out of the cell directly into the atmosphere. The atmosphere exerts a pressure of 760 mm Hg at sea level and is composed primarily of nitrogen and oxygen. Oxygen constitutes 21% of the atmosphere and, according to *Dalton's law*, will exert 21% of the barometric pressure, which means the partial pressure of oxygen in the atmosphere at sea level will be equal to 760 × 0.21, or 160 mm Hg. Oxygen will move by diffusion from the atmosphere directly into the single-cell organism, and carbon dioxide will diffuse out of the cell into the atmosphere, thereby maintaining acceptable levels of the two gases within the cell (see Fig 18–1). The level of oxygen within the cell will be a direct result of the atmospheric P_{O_2}, whereas the level of carbon dioxide within the cell will be a direct result of the rate of CO_2 produced by the cell.

Compared with a single-cell organism, a *multicell organism* requires more complex mechanisms for supplying oxygen and removing carbon dioxide. In humans, for example, the thoracic pump, lungs, heart, blood vessels, and blood are all involved in the process of supplying oxygen and removing carbon dioxide. The increased complexity of the gas supply system in humans brings an increased potential for complications. Events that affect any one of the elements in the gas supply system will have an

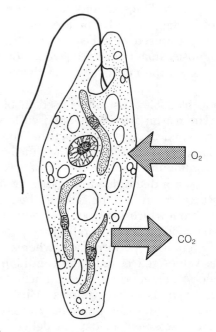

FIG 18–1.
Schematic of a single-cell organism.

impact on the levels of oxygen and carbon dioxide within the body.

The exchange of oxygen and carbon dioxide is referred to as *respiration*. *External respiration* is defined as the exchange of oxygen and carbon dioxide between the blood in the lungs and the gas in the alveoli. *Internal respiration* is defined as the exchange of oxygen and carbon dioxide between the blood in the tissue capillaries and the metabolizing cell.

ARTERIAL OXYGENATION

The three indices of arterial oxygenation are (1) arterial P_{O_2} (Pa_{O_2}), (2) percent saturation, and (3) oxygen content.

The previous example of the single-cell organism demonstrated that atmosphere P_{O_2} determined the level of oxygen within this organism. In humans, the Pa_{O_2} is also influenced by the atmospheric P_{O_2} in as much as the atmospheric P_{O_2} determines the alveolar P_{O_2} (PA_{O_2}), which, in turn, sets the maximum Pa_{O_2}. The addition of water vapor and carbon dioxide to the air as it is inhaled decreases the concentration of oxygen in the lungs compared with the atmosphere, which decreases the partial pressure exerted by oxygen within the alveoli. Although it is difficult to directly measure the PA_{O_2}, it can be calculated by the *alveolar gas equation*, which states[14]:

$$PA_{O_2} = (PB - PH_2O)FI_{O_2} - PA_{CO_2}\left[FI_{O_2} + \frac{(1 - FI_{O_2})}{R}\right]$$

The alveolar gas equation has been modified for clinical use to:

$$PA_{O_2} = (PB - 47)FI_{O_2} - \frac{Pa_{CO_2}}{0.8}$$

The alveolar gas equation demonstrates that changes in barometric pressure and FI_{O_2} have a corresponding impact on the PA_{O_2}. For example, if either of these two variables increase, the PA_{O_2} will also increase, and if either decrease, the PA_{O_2} will do likewise. The alveolar gas equation also demonstrates that an increase in the Pa_{CO_2} will be accompanied by a decrease in the PA_{O_2}, whereas a decrease in Pa_{CO_2} will be accompanied by an increase in PA_{O_2}.

The alveolar gas equation is used to calculate the PA_{O_2} for any combination of FI_{O_2}, barometric pressure, and Pa_{CO_2} (Table 18–2). The PA_{O_2} increases

TABLE 18–2.

PA_{O_2} of a Patient With Pa_{CO_2} of 40 mm Hg at a Barometric Pressure of 760 mm Hg for Various FI_{O_2}

FI_{O_2}	PA_{O_2}
0.30	164
0.40	235
0.50	306
0.60	377
0.70	450
0.80	520
0.90	591
1.00	663

above 100 mm Hg at a rate of approximately 7 mm Hg for 0.01 increase in FI_{O_2} above 0.21. For example, the PA_{O_2} of a patient on an FI_{O_2} of 0.40 would be estimated as follows:

$$PA_{O_2} = 100 \text{ mm Hg} + (FI_{O_2} - 0.21) \times 7 \text{ mm Hg}$$
$$= 100 + (0.40 - 0.21) \times 7$$
$$= 100 + 133$$
$$= 233 \text{ mm Hg.}$$

Comparison of the PA_{O_2} estimated in this example with the PA_{O_2} calculated using the alveolar gas equation shows the usefulness of this technique in the clinical setting (see Table 18–2). Knowledge of the PA_{O_2} is important to the clinician because it establishes a standard against which the Pa_{O_2} can be compared. In an ideal situation, the lungs would act as a perfect exchange system, and the Pa_{O_2} would be the same as the PA_{O_2}. In real life we do not find ideal situations, and the lungs do not act as a perfect exchange system. Therefore, there is a difference between the partial pressure of oxygen in the alveolus and the partial pressure of oxygen in the arterial blood. This difference is known as the alveolar-arterial oxygen pressure difference [$P(A-a)O_2$]. The $P(A-a)O_2$ is calculated as follows:

$$P(A-a)O_2 = PA_{O_2} - Pa_{O_2}$$

The $P(A-a)O_2$ is an index of the lungs' efficiency as an oxygenator. There is an inverse relationship between $P(A-a)O_2$ and oxygenation efficiency. The greater the $P(A-a)O_2$, the less efficient the lungs are in oxygenating the blood.

The normal $P(A-a)O_2$ when one breathes room air is in the range of 4 to 12 mm Hg. The $P(A-a)O_2$ increases with age to about 16 mm Hg in normal persons 61 to 75 years of age. A room air $P(A-a)O_2$ greater than normal indicates the presence of either ventilation-perfusion mismatch, diffusion defect, or shunt.

The oxygen in the alveolus diffuses into the pulmonary capillary and is transported by the blood in two ways: (1) dissolved in the plasma and (2) chemically combined with hemoglobin. The amount of oxygen that dissolves in plasma is governed by *Henry's law*. Henry's law states that the mass of a soluble gas that can be dissolved in a volume of liquid at a given termperature is proportional to the partial pressure of that gas. At normal body termperature, 100 ml of blood (vol%) will hold 0.003 ml of oxygen for each 1 mm Hg of pressure (Fig 18–2). At a P_{O_2} of 100 mm Hg, each vol% of plasma will transport 0.3 ml of dissolved oxygen. The amount of oxygen dissolved in the plasma is calculated as follows:

$$\text{Dissolved } O_2 \text{ (vol\%)} = 0.003 \times P_{O_2}.$$

The normal range for Pa_{O_2} in adults breathing room air at sea level is 80 to 100 mm Hg. The Pa_{O_2} usually decreases below 80 mm Hg in adults over the age of 60 years due to the degeneration of the lungs that takes place in the normal aging process. Shapiro et al. suggest that subtracting 1 mm Hg for each year over 60 years from 80 mm Hg will approximate the lower end of normal in older patients.[20] Using this approach, Pa_{O_2} of 75 mm Hg would be considered normal in a 65 year old. The normal range for Pa_{O_2} in newborns is 40 to 70 mm Hg.

The presence of a Pa_{O_2} less than normal is called *hypoxemia*. Hypoxemia signals the potential of an inadequate supply of oxygen for the tissues. *Hyperoxemia* is the presence of a Pa_{O_2} greater than normal.

To understand how a low Pa_{O_2} will influence the supply of oxygen to the tissue, one must understand the dynamics of the reaction between oxygen and hemoglobin. Oxygen is transported chemically combined with hemoglobin in the red blood cell (RBC). Oxygen and hemoglobin reversible combine to form oxyhemoglobin.

Hemoglobin is a conjugate protein made up of a protein called *globin* and a ferrous-protoporphyrin complex called *ferroheme*.[16] It has been experimentally shown that the maximum theoretical combining power of hemoglobin for oxygen is 1.39 ml of oxygen per gram of hemoglobin (Huffner factor). However, because it has also been demonstrated that the full potential combining power of hemoglobin for oxygen is not realized in the cliniical setting due to the universal presence of carboxyhemoglobin, an abnormal hemoglobin that results from exposure to smoking and other air pollution (e.g., exhaust fumes), a slightly lower value of 1.34 ml of oxygen per gram of hemoglobin is used in clinical practice.[1] Therefore, a patient with 15 gm of hemoglobin/100 ml of blood (gm%) has the potential to transport 1.34 × 15, or 20.1 vol%, of oxygen in the form of oxyhemoglobin.

The reaction between hemoglobin and oxygen is dependent on the amount of oxygen present relative to the hemoglobin. The relationship between the level of oxygen and the reaction with hemoglobin is graphically described by the oxyhemoglobin dissociation curve (Fig 18–3). The curve shows that as the amount of oxygen is increased, as reflected in an increased P_{O_2}, the amount of oxyhemoglobin increases

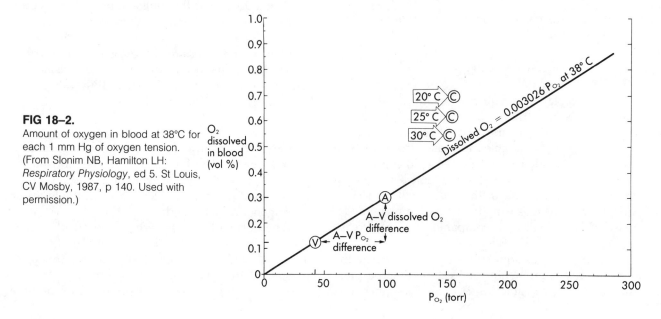

FIG 18–2.
Amount of oxygen in blood at 38°C for each 1 mm Hg of oxygen tension. (From Slonim NB, Hamilton LH: *Respiratory Physiology*, ed 5. St Louis, CV Mosby, 1987, p 140. Used with permission.)

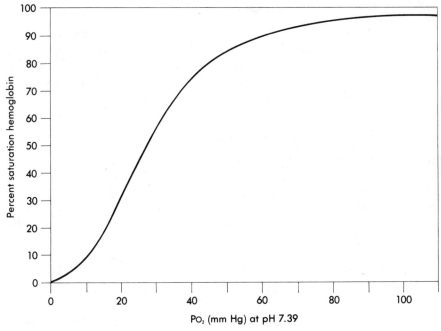

FIG 18–3.
Oxyhemoglobin dissociation curve. (From Lane EE, Walker JE: *Clinical Arterial Blood Gas Analysis.* St Louis, CV Mosby, 1978, p 48. Used with permission.)

until the hemoglobin becomes 100% saturated and can no longer react with oxygen. At this point, additional oxyhemoglobin will not be formed regardless of any increase in the partial pressure of oxygen.

The oxyhemoglobin dissociates curve has an s, or sigmoid, shape. The shape of the curve has important clinical implication because the upper flat portion (plateau) allows the oxyhemoglobin level to remain relatively constant in the face of fluctuation in the PA_{O_2}, whereas the step segment allows large quantities of O_2 to be released to the tissue for relatively small charges in the tissue capillary P_{O_2}.

The quantity of oxygen transported in the form of oxyhemoglobin is calculated as follows:

O_2 combined with hemoglobin
$$= (Hb \times 1.34) \times \% \text{ saturation.}$$

The percent saturation is determined in the blood gas laboratory by either indirect or direct techniques. Indirect techniques utilize nomograms and graphs, while the direct techniques measure the percent saturation through volumetric methodologies and colorimetry.[1] One can use the oxyhemoglobin dissociation curve to approximate the percent saturation. For example, in a patient with a Pa_{O_2} of 100 mm Hg, one can use the curve to find that the percent saturation is 97% (see Fig 18–3). Therefore, the quantity of oxygen transported as oxyhemoglobin in a patient with a hemoglobin concentration of 15 gm% and a Pa_{O_2} of 100 mm Hg would be calculated as follows:

O_2 combined with hemoglobin
$$= (15 \text{ gm\%} \times 1.34 \text{ ml } O_2/\text{gm})0.97$$
$$= (20.1 \text{ vol\%})0.97$$
$$= 19.5 \text{ vol\%.}$$

The reaction between oxygen and hemoglobin is influenced by both physical and chemical changes within the blood and the RBC (Table 18–3).[9] Changes in the reaction between oxygen and hemoglobin, known as the *affinity of hemoglobin for oxygen,* are represented by changes in the position of the oxyhemoglobin dissociation curve. Compared with the normal position of the oxyhemoglobin dissociation curve, factors that increase the affinity of he-

TABLE 18–3.

Factors That Influence the Affinity of Hemoglobin for Oxygen

FACTOR	EFFECT ON AFFINITY	P_{50}
P_{CO_2}		
Increased	Decreased	Increased
Decreased	Increased	Decreased
Temperature		
Increased	Decreased	Increased
Decreased	Increased	Decreased
Plasma pH		
Increased	Increased	Decreased
Decreased	Decreased	Increased
2-3-Diphosphoglycerate		
Increased	Decreased	Increased
Decreased	Increased	Decreased
Carbon monoxide		
Increased	Increased	Decreased

moglobin for oxygen are represented by curves in positions to the left of normal, whereas factors that decrease the affinity of hemoglobin for oxygen are represented by curves in position to the right of normal (Fig 18–4).

Different levels of carbon dioxide affect the reaction between oxygen and hemoglobin. As the P_{CO_2} increases, the affinity of hemoglobin for oxygen is less and the oxyhemoglobin dissociation curve is in a position to the right of normal. The new position of the curve shows that compared with normal, less oxygen will have combined with the hemoglobin at any given P_{O_2}. The impact of carbon dioxide on the reaction of oxygen and hemoglobin is called the *Bohr effect*.[21]

The standard measure of the position of the oxyhemoglobin dissociation curve is called the P_{50}. The P_{50} is the P_{O_2} at which the hemoglobin is 50% saturated with oxygen at a temperature of 37°C and a pH of 7.40. The normal P_{50} of human blood is 26.6 mm Hg but varies in normal patients.[15] An elevated P_{50} signifies that the affinity of hemoglobin for oxygen has been decreased and the curve has shifted to the right. A decreased P_{50} signifies that the affinity of hemoglobin for oxygen has increased and the position of the curve has been shifted to the left (see Table 18–3).

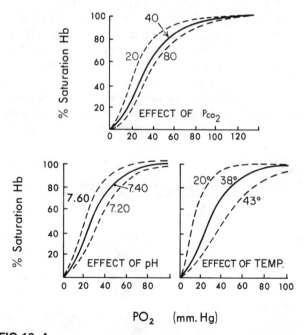

FIG 18–4.
Changes in the reaction between oxygen and hemoglobin are represented by changes in the position of the oxyhemoglobin dissociation curve. (From Cherniak RM, Cherniak L: *Respiration in Health and Disease*, ed 3. Philadelphia, WB Saunders, 1983, p 79. Used with permission.)

Oxygen Content

The oxygen content is the total amount of oxygen carried in the blood and is equal to the sum of the oxygen dissolved in the plasma added to the oxygen combined with hemoglobin. Oxygen content is calculated in the three steps:

Given:
$$P_{aO_2} = 100 \text{ mm Hg}$$
$$S_{aO_2} = 97\%$$
$$Hb = 15 \text{ gm}\%$$

Calculate: C_{aO_2}

1. *Calculate the quantity of oxygen dissolved in the plasma:*
   $$P_{aO_2} \times \text{solubility coefficient}$$
   $$100 \text{ mm Hg} \times 0.003 \text{ vol}\%/\text{mm Hg}$$
   $$= 0.3 \text{ vol}\% \text{ dissolved in plasma}$$

2. *Calculate the quantity of oxygen combined with hemoglobin:*
   a. Hb concentration × amount of O_2 held by 1 gm of hemoglobin (assume 100% saturation):
   $$15 \text{ gm}\% \times 1.34 \text{ ml } O_2/\text{gm} = 20.1 \text{ vol}\%$$
   b. Correct for actual Hb saturation:
   $$20.1 \times 0.97 = 19.5 \text{ vol}\% \text{ combined}$$
   with hemoglobin

3. *Add the quantity dissolved to the quantity combined:*
   $$C_{aO_2} = \text{Dissolved } O_2 + \text{Combined } O_2$$
   $$= 0.3 \text{ vol}\% \text{ (dissolved)}$$
   $$+ 19.5 \text{ vol}\% \text{ (combined)}$$
   $$= 19.8 \text{ vol}\%.$$

Comparison of the amount of oxygen transported as oxyhemoglobin with the amount transported as dissolved oxygen shows that approximately 65 times more oxygen is transported combined with hemoglobin than is dissolved in the plasma. This example demonstrates the importance of the hemoglobin concentration in oxygen transport. Two patients with similar P_{aO_2} but different hemoglobin levels would have different oxygen contents (Table 18–4). Although two patients may have an identical P_{aO_2}, the patient with an increased hemoglobin concentration will have a substantially higher oxygen content.

The degree of hemoglobin saturation determines the relationship between changes in P_{O_2} and changes in the oxygen content. The quantity of ox-

TABLE 18–4.

Calculation of the Oxygen Content of Two Patients With Similar PaO_2 But Different Hemoglobin Levels

PARAMETER	PATIENT A (ANEMIA)	PATIENT B (POLYCYTHEMIA)
Hemoglobin	7 gm%	18 gm%
PaO_2	100 mm Hg	100mm Hg
SaO_2	97%	97%
Oxygen dissolved ($PaO_2 \times 0.003$)	0.30 vol%	0.30 vol%
Oxygen combined with hemoglobin (gm% $\times$ 1.34 $\times$ SaO_2)	9.10 vol%	23.40 vol%
Oxygen content (dissolved + combined)	9.40 vol%	23.70 vol%

ygen in the dissolved phase changes in a linear fashion over the range of PO_2 present and the quantity of oxygen in the combined phase changes in a nonlinear manner (Table 18–5). The fact that the quantity of oxygen combined with hemoglobin changes most rapidly at PO_2 less than 60 mm Hg means that changes in a patient's PO_2 results in a greater change in oxygen content when the PO_2 is less than 60 mm Hg. For example, when a patient's PO_2 increased from 40 to 50 mm Hg, the oxygen content would increase by 1.73 vol%, but when the PO_2 increased from 90 to 100 mm Hg, the O_2 content would increase only 0.43 vol%. This observation demonstrates that PO_2 change in the range of less than 60 mm Hg signifies dramatic changes in the oxygen content, whereas changes in the PO_2 in the range above 100 mm Hg signifies minimal changes in oxygen content.

TABLE 18–5.

The Quantity of Oxygen Carried by the Blood With Various PO_2 Values

PO_2, MM HG	DISSOLVED, VOL%	COMBINED WITH HEMOGLOBIN, VOL%	OXYGEN CONTENT, VOL%	OXYGEN CHANGES PER MM HG, VOL%
10	0.03	2.70	2.73	0.273
20	0.06	7.00	7.06	0.433
30	0.09	11.40	11.49	0.443
40	0.12	15.00	15.12	0.363
50	0.15	16.70	16.85	0.173
60	0.18	17.80	17.98	0.113
70	0.21	18.54	18.75	0.077
80	0.24	18.90	19.14	0.040
90	0.27	19.30	19.57	0.043
100	0.30	19.50	19.80	0.023
150	0.45	20.1	20.55	0.015
200	0.60	20.1	20.70	0.003
300	0.90	20.1	21.0	0.003
400	1.2	20.1	21.3	0.003
500	1.5	20.1	21.6	0.003
600	1.8	20.1	21.9	0.003
700	2.1	20.1	22.2	0.003

OXYGEN DELIVERY TO THE TISSUE

The prime objective of oxygen transport is to deliver oxygen to the cells to meet their metabolic needs. *Hypoxia* is a state in which the oxygen demands of the tissue exceed the oxygen supply. There are four different forms of hypoxia:
1. *Hypoxemic hypoxia*: Hypoxia caused by the presence of hypoxemia.
2. *Anemic hypoxia*: Hypoxia caused by low hemoglobin levels.
3. *Circulatory hypoxia*: Hypoxia caused by a decrease in tissue perfusion.
4. *Histotoxic hypoxia*: Hypoxia caused an inability of the tissue cells to utilize oxygen (e.g., cyanide poisoning).

Blood gas data are used to assess for the presence of hypoxia. We know from our previous calculations that a person with a PaO_2 of 100 mm Hg and 15 gm% of hemoglobin will have an oxygen content of 19.5 vol%. The oxygen is carried in the blood by the cardiovascular system from the lungs to the tissue where it can be used by the cells. Therefore, the quantity of oxygen delivered to the tissue is determined by (1) the partial pressure of oxygen in the blood and the cells, (2) the quantity of hemoglobin, (3) the affinity of the hemoglobin for oxygen, and (4) blood flow to the tissue.

A shift of the oxyhemoglobin dissociation curve can result in normal, high, and low affinity states (Fig 18–5). If the PO_2 drops from 100 mm Hg in the artery to 40 mm Hg in the tissue capillary, normally hemoglobin is able to deliver 22% of capacity. Blood with hemoglobin that has increased affinity for oxygen will be able to deliver 15% of capacity, and the blood with decreased affinity can deliver 34% of capacity. Factors that influence the affinity of hemoglobin for oxygen have an impact on the ability of blood to deliver oxygen to the tissue (see Table 18–3).

A shift of oxyhemoglobin dissociation curve to the right promotes the release of oxygen by the hemoglobin, whereas a shift to the left inhibits the process. Although a shift of the oxyhemoglobin dissociation curve to the left is usually looked on as detrimental to tissue oxygenation, experimental and clinical evidence suggests that at a PaO_2 of less than 36 mm Hg, a shift to the left is, in fact, advantageous.[12, 24] The benefits of a leftward shift in severe hypoxemia are due to the fact that the arterial blood is better able to transport and deliver more oxygen

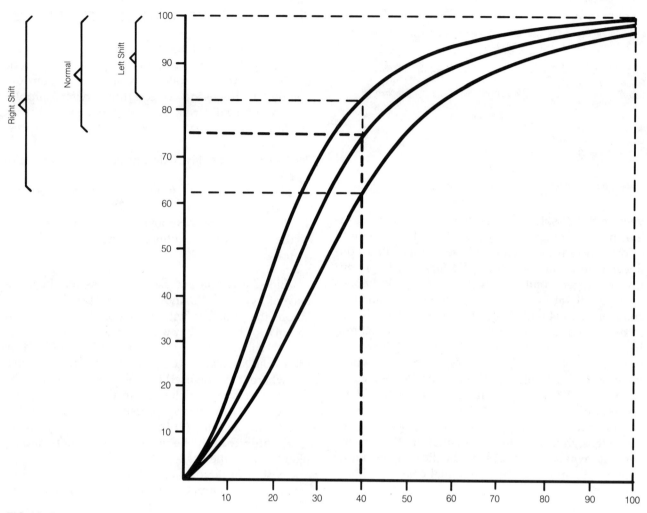

FIG 18–5.
A shift of the oxyhemoglobin curve can result in normal (unload 22% of capacity), high (unload 15% of capacity), or low (unload 34% of capacity) affinity states.

at a PaO$_2$ less than 36 mm Hg when the affinity of hemoglobin for oxygen is increased. It is important to remember that the advantage of the leftward shift is found only when the PaO$_2$ is 36 mm Hg or less.

The quantity of O$_2$ delivered to the tissue is also a function of the cardiac output. The total O$_2$ available to the tissue is called the *systemic oxygen transport (SO$_2$T)*. The SO$_2$T is equal to the cardiac output multiplied by the O$_2$ content. A patient with a cardiac output of 5 L/min and an O$_2$ content of 19.8 vol% will have a total SO$_2$T of 990 ml/min, whereas a patient with the same content but a cardiac output of 2.5 L/min will have a total SO$_2$T of only 495 ml/min. A normal SO$_2$T of 990 ml/min is well in excess of the normal O$_2$ demands of the body of 250 ml/min; however, this is not to say that all organs within the body have the same level of excess oxy-

gen. The heart, for example, uses most of the O$_2$ that it receives, whereas the kidneys and skin use a much smaller proportion of the O$_2$. The concept of SO$_2$T shows that changes in cardiac output can have a profound effect on the quantity of O$_2$ delivered to the tissue. As cardiac output decreases, the quantity of oxygen delivered to the tissue also decreases. The assessment of O$_2$ delivery must take into consideration the cardiac output of the patient and the perfusion state of the various organs.

The partial pressure of oxygen in the mixed venous blood (P$\bar{v}$O$_2$) is used as a nonspecific index of oxygen delivery. Mixed venous blood is sampled from the pulmonary artery by way of a pulmonary artery catheter. Because of the technical difficulty of placing and maintaining a pulmonary artery catheter, this test is reserved for patients found in intensive care units. A P$\bar{v}$O$_2$ of 40 mm Hg and greater is believed to indicate adequate tissue oxygenation in most clinical states, and a P$\bar{v}$O$_2$ less than 20 mm Hg indicates inadequate tissue oxygenation.[6, 18] It is important to note that a normal P$\bar{v}$O$_2$ does not always indicate that tissue oxygen delivery is adequate. Patients in septic shock, for example, have severe impairment of their oxygen delivery mechanisms but often have normal or even elevated P$\bar{v}$O$_2$. Recent clinical and theoretical evidence indicates that the P$\bar{v}$O$_2$ is not always reflective of oxygen delivery.[7, 22] Therefore, the use of P$\bar{v}$O$_2$ as a clinical assessment index of oxygen delivery should be used with discretion.

CARBON DIOXIDE TRANSPORT AND ALVEOLAR VENTILATION

The Pa$_{CO_2}$ is determined by the quantity of CO$_2$ produced by the body per minute ($\dot{V}$CO$_2$) relative to the minute alveolar ventilation ($\dot{V}$A). The relationship of Pa$_{CO_2}$, $\dot{V}$CO$_2$, and $\dot{V}$A is shown by the following equation, where K is a constant[22]:

$$Pa_{CO_2} = \frac{\dot{V}_{CO_2}}{\dot{V}_A} \times K.$$

This equation shows that if the production of carbon dioxide remains constant, the Pa$_{CO_2}$ will decrease when the alveolar ventilation increases and will increase when the alveolar ventilation decreases.

A Pa$_{CO_2}$ in the range of 35 to 45 mm Hg is considered normal. *Hypercapnia* is a condition in which the Pa$_{CO_2}$ is more than 45 mm Hg, and *hypocapnia* is a condition in which the Pa$_{CO_2}$ is less than 35 mm Hg.

Pa$_{CO_2}$ is the best index of alveolar ventilation. A Pa$_{CO_2}$ less than 35 mm Hg signifies that the patient has ventilation in excess of the CO$_2$ elimination needs of his or her body, which is known as *hyperventilation*. A Pa$_{CO_2}$ greater than 45 mm Hg signifies that the patient has ventilation inadequate to meet the CO$_2$ elimination needs of his or her body, which is known as *hypoventilation*. Factors with an impact on alveolar ventilation, such as respiratory rate, tidal volume, and dead space volume, will affect the Pa$_{CO_2}$. It is important to note that the adequacy of ventilation can be assessed only by measuring the Pa$_{CO_2}$.

Carbon dioxide is transported by the blood in three forms: (1) dissolved, (2) as bicarbonate (HCO$_3^-$), and (3) combined with proteins in the form of carbamino compounds. The relationship between the P$_{CO_2}$ and the total amount of CO$_2$ present in the blood is graphically described by the CO$_2$ dissociation curve (Fig 18–6). The CO$_2$ dissociation curve is more linear than the O$_2$ dissociation curve. The linear relationship between the P$_{CO_2}$ and the CO$_2$ content means that changes in the P$_{CO_2}$ characterize a proportionate change in the CO$_2$ content of the blood. Carbon dioxide is approximately 20 times more soluble in blood than O$_2$. As a result, a significant proportion of the CO$_2$ removed by the lungs (10%) is transported in the dissolved form.

Most of the CO$_2$ (60%) is transported in the form of plasma HCO$_3^-$. Bicarbonate is formed by the reaction of CO$_2$ and H$_2$O as follows:

$$CO_2 + H_2O \leftrightarrow H_2CO_3 \leftrightarrow H^+ + HCO_3^-.$$

Under normal conditions, the reaction between CO$_2$ and H$_2$O is very slow. However, in the RBC an enzyme *carbonic anhydrase* is present. The carbonic anhydrase increases the rate of the reaction between CO$_2$ and H$_2$O. As the concentration of HCO$_3^-$ increases in the RBC, the HCO$_3^-$ diffuses out of the cell into the plasma. The HCO$_3^-$ with its negative charge can easily pass through the RBC membrane; however, the hydrogen ion with its positive charge (H$^+$) cannot pass through the cell membrane and therefore remains within the erythrocyte. To maintain an electrical neutral state, chloride (Cl$^-$), the most abundant plasma anion, diffuses into the RBC.

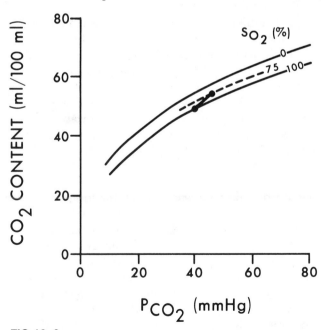

FIG 18–6.
Carbon dioxide dissociation curve. (From Murray JF: *The Normal Lung*, ed 2. Philadelphia, WB Saunders, 1986, p 180. Used with permission.)

The process of HCO_3^- moving out of the RBC and Cl^- moving in is known as the *chloride shift*.

Some of the hydrogen ions produced by the reaction of CO_2 and H_2O combine with hemoglobin. The H^+ more readily binds with the hemoglobin that has not reacted with O_2 (reduced hemoglobin); therefore, the level of O_2 in the RBC will influence the ability of blood to transport CO_2. More CO_2 can be transported at a given P_{CO_2} at low levels of O_2 than can be transported at higher levels of O_2. The fact that blood can transport more CO_2 in the deoxygenated state than in the oxygenated state is known as the *Haldane effect*.[10]

ACID-BASE BALANCE

Blood gases, primarily the CO_2, have an impact on the patient's acid-base status. Changes in the level of plasma CO_2 will affect the pH of the blood because, as we have already seen, CO_2 is transported in the form of HCO_3^- and H_2CO_3 (carbonic acid), and as such influences the hydrogen ion concentration of the blood.

An *acid* is defined as a hydrogen ion donator, whereas a *base* is defined as a hydrogen ion acceptor. The acidity of a solution is measured by its pH. The pH is the negative logarithm of the hydrogen ion concentration. A decreasing pH signifies an increase in the hydrogen ion concentration, and an increasing pH signifies a decrease in the hydrogen ion concentration.

Body acids can be classified as falling into one of two categories: volatile acids and nonvolatile acids. A volatile acid is one that can either physically or chemically change between a liquid and a gaseous state. Carbonic acid is the most important volatile acid in the body and, as previously discussed, can dissociate into CO_2 and H_2O. Carbonic acid is eliminated from the body as CO_2 by the lungs. Approximately 15,000 to 24,000 mEq of volatile acid is eliminated from the body each day by the lungs.

The nonvolatile acids are eliminated from the body by the kidneys. The nonvolatile acids are a byproduct of (1) incomplete oxidation of metabolites, (2) metabolism of protein, (3) anerobic metabolism, and (4) nonglucose aerobic pathways. Approximately 50 to 100 mEq of nonvolatile acids are eliminated by the kidneys each day. The kidneys are also responsible for the reabsorption of 5,000 mEq of HCO_3^- each day. Whereas the lungs contribute to acid-base balance through the elimination of volatile acids, the kidneys contribute through both the elim-

ination of nonvolatile acids and the reabsorption of HCO_3^-. A change in the lungs' ability to remove CO_2 from the blood or the kidneys' ability to either remove nonvolatile acids or reabsorb HCO_3^- will have a profound effect on the pH of the blood.

The relationship between H_2CO_3 and HCO_3^- and the plasma pH is described by the Henderson-Hasselbalch equation. This equation is as follows:

$$pH = pK + \log \frac{[HCO_3^-]}{[H_2CO_3]}.$$

The value of pK is 6.1, the normal HCO_3^- concentration in arterial blood is 24 mEq/L, and the H_2CO_3 level is equal to the $P_{CO_2} \times 0.03$. Substituting these normal values in the Henderson-Hasselbalch equation gives the following:

$$
\begin{aligned}
pH &= 6.1 + \log \frac{[24]}{[40 \times 0.03]} \\
&= 6.1 + \log \frac{24}{1.2} \\
&= 6.1 + \log 20 \\
&= 6.1 + 1.3 \\
&= 7.40.
\end{aligned}
$$

It is important to recognize that as long as the ratio of HCO_3^- to H_2CO_3 remains 20:1, the pH of the blood will stay at 7.40.

The plasma HCO_3^- concentration is regulated primarily by the kidneys (metabolic pathway), whereas the concentration of CO_2 is regulated by the alveolar ventilation (respiratory pathway). The Henderson-Hasselbalch equation can be rewritten to illustrate the relationship of the metabolic and respiratory pathways on the plasma pH:

$$pH = pK + \log \frac{[Metabolic]}{[Respiratory]}$$

The rewritten Henderson-Hasselbalch equation demonstrates that the pH is determined by a balance of metabolic and respiratory conditions. As long as the metabolic and respiratory factors maintain the ratio of HCO_3^- to H_2CO_3 at 20:1, the pH will be 7.40. For example, if the HCO_3^- level increased from a normal of 24 to 48 mEq/L, and the H_2CO_3 increased from 1.2 to 2.4 mEq/L, the ratio of HCO_3^- to H_2CO_3 would remain 20:1, and the pH would stay at 7.40 even though the absolute concentration of HCO_3^- and H_2CO_3 had doubled.

The fact that the pH is determined by the ratio of base to acid provides an important mechanism for the maintenance of plasma pH. The body attempts to maintain the plasma pH in the normal range of

7.35 to 7.45. The presence of a plasma pH less than 7.35 is called *acidemia*. Acidemia signifies the presence of a greater than normal hydrogen ion concentration. The presence of a plasma pH greater than 7.45 is called *alkalemia*, which signifies a less than normal hydrogen ion concentration. An abnormal process that would tend to increase the plasma pH is referred to as an *alkalosis*, whereas an abnormal process that would tend to decrease the plasma pH is referred to as an *acidosis*. Two types of events can lead to a decrease in the pH: (1) an increase in the hydrogen ion concentration and (2) a decrease in the HCO_3^- concentration. In the same light, two types of events can lead to an increase in the pH: (1) a decrease in the hydrogen ion concentration and (2) an increase in the HCO_3^- concentration.

The Henderson-Hasselbalch equation demonstrates that the plasma pH is regulated by the balance of metabolic and respiratory factors. Acid-base disturbances are usually differentiated into those of respiratory origin and those of metabolic origin. Processes that cause the pH to decrease can be categorized as being either a *metabolic acidosis* or a *respiratory acidosis*. Processes that cause the pH to increase can be categorized as being either a *metabolic alkalosis* or a *respiratory alkalosis*. The respiratory contribution to acid-base balance is solely through the elimination of volatile acid, whereas the metabolic processes can impact hydrogen ion concentration through nonvolatile acid excretion and HCO_3^- reabsorption (Fig 18–7).

The area of acid-base balance is often viewed by the clinician as the most difficult aspect of blood gas interpretation. Part of the difficulty arises from the fact that the acid-base literature is full of in vitro and in vivo parameters that, though intended to clarify the process, often create an aura of complexity that is unwarranted. Schwartz and Relman's conclusion that "traditional measures of pH, P_{CO_2}, and plasma bicarbonate level continue to be the most reliable biochemical guides in the analysis of acid base disturbances" is as true today as it was when written in 1963.[19] The clinician must master the interrelationship of pH, P_{CO_2}, and plasma bicarbonate before attempting to understand more complex values.

The acid-base state is determined by the pH. A pH greater than 7.45 means that the patient has an alkalemia. A pH less than 7.35 means that the patient has an acidemia. A pH between 7.35 and 7.45 is considered normal. It is important to note that the presence of a normal pH does not rule out the possibility of an acid-base disturbance. Once the acid-base state of the blood is determined, the clinician

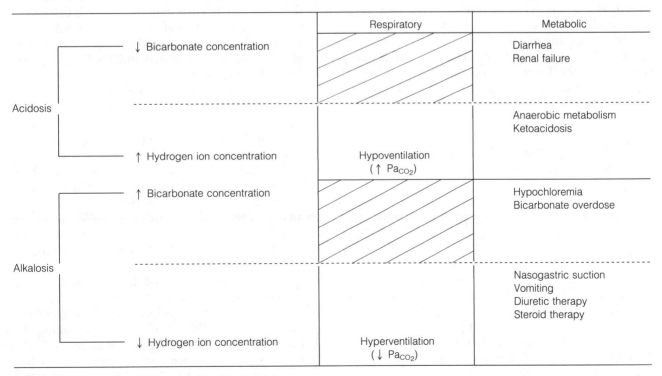

FIG 18–7.
Common respiratory and metabolic acid-base disturbances.

must next identify the presence of any respiratory or metabolic abnormalities.

The identification of a respiratory acid-base abnormality is straightforward. If the Pa_{CO_2} is outside the normal range (35–45 mm Hg), a respiratory acid-base disturbance exists. A respiratory acidosis is present when the Pa_{CO_2} is more than 45 mm Hg, and a respiratory alkalosis exists when the Pa_{CO_2} is less than 35 mm Hg.

The plasma bicarbonate level is used to determine the presence of a metabolic acid-base abnormality. In general, plasma bicarbonate levels more than 26 mEq/L signify the presence of a metabolic alkalosis, whereas plasma bicarbonate levels less than 22 mEq/L signify the presence of a metabolic acidosis. It is important to note that identification of the presence of a metabolic acid-base abnormality is not quite as clean cut as the method used to identify the presence of respiratory acid-base abnormalities. The reason is due to the fact that although the plasma bicarbonate is the index of the metabolic contribution to acid-base balance, some carbon dioxide is transported in blood as plasma bicarbonate. Therefore, changes in the arterial Pa_{CO_2} will cause slight changes in the plasma bicarbonate over and above the metabolic processes.

Ideally the plasma bicarbonate level should be corrected for any changes caused by the Pa_{CO_2} before it is used to assess for the presence of a metabolic acid-base process. The plasma bicarbonate increases approximately 0.07 mEq/L for each 1 mm Hg increase in P_{CO_2} above 40 mm Hg and decreases 0.2 mEq/L for each 1 mm Hg decrease in P_{CO_2} below 40 mm Hg.[4] Therefore, in a patient with a Pa_{CO_2} of 70 mm Hg, it can be estimated that:

Given:
Initial Pa_{CO_2} = 40 mm Hg,
Increased Pa_{CO_2} = 70 mm Hg,
Change in $[HCO_3^-]$ = (70 − 40 mm Hg)
$\times$ 0.07 mEq/L/mm Hg
= 30 mm Hg
$\times$ 0.07 mEq/L/mm Hg
= 2.1 mEq/L.

In this case, 2.1 mEq/L would be subtracted from the reported bicarbonate value. This new bicarbonate value would be used to determine the presence of a metabolic acid-base process as previously described. In another example, if the patient had a Pa_{CO_2} of 20, it can be estimated that:

Given:
Initial Pa_{CO_2} = 40 mm Hg
Decreased Pa_{CO_2} = 20 mm Hg
Change in $[HCO_3^-]$ = (40 − 20 mm Hg) $\times$
0.20 mEq/L/mm Hg
= 20 mm Hg $\times$
0.20 mEq/L/mm Hg
= 4.0 mEq/L.

In this example, 4.0 mEq/L would be added to the reported bicarbonate value, and this new bicarbonate value would be used to determine the presence of a metabolic acid-base process as described earlier.

Physiologists have developed several calculations that allow the clinician to correct for the respiratory impact on the bicarbonate level. These derived parameters are used to quantitate the metabolic contribution to the acid-base imbalance. Two of the most commonly used parameters are the *standard bicarbonate* and *base excess.*

Standard bicarbonate is a calculated bicarbonate value that would exist if the patient's Pa_{CO_2} was 40 mm Hg and hemoglobin was 100% saturated with oxygen. In theory, the standard bicarbonate eliminates the impact of changes in the Pa_{CO_2} on the bicarbonate level and therefore is used as a measure of the metabolic contribution to acid-base balance. A standard bicarbonate level in excess of 26 mEq/L is a sign of the presence of a metabolic alkalosis. A standard bicarbonate level less than 22 mEq/L is a sign of a metabolic acidosis.

The concept of the standard bicarbonate, as introduced by Jorgensen and Astrup in 1957, was based on data collected under in vitro conditions (in a test tube).[11] Other data have since shown that the standard bicarbonate does not always represent what the plasma bicarbonate would be if the blood was brought to a P_{CO_2} of 40 mm Hg while it was still in the body (in vivo).[4] The discrepancy between the standard bicarbonate and in vivo studies is due to the fact that the blood vessels are permeable to bicarbonate, and therefore in the body some of the bicarbonate diffuses between the blood and the extra vascular fluid. The data used to calculate the standard bicarbonate were generated from blood studies in test tubes. The test tubes caused all the bicarbonate to stay within the sample, thereby making the results somewhat higher than would be found in the body. The standard bicarbonate works best when there is little or no metabolic acid-base abnormality.[5]

Base excess is an index of the magnitude of the metabolic contribution to an acid-base disturbance. It is a measure of the quantity of acid or base in milliequivalents needed to titrate 1 L of blood to a pH of 7.40 at a temperature of 37°C and a P_{CO_2} of 40 mm Hg. The normal base excess is in the range of -2 to $+2$ mEq/L. A base excess less than -2 signifies the presence of a metabolic acidosis, whereas a base excess more than $+2$ signifies the presence of a metabolic alkalosis. The larger the base excess value, the more severe the metabolic acid-base disturbance.

A patient's acid-base state is classified as being in one of four categories: (1) normal, (2) acute, (3) compensatory, and (4) mixed. The normal condition is a state in which a normal plasma pH is accompanied by normal levels of HCO_3^- and P_{CO_2}. The acute condition is a state in which the plasma pH is outside the normal range, and the cause (either metabolic or respiratory) is accompanied by a normal process. For example, a patient with a pH of 7.27, a Pa_{CO_2} of 55 mm Hg, and a HCO_3^- of 25 mEq/L would have an acute acid-base condition. In this case, the patient would have an acidemia caused by an acute respiratory acidosis.

In the face of an acute acid-base disturbance, the body will try to compensate for the primary disturbance (bring the pH back into the normal range) by returning the ratio of HCO_3^- to H_2CO_3 to 20:1. The compensation is accomplished by altering the unaffected process. In our example of the patient with a Pa_{CO_2} of 55 mm Hg and a HCO_3^- of 25 mEq/L, the body would attempt to compensate for the primary respiratory acidosis by way of a metabolic alkalosis (Fig 18–8). The degree of compensation is classified by the pH of the blood. In the compensation process, the condition is said to be *partially compensated* if the pH has not been returned to the normal range and *fully compensated* when the compensatory process has returned the pH to the normal range.

The likelihood of full compensation is inversely related to the severity of the primary disturbance. In other words, it is unlikely that full compensation will occur if the acute disturbance was very severe; however, full compensation would be likely if the primary disturbance was minor. Arbus et al.[3] and Brackett et al.[5] have presented data that establish expected compensation limits. The fact that full compensation is unlikely to occur in severe acid-base disturbances has led to an alternate classification of the compensatory process. The compensation process can be classified as being *maximal* or *less than maximal*. Maximal compensation describes a state in which the pH, though not in the normal range, has

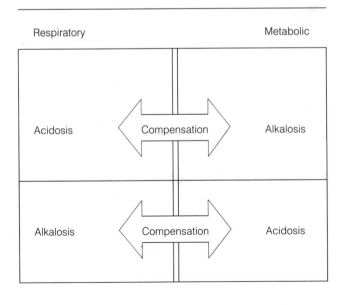

FIG 18–8.
Acid-base compensation matrix.

TABLE 18–6.

The Four Acid-Base States

	Pa_{CO_2}	HCO_3^-	pH
I. Normal	N	N	N
II. Primary			
Respiratory			
Acidosis	↑	N	↓
Alkalosis	↓	N	↑
Metabolic			
Acidosis	N	↓	↓
Alkalosis	N	↑	↑
III. Compensatory			
Partially compensated			
Respiratory			
Acidosis	↑	↑	↓
Alkalosis	↓	↓	↑
Metabolic			
Acidosis	↓	↓	↓
Alkalosis	↑	↑	↑
Fully compensated			
Respiratory			
Acidosis	↑	↑	N
Alkalosis	↓	↓	N
Metabolic			
Acidosis	↓	↓	N
Alkalosis	↑	↑	N
IV. Mixed			
Acidosis	↑	↓	↓
Alkalosis	↓	↑	↑

TABLE 18–7.

Data Used in the Evaluation of Blood Gas Results

ARTERIAL OXYGENATION	OXYGEN DELIVERY	ALVEOLAR VENTILATION	ACID-BASE BALANCE
PaO_2	PaO_2	$PaCO_2$	$PaCO_2$
FI_{O_2}	FI_{O_2}	Tidal volume	pH
	Hemoglobin level	Respiratory rate	HCO_3^-
	Cardiac output		
	P_{50}		
	$P\bar{v}O_2$		

been restored as close to normal as the compensatory mechanisms of the body are expected to achieve. Less than maximal compensation is a state in which compensation has begun, but the compensation process has not achieved its maximum effect.

A *mixed acid-base* disturbance is a state in which two acute disturbances are present. For example, a patient with both a metabolic acidosis and a respiratory acidosis (e.g., during cardiopulmonary arrest) has a mixed acid-base state. Of all the acid-base states, the mixed disturbances are often the most difficult to diagnose (Table 18–6).

The clinician, by interpreting clinical and laboratory data, is, in fact, answering questions about the patient's clinical status. Therefore, to be able to interpret blood gas results, the clinician needs to know both the questions to ask and the data required to derive the correct answers. Blood gas data are most often used to formulate answers to the clinical questions listed in Figure 18–9. The data required to evaluate arterial oxygenation, tissue oxygenation, alveolar ventilation, and acid-base balance are presented in Table 18–7. The clinicians use these data to formulate answers to the questions presented in Figure 18–9. A systematic approach to analyzing blood gas results is very important. One approach is to use a decision matrix like the one in Figure 18–9 to interpret blood gas results.

A. *Arterial Oxygenation*
  1. What is the patient's arterial oxygenation state?

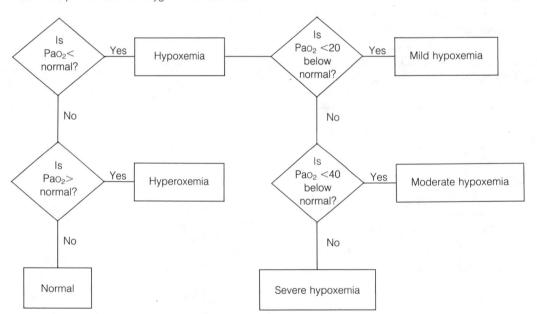

2. How efficient are the patient's lungs functioning as oxygenators?

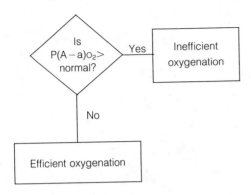

3. What is the patient's acid-base state?

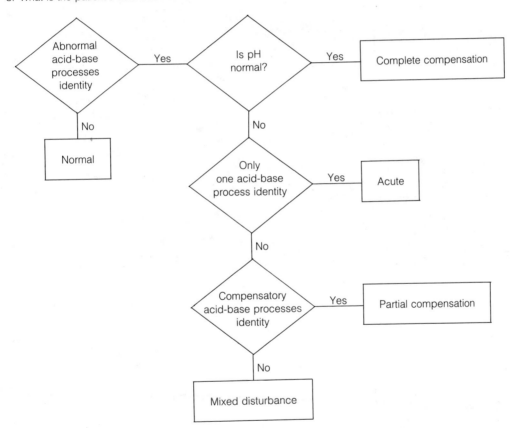

B. *Tissue Oxygenation*
Does the patient have the *potential* for tissue hypoxia?

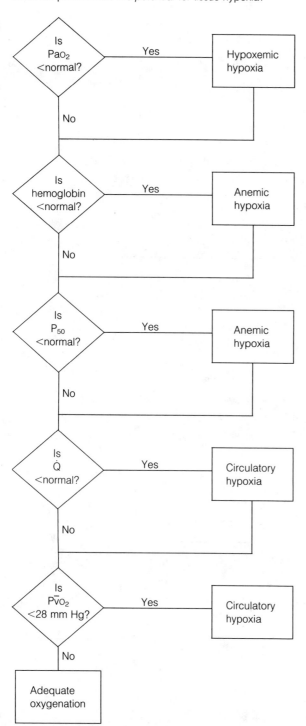

C. *Alveolar Ventilation*

Is alveolar ventilation adequate to meet the patient's CO_2 elimination curve?

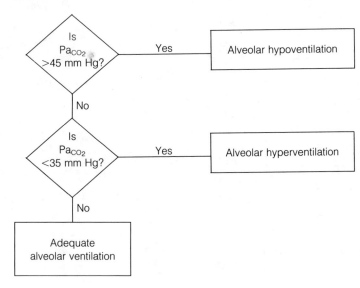

D. *Acid-Base Balance*

1. What is the state of the patient's arterial pH?

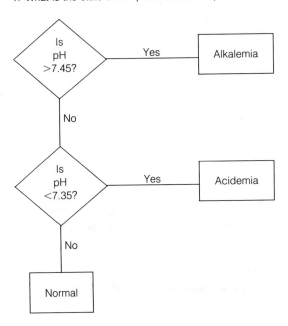

2. Are there any abnormal acid-base processes present?

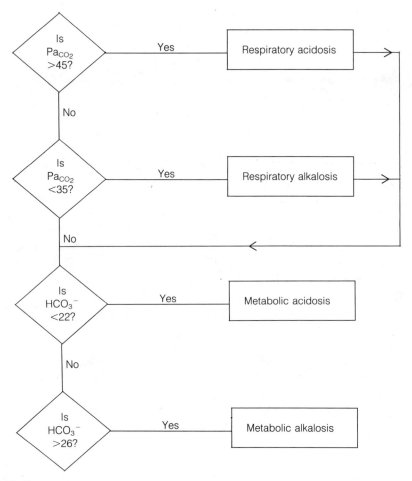

FIG 18–9.
A–D, decision matrices for interpreting blood gas results.

REFERENCES

1. Adams AP, Hahn CEW: Principles and practice of blood-gas analysis. *Franklin Sci Projects* 1979; 40:85–91.
2. Allen EV: Thromboangiitis obliterans: Methods of diagnosis of chronic occlusive arterial lesions distal to the wrist with illustrative cases. *Am J Med Sci* 1929; 178:237.
3. Arbus GS, Hebert LA, Levesque PR, et al: Characterization and clinical application of the "significance band" for acute respiratory alkalosis. *N Engl J Med* 1969; 280:117.
4. Armstrong BS, Mohler JG, Jung RC, et al: The in vivo carbon dioxide titration curve. *Lancet* 1966; 1:759.
5. Brackett NC, Wingo CF, Muren O, et al: Acid-base response to chronic hypercapnia in man. *N Engl J Med* 1969; 280:124.
6. Bryan-Brown CW, Baek SM, Makabali G, et al: Consumable oxygen: Availability of oxygen in relation to oxyhemoglobin dissociation. *Crit Care Med* 1973; 1:17.
7. Danek SJ, Lynch JP, Weg JG, et al: The dependence of oxygen uptake on oxygen delivery in the adult respiratory distress syndrome. *Am Rev Respir Dis* 1980; 122:387–395.
8. Eriksen HC, Sorensen HR: Arterial injuries: Iatrogenic and noniatrogenic. *Acta Chir Scand* 1969; 135:133.
9. Finch CA, Lenfant C: Oxygen transport in man. *N Engl J Med* 1972; 286:407–415.
10. Grant BJB: Influence of Bohr-Haldane effect on steady-state gas exchange. *J Appl Physiol* 1982; 52:1330–1337.
11. Jorgensen K, Astrup P: Standard bicarbonate, its clinical significance and a new method for its determination. *Scand J Clin Lab Invest* 1957; 9:122.
12. Lund T, Koller ME, Kofstad J: Severe hypoxia without evidence of tissue hypoxia in adult respiratory distress syndrome. *Crit Care Med* 1984; 12:75–76.
13. Martensen JD: Clinical sequelae from arterial needle puncture cannulation and incision. *Circulation* 1967; 35:118.
14. Martin J: Abbreviating the alveolar gas equation: An argument for simplicity. *Respir Care* 1986; 31:40.

15. Murray JF: *The Normal Lung.* Philadelphia, WB Saunders Co, 1986, pp 163–231.
16. Perutz MF: Structure and mechanisms of hemoglobin. *Br Med Bull* 1976; 32:195–208.
17. Sackner MA, Avery WG, Sokolowski J: Arterial puncture by nurses. *Chest* 1971; 59:97.
18. Schmidt CR, Frank LP, Forsythe SB, et al: Continuous $S\bar{v}O_2$ measurement and oxygen transport patterns in cardiac surgery patients. *Crit Care Med* 1984; 12:523.
19. Schwartz WB, Relman AS: A critique of the parameters used in the evaluation of acid-base disorders. *N Engl J Med* 1963; 268:1382.

20. Shapiro BA, Harrison RA, Walton JR: *Clinical Application of Blood Gases.* Chicago, Year Book Medical Publishers, 1982, p 125.
21. Slonim NB, Hamilton LH: *Respiratory Physiology.* St Louis, CV Mosby Co, 1987, p 151.
22. Tenney SM, Mithoefer JC: The relationship of mixed venous oxygenation to oxygen transport: With special reference to adaptation to high altitude and pulmonary disease. *Am Rev Respir Dis* 1982; 125:474–479.
23. West JB: *Respiratory Physiology—the Essentials.* Baltimore, Williams & Wilkins Co, 1985, pp 17–18.
24. Willford DC, Hill EP, Moores WY: Theoretical analysis of optimal P_{50}. *J Appl Physiol* 1982; 52:1043–1048.

Systematic Modification of Ventilatory Support

Robert M. Kacmarek, Ph.D., R.R.T.

Of central importance to the practice of respiratory care is the maintenance of patients requiring mechanical ventilatory support. Evaluating patient response to mechanical ventilation, monitoring the function of the mechanical ventilator, and appropriately modifying ventilatory support based on patient response are the primary elements of appropriate ventilator care. Respiratory care practitioners are highly involved with the technical aspects of critical care and tend to be programmed to focus more on the ventilator than the patient. This chapter is intended to draw that focus more to the patient by presenting clinical information related to the practitioner's role in the monitoring and modification of the patient-ventilator system.

First, the most important element of the system, the patient, will be discussed in terms of his or her response to mechanical ventilation. Next, periodic evaluation of the patient-ventilator system and troubleshooting of technical malfunctions are presented. Finally, topics covering alterations of the level of oxygenation and ventilation, application of various inspiratory-expiratory (I/E) ratios, inspiratory waveforms, modes of ventilation, and weaning from ventilatory support are presented.

PATIENT RESPONSE TO MECHANICAL VENTILATION

Most respiratory care practitioners rapidly develop the ability to ensure appropriate function of the mechanical ventilator. However, because of a technical orientation, the evaluation of the patient may be slighted. Any systematic evaluation of the patient-ventilator system must have the patient as its primary concern. Appropriate operation of the ventilator is essential, but appropriate response of the patient to the insult of the mechanical ventilator is critical.

Mechanical ventilation is instituted to maintain appropriate gas exchange. However, in addition to monitoring the effects of mechanical ventilation on gas exchange, pulmonary mechanics, and breath sounds, the effect of mechanical ventilation on the cardiovascular system must be periodically assessed (Table 19–1).

Gas Exchange

The primary method of assessing adequacy of gas exchange is arterial blood gas (ABG) analysis. The frequency with which analysis should be performed is highly variable. In acutely ill, unstable patients, analysis of ABGs may be required as frequently as every 15 minutes, whereas in chronic ventilator-assisted patients, weekly, monthly, or

TABLE 19–1.
Monitoring Patient Response to Mechanical Ventilation

Gas exchange
Pulmonary mechanics
Breath sounds
Cardiovascular system

even less frequent analysis may be acceptable. A general rule that can be applied to most acute settings is that arterial blood gas analyses should be obtained whenever a patient's status is markedly altered or when significant changes are made in the approach used to ventilate or oxygenate. Most patients in intensive care units require the analysis of one or two ABGs per shift.

Arterial blood gas data are always evaluated with respect to the level of ventilatory and oxygenation support a patient is receiving. An alteration in Pa_{CO_2} is normally a direct reflection of a change in alveolar ventilation. Increased Pa_{CO_2} indicates decreased alveolar ventilation, whereas decreased Pa_{CO_2} indicates increased alveolar ventilation. Whenever the Pa_{CO_2} increases, a hierarchy of possibilities should be formulated. What pathophysiologic changes result in a decreased alveolar ventilation? Atelectasis, pneumothorax, retained secretions, or partial airway obstruction can cause maldistribution of ventilation. Thus, some areas of the lung are poorly ventilated, preventing gas exchange, whereas others may be overventilated, decreasing perfusion and increasing dead space and inhibiting gas exchange. The Pa_{CO_2} also increases when the patient's metabolic rate increases. Fever, pain, anxiety, and fear may all increase metabolic rate. Last, but frequently a very common cause, the patient fighting the ventilator's delivery of a positive pressure breath or the patient breathing through a poorly designed ventilator circuit may increase metabolic rate and increase Pa_{CO_2}.[22]

Increased work of breathing is present whenever the following are noted:

1. Baseline pressures drop more than 1 to 2 cm H_2O during initiation of an assisted breath or during the spontaneous breathing phase of intermittent mandatory ventilation/synchronized intermittent mandatory ventilation (IMV/SIMV).[18, 44]
2. Multiple spontaneous breaths are attempted during the delivery of a positive pressure breath.[38]
3. The patient attempts to exhale during the inspiratory positive pressure phase.[55]

Fighting the delivery of a positive pressure breath can have significant sequelae. Specifically, peak airway pressures markedly rise, increasing intrathoracic pressure, causing a decrease in cardiac output and gas exchanges, and may precipitate the development of air leaks.[55]

An increase in Pa_{CO_2} normally requires that one or more of the following be instituted: (1) performance of bronchial hygiene if secretion accumulation or atelectasis is present; (2) increased level of mechanical ventilation (increased rate and tidal volume) whenever a change in pulmonary pathologic condition alters gas exchange capabilities; (3) intravenous fluid therapy or pharmacologic support if the altered Pa_{CO_2} is a result of decreased cardiac output; (4) administration of aerosolized sympathomimetics if bronchospasm or mucosal edema are present; (5) sedation if the patient is anxious, fearful, or frightened by mechanical ventilation; or (6) adjustment of the ventilator settings if fighting the ventilator is a result of the sensitivity setting, inadequate IMV flow, or lengthy inspiratory time (Table 19–2).

A decrease in the Pa_{CO_2} is an indication of improved alveolar ventilation. It may be noted following suctioning, the administration of a sympathomimetic, the insertion of a chest tube, improvement in pulmonary perfusion by the administration of fluid or pharmacologic agents, or resolution of the pulmonary pathologic condition. Patients maintained in *assist/control* or *IMV/SIMV modes* may alter their level of ventilation because of fear, pain, or increased work of breathing caused by technical limitations of the system, as previously discussed.

Decreases in Pa_{CO_2} require that one or more of the following be instituted: (1) a decrease in the level of alveolar ventilation, decreasing either the rate or the tidal volume; (2) sedation, if a result of fear, anxiety, or pain; or (3) alteration in system design if increased level of ventilation is a result of technical problems (Table 19–3). In patients with increased intracranial pressure, periodic or short periods of hyperventilation reduce cerebral blood flow by indirectly causing vascular constriction.[47, 48] If increased intracranial pressure is a concern, hyperventilation may be indicated.[60]

It is always important to identify the cause of a Pa_{CO_2} change before making ventilator adjustments. Remember, the Pa_{CO_2} may be returned to baseline

TABLE 19–2.

Responses to Increased Pa_{CO_2}

Bronchial hygiene: if excess secretion or atelectasis present
Increased mechanical ventilation: if altered gas exchange capabilities
Fluid or pharmacologic support: if cardiac output decreased
Sympathomimetics: if bronchospasm or mucosal edema present
Sedation: if anxious or fearful
Adjustment of inspiratory phase: if system increasing work of breathing

TABLE 19–3.

Responses to Decreased Pa_{CO_2}

Decrease in level of ventilation: if pathologic condition resolving
Sedation: if a result of fear, pain, or anxiety
Alteration in system design: if a result of resistance to spontaneous
 inspiration

by technical adjustments of the system or by sedation, fluids, pharmacologic support, bronchial hygiene, as well as an alteration in the mechanical tidal volume and rate.

Changes in arterial pH, if of pulmonary origin, are reflected in changes in Pa_{CO_2}. However, pH changes in ventilator-dependent patients may be of metabolic origin. One of the primary causes of metabolic acidosis is tissue hypoxia, resulting from insufficient delivery of oxygen.[56] Whenever a metabolic acidosis is noted, oxygen content, cardiac output, and tissue perfusion should be evaluated. If the cause is lactic acidosis, an increase in the $F_{I_{O_2}}$, positive end-expiratory pressure (PEEP) level, or cardiovascular support may be indicated. Metabolic alkalosis is the most common blood gas alteration in critically ill ventilator-dependent patients.[24] Because of a lack of intake of solid food and the administration of diuretics, vasoactive agents, and steroids, development of electrolyte imbalance is common. Many of these patients suffer from Cl^- or K^+ deficiencies, which directly lead to the development of a metabolic alkalosis. Appropriate medical steps should be taken to correct the cause of the alkalosis, because an alkalosis of any origin inhibits muscle function and increases the likelihood of cardiac arrhythmias.[24, 43]

Normally, metabolic problems are addressed by reversing the pathophysiologic alteration causing the problem. However, if a severe pH change is present and the correction of the underlying pathologic condition is time consuming, alteration in the level of mechanical ventilation in an attempt to normalize the pH may be necessary.

Alterations in arterial oxygenation are normally a direct result of a change in total physiologic shunt or ventilation-perfusion relationships. Decreases in Pa_{O_2} result when perfusion is present but ventilation is limited. Patients developing retained secretions, atelectasis, bronchospasm, pneumothorax, and adult respiratory distress syndrome (ARDS) frequently demonstrate decreases in Pa_{O_2}. Increased Pa_{O_2} often occurs when these pathophysiologic problems are reversed. It is not uncommon to see Pa_{O_2} rise after suctioning, the administration of a bronchodilator, chest physical therapy, or the elimination of a pneumothorax. As with changes in Pa_{CO_2}, ventilator adjustments may be required. However, in the case of a decreased Pa_{O_2}, the cause of the altered Pa_{O_2} should be determined and appropriate therapy directed toward its resolution, along with increasing the $F_{I_{O_2}}$ or PEEP levels (Table 19–4).

Recently, noninvasive methods of monitoring gas exchange have become increasingly popular. Capnography is used to continuously monitor end-tidal CO_2 levels, pulse oximeters are used to monitor oxyhemoglobin percent saturation, and transcutaneous electrodes are used to monitor transcutaneous P_{O_2} and P_{CO_2}.[7, 26, 41] Transcutaneous electrodes have been used extensively in infants to reflect arterial blood gases; however, their application to adults has been limited because of poor reliability with arterial blood gas data in low flow states.[19, 37, 50] However, capnography and oximetry have demonstrated usefulness in monitoring adults. Both technologies are particularly effective in monitoring patients during transit, the initial application of mechanical ventilation where frequent adjustment in level of ventilation and oxygenation are necessary, and during weaning.[8, 21, 27, 49] They provide a rapid real time indication of blood gas changes and may reduce the frequency of ABG analysis. However, blood gas analysis is still necessary because both measurements are indirect, and neither reflects arterial pH. An additional problem with oximetry is the understanding by other health care professionals that oximetry provides oxyhemoglobin percent saturation, not Pa_{O_2} (Table 19–5).

TABLE 19–4.

Responses to Decreased Pa_{O_2}

Suctioning
Administration of sympathomimetics
Chest physical therapy
Increased $F_{I_{O_2}}$
Increased PEEP

TABLE 19–5.

Noninvasive Methods of Monitoring Gas Exchange

Capnography
 Mean exhaled CO_2
 End-tidal CO_2
Pulse oximetry
 Oxyhemoglobin saturation
 Pulse
Transcutaneous method
 P_{O_2}
 P_{CO_2}

Pulmonary Mechanics

Even though a patient is being mechanically ventilated, periodic evaluation of spontaneous ventilatory capability and pulmonary mechanics is essential. These variables can provide direct data on the status of the pulmonary system and, if monitored regularly, help in determining when ventilatory support can be decreased or discontinued.

Patients maintained in the IMV/SIMV mode require evaluation and documentation of spontaneous tidal volume and rate whenever the patient-ventilator system is evaluated. Increased spontaneous tidal volume may be the first indication that the patient is capable of assuming a greater role in the maintenance of ventilation. Decreases in the tidal volume, with an increase in respiratory rate, usually indicate increased effort is required to maintain gas exchange and should alert the practitioner to the possible need for increased ventilatory support. Decreased respiratory rate in the IMV/SIMV mode occurs when patients sleep or are sedated but may also be an indication of greater spontaneous ventilatory capability if associated with an increased tidal volume. In the assist/control mode, spontaneous tidal volume and rate should also be periodically evaluated. However, the true capabilities of the patient may not be noted in the short time necessary to evaluate the tidal volume and rate. Evaluation of spontaneous tidal volume and rate is normally not attempted in the control mode because in this mode patients are not expected to ventilate spontaneously. Stimulating them to do so may cause fighting of the ventilator.

Tidal volume and rate do provide data on a patient's spontaneous breathing capabilities; however, the best indicator of ventilatory reserve is the ability to breathe deeply.[3] Thus, careful monitoring of vital capacity or inspiratory force (see weaning section of this chapter for details) provides a useful index. Increases in these values are associated with an increase in ventilatory reserve and a greater probability of sustained spontaneous ventilation.[55] If ventilatory reserve is improving, a decrease in ventilatory support may be indicated, such as decreasing IMV/SIMV rate, switching from assist/control to IMV/SIMV mode, or beginning weaning (Table 19–6).[42]

Compliance and Resistance

Estimations of system compliance and resistance provide quantitative data on the progression of pulmonary pathologic conditions.[5] They reflect the *stiffness* of the system and gas flow resistance. Compliance and airway resistance should be periodically

TABLE 19–6.

Monitoring Pulmonary Mechanics

Spontaneous tidal volume and rate
Vital capacity
Inspiratory force
System compliance
System resistance

evaluated in all mechanically ventilated patients. Of course, values consistent with those obtained in the pulmonary function laboratory are impossible; however, when measurements are consistently determined, changes over time reflect changes in elastic or nonelastic resistance to ventilation.

An inspiratory positive pressure curve with a 1.5-second inflation hold (Fig 19–1) provides a gross estimate of:

1. The amount of pressure required to overcome *total patient–ventilator resistance* to ventilation (peak pressure)
2. *Total system elastic resistance* to ventilation (plateau press)
3. *Total system nonelastic resistance* to ventilation (peak minus plateau pressure)

It must be remembered that these pressures are reflective of the total patient–ventilator system and thus may markedly differ from true patient values.

Effective static compliance (C$_{ES}$) is determined by dividing the measured exhaled, or expired, mechanical tidal volume (VT$_{measured}$) by the plateau pressure minus the PEEP level. A measured mechanical tidal volume is used because it is a more

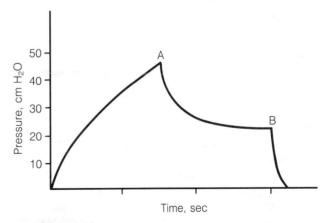

FIG 19–1.
An inspiratory positive pressure curve with a 1.5-second inflation hold: *A*, peak airway pressure; *B*, plateau pressure.

accurate estimation of the volume received on the previous breath than the machine volume setting:

Given:
    Exhaled tidal volume ($VT_{measured}$) = 1,000 ml
    Plateau pressure = 50 cm H_2O
    PEEP = 10 cm H_2O
Calculate: Effective static compliance (C_{ES}):

$$C_{ES} = \frac{VT_{measured}}{\text{plateau pressure} - PEEP}$$

$$= \frac{1,000 \text{ ml}}{50 - 10 \text{ cm } H_2O}$$

$$= 25 \text{ ml/cm } H_2O.$$

The term effective static compliance is used in this calculation since the value determined is an estimate of total system static compliance. The PEEP level is subtracted from the plateau pressure because the PEEP is not reflective of the amount of pressure required to maintain the static tidal volume in the system. Including PEEP in the determination of compliance increases the error in the calculation. If this error were constant, it could be tolerable; however, since PEEP levels change or are eliminated, the magnitude of the error also changes. Some practitioners also correct measured exhaled tidal volumes for the compressible volume loss (V_{loss}) of the system and thus use the following formula to calculate C_{ES}:

Given:
    Exhaled tidal volume ($VT_{measured}$) = 1,000 ml
    Plateau pressure = 50 cm H_2O
    PEEP = 10 cm H_2O
V_{loss} = 120 ml (3 ml/cm H_2O × 40)
Calculate: Effective static compliance (C_{ES}):

$$C_{ES} = \frac{VT_{measured} - V_{loss}}{\text{plateau pressure} - PEEP}$$
$$= \frac{1,000 - 120 \text{ ml}}{50 - 10 \text{ cm } H_2O}$$
$$= 22 \text{ ml/cm } H_2O.$$

The correction for compressible volume loss provides a more accurate estimate of C_{ES}; however, since the volume loss factor is a constant, the error in C_{ES} when it is not included is also constant. Thus, a reliable estimate of C_{ES} can be determined without correcting for compressible volume loss as long as the same type of ventilator circuit is always used on a particular patient (Table 19–7).

Dynamic compliance (Cdyn) is an estimate of total patient-ventilator system resistance to ventilation and is based on peak airway pressure instead of plateau pressure:

Given:
    Exhaled tidal volume ($VT_{measured}$) = 1,000 ml
    Peak pressure = 70 cm H_2O
    PEEP = 5 cm H_2O
Calculate: Dynamic compliance (Cdyn):

$$Cdyn = \frac{VT_{measured}}{\text{Peak pressure} - PEEP}$$

$$= \frac{1,000 \text{ ml}}{70 - 5 \text{ cm } H_2O}$$

$$= 15 \text{ ml/cm } H_2O.$$

Dynamic compliance is less useful than C_{ES} because it does not differentiate if alterations in values are a result of changes in elastic or nonelastic system resistance to ventilation. For this reason, the determination of C_{ES} along with an estimate of system resistance is recommended.

A decrease in C_{ES} indicates the system is stiffer. Decreased C_{ES} occurs with endobronchial intubation, total airway obstruction, atelectasis, consolidation, pneumothorax, or ARDS.[33] Basically, any change that limits the expandability of the system decreases C_{ES}. An increase in C_{ES} signals an improvement of pulmonary pathologic conditions, expansion of an atelectatic area, the resolution of a consolidation, decompression of a pneumothorax, or the reversal of ARDS. Increased C_{ES} may signal the need to evaluate the level of ventilatory support provided, whereas a decrease in C_{ES} may indicate the need for greater ventilatory support, increased PEEP levels, or bronchial hygiene.

It is important to note that single values for C_{ES} have limited usefulness, although markedly decreased values do indicate a stiff system. More appropriately, the trend in C_{ES} should be followed. If

TABLE 19–7.

Causes of Static Compliance and Airway Resistance Changes

C_{ES} decreased: System stiffer
Atelectasis
Consolidation
Pneumothorax
ARDS
Endobronchial intubation
Total airway obstruction
C_{ES} increased: System more elastic
Resolution of above problems
R_A increased: Lumen of airway decreased
Bronchospasm
Mucosal edema
Partial airway obstruction
R_A decreased: Lumen of airway increased
Resolution of above problems

the Cɛs is decreasing, the cause should be determined and appropriate action taken. When Cɛs increases again, appropriate steps to decrease therapy or level of support should be taken.

Nonelastic resistance to ventilation or system airway resistance (Rᴀ) can be estimated by dividing the difference between the peak and plateau pressure by the peak flow rate:

Given:
    Peak pressure = 70 cm H_2O
    Plateau pressure = 50 cm H_2O
    Peak flow = 60 L/min
Calculate: Airway resistance (Rᴀ):

$$R_A = \frac{\text{Peak pressure} - \text{plateau pressure}}{\text{Peak flow}}$$
$$= \frac{70 - 50 \text{ cm } H_2O}{60 \text{ L/min}}$$
$$= 0.33 \text{ cm } H_2O/L/min.$$

This calculation is a very gross estimate of airway resistance because the flow rate delivered by ventilators is inconsistent. Even if the ventilator is designed to provide a square wave flow, all ventilator flows taper at end inspiration. For this reason, many practitioners simply record the peak and plateau pressures but do not actually calculate airway resistance.

Increases in airway resistance are caused by pathophysiologic changes that decrease airway lumen: edema, partial airway obstruction, or bronchospasm. Thus, bronchial hygiene therapy or aerosolized sympathomimetics may be indicated when estimates of airway resistance increase. In addition, the pressure necessary to overcome airway resistance can be decreased by one of two alterations in gas delivery. First, inspiratory flow rate can be decreased. Since the magnitude of peak pressure is dependent on flow, decreased flow lowers peak pressure. However, a decrease in peak flow increases inspiratory time:

Given:
    Tidal volume (V_T) = 1,000 ml (1.0 L)

    Peak flow ($\dot{V}$) = 60 L/min (1.0 L/sec)
Calculate: Inspiratory time (t_I):

$$\dot{V} = \frac{V_T}{t_I}$$
$$t_I = \frac{V_T}{\dot{V}}$$
$$= \frac{1.0 \text{ L}}{1.0 \text{ L/sec}}$$
$$= 1.0 \text{ sec.}$$

However, if the peak flow is decreased to 30 L/min:

Given:
    Tidal volume (V_T) = 1,000 ml (1.0 L)

    Peak flow ($\dot{V}$) = 30 L/min (0.5 L/sec)

$$\dot{V} = \frac{V_T}{t_I}$$
$$t_I = \frac{V_T}{\dot{V}}$$
$$= \frac{1.0 \text{ L}}{0.5 \text{ L/sec}}$$
$$= 2.0 \text{ sec.}$$

The change in flow rate may have markedly decreased peak airway pressure, but because of the increased inspiratory time, the mean airway pressure and mean intrathoracic pressure may have increased. Caution must be exercised whenever a change such as this is performed. Second, the peak airway pressure can also be decreased by decreasing the tidal volume and increasing the rate but maintaining a consistent minute volume. Again, if this maneuver is performed, care must be taken to evaluate the effect on gas exchange and cardiovascular status. In general, the source of the increased airway resistance should be treated with minor alterations in the relationship between flow rate, tidal volume, and rate. As with effective static compliance, airway resistance measurements evaluated over time are more valuable an index of change in the system than a single value.

Breath Sounds

Every respiratory care practitioner should be skilled in the art of auscultation of the chest. Identification of atelectasis or consolidation, endobronchial intubation, esophageal intubation, and pneumothorax are all facilitated by the evaluation of breath sounds. As with other assessment techniques, chest auscultation should be performed every time a patient-ventilator system evaluation is done. Increased peak airway pressure occurs with all of the previously mentioned problems; however, findings of chest auscultation differ with each. Diminished or absent breath sounds on the left side usually can be noted with right endobronchial intubations, or left-sided pneumothorax; whereas breath sounds with right-sided pneumothorax usually are greatly diminished or absent on the right and normal or decreased on the left. Auscultation of the chest and abdomen immediately after intubation is necessary to rule out endobronchial or esophageal intubations. Auscultation of the trachea is also important when the minimal leak or minimal occluding volume technique is used to inflate airway cuffs.

Cardiovascular Status

The system most frequently adversely affected by mechanical ventilation is the cardiovascular system. As a result, this sytem requires careful monitoring whenever ventilatory support is required. Evaluation of the cardiovascular system should occur with routine patient-ventilator evaluations and any time alterations are made in the provision of ventilatory support.

Heart rate, rhythm, and blood pressure are the most important variables to monitor. The heart is highly sensitive to changes in acid-base status and oxygenation state, as well as altered intrathoracic pressures. Increasing levels of mechanical ventilation usually result in increased mean intrathoracic pressure. This increased mean pressure may inhibit venous return, resulting in an increase in heart rate and decrease in blood pressure. If a significant change in heart rate does occur, a reevaluation of methods used to increase ventilatory support should be made. For example, increasing the rate normally increases mean airway pressure more than increasing the tidal volume. In addition, whenever the level of ventilatory support cannot be altered because of cardiovascular response, fluid or pharmacologic support of the cardiovascular system may be indicated.

The first organ to respond to hypoxemia is the heart.[56] Hypoxemia normally causes the heart rate to increase; however, the severely compromised heart may become bradycardic. In addition, hypoxemia may precipitate cardiac arrhythmias. When ventricular arrhythmias develop, steps to improve tissue oxygenation and assurances of continued ventilation should be made.

Cardiac output and peripheral perfusion are also affected by mechanical ventilation and oxygenation. Alterations in oxygen delivery or extraction may be reduced by alterations in peripheral perfusion. The development of cyanosis, the loss of skin turgor, decreased skin temperature, and a decrease in urinary output are all reflections of decreased peripheral perfusion and cardiac output.

PERIODIC EVALUATION OF THE PATIENT-VENTILATOR SYSTEM

The sophistication of mechanical ventilators has increased exponentially over the past 10 years. Today's generation of ventilators give practitioners the false sense that the ventilator is performing as indicated without the need of an independent assurance of its function. However, as a result of miscalibration, inadvertent alterations of setting, or technical problems or limitations, any ventilator system may malfunction.

To ensure proper function of the patient-ventilator system, one must perform independent periodic evaluation of this system, even when using machines that provide graphic or digital displays of parameters. The frequency of system evaluation is dependent on the clinical status of the patient and the activity in the area of the ventilator. In acutely unstable patients, constant evaluation of the patient-ventilator system may be necessary, whereas in chronic ventilator-assisted patients, one check per shift may be adequate. In general, two- to four-system evaluations per shift are required.[31]

Protocol

It is important to realize that whenever a system evaluation is made, the patient's cardiopulmonary status should be evaluated. Alteration in a patient's clinical status (e.g., pneumothorax, hypotension, airway obstruction) do have a profound effect on the ventilator system as well as on the patient.

A ventilator flow sheet used by the Massachusetts General Hospital Respiratory Care Department to monitor the function of puritan-Bennett 7200 ventilators is shown in Figure 19–2. Because of the complexity of today's systems, this institution has designed different flow sheets for each type of ventilator. In addition to ventilator parameters, information concerning the type and size of artificial airway used, the volume of gas and the gas pressure in the cuff of the artificial airway, arterial blood gas data, and the patient's spontaneous tidal volume, respiratory rate, vital capacity, and inspiratory force are included.

Whenever a ventilator check is performed, the practitioner should first verify that all variables on the ventilator are set as ordered. When this check is done, it is important to review the previous practitioner's notes to identify machine calibration problems. That is, the machine rate may be set at 12

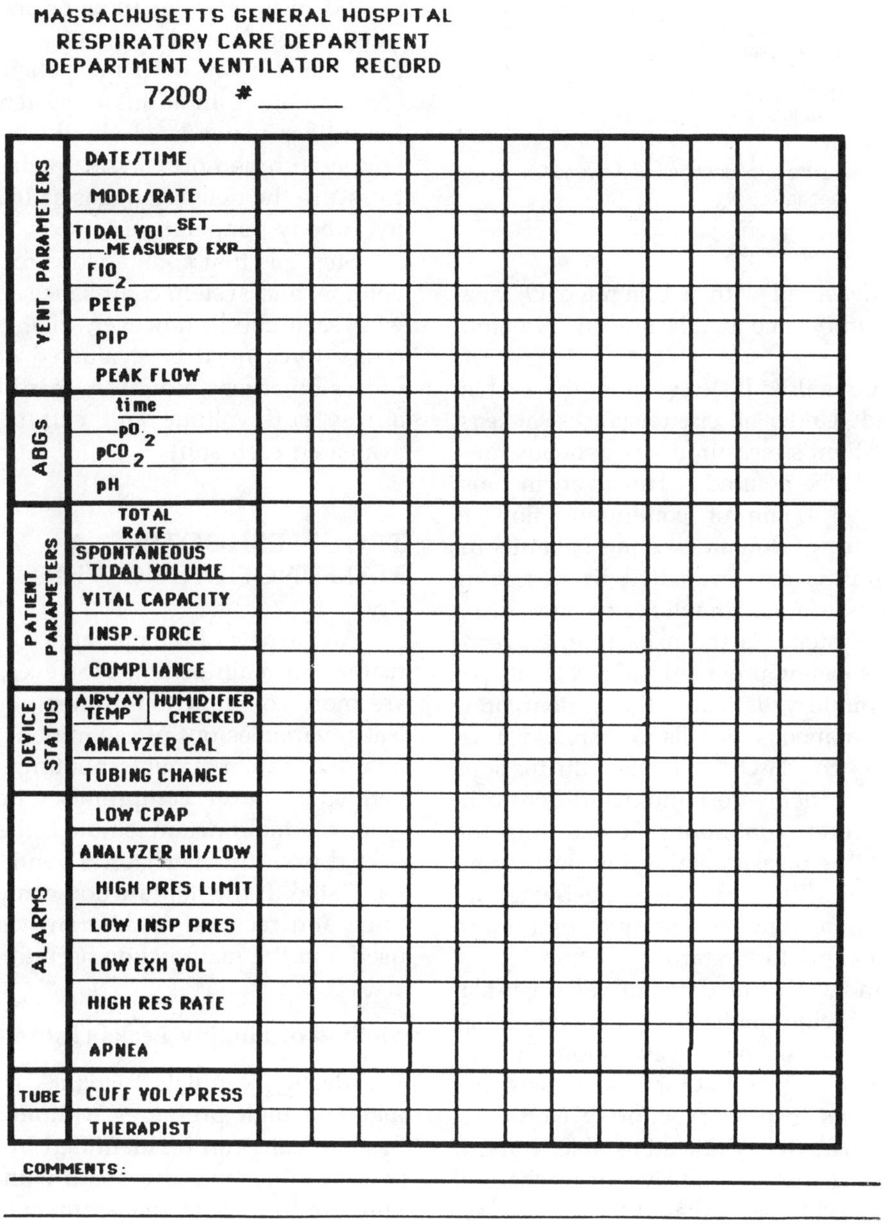

MASSACHUSETTS GENERAL HOSPITAL
RESPIRATORY CARE DEPARTMENT
DEPARTMENT VENTILATOR RECORD
7200 #_____

VENT. PARAMETERS	DATE/TIME													
	MODE/RATE													
	TIDAL VOL—SET ___ —MEASURED EXP													
	FIO₂													
	PEEP													
	PIP													
	PEAK FLOW													
ABGs	time ___ —pO₂— pCO₂—													
	pH													
PATIENT PARAMETERS	TOTAL RATE													
	SPONTANEOUS TIDAL VOLUME													
	VITAL CAPACITY													
	INSP. FORCE													
	COMPLIANCE													
DEVICE STATUS	AIRWAY TEMP | HUMIDIFIER CHECKED													
	ANALYZER CAL													
	TUBING CHANGE													
ALARMS	LOW CPAP													
	ANALYZER HI/LOW													
	HIGH PRES LIMIT													
	LOW INSP PRES													
	LOW EXH VOL													
	HIGH RES RATE													
	APNEA													
TUBE	CUFF VOL/PRESS													
	THERAPIST													

COMMENTS:

FIG 19–2.
Ventilator flow sheet for the Puritan-Bennett 7200 ventilator. Used by the Massachusetts General Hospital Respiratory Care Department.

breaths/min; however, the machine at this setting delivers only 10 breaths/min. Or, the tidal volume may be set at 800 ml, but the machine is delivering 1,000 ml. Ideally, the machine should deliver what is indicated on the control panel; however, in the real world many ventilators do not always function as designed. Any machine that is significantly out of calibration should be removed from the clinical area and scheduled for preventive maintenance (Table 19–8).

Step 2 is the evaluation of what the patient is actually receiving. A discrepancy between findings in step 1 and step 2 identifies variables out of calibration and possible machine malfunctions. Machine rate is counted, and exhaled tidal volume is measured with an independent spirometer. (Remember, because of compressible volume loss, the setting of tidal volume on the machine and the actual delivered tidal volume will differ.) *Assurance that exhaled tidal volume is consistent with ordered tidal volume is es-*

TABLE 19–8.

Protocol for Patient-Ventilator System Evaluation

1. Verify that all variables are set as ordered.
2. Determine what the patient is actually receiving.
3. Verify the alarm setting.
4. Check system temperature and functioning of humidifier.
5. Evaluate pulmonary mechanics.

sential. FI_{O_2} is measured with a calibrated O_2 analyzer, and inspiratory time is measured with a stopwatch.

With continuous-flow IMV systems, the system flow is evaluated. Under all circumstances, at least four times the patient's measured spontaneous minute volume should be assured.[34] However, in most patients, 60 to 90 L/min of continuous flow is needed.[34] Adequacy of flow in meeting patient's inspiratory demands is also evaluated by observing the machine pressure manometer and measuring flow exiting the system via the exhalation valve. If adequate flow is being provided to meet the patient's peak inspiratory demand, the system pressure during spontaneous ventilation should fluctuate only $\pm$ 2 cm H_2O.[32] Greater fluctuations indicate increased patient effort and insufficient continuous flow. Second, continuous flow exiting the exhalation should be measurable during peak spontaneous inspiration.[31] If flows are inadequate, increase continuous gas flow rate, being careful not to create significant expiratory retard.

When demand valves or demand valve ventilators are used to provide spontaneous inspiratory gas flow during SIMV or IMV mode ventilation, fluctuation of greater than ± 2 cm H_2O indicates increased patient spontaneous inspiratory effort.[32] Normally, demand valve sensitivity is not adjustable; thus, if increased work is suspected, the level of mechanical ventilation may need to be increased, the patient sedated, or the ventilator changed to a continuous-flow IMV system where the spontaneous inspiratory work of breathing is lower.[20, 22, 36, 59]

Step 3 is the evaluation of alarm settings (refer to the section on *false alarm warning* for details). All patient-ventilator systems usually have a minimum of two alarms: ventilator disconnect and high airway pressure. In addition, continuous use of an inline oxygen analyzer is highly recommended, as well as a loss of pressure alarm when PEEP is employed.

Step 4 is the assurance of proper function of the system's humidification device. Accumulation of water in system tubing can affect peak airway pressure and delivered tidal volume. Thus, circuits should include water traps or should have condensated water drained frequently. Fluid should always be drained away from the patient to prevent auto-contamination. In addition, system temperature and humidifier water level should be checked. System temperature is normally maintained at 33°C to 37°C to assure the delivery of gas at 100% relative humidity at body temperature.

Step 5 is that spontaneous respiratory rate, tidal volume, and system compliance should be evaluated with each check; however, vital capacity and inspiratory force need be evaluated only once per shift unless otherwise indicated. In addition, the artificial airway cuff volume and cuff pressure should be evaluated each shift.

TROUBLESHOOTING A MALFUNCTIONING VENTILATOR

Any aspect of the operation of a mechanical ventilator can malfunction. However, certain problems are more common than others, specifically, system leaks, variables out of calibration, and alarm system failures. When troubleshooting a malfunctioning ventilator, never compromise the patient's status. Once the malfunction is noted, the patient is disconnected from the mechanical ventilator and manually ventilated. If the malfunction cannot be readily identified and rectified, a different ventilator should be used and the malfunctioning unit sent for repair.

Method of Finding Leaks (Table 19–9)

Ideally, ventilator circuits should be able to maintain high pressures without system gas leaks. System leaks can be identified by delivering a fixed volume of gas into the circuit with the high-pressure limit control set at maximum while preventing exhalation and occluding the patient wye. Pressures to 80 cm H_2O held for 2 to 4 seconds should be obtainable with every ventilator circuit. If the peak pres-

TABLE 19–9.

Test for System Leaks*

First:	Set high-pressure alarm at maximum.
Second:	Set tidal volume at 1.0 L.
Third:	Occlude patient wye and prevent exhalation.
Fourth:	Deliver tidal volume.

*Pressures to 80 cm H_2O should be held for 2 to 4 seconds; if not, leak exists.

sure rapidly drops from its maximum while the system is occluded, a leak exists. The most common source of leaks is the humidifier and other points of connection, particularly if the humidifier is periodically opened for refilling. Second, diaphragms on exhalation valves wear out, causing system leaks. Third, small holes in both disposable and permanent large-bore tubing is common. If the presence of a leak is established and the source cannot be identified, the complete circuit should be changed. If this change does not correct the problem, the leak may be internal, and the machine should be removed from the patient area to be serviced (Table 19–10).

Machine Calibration

Theoretically, if a ventilator is to deliver 10 breaths/min, an independent assessment should verify 10 breaths/min are delivered. Such verification, however, may not always occur clinically. Each manufacturer lists a tolerance range for all variables on mechanical ventilators. Specifically, the rate setting may have a ± 10% error, or the tidal volume setting may have a ± 5% error. Whenever the difference between a set and delivered variable exceeds the manufacturer's tolerance ranges, the ventilator should be removed from patient care and sent for servicing.

Alarm Systems

Patient-ventilator alarm systems are designed to notify practitioners of system malfunctions or changes in patients' clinical status. Alarms should always be set to identify even the slightest of system changes (Table 19–11).

System pressure alarms are generally one of three types: (1) high pressure, (2) low pressure, and (3) loss of PEEP. High-pressure alarms are designed to identify an acute increase in system pressure and should be set about 10 cm H_2O above average peak airway pressure. The actual level above peak airway pressure is dependent on the patient's clinical status. In patients tolerating ventilation well, with fairly stable peak airway pressure, setting the alarm less

TABLE 19–10.

Primary Causes of System Leaks

Humidifier
Exhalation valve diaphragm
Connections and tubing
Internal machine leak

TABLE 19–11.

Setting of System Alarms

High-system pressure
    About 10 cm H_2O above average peak airway pressure
Low-system pressure
    5–10 cm H_2O below average peak airway pressure
Loss of PEEP
    3–5 cm H_2O below PEEP level
Oxygen analyzer
    0.05 above F_{IO_2}
    0.05 below F_{IO_2}

than 10 cm H_2O above peak airway pressure may be appropriate. However, in the agitated patient whose peak airway pressure fluctuates considerably, the high-pressure alarm may have to be set 10 cm H_2O above peak airway pressure, or greater, to prevent periodic alarming simply because of agitation. In most ventilators, the high-pressure alarm, venting of additional pressure and volume, and the termination of inspiration coincide. However, in a few ventilators these characteristics may not apply. If using machines with independent controls for the high-pressure alarm and pressure release, be sure they are set with the alarm sounding 2 or 3 cm H_2O before gas is vented. If the high-pressure popoff is set at a level lower than the high-pressure alarm, practitioners may not be alerted to the presence of increased peak airway pressures. This increase may result in a significant decrease in ventilation if the majority of the tidal volume is vented. This scenario is particularly serious if a pneumothorax or endobronchial intubation should occur.

The low-system pressure alarm is designed to identify system leaks, resulting in a decrease in peak airway pressure. This alarm should be set 5 to 10 cm H_2O below average peak airway pressure.

Loss of PEEP alarm is used to identify minor leaks in the system causing PEEP levels to decrease or to identify circumstances where increased patient spontaneous inspiratory effort causes PEEP level to fall significantly. Generally, the loss of PEEP alarm is set 3 to 5 cm H_2O below PEEP level. The actual setting is dependent on patient spontaneous inspiratory effort. The greater the fluctuation in PEEP level during inspiration, the lower the setting.

Continuous monitoring of F_{IO_2} with an independent O_2 analyzer is highly recommended. This alarm should be able to recognize increased or decreased F_{IO_2}. Generally, the alarm is set to sound if F_{IO_2} increases or decreases by 0.05.

The function of all alarms should be evaluated

with each ventilator check. This evaluation is accomplished by creating the circumstance under which the alarm should sound, specifically, causing the system pressure to increase, creating system leaks, and exposing the O_2 analyzer to increased and decreased F_{IO_2}.

Care must always be taken to ensure that alarms do not frequently sound when no clinical problem exists. The alarm will frequently sound if the alarm level is set too close to the parameter being monitored. As mentioned previously, agitated patients are of greatest concern. When alarms sound frequently for no apparent reason, personnel have a tendency to ignore the alarm and thus not respond when an actual problem does exist.

As a final note, even the most sophisticated alarm will function only when activated. Thus, as a general rule, patient-ventilator system alarms should *never* be turned off. When patients are disconnected from the ventilator for short periods (e.g., for suctioning), time delays should be activated. This delay in activation should help prevent the primary alarm identifying ventilator discontinuance from being the cardiac monitor.

SYSTEMATIC ALTERATION IN LEVEL OF OXYGENATION

Tissue oxygenation is based on a number of variables but can be simplified for general discussion to two primary factors: oxygen delivery and oxygen content. Oxygen delivery is based primarily on cardiac output, acid-base status, blood volume, and tissue perfusion. If we assume that acid-base balance is normalized, the major ventilatory concern regarding oxygen delivery is cardiac output. For this reason, alterations in level of ventilation should always be made with their impact on cardiac output considered. That is, alterations in tidal volume, rate, minute ventilation, I/E ratios, inspiratory times, inspiratory pauses, and PEEP level should be made only after consideration of their effect on cardiovascular stability.

Oxygen content is based on hemoglobin content, oxyhemoglobin saturation, and PaO_2. Of these variables, PaO_2 is the only one directly affected by manipulation of respiratory care equipment. (It is true that oxyhemoglobin percent saturation is affected, but indirectly, by changes in Pa_{CO_2}.) PaO_2 is affected essentially by the adjustment of two variables, F_{IO_2} and PEEP. Improvement in venous return does reduce to some extent the hypoxemic effects of

shunting and venous admixtures; however, F_{IO_2} and PEEP are the primary variables normally manipulated.

Increasing a Decreased PaO_2

In general, in most critically ill patients, a decreased PaO_2 is a PaO_2 below 60 to 70 mm Hg.[53] Arterial hypoxemia is caused primarily by intrapulmonary shunting or venous admixture (shunt effect) and is increased by a decreased venous return. If we assume that venous return and cardiac output are adequate, two alterations to increase PaO_2 are possible: increasing F_{IO_2} or increasing PEEP. If the F_{IO_2} is 0.40 or less, and the pulmonary problem is not a result of a generalized disease process causing increased intrapulmonary shunting, the F_{IO_2} is normally the first variable to be increased; whereas if the F_{IO_2} is greater than 0.40, and the disease process has caused generalized intrapulmonary shunting, applying PEEP or increasing its level should be considered. Whenever F_{IO_2} is above 0.40 and the problem is localized, or it is a result of venous admixutre, increasing the F_{IO_2} is normally considered first, since the addition of PEEP in this circumstance may foster $\dot{V}/\dot{Q}$ inequalities.[11, 23] The use of PEEP is indicated primarily when a generalized disease process is present.[17, 58] However, PEEP may be useful with localized problems that are not responsive to increase in F_{IO_2} (Table 19–12).

In general, PEEP levels are increased in increments of 2 to 5 cm H_2O, followed by careful assessment of the cardiovascular impact of the change. F_{IO_2} changes are normally 0.05 to 0.10. However, F_{IO_2} is increased more rapidly in the face of severe hypoxemia. The long-term use of F_{IO_2} at or near 1.0 should always be discouraged because it increases

TABLE 19–12.

Increasing a Decreased PaO_2*

F_{IO_2} <0.40
Localized or generalized disease
First: Increase F_{IO_2}
Second: Add or increase PEEP
F_{IO_2} >0.40
Localized disease
First: Increase F_{IO_2}
Second: Add or increase PEEP
Generalized disease
First: Add or increase PEEP
Second: Increase F_{IO_2}

*An adequately functioning cardiovascular system is assumed.

intrapulmonary shunt and has toxic effects on lung parenchyma.[4, 15, 39,54]

However, 100% oxygen should be used immediately in the presence of cardiopulmonary instability where severe hypoxemia is anticipated, remembering that once stability has been obtained, $F_{I_{O_2}}$ should be returned to appropriate levels.

Decreasing an Increased Pa_{O_2}

Whether to decrease the $F_{I_{O_2}}$ or PEEP when Pa_{O_2} is elevated is dependent on the actual $F_{I_{O_2}}$ and PEEP level. If the $F_{I_{O_2}}$ is above 0.50, the primary concern is decreasing the $F_{I_{O_2}}$ because of the toxic effects of O_2 at high concentrations.[4, 15] Once the $F_{I_{O_2}}$ is below 0.50, the PEEP level can be slowly decreased, alternating with further decreases in the $F_{I_{O_2}}$. PEEP is decreased in 5 cm H_2O increments, whereas $F_{I_{O_2}}$ may be decreased by 0.05 to 0.10 or more each alteration. Decreasing the PEEP level may result in increased venous return; therefore, careful monitoring of the cardiovascular system should occur whenever PEEP is decreased as well as increased. Following changes in either $F_{I_{O_2}}$ or PEEP, the patient's cardiopulmonary status should be completely evaluated (Table 19–13).

SYSTEMATIC ALTERATION IN LEVEL OF VENTILATION

Alterations in level of ventilation should be made only after consideration of the cardiovascular effects of each alternative. In general, changes that least affect cardiovascular status (increase mean intrathoracic pressure) should be considered first, followed by those with a more profound effect.

Increasing a Decreased Pa_{CO_2}

Prior to making ventilator adjustments on a patient with a respiratory alkalosis, one must determine the cause of the alkalosis. In the assist/control,

IMV, or SIMV modes, patients hyperventilate because of pain, anxiety, fear, hypoxemia, metabolic acidosis, and central nervous system trauma. If one of these problems is noted to be the cause of the hyperventilation, correction of the primary problem should eliminate the hyperventilation. If true mechanical hyperventilation exists, regardless of mode, hyperventilation may be corrected by decreasing the ventilatory rate, which is normally the first choice in all but the assist/control mode. Tidal volume is usually not decreased unless volumes greater than 15 ml/kg of ideal body weight are used. Remember, decreasing the rate helps most to decrease the mean intrathoracic pressure. In the assist/control mode, alterations in rate and tidal volume do little to correct mechanical hyperventilation. If the tidal volume is excessive, it can be decreased. However, in most circumstances, patients in assist/control mode ventilation require sedation to eliminate mechanical hyperventilation because it is the patient who is selecting the higher mechanical rate, not the machine (Table 19–14).

Mechanical dead space should *never* be used in anything but control mode ventilation; even in this mode it is usually not indicated.[33] In IMV, SIMV, and assist/control modes, mechanical dead space is likely to increase the patient's spontaneous ventilatory efforts. Dead space stimulates the patient to work harder to reduce the Pa_{CO_2} to a desired level but usually does not correct the mechanical hyperventilation. In control mode, mechanical dead space is useful only when very large tidal volumes are required to satisfy a patient's sense that he or she is being adequately ventilated. Typically, patients ventilated for neuromuscular or neurologic diseases who require a very large tidal volume to satisfy their

TABLE 19–13.

Decreasing an Increased Pa_{O_2}

$F_{I_{O_2}}$ >0.50
   First: Decrease $F_{I_{O_2}}$
   Second: Decrease PEEP
$F_{I_{O_2}}$ <0.50
   First: Decrease PEEP
   Second: Decrease $F_{I_{O_2}}$

TABLE 19–14.

Increasing a Decreased Pa_{CO_2}

Determine cause
Correct primary problem
   Sedate for anxiety, pain, fear
   Increase $F_{I_{O_2}}$ or PEEP if hypoxemic
   Treat metabolic acidosis
   If central nervous system problem, manage
      appropriately
If simply mechanical hyperventilation
   IMV/SIMV or control mode
      First: Decrease rate
      Second: Decrease tidal volume
   Assist/control mode
      Decrease tidal volume if excessive
      Normally, sedation is required

need to feel ventilated may require the use of dead space.

Decreasing an Increased Pa$_{CO_2}$

An increased Pa$_{CO_2}$ in patients mechanically ventilated is normally caused by mechanical hypoventilation. It is essentially corrected by increasing the level of ventilation by increasing either the mechanical rate or the tidal volume. The decision of which to increase depends on the actual rate and tidal volume. Always attempt to adjust the variable that has the least effect on mean intrathoracic pressure (Table 19–15).

As a general guideline, 12 to 15 ml/kg of ideal body weight is the tidal volume required by most patients mechanically ventilated.[25, 33, 55] This level, however, may be modified for each patient. For example, obese patients may require a much larger tidal volume, whereas patients with chronic restrictive pulmonary disease may require a much smaller tidal volume. In patients who are mechanically hypoventilated with a mechanical rate of 8/min or greater, the practitioner should first ensure that the tidal volume is appropriate. If the tidal volume is low, it should be increased before changes in mechanical rate are made. If the tidal volume is set appropriately, the rate should be increased.

Tidal volume is usually increased before rate, because a change of 100 to 200 ml normally does not cause as great an increase in mean intrathoracic pressure as a 1 to 2/min increase in rate.[5] This observation is true only if the tidal volume delivered is on the steep aspect of the patient's compliance curve. Once the tidal volume extends into the flat part of the compliance curve, increases in tidal volume will markedly increase peak airway pressure.

It is always difficult to apply any hard and fast rules to altering ventilator parameters; however, the following does always apply: Whenever any change in the level of ventilation is made, concern for its cardiovascular effects must be foremost, and a careful evaluation of the cardiovascular system before and after making the change is essential.

Inflation Hold

Since the advent of IMV/SIMV mode ventilation, the need for maintaining a fixed 1:1.5 or 1:2 I/E ratio has changed considerably. With IMV/SIMV, expiratory times are normally lengthy and mechanical rates slow, 12/min or fewer. To allow a patient to breathe in this manner would require an inspiratory time of about 2.5 seconds. Mechanical inspiratory times of this length are rarely tolerated by spontaneously ventilating patients.

Underlining the desire to maintain I/E ratios at a specific level is a primary concern about inspiratory time. In adults, unless the presence of regional variations in ventilation exist, inspiratory times should be kept between about 1 and 1.5 sec.[25] Lengthy inspiratory times do improve level of ventilation but may also increase work of breathing, and thus CO_2 production, by not delivering tidal volume as rapidly as needed.[38] When ventilatory rates are high (>20/min) regardless of mode, I/E ratio does become the more important variable. Here, care should be taken to ensure I/E ratios are always 1:1.5 or less (1:2). Remember, inspiratory time must be less than expiratory time to prevent air trapping and increased functional residual capacity (Table 19–16).

Inspiratory Wave Flow Pattern

Little clinical effect of varying inspiratory wave patterns has been demonstrated.[28–30] The use of a square wave, sine wave, or decelerating or accelerating pattern appears academic under most clinical situations, the one exception being patients with increased airway resistance.[28] In these patients, better gas exchange appears to be achieved with a decelerating waveform. However, the same effect can be

---

TABLE 19–15.

Decreasing an Increased Pa$_{CO_2}$*

If rate is 8/min or greater
  First: Increase tidal volume
  Second: Increase rate
If rate is less than 8/min
  First: Increase rate
  Second: Increase tidal volume

*It is assumed that tidal volume is not excessive, e.g., about 12 to 15 ml/kg.

TABLE 19–16.

Inflation Hold

Indication
  Regional variation in pulmonary mechanics
Function
  Improvement in ventilation
Application
  Prevent total inspiratory time from exceeding 2 seconds by adjusting inspiratory flow rate
Length
  0.25–1.0 sec

achieved with inflation holds and lengthened inspiratory times.

The use of an accelerating inspiratory waveform does seem to cause minor increases in mean intrathoracic pressure and decreases the effectiveness of gas exchange without any demonstrable advantage.[29] In most clinical situations, the use of either square or sine wave gas flow patterns would seem appropriate, with the specific selection based purely on bias.

Mode of Ventilation

Technically, there are four basic modes of ventilation: (1) control, (2) assist/control, (3) IMV, and (4) SIMV. However, clinically, two general approaches are normally used. Either the patient is capable, and it is desirable for the patient to actively participate in the process of mechanical ventilation, or the patient should not be allowed to participate and frequently is pharmacologically controlled during mechanical ventilation.[51, 52]

Thus, a spectrum is established from spontaneous ventilation to pharmacologically controlled mechanical ventilation. The only modes of ventilation that allow selection of any point on this spectrum are IMV and SIMV (Table 19–17). With the assist/control mode, the patient can participate in the initiation of inspiration but cannot take a primary role in gas movement. The use of the control mode usually requires complete pharmacologic suppression of ventilation or patients are likely to fight the ventilator and attempt to breathe between control breaths. Accordingly, the use of the control mode setting is discouraged.

The practitioner thus has the choice between IMV/SIMV and assist/control modes of ventilation. With the IMV/SIMV mode, rapid and easy adjust-

TABLE 19–17.

Technical Modes of Ventilation

Control
Always requires sedation
Infrequently used
Assist/control
Control available with sedation
Patient-initiated breath
Minimal patient role in ventilation
Recommended in severe COPD patients
IMV/SIMV
Allow patient interaction
Any mechanical rate possible
Control available with sedation
Technical problems

ment across the full spectrum is possible, whereas with the assist/control mode, only minimal patient interaction is feasible.

In most patients the decision to use IMV (continuous flow) or SIMV (demand flow) is purely academic. However, in patients requiring mechanical ventilation for primary pulmonary abnormalities or multiorgan system failure, the use of continuous-flow systems is recommended.[34] Decreased work of breathing with these systems when compared to demand flow systems has been demonstrated.[36, 59] However, in the short-term, mechanically ventilated postoperative patient, SIMV does seem appropriate.

The problems with demand-flow systems are being addressed by manufacturers. Improved demand valves are being developed and the incorporation on some ventilators of an adjunct mode to SIMV or continuous positive-airway pressure, referred to as *inspiratory assist*, or pressure support has been developed.[12, 46, 57] This adjunct rapidly pressures the system to a plateau level during spontaneous inspiration and appears to assist in overcoming the resistance of the demand valve, the ventilator circuit, and the artificial airway.[35, 45] However, greater clinical experience is necessary before guidelines for its use can be defined.

The use of assist/control mode ventilation is preferred by many and may be particularly advantageous in patients where resting of ventilatory muscles is indicated.[9] However, outside its use in the patient with severe COPD, there seems to be no clinical advantage over IMV/SIMV. The single disadvantage of assist/control ventilation is its inability to allow significant patient interaction in the process of ventilation.

A great debate over the most appropriate mode of ventilation has existed for years and has yet to be completed. At best, it can be stated that the selection of specific modes of ventilation is arbitrary and determined primarily by bias and experience, except in a few circumstances. In general, the use of the control mode is discouraged. When patients are maintained at relatively high (>8–10/min) mechanical rates, no significant benefit from either the IMV, SIMV, or assist/control mode has been established. At lower mechanical ventilatory rates (≤7/min), IMV and SIMV modes allow the patients a primary role in the process of ventilation. The SIMV mode, because of the resistance of demand values, is not recommended when patients with primary pulmonary problems or multiorgan system failure are ventilated, and assist/control mode ventilation may be most appropriate in patients with severe COPD.

Weaning From Mechanical Ventilatory Support

Patients are weaned from mechanical ventilatory support when they are physiologically capable of ventilating spontaneously. As simple as it may sound, it is important to be constantly aware of this fact when you are evaluating a patient's capability to wean. Although adequacy of spontaneous ventilatory capabilities and gas exchange are essential to weaning, it is also essential to ensure that other organ systems are capable of tolerating the increased stress of spontaneous ventilation prior to discontinuing ventilatory support.

Clinical judgment is normally the most accurate variable evaluating readiness and adequacy of spontaneous ventilatory capabilities. Many patients who meet the following criteria do not wean, and many who do not meet these criteria readily assume spontaneous ventilation (Table 19–18).

Pathophysiologic Condition Necessitating Ventilation

The single most important variable to evaluate when determining readiness to wean is the reversal of the pathophysiologic condition necessitating the institution of ventilatory support. If the pathologic condition necessitating ventilatory support is not reversed, the probability of assumption of spontaneous ventilation is small whether the precipitating pathologic condition is an exacerbation of COPD, neuromuscular disease, or ARDS.

Ventilatory Reserve

Patients must possess an adequate ventilatory reserve to sustain the increased stress of prolonged spontaneous ventilation.[40] In addition, the patient's spontaneous tidal volume and respiratory rate must be acceptable. Spontaneous respiratory rate should not be excessive, normally less than 25/min. Greater rates are normally associated with a smaller tidal volume, greater dead space ventilation, and increased ventilatory work and therefore are unlikely to sustain gas exchange over a prolonged period.

Spontaneous tidal volume should be 2 to 3 ml/kg of ideal weight or greater.[33] Normal tidal volume is about 7 to 9 ml/kg; however, it is unlikely that patients maintained on mechanical ventilation will have volumes in this range. Two to 3 ml/kg is normally greater than dead space volume and is the minimal value established as an acceptable level.

The most important variable to evaluate is the capability of the patient to take a deep breath. Remember, the greater the patient's vital capacity, the greater his or her ventilatory reserve, that is, the greater the patient's ability to withstand additional cardiopulmonary stress. Normal vital capacities are about 70 to 90 ml/kg; however, 10 to 15 ml/kg of ideal body weight is normally the minimal level acceptable when the patient is evaluated for weaning.[6] If values fall below this range, most patients will not have the reserves to maintain prolonged spontaneous ventilation. Intubated and mechanically ventilated patients may not be cooperative enough to provide a maximal vital capacity. However, the measurement of inspiratory force also provides an excellent estimate of ventilatory reserve. Most normal subjects can generate an inspiratory force of -100 cm H_2O or greater. The minimal acceptable level when one is evaluating weaning capabilities is -20 to -25 cm H_2O within 20 seconds (Table 19–19).[56]

Evaluation of spontaneous ventilatory capabilities is frequently difficult in patients receiving significant ventilatory support. Patients ventilated at a rate of 12/min with a mechanical tidal volume of 1,000 ml may not have the stimulus to ventilate spontaneously. Thus, in patients who fail to meet these criteria, and if clinical judgment indicates they should be able to ventilate spontaneously, a trial at spontaneous ventilation is frequently indicated. After 10 minutes of spontaneous ventilation, increased CO_2 levels may stimulate ventilation. Reassessment of ventilatory reserve at this time may prove acceptable. Again, clinical judgment should always be the final determinant.

TABLE 19–18.

Criteria for Ventilator Weaning

Reversal of pathology requiring mechanical ventilation
Adequate ventilatory reserve
Adequate gas exchange capabilities
Absence of acute pulmonary pathologic conditions
Adequate cardiovascular reserves
No major organ system failures
Normal fluid and electrolyte balance
Appropriate nutritional status
Psychologic support

TABLE 19–19.

Ventilatory Reserve

Spontaneous rate ≤25/min
Spontaneous tidal volume ≥2 to 3 ml/kg
Vital capacity ≥10 to 15 ml/kg
Inspiratory force ≥ -20 to -25 cm H_2O in 20 seconds

Gas Exchange Capabilities

In addition to spontaneous ventilatory capabilities, adequate gas exchange mechanisms must be intact. Arterial blood gases should be acceptable considering the patient's history. Pa_{O_2} should be above 60 to 70 mm Hg at a $F_{I_{O_2}}$ of 0.40 or less, and the pH should be within the normal range (7.35–7.45) and the Pa_{CO_2} normal for the particular patient. For most patients, a normal level is a Pa_{CO_2} of about 40 mm Hg. However, for chronic CO_2 retainers, this level may be 50 to 60 mm Hg. If a patient is a chronic CO_2 retainer but has been maintained with mechanical ventilation at a Pa_{CO_2} of 40 mm Hg, it is unlikely that this patient will be capable of maintaining a Pa_{CO_2} of 40 mm Hg while breathing spontaneously. Time must be taken to return the patient's acid-base status to its chronic normal before the attempt to wean (Table 19–20).

Intrapulmonary shunting should be acceptable. For most patients receiving mechanical ventilation, this amount would be a shunt of less than 15% to 20%, or an alveolar-arterial oxygen $P(A-a)_{O_2}$ gradient of ≤ 300 mm Hg or a $Pa_{O_2}/F_{I_{O_2}}$ ratio of greater than 2.[13, 56]

In addition, no indication of excessive dead space should be noted, because the greater the dead space, the harder the patient must work to maintain gas exchange. In general V_D/V_T ratios while the patient is ventilated should be less than 0.60, and no significant discrepancy between the expected minute volume and Pa_{CO_2} should be noted.[14]

Pulmonary and Cardiovascular System

In general, patients with acute pulmonary pathologic conditions are incapable of weaning from ventilatory support. That is, no acute pneumonia, atelectasis, pleural effusion, or pneumothorax should be present. In addition, patient temperature should be normal. As temperature increases, oxygen consumption and carbon dioxide production is increased, thus increasing the stress of ventilating spontaneously.

TABLE 19–20.

Gas Exchange Capabilities

Pa_{O_2}, 60 to 70 mm Hg at an $F_{I_{O_2}}$ of ≤ 0.40
Intrapulmonary shunt, $\leq 20\%$
$P(A-a)_{O_2}$, <300 mm Hg
$Pa_{O_2}/F_{I_{O_2}}$, >2
pH normal, 7.35–7.45
Pa_{CO_2} normal, 35–45 mm Hg
COPD patients at their normal range
V_D/V_T, $<60\%$

Cardiovascular reserves must be acceptable; the increased work of spontaneous ventilation will add additional stress to the cardiovascular system. Cardiac output should be normal; pulmonary and systemic hemodynamics must be acceptable. Heart rate should be normal, and no significant ventricular or atrial arrhythmias should be present.

Other Organ Systems

Spontaneous ventilatory capability is also dependent on all other major organ systems. Renal failure, central nervous system disturbances, gastrointestinal problems, and liver failure can all affect weaning. Thus, the status of these systems must be considered prior to weaning.

Most important, the patient's nutritional status and fluid and electrolyte balance must be appropriate.[2] Long-term, ventilator-dependent patients inappropriately maintained nutritionally may not have the capabilities to perform the increased work of spontaneous ventilation. Their CO_2 production may be increased, compromising their spontaneous ventilatory capabilities. Finally, electrolyte balance is essential for proper voluntary muscle function. Specifically, K^+, Cl^-, CA^{++}, PO_4^{---}, Mg^{++} should be within normal limits.[1, 10]

Psychologic Preparation

Last, and all too often forgotten, is the patient's psychologic preparation for the transition from mechanical ventilation to spontaneous ventilation. In short-term mechanical ventilation it is usually not a major concern; however, in patients maintained over a lengthy period on mechanical ventilation, it becomes an increasingly important factor.

Why, when, and how you are going to wean the patient should be carefully explained. Long-term, ventilator-dependent patients are understandably going to be frightened and anxious about the elimination of support that has been keeping them breathing. Explain the procedure in detail, reassure the patient of your continued presence, establish the patient's confidence in himself or herself by reinforcing the patient's progress. However, never tell patients they will not need to have mechanical ventilation restarted. If they repeatedly fail weaning, they will begin to lose confidence in themselves and to mistrust you. Simply inform them that you are evaluating how well they can breathe spontaneously and will reinstitute ventilation at a specific time, or when they start to fatigue. If they are capable of continuously maintaining spontaneous ventilation, let them do so.

Appropriate psychologic preparation can be a critical variable, especially with long-term, ventilator-dependent patients who have underlying chronic disease states, especially COPD patients, and should never be overlooked when you are preparing a patient for weaning.

Process of Weaning

Patients requiring short-term mechanical ventilation usually assume spontaneous ventilation very rapidly when physiologically prepared. Decreases in IMV/SIMV rates over a short period of time (4–8 hours) or simply complete discontinuance with close monitoring is acceptable in most cases. In patients requiring long-term mechanical ventilation, no cookbook approach that consistently works is available. Each patient must be considered an individual, and weaning protocols must be tailored to the patient's needs. In some, slowly decreasing IMV/SIMV rates over a number of days is appropriate. In others, alternating periods of spontaneous ventilation and mechanical ventilation are best. In many circumstances, weaning the long-term, ventilator-dependent patient becomes more of an art than a science. The patient must develop a rapport with the practitioner, and the practitioner must gain the patient's confidence and trust for weaning of this type of patient to be successful.

Weaning of long-term, ventilator-dependent patients requires very precise guidelines: specifically, what $F_{I_{O_2}}$, what rate if the IMV mode is used, how long spontaneously ventilating during periods off the ventilator? In addition, precise definition of when mechanical ventilation should be reinstituted must be written. For instance, if the Pa_{CO_2} is more than 60 mm Hg, the pulse rate more than 120/min, and respiratory rate greater than 25/min, mechanical ventilation should be immediately reinstituted. Finally, a respiratory therapist should be at the bedside throughout the weaning period if the patient can tolerate spontaneous ventilation for only short periods (<45 min). For long weaning periods, clinical judgment must be employed.

SUMMARY

This chapter has attempted to establish guidelines within an area of respiratory care filled with controversy. Guidelines presented are based on physiologic and scientific data. However, the scientific basis of this area is continually evolving; today's guidelines rapidly become tomorrow's history. Man-

agement of the mechanically ventilated patient is as much an art as it is a science, and all guidelines must be continually scrutinized and always tempered by clinical judgment.

REFERENCES

1. Agusti AH, Torres A, Estopa R: Hypophosphatemia as a cause of failed weaning—the importance of metabolic factors. *Crit Care Med* 1982; 12:142–143.
2. Barrocas A, Trotola R, Alonso A: Nutrition and the critically-ill pulmonary patient. *Respir Care* 1983; 28:50–61.
3. Bendixen H, Egbert LD: *Respiratory Care.* St Louis, CV Mosby Co, 1965.
4. Block ER: Recovery from hyperoxic depression of pulmonary 5-hydroxytryptamine clearance—effect of inspired PO_2 tension. *Lung* 1978; 155:131–140.
5. Bone R: Monitoring ventilatory mechanics in acute respiratory failure. *Respir Care* 1983; 28:597–603.
6. Brown AG, Pontoppidan H, Chiang H: Physiological criteria for weaning patients from prolonged artificial ventilation. Abstracts of Scientific Papers, Annual Meeting of the ASA, Boston, 1972.
7. Chaudhary BA, Burke NK: Ear oximetry in clinical practice. *Am Rev Respir Dis* 1978; 117:173–175.
8. Cheng EY, Renschler MF, Mihm FG: Noninvasive respiratory monitoring of patients during weaning from mechanical respiratory support. *Anesth Analg* 1986; 65:S29.
9. Cropp AJ, DiMarco AF, Attose MD: Effects of intermittent assisted ventilation in patients with severe chronic obstructive pulmonary disease. *Am Rev Respir Dis* 1984; 129:A34.
10. Dhingra S, Solven F, Wilson A: Hypomagnesemia and respiratory muscle power. *Am Rev Respir Dis* 1984; 129:497–498.
11. Douglas ME, Downs JB: Cardiopulmonary effects of PEEP and CPAP. *Anesth Analg* 1978; 57:347–350.
12. Engstrom Division of Gambro, Inc: *Engstrom Erica,* product literature. Engstrom Division of Gambro, Lincolnshire, Ill, 1983.
13. Feeley TW, Hedley-Whyte J: Weaning from controlled ventilation and supplemental oxygen—weaning from intermittent positive-pressure ventilation. *N Engl J Med* 1975; 292:903–906.
14. Fitzgerald LM, Huber GL: Weaning the patient from mechanical ventilation. *Heart Lung* 1976; 5:228–234.
15. Frank L, Massaro D: The lung and oxygen toxicity. *Arch Intern Med* 1979; 139:347–350.
16. Fuleihan SF, Wilson RS, Pontoppidan H: Effects of mechanical ventilation with end-inspiratory pause on blood-gas exchange. *Anesth Analg* 1976; 55:122–130.
17. Gallagher TJ, Civetta JM: Goal-directed therapy of acute respiratory failure. *Anesth Analg* 1980; 59:831–836.

18. Gherini S, Peters RM, Virgilio RW: Mechanical work on the lungs and work of breathing with positive end-expiratory pressure and continuous positive airway pressure. *Chest* 1979; 76:251–256.

19. Gibbons PA, Sedlow DB: Changes in oxygen saturation during elective tracheal intubation in infants [abstract]. *Anesth Analg* 1986; 65:S58.

20. Gibney RTN, Wilson RS, Pontoppidan H: Comparison of work of breathing on high gas flow and demand value continuous positive airway pressure systems. *Chest* 1982; 82:692–695.

21. Graham TM, Chang KSK, Stevens WC: Arterial oxygen desaturation and effect of supplemental O_2 during transit from OR to PAR utilizing a pulse oximeter [abstract]. *Anesth Analg* 1986; 65:S62.

22. Henry WC, West GA, Wilson RS: A comparison of the oxygen cost of breathing between a continuous-flow CPAP system and a demand-flow CPAP system. *Respir Care* 1983; 28:1273–1281.

23. Hobelmann CF, Smith DE, Virgilio RW, et al: Mechanics of ventilation with positive end-expiratory pressure. *Ann Thorac Surg* 1977; 24:68–74.

24. Hodgkin JE, Soeprono FF, Chan DM: Incidence of metabolic alkalemia in hospitalized patients. *Crit Care Med* 1980; 8:725–728.

25. Hotchkiss RS, Wilson RS: Mechanical ventilatory support. *Surg Clin North Am* 1983; 63:417–437.

26. Hutch R, Hutch A, Albani M, et al: Transcutaneous PO_2 monitoring in routine management of infants and children with cardiorespiratory problems. *Pediatrics* 1976; 57:681–686.

27. Ishikawa S, Linzmayer I, Segal MS: Clinical use of noninvasive method for determining oxygen saturation: Ear oximetry. *Ann Allergy* 1978; 41:17–20.

28. Jansson L, Jonson B: A theoretical study on flow patterns of ventilators. *Scand J Respir Dis* 1972; 53:237–246.

29. Johansson H: Effects of different gas flow patterns on central circulation during respiratory treatment. *Acta Anaesth Scand* 1975; 19:96–103.

30. Johansson H: Effects of different inspiratory gas flow patterns on thoracic compliance during respiratory treatment. *Acta Anaesth Scand* 1975; 19:89–95.

31. Kacmarek RM: To forestall ventilator trouble, first verify accuracy of settings. *Crit Care Mon* 1984; 4:1,6.

32. Kacmarek RM, Dimas S, Reynolds J, et al: Technical aspects of positive end-expiratory pressure: II. PEEP with positive pressure ventilation. *Respir Care* 1982; 27:1490–1504.

33. Kacmarek RM, Mack CM, Dimas S: *The Essentials of Respiratory Therapy*, ed 2. Chicago, Year Book Medical Publishers, 1985.

34. Kacmarek RM, Wilson RS: IMV systems: Do they make a difference [editorial]? *Chest* 1985; 87:557.

35. Kanak R, Fahey PJ, Vanderwarf C: Oxygen cost of breathing: Changes dependent upon mode of mechanical ventilation. *Chest* 1985; 87:126–127.

36. Katz JA, Kraemer RW, Gjerde GE: Inspiratory work and airway pressure with continuous positive airway pressure delivery systems. *Chest* 1985; 88:519–526.

37. Krauss AN, Waldman S, Frayer WW, et al: Noninvasive estimates of arterial oxygenation in newborn infants. *J Pediatr* 1978; 93:275–278.

38. Marini JJ, Capps JS, Culver BH: The inspiratory work of breathing during assisted mechanical ventilation. *Chest* 1985; 87:612–618.

39. McAslan TC, Matjasko-Chiu J, Turney SZ, et al: Influence of inhalation of 100% oxygen on intrapulmonary shunt in severely traumatized patients. *J Trauma* 1973; 13:811–821.

40. Michel L, McMichan JC, Marsh HM, et al: Measurement of ventilatory reserve as an indicator for early extubation after cardiac operation. *J Thorac Cardiol Surg* 1979; 78:761–764.

41. Mihn FG, Halperin BD: Non-invasive monitoring of respiratory failure with pulse oximetry and capnography [abstract]. *Anesthesiology* 1983; 59:A136.

42. Millbern SM, Downs JB, Junper LC, et al: Evaluation of criteria for discontinuing mechanical ventilatory support. *Arch Surg* 1978; 113:1441–1443.

43. Nunn JF: *Applied Respiratory Physiology*, ed 2. Stoneham, Mass, Butterworth, 1977.

44. Op't Holt TP, Hall MW, Bass JB, et al: Comparison of changes in airway pressure during continuous positive pressure (CPAP) between demand value and continuous flow devices. *Respir Care* 1982; 27:1200–1209.

45. Prakash O, Meij S: Cardiopulmonary response to inspiratory pressure support during spontaneous ventilation vs. conventional ventilation. *Chest* 1985; 88:403–408.

46. Puritan-Bennett Corporation: *7200 Ventilator*. Product literature. Overland Park, Kans, Puritan-Bennett Corp, 1985.

47. Rehder K, Sessler AD, Marsh HM: General anesthesia and the lung. *Am Rev Respir Dis* 1975; 112:541–563.

48. Reivich M: Arterial PCO_2 and cerebral hemodynamics. *Am J Physiol* 1964; 25:206–215.

49. Saunders NA, Powles ACP, ReBuck AS: Ear oximetry: Accuracy and practicability in the assessment of arterial oxygenation. *Am Rev Respir Dis* 1976; 113:745–749.

50. Scacci R, McMahon JL, Miller WF: Oxygen tension monitoring with cutaneous electrodes in adults. *Med Instrum* 1976; 10:192–196.

51. Shah DM, Newell JC, Dutton RE, et al: Continuous positive airway pressure versus positive end-expiratory pressure in respiratory distress syndrome. *J Thorac Cardiovasc Surg* 1977; 74:557–562.

52. Shapiro BA, Cane RD: The IMV-AMV controversy: A plea for clarification and redirection [editorial]. *Crit Care Med* 1984; 12:472–473.

53. Shapiro BA, Cane RD, Harrison RA: Positive end-expiratory pressure in acute lung injury. *Chest* 1983; 83:558–563.

54. Shapiro BA, Cane RD, Harrison RA, et al: Changes in intrapulmonary shunting with administration of 100% oxygen. *Chest* 1980; 77:138–144.

55. Shapiro BA, Harrison RA, Kacmarek RM, et al: *Clinical Application of Respiratory Care*, ed 3. Chicago, Year Book Medical Publishers, 1985.

56. Shapiro BA, Harrison RA, Walton JR: *Clinical Application of Blood Gases*, ed 3. Chicago, Year Book Medical Publishers, 1982.

57. Siemens-Elema Ventilator Systems: *Servo 900C*. Product literature. Schaumburg, Ill, Siemens-Elema, 1982.

58. Suter PM, Fairly HB, Isenberg MD: Optimal end-expiratory airway pressure and patients with acute pulmonary failure. *N Engl J Med* 1975; 292:284–290.

59. Viale JP, Annat G, Bertrand O: Additional inspiratory work in intubated patient breathing with continuous positive airway pressure systems. *Anesthesiology* 1985; 63:536–539.

60. Wollman H, et al: Effects of extremes of respiratory and metabolic alkalosis on cerebral blood flow in man. *J Appl Physiol* 1968; 24:60–72.

Deterioration Despite Intensive Respiratory Care

George G. Burton, M.D.

The reader will by now have learned the indications for starting (and, indeed, stopping) mechanical ventilation in patients with respiratory failure. The quantitative data that support these clinical decisions are fairly well established and, when they are intelligently used, generally ensure a smooth transition between the spontaneously breathing and mechanically ventilated states.

The purpose of this chapter is to discuss the patient who does not do well in the interval, who, despite what appears to be a correct initial diagnosis and good subsequent respiratory care, still has clinical deterioration of his condition rather than improvement, with therapy. Such patients will demonstrate worsening and oxygen-refractory hypoxemia, evidence of persistently abnormal pulmonary mechanics, unresolved or worsening chest radiographs, and difficulty in ventilator weaning, either singly or in combination. Laboratory data will show persistent elevation of the alveolar-arterial oxygen gradient ($P(A-a)O_2$) or decrease in the arterial/alveolar oxygen ratio as evidence of the patient's worsening status in addition to the disease- or condition-specific abnormalities to be discussed.

A myriad of pathophysiologic and mechanical factors can (and do) explain these phenomena.[2, 4] It may be difficult for the therapist to keep all the possibilities for such deterioration in mind. I have found it helpful to use a simple mnemonic (C-A-P P-N-E-U-M-O-N-I-A) to prod my memory. The therapist will do well to consider each of the possibilities suggested by the mnemonic, as he or she attempts to identify the etiology of the persisting or worsening respiratory failure (Fig 20–1).

Each of these conditions will be discussed separately, with an emphasis on the diagnosis rather than the therapy of each of these conditions. The reader is referred elsewhere for a discussion of the specific pertinent therapies.[2]

CARDIOVASCULAR COMPLICATIONS

Instability of cardiovascular function is an unfortunate, but not uncommon, complication or concomitant of respiratory care in critically ill patients. For this reason, most ventilator patients are as tightly, or even more closely, monitored than patients in coronary care units. Cardiac rate, cardiac rhythm, ECG morphology, and vascular pressures are usually all monitored in such patients, given the potential for arrhythmias, congestive heart failure (CHF), hydrostatic pulmonary edema, and systemic arterial hypotension or hypertension. Finally, the occurrence of acute myocardial infarction (AMI) while the patient is being artificially ventilated for another reason has recently been reported.[1]

Cardiac Arrhythmias

Almost any type of cardiac arrhythmia may occur in the critically ill patient. Contributing factors, in addition to myocardial ischemia, may include hypoxia, electrolyte disturbances, anxiety, and drug toxicity (theophylline and digitalis preparations).

Cardiovascular complications
Adult respiratory distress syndrome
Pulmonary emboli

Pneumothorax
Neuropsychiatric events
Electrolyte and fluid balance abnormalities
Upper airway obstruction
Malnutrition
Oxygen toxicity
Nonsense data
Infection
Atelectasis

FIG 20–1.
Mnemonic: causes of deterioration, or failure to respond, under intensive respiratory care.

The physiologic impact of such arrhythmias occurs when the filling (diastolic) volume of the left ventricle is reduced or the pump function of the heart is reduced (or both), leading to CHF and systemic hypotension. It is beyond the scope of this chapter to describe each of these arrhythmias in detail, but the reader should be able to recognize the basic rhythms listed in Table 20–1.

Should any of these arrhythmias be detected, prompt nursing and physician intervention should be sought. In the interval before normal cardiac function can be restored, the therapist may wish to temporarily increase the F_{IO_2} to 1.0 and to terminate the medication nebulization or tracheal suctioning that may have precipitated the arrhythmia.

Congestive Heart Failure

This complication of intensive respiratory care is not invariably evidenced by foaming pulmonary edema. A decrease in pulmonary compliance, widening of the $P(A-a)O_2$, and progressive pulmonary infiltrates may herald the development of either congestive heart failure (CHF) or the adult respiratory distress syndrome (ARDS), discussed in the next section. Differentiation between these two con-

TABLE 20–1.

Common Life-Threatening Cardiac Arrhythmias

Ventricular ectopy (extrasystoles)
Ventricular tachycardia and fibrillation
Complete heart block
Atrial fibrillation with ventricular rate > 130–150
Paroxysmal atrial tachycardia
Severe sinus bradycardia
Cardiac standstill (arrest)

---

ditions is made by history and by the finding of an elevated *pulmonary capillary wedge pressure* (PCWP) in CHF.

Fluid overload is a common cause of iatrogenic CHF, and intake and output records must be carefully examined when this condition is suspected. Other causes of hydrostatic pulmonary edema include decreased ventricular contractility (e.g., following an acute myocardial infarction), mitral stenosis or regurgitation, pericardial effusion, use of myocardial depressant drugs (e.g., the beta-blockers), systemic hypertension, and the cardiac arrhythmias as previously discussed. Other causes are sufficiently rare as to not warrant discussion here.

Systemic Hypotension

Tissue hypoxia will develop whenever the perfusion of blood falls below critical minima, no matter what the oxygen content of the perfusate. Most authorities currently agree that a systemic blood pressure less than 80 mm Hg, or a mean arterial pressure less than 60 mm Hg is critical. Hypotension may be cardiogenic (see earlier discussion), septic (e.g., in gram-negative septicemia), drug-induced (particularly with beta-blockers, hydralazine, and sodium nitroprusside), or as a result of high transpulmonary pressures (particularly with high positive end-expiratory pressures, or PEEP). The therapist should suspect hypotension or hypovolemia as the cause of tissue hypoxia when the cardiac output is normal or high, the PCWP is normal, and the mixed venous oxygen saturation ($S\bar{v}O_2$) is low.

In summary, the therapist should recall that the metabolic function of oxygen is at the cellular (indeed, the *mitochondrial* level). If examination of the lungs as a gas exchanger fails to indicate the source of difficulty, immediate attention should be given to the cardiovascular system and its contents (blood containing hemoglobin) as the possible culprit. The use of monitoring oxygen content (Hg [gm%] × SaO_2 × 1.34) and oxygen transport (cardiac output × oxygen content) has been discussed elsewhere in this volume.

Acute Myocardial Infarction

When one thinks about it, the clinical setting is right for acute myocardial infarction (AMI) complicating intensive respiratory care, especially when it may coexist with respiratory failure in chronic obstructive pulmonary disease (COPD). Stress, tobacco smoking, and obesity may preexist in both conditions. The intubated patient cannot complain of typical anginal chest pain, and the first indication of AMI developing in the intensive care unit (ICU) may be unexplained arrhythmias, hypotension, or CHF. The diagnosis is made by comparison of serial ECGs and cardiac enzyme determinations.

In the immediate peri-infarction period, care must be taken in the use of agents that enhance cardiac irritability, notably theophylline-containing products and beta-adrenergic stimulants.

ADULT RESPIRATORY DISTRESS

The high-permeability pulmonary edema (HPPE) of the adult respiratory distress syndrome (ARDS) frequently is the cause of respiratory insufficiency. Not so well recognized is the fact that ARDS may develop while the patient is being ventilated for an altogether different reason! Conditions that underlie ARDS do not disappear in the ICU, and infection, hypotension, transfusion of blood, and aspiration may certainly occur in the best of hands.

Many signs of deterioration will be present in full-blown ARDS. The only important differentials are widespread pneumonitis and hydrostatic pulmonary edema (already discussed). In ARDS and pneumonitis, the PCWP is normal, in hydrostatic pulmonary edema, it will be elevated, and, thus, measurement of the PCWP will guide diagnosis as well as therapy. The student is urged to refer to standard textbooks to review the diagnosis and therapy of this serious and common condition.[2, 4]

PULMONARY EMBOLI

Pulmonary embolism arising from systemic venous thrombi still complicates the prolonged immobilization of critically ill patients, although there is some evidence that the incidence of this significant cause of morbidity and mortality is decreasing.[9] A sudden, precipitous deterioration in the ventilator patient's condition may herald the occurrence of this event.

The alert therapist will recognize tachypnea, tachycardia, a right ventricular gallop rhythm, and hypotension as possible indications of a pulmonary embolic event. Awareness of the patient's increased dead space/tidal volume ratio (V_D/V_T) with use of a nomogram developed by Selecky et al. will also be helpful.[10]

The chest radiographic signs of pulmonary em-

bolism are nonspecific at best and must not be relied on to make the diagnosis. Results of bedside perfusion lung scans using radionuclide may be abnormal, but interpretation of this test may be difficult without a simultaneous ventilation lung scan. The gold standard diagnostic test is pulmonary angiography, where the emboli will appear as filling defects in the pulmonary arterial tree.

There is no respiratory therapy technique specific to the treatment of pulmonary emboli disease. Maintenance of oxygenation is important, usually delivered in this situation by temporarily increasing the FI_{O_2}. Anticoagulant therapy with heparin or thrombolytics is not without hazard, particularly in the traumatized or postsurgical patient, in whom bleeding may occur.

PNEUMOTHORAX

The intubated patient cannot complain of anything, let alone the chest pain and severe air hunger that may reflect the development of a pneumothorax in the classic, nonintubated setting. Indeed, the development of pneumothorax in the ICU is being recorded more and more frequently as a result of both disease processes and iatrogenically (Table 20–2).[6] The mortality of pneumothorax and other types of barotrauma complicating respiratory failure is not insignificant.

The sudden onset of a pneumothorax may be recognized by a rapid decrease in dynamic compliance requiring higher ventilator cycling pressures, sudden onset of tachycardia or bradycardia, evidence of mediastinal shift at the bedside or by chest radiograph, evidence of hyperresonance over the affected pneumothorax, or any combination thereof.

Treatment consists of the prompt, expert placement of a chest tube (tube thoracostomy). The use of *prophylactic chest tubes* to prevent pneumothorax in

TABLE 20–2.

Causes of Pneumothorax in the Intensive Care Unit

DISEASE CONDITIONS	IATROGENIC
Bullous emphysema	After thoracotomy
Necrotizing pneumonia, tuberculosis	After bronchoscopy (usually with biopsy)
ARDS	Positive end-expiratory pressure
Sepsis, hypovolemia	Central vascular catheterization
Bronchopleural fistula	High ventilator cycling pressures and rates (pulmonary barotrauma)

high PEEP and in lungs requiring high peak inspiratory cycling pressures is still open to debate.[6]

NEUROPSYCHIATRIC EVENTS

Intracranial Catastrophies

Intracranial catastrophies (e.g., ruptured cerebral aneurysms) can complicate respiratory care of ventilator patients. Use of *sedatives, anesthetic agents,* and *muscular relaxants* can decrease the utility of the periodic neurologic examinations in critically ill patients. *Cephalogenic pulmonary edema* as a sequela of sudden increases in intracranial pressure (ICP) is well known, as are the deleterious effects of *hypoxemia* (PaO$_2$ of <60 mm Hg) on cerebral blood flow.

The so-called *ICU syndrome* is well known to any therapist working for long with critically ill patients, though its scientific basis is far from clear. The syndrome, which evidences itself as patient irritability, confusion, fear, anger, and even frank psychosis interferes with many aspects of respiratory care, particularly that of ventilator weaning.

Often forgotten is the fact that blood gas changes in themselves may produce neuropsychiatric effects. In this context *psychiatric complaints* such as depression, irritability, loss of judgment, nonspecific confusion, lack of concentration, *free-floating anxiety*, and frank paranoia have been reported in normal volunteers made experimentally hypoxemic.[2, 5] On the other hand, changes in *neurologic status*, such as tetany and convulsions with alkalemia, and asterixis, somnolence, and frank coma with acidosis, as a result of pH aberrations are also well recognized.

Thus, we see that neuropsychiatric events can be either the cause or effect of abnormalities in respiratory gas exchange. An increasingly sophisticated literature documents the use of invasive and noninvasive techniques in the diagnosis and monitoring of intracranial function, such as continuously monitored EEG, ICP, cerebral blood flow (CBF) by positron emission tomography (PET), bedside computed tomography (CT), and sensory evoked potential determinations.[5]

ELECTROLYTE AND FLUID BALANCE ABNORMALITIES

Recent literature has stressed meticulous attention to fluid and electrolyte balance as essential to the success of processes as diverse as weaning the COPD patient from ventilator support to optimal management of patients with ARDS.[4] For purposes of convenience, the two will be considered separately here.

Electrolyte Balance

The cations sodium (Na$^+$) and potassium (K$^+$) are essential to neuromuscular metabolism. Hyponatremia frequently causes confusion and muscular weakness when the serum sodium concentration falls below 125 to 130 mEq/L. Hypokalamia causes cardiac arrhythmias and reduced skeletal and smooth muscle contraction when serum potassium levels fall below 3.0 mEq/L. Thus, cardiac arrhythmias, abdominal ileus, and muscle weakness (both diaphragm and skeletal muscle) should alert the respiratory care worker to check these laboratory parameters in the difficult to wean patient.

The anions bicarbonate (HCO$_3^-$), phosphate (PO$_4^=$), and chloride (Cl$^-$) are important in the body acid-base and energy economy. Metabolic alkalemia is the most common acid-base abnormality seen in our blood gas laboratory. The reader will recall that respiratory compensation for this abnormality consists of alveolar hypoventilation, not at all desired in the weaning process.

Furthermore, alkalotic blood has an increased affinity for oxygen, again, not as a desired situation in the already hypoxic patient. Recent work has stressed the importance of phosphate in muscular metabolism and the not infrequent association of malnutrition-induced hypophosphatemia and difficulty in discontinuing ventilation support.[8]

Fluid Balance

No one has worked in an ICU for long before he or she becomes aware of the hazards of both overhydration and underhydration in the ventilated patient. Although the judicious use of the pulmonary artery (Swan-Ganz) catheter has helped bring a more rational physiologic basis to the use of fluids and vasoactive drugs, mistakes are still made that could have been avoided by nothing more complicated than at least daily attention to intake and output records.

Ventilator patients who are overhydrated will demonstrate falling pulmonary compliance, widening of the A-aDO$_2$, evidence of CHF on the chest radiograph, and elevation of the PCWP above the normal 6 to 12 mm Hg. Clearly such patients will meet our criteria of deterioration under intensive respiratory care. Therapy will consist of reduction in the infusion rate of parenteral fluids, restriction of oral fluid intake, and prudent use of diuretic medication.

Underhydration in ventilated patients may present as cardiovascular instability (hypotension) with the use of PEEP, thickening of respiratory mucus, and oliguria. The therapist should recall the adage that "there is no mucolytic like water" and always consider dehydration as a cause for thick tenacious respiratory secretions. By way of treatments, hydration of the airway by direct instillation of normal saline, humidification of inspired gases, or ultrasonic nebulization of fluids should all be considered.

UPPER AIRWAY OBSTRUCTION

The simple fact that the ventilator patient is intubated or has a tracheotomy does not preclude the possibility of upper airway obstruction. The presence of this complication may be first suggested by the observation of "suctioning difficulty," though it may not always be the case (see discussion that follows). A sudden increase in dynamic airway resistance may be reflected in an elevation of peak airway pressure on the ventilator or by an increase in the frequency of nonmandated spontaneous breaths in the patient on intermittent mandatory mode of ventilation (IMV mode). Cough and substernal discomfort may represent the development of tracheitis.

Large airway mucus plugging (Fig 20–2), gastric content or foreign body aspiration, previously unrecognized tracheal stenosis, hemorrhage, and herniation of balloon cuffs over the distal end of the tracheostomy or endotracheal tube may manifest in this manner. Inadvertent intubation of the right mainstem bronchus or esophagus and kinking of the endotracheal tube may also be thought of as large airway complications of ventilator care.

In all of these situations, a ball-valve type of mechanism may be present in that a suction catheter may push aside the obstruction on insertion. Accordingly, bronchoscopy through the endotracheal tube may be necessary to diagnose and treat these complications of intensive respiratory care.

MALNUTRITION

Recent surveys have indicated a 10% to 20% incidence of clinically significant malnutrition in hospitalized patients in the United States.[8] In ventilator patients, malnutrition significantly contributes to overall morbidity and mortality by (1) reducing the competence of both cellular and humoral defense

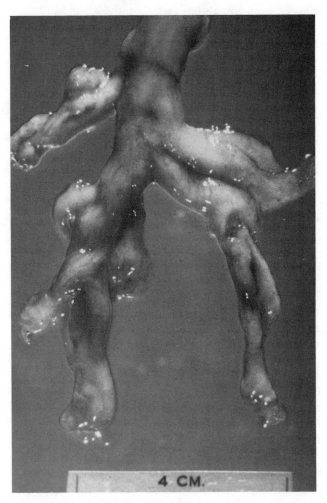

FIG 20–2.
A mucus plug, a perfect cast of the first three generations of airway, removed at the time a tracheotomy was performed in a dehydrated patient with chronic bronchitis.

mechanisms; (2) causing weakness of the respiratory muscles, thus causing alveolar hypoventilation and difficulty in ventilator weaning; and (3) causing decreased mobility resulting in a progressive deconditioning dyspnea–immobility-deconditioning vicious cycle.

Brief physical examination should compare the patient's observed weight with normal standards for sex, age, and height. Clinical evidence of weakness, muscle wasting, loss of fat stores, glossitis, easy bruisability, and edema should also be observed. More precise determinations include the midarm muscle circumference and the creatinine excretion index.

Laboratory studies may reveal anemia, lymphocytopenia, and hypoalbuminuria or a reduction in transferrin and serum cholesterol. Delayed or reduced hypersensitivity to various recall antigens (mumps, *Candida*, histoplasmin, *Trichophyton*, purified protein derivative, and streptokinase/streptodornase) may also be present.

Treatment is relatively specific to the identified component deficiencies and may be achieved by oral-gastric hyperalimentation or intravenous total parenteral nutrition (TPN). Patients who have good gastric emptying and who have neither ileus nor diarrhea should probably receive a trial of hyperalimentation before resorting to TPN.[8]

OXYGEN TOXICITY

Although clinically significant pulmonary oxygen toxic effects are rare, they certainly must be considered in our differential diagnosis of the seriously ill, ventilated patient. The toxic effects of the oxygen metabolites (superoxides, peroxides, and hydroxy radicals have been studied extensively in experimental animals).[1, 2] There, one sees an acute exudative phase with alveolar edema, atelectasis, and hemorrhage and a later chronic proliferative phase with fibroblastic proliferation and hyaline membrane formation. The time course of symptoms and laboratory findings in human volunteers breathing humidified 100% oxygen is seen in Table 20–3.

At the bedside, these effects may be perceived as decreasing pulmonary compliance requiring higher and higher ventilator peak pressures, widening of the $P(A-a)O_2$, and progressive infiltrates in the chest radiograph. In themselves, these changes are nonspecific (see the section on ARDS).

It should be stressed that no changes in pulmonary function or gas exchange have been documented in human subjects breathing 60% oxygen or less for days or weeks.[1, 2] There is, however, some evidence to support the notion that pulmonary infection, other preexisting pulmonary diseases, and use of high ventilator cycling pressures may accelerate the effects outlined in Table 20–3.

There is no specific therapy at present for pulmonary oxygen toxicity, and prevention is the best cure. In patients with normal oxygen-carrying capacity, cardiac output, and preserved regional blood flow, there is no need for oxygen therapy that will result in PaO_2 tensions above 50 to 60 mm Hg.

The fear of oxygen toxicity is almost worse than the condition itself. There is absolutely no evidence that short (<5 hours) periods of 100% oxygen would result in parenchymal oxygen toxicity.[1] In critical situations, this therapeutic window may be used to sort out and treat other causes of abnormal or deteriorating pulmonary gas exchange. Alveolar hypoventilation as an effect of oxygen therapy is related to supplemental oxygen satisfying a patient's hypoxic drive. Termed "carbon dioxide narcosis" in earlier literature, it is not a form of oxygen toxicity.

NONSENSE DATA

There is no place in the hospital where more data generators, data collectors, and data interpreters vector their skills than on the ventilator patient in the ICU. Thus, the possibility exists that some information may be, quite simply, *wrong*; a clinical response to such erroneous data may be more wrong still. Erroneous response to nonsense data is a real enough possibility to be worth a moment's consideration. Some examples may be illustrative.

Wrong Patient
Could there be two Mary Kellys, both on ventilators in one 500-bed hospital at the same time? Yes, and their laboratory data got hopelessly mixed up for the first 24-hours! Can a hospitalized, nonsmoking patient have a carboxyhemoglobin level of 10 vol%? No, it was a blood gas drawn from a smoker in the next room.

Wrong Intake and Output Data
The clinical importance of intake and output records for optimal fluid and ventilator management has already been discussed. Errors in addition and lost (or thrown away) urine specimens present significant errors in therapeutic management. A plea can be made for frequent daily patient weights and prudent use of pulmonary artery catheters as independent cross-references.[9]

Erroneous Blood Gas Determinations
There is no single laboratory value of more importance in the management of ventilator patients

TABLE 20–3.

Oxygen Toxicity Effects in Normal Human Volunteers

TIME COURSE, HR*	LABORATORY FINDINGS
6–12	Nonproductive cough, tracheobronchitis, substernal pain, paresthesias, nausea
24	Reduction in pulmonary compliance
30	Decrease in pulmonary diffusion capacity
60	Progressive decrease in vital capacity

*All times are approximate.

than the correctly performed arterial blood gas (ABG) determination. Errors that may arise include wrong patient (already discussed), input data error, sampling error, timing error, analysis error, and charting error.

Input Error.—Blood gas analysis depends on a knowledge of patient temperature, whereas blood gas interpretation requires a precise knowledge of FI_{O_2}, if known, as well as hemoglobin. Data input errors will result in nonsensical aberrations in patient data. For example, a PaO_2 of 150 mm Hg is possible if a patient with pulmonary disease is breathing 100% O_2; it is nonsense data by virtue of the alveolar air equation if he or she is breathing room air.

Sampling Error.—Contrary to popular belief, venous blood can pulsate into a syringe and thus be erroneously reported as arterial blood. In the non-cyanotic patient who is not tachycardic or tachypnic on room air at rest and whose PaO_2 is reported at 20 mm Hg, the therapist should suspect venous blood!

Analysis Error.—Even in the best of laboratories, direct analysis errors may occasionally happen. Any laboratory measurement, as well as blood gas measurements, can be subject to analysis error. Again, if the laboratory data do not agree with clinical observation of the patient, a repeat blood gas sample should be analyzed.

Timing Error.—If arterial blood gases are sampled too soon or too long after a ventilator parameter change, another sort of error may occur. For example, if PEEP has just been added to a ventilator setting, 10 to 20 minutes should elapse before blood gas determinations may accurately be performed for areas of lung with long time constants to be affected by the PEEP addition. However, arterial blood gases can and do change within seconds. A patient with normal blood gases one minute may be profoundly hypoxemic the next, as a result of massive pulmonary emboli or extensive atelectasis. Again, the caution should be that if the blood gas does not agree with the clinical findings, the blood gas determination should be repeated.

Charting Error.—When data need to be electronically or manually transferred from one piece of paper (e.g., a laboratory slip) to another (e.g., the patient chart), another source of error is present. Charting error may take the wrong patient track previously mentioned or may simply consist of inverted numbers, such as a PaO_2 of 47 instead of 74 mm Hg or a Pa_{CO_2} of 36 being reported as a PaO_2 of 36 mm Hg.

Radiographic Error

Chest radiographic findings impact on care of the ventilator patient nearly as strongly as blood gas results. Care must be taken to neither underread nor overread portable chest x-rays, which have similar potential errors of wrong patient, timing, and charting as previously discussed. In addition, technique differences (exposure, phase of respiration), patient position difference, and film labeling errors (left, right, erect, supine, decubitus) are potential sources of error.

Erroneous Sputum Analyses

Careful bacteriologic monitoring of respiratory secretions is a vital part of good respiratory care. The therapist should attempt to ascertain the clinical relevance of sputum analysis and not overreact to a laboratory finding that may suggest colonization rather than infection of the airways.[7] This topic is discussed further in the next section.

Medication Error

Regrettably, even in the best intensive care units, medication errors can occur. *Polypharmacy* is a term that reflects the large number of pharmacologic agents used in the care of the critically ill patient. If this type of error is suspected, the therapist should check the nurse's record of drugs *given* rather than spending too much time inquiring as to what medication was *ordered*.

Respiratory Therapy Error

Respiratory care practitioners are not themselves immune from performance as well as knowledge errors. Respiratory therapy errors may be of commission or omission, but both contribute to the generation of nonsense data.

Physicians do not usually differentiate between the error hazard in the use of intravenous and inhaled pharmacologic agents; they expect that an ultrasonic aerosol treatment will be given (if ordered) just as certainly as intravenous digoxin or penicillin. The alleged reason or reasons that therapy sessions are missed are numerous.

It is the responsibility of the therapist to ensure that the record of his or her therapeutic interaction with the patient is legibly charted, accurate, concise, and available for review by physicians and nursing staff. Also, he or she must not contribute to the potential problem of nonsense data in anyway whatsoever.

INFECTION

Pulmonary infection is a frequent cause of respiratory failure. Infection may also be a cause of deterioration in ventilated patients, even with bronchial hygiene practices that are excellent, particularly in the immune-suppressed patient. Though development of acute or subacute *bronchitis* and *pneumonia* are perhaps the most common nosocomial infections in ventilator patients, one must also suspect *sinusitis*, infected *decubitus ulcers* of the skin, and *urinary tract infections* as causing the observed changes. Associated with any of these conditions, sepsis and the hypermetabolic state may complicate the situation still further.

Patients with pulmonary infection may have a fever, a change in color or viscosity of sputum, an infiltrate on the chest radiograph, peripheral sputum leukocytosis (or both), and a change in the bacteriologic flora of respiratory secretions. Septicemia, with or without hypotension, may occur in as many as 20% of infected patients.[7] The respiratory care worker must be careful to differentiate between no-

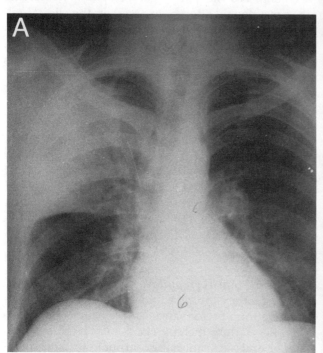

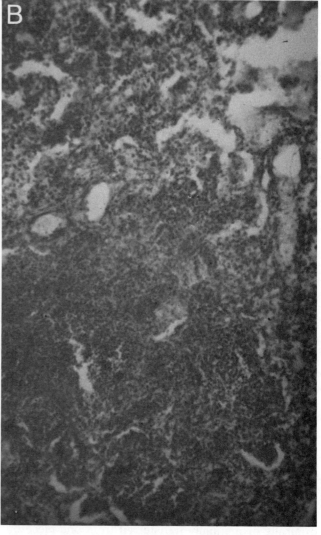

FIG 20–3.
Lobar pneumonia in a 38-year-old male smoker with diabetes melitus. Classic lobar consolidation is seen on the chest radiograph **(A).** Diffuse alveolar filling with bacteria leukocytes and fibrina-ceous debris are seen in the photomicrograph **(B)** of tissue removed at autopsy.

socomial colonization and nosocomial infection; only in the latter will two or more of the classic findings just listed be present.

The fact that not all significant respiratory infections manifest as significant radiographic infiltrates is illustrated in Figures 20–3 and 20–4. In Figure 20–4,A, a pneumonic infiltrate was never seen, although significant bronchopneumonia was present at autopsy. Failing prevention, the accurate determination of the offending pathogen is the key to successful therapy, and bronchoscopy with shielded brush washing, alveolar lavage, and even transthoracic needle biopsy may be necessary to achieve this

end. The interested reader is urged to study this important subject in more detail.[3]

ATELECTASIS

Mucus plugging of large or small airways is a well-recognized complication of acute respiratory care. When it occurs, lung segments distal to the obstructed airways will become airless (atelectatic) and blood passing through them will not participate in the gas exchange oxygenation progress. This shunt-like effect will be appreciated as oxygen-refractory

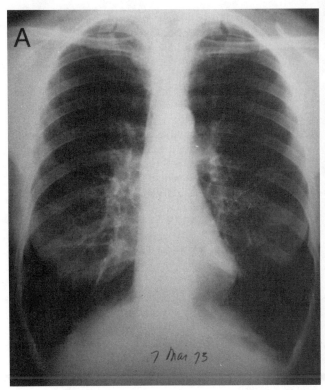

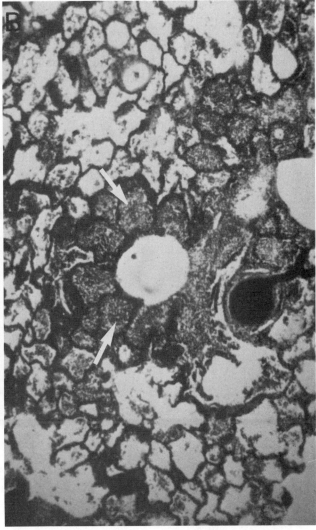

FIG 20–4.
Chest radiograph **(A)** and photomicrograph **(B)** of lung tissue removed at autopsy in a 55-year-old woman with antitrypsin deficiency. Note that hyperaeration of the lungs is easily seen in the radiograph *(left)* but that no clear evidence of pneumonitis is present despite the clear involvement of peribronchial alveoli *(arrow)* with inflammatory infiltrate (bronchopneumonia) in the autopsy specimen.

hypoxemia, with widening of the $P(A-a)O_2$ difference. Pulmonary compliance may decrease, and lobar, segmental, subsegmental, or widespread diffuse infiltrates may be seen in the chest radiograph. Atelectasis may, of course, occur at the level of the terminal respiratory unit (so-called microatelectasis), in which case it will not be radiographically visible at all.

Development of atelectasis is particularly common in the postoperative period, in patients with thick, tenacious secretions, in patients in whom the ventilator tidal volume is small (<10 to 12 ml/kg), in ventilated patients in whom periodic ventilator sighs are not provided, in obese patients and patients with pulmonary emboli, and in patients with fluid volume overload. Treatment includes chest physical therapy, bronchial suctioning, bronchoalveolar lavage, therapeutic bronchoscopy, and reworking of ventilator orders to include sighs, larger tidal volumes, and, if appropriate, PEEP.

SUMMARY

Some order can be brought out of the chaos that turns around the critically ill ventilator patient who, despite efforts to the contrary, is not doing well. More often than not, the errors that are made are those of cognitive omission rather than diagnostic or therapeutic commission. I hope that the approach outlined herein will be helpful to the readers who find themselves and their patients in such situations.

REFERENCES

1. Brown DL: Pulmonary barotrauma, in Kirby RR, Taylor RW (eds): *Respiratory Failure*. Chicago, Year Book Medical Publishers, 1986, pp 602–611.
2. Burton GG, Hodgkin JE: *Respiratory Care: A Guide to Clinical Practice*, ed 2. Philadelphia, JB Lippincott & Co, 1984, section 3.
3. Crawford GE: *Infectious Disease Problems in Respiratory Failure*, in Kirby RR, Taylor RW (eds): *Respiratory Failure*. Chicago, Year Book Medical Publishers, 1986, pp 365–386.
4. Kirby RR, Taylor RW (eds): *Respiratory Failure*. Chicago, Year Book Medical Publishers, 1986.
5. Luce JM: Neurologic monitoring. *Respir Care* 1985; 30:471.
6. Miller KS, Sahn SA: Chest tubes—indications, technique, management and complications. *Chest* 1987; 91:258.
7. Pennington JE: *Respiratory Infections: Diagnosis and Management*. New York, Raven Press, 1983.
8. Proctor CO Sr: Nutritional support, in Kirby RR, Taylor RW (eds): *Respiratory Failure*. Chicago, Year Book Medical Publishers, 1986, pp 496–514.
9. Robin ED: The cult of the Swan-Ganz catheter: Overuse and abuse of pulmonary-flow catheters. *Ann Intern Med* 1985; 102:445.
10. Selecky PA, Wasserman K, Klein M, et al: A graphic approach to assessing interrelationships among minute ventilation, arterial carbon dioxide tension, and ratio of physiologic dead space to tidal volume in patients on respirators. *Am Rev Respir Dis* 1978; 117:185.

Appendix A

Major Drug Families

Joseph L. Rau, Jr., Ph.D., R.R.T.

A useful learning technique as well as memory aid with drugs is to group the numerous agents by class. Instead of attempting to remember each drug's purpose, the reader is better off learning the purpose of an entire class and then becoming familiar with the specific agents in that class. New drugs can be understood by locating their class. As knowledge increases, different modes of action within a class can be identified. Such an organizational hierarchy is presented in this appendix. The first section lists some helpful sources of drug information for those seeking a better understanding of clinical pharmacology.

SOURCES OF DRUG INFORMATION

Reference Texts

The United States Pharmacopeia, rev 21: *The National Formulary*, ed 16 [USP-NF]. Rockville, Md, United States Pharmacopeial Convention, 1985.

Physicians' Desk Reference [PDR], ed 41. Oradell, NJ, Medical Economics Co, 1987 (or current year's edition).

Drug Facts and Comparisons. St Louis, Facts and Comparisons, Division of JB Lippincott Co, 1987.

General Texts

Gilman AG, Goodman LS, Rall TW, et al (eds): *Goodman and Gilman's The Pharmacological Basis of Therapeutics*, ed 7. New York, Macmillan Publishing Co, 1985.

Respiratory Pharmacology Texts

Cherniack RM (ed): *Drugs for the Respiratory System*. New York, Grune & Stratton, 1986.

Lehnert BE, Schachter EN: *The Pharmacology of Respiratory Care*. St Louis, CV Mosby Co, 1980.

Rau JL Jr: *Respiratory Therapy Pharmacology*, ed 2. Chicago, Year Book Medical Publishers, 1984.

Ziment I: *Respiratory Pharmacology and Therapeutics*. Philadelphia, WB Saunders Co, 1978.

RESPIRATORY CARE (BRONCHOACTIVE) DRUGS

Sympathomimetic (Adrenergic) Bronchodilators
Epinephrine
Isoproterenol (Isuprel)
Isoetharine (Bronkosol)
Metaproterenol (Alupent, Metaprel)
Terbutaline (Brethine, Bricanyl)
Albuterol (Proventil, Ventolin)
Bitolterol (Tornalate)

Parasympatholytic (Anticholinergic) Bronchodilators
Atropine
Glycopyrrolate (Robinul)
Ipratopium (Atrovent)

Xanthine Bronchodilators
Theophylline
Aminophylline

Mucolytics and Expectorants
Acetylcysteine (Mucomyst)
Sodium bicarbonate
Saline (isotonic, hypotonic, hypertonic)
Distilled water

Surface-active Agent
Ethyl alcohol

Corticosteroids
Dexamethasone (Decadron)
Beclomethasone (Vanceril, Beclovent)
Triamcinolone (Azmacort)
Flunisolide (AeroBid)

Antiasthmatics
Cromolyn sodium (Intal, Aarane)

RELATED DRUG CLASSES

In addition to bronchoactive agents, many of which are given by aerosol, the following drug classes are of interest to respiratory care personnel.

Antibiotics, Antibacterial, and Antiviral Agents

Penicillins
Penicillin G
Penicillin V
Oxacillin (Prostaphlin)
Cloxacillin (Tegopen)
Methicillin (Staphcillin)
Ampicillin (Omnipen)
Amoxicillin (Polymox)
Carbenicillin (Geopen)

Cephalosporins
Cephalexin (Keflex)
Cephalothin (Keflin)
Cephaloridine (Loridine)
Cephradine (Velosef)
Cephaloglycin (Kafocin)
Cefaclor (Ceclor)
Cefotaxime (Claforan)
Ceftizoxime (Cefizox)
Cefoperazone (Cefobid)

Aminoglycosides
Streptomycin
Gentamicin (Garamycin)
Tobramycin (Nebcin)
Kanamycin (Kantrex)
Amikacin (Amikin)
Neomycin (Neosporin)
Netilmicin (Netromycin)

Tetracyclines
Tetracycline (Achromycin)
Oxytetracycline (Terramycin)
Chlortetracycline (Aureomycin)
Demeclocycline (Declomycin)

Methacycline (Rondomycin)
Doxycycline (Vibramycin)
Minocycline (Minocin)

Miscellaneous Antibiotic Agents
Chloramphenicol (Chloromycetin)
Erythromycin (E-Mycin, Ilotycin)
Clindamycin (Cleocin)
Spectinomycin (Trobicin)
Polymyxin B sulfate
Colistin sulfate (Coly-Mycin S)
Vancomycin (Vancocin)
Bacitracin (Baciguent)
Metronidazole (Flagyl)
Trimethoprim-sulfamethoxazole (Bactrim)
Pentamidine (Pentam)

Antifungal Agents
Amphotericin B (Fungizone)
Nystatin (Mycostatin)
Griseofulvin (Grisactin, Fulvicin-U/F)

Antituberculosis Agents
Isoniazid (INH)
Rifampin (Rifadin, Rimactane)
Ethambutol (Myambutol)
Streptomycin
p-Aminosalicylic acid (PAS)
Cycloserine (Seromycin)

Antiviral Agents
Acyclovir (Zovirax)
Amantadine (Symmetrel)
Rimantadine
Ribavirin (Virazole)
Idoxuridine (Herplex)
Vidarabine (Vira-A)
Interferon
Zidovudine (Retrovir)

CARDIOVASCULAR AGENTS

Cardiac Agents

Cardiac Glycosides
Digitoxin
Digoxin (Lanoxin)
Ouabain

Antiarrhythmics
Quinidine
Lidocaine (Xylocaine)
Procainamide (Pronestyl)

Phenytoin (Dilantin)
Propranolol (Inderal)
Bretylium (Bretylol)
Verapamil (Calan)
Calcium chloride
Atropine
Disopyramide (Norpace)
Mexiletine (Mexitil)
Encainide (Enkaid)
Flecainide (Tambocor)
Esmolol (Brevibloc)

Cardiac Stimulants
Epinephrine
Isoproterenol
Dobutamine (Dobutrex)

Antihypertensives
Hydralazine (Apresoline)
Methyldopa (Aldomet)
Clonidine (Catapres)
Guanethidine (Ismelin)
Reserpine (Serpasil)
Sodium nitroprusside (Nipride)
Diazoxide (Hyperstat)
Guanfacine (Tenex)

β_1-Blockers
Metoprolol (Lopressor)
Atenolol (Tenormin)

β_1- and β_2-Blockers
Propranolol (Inderal)
Nadolol (Corgard)
Timolol (Blocadren)
Pindolol (Visken)

α-Blockers
Prazosin (Minipress)
Phentolamine (Regitine)
Tolazoline (Priscoline)

Coronary Vasodilators

Organic Nitrates
Amyl nitrite
Nitroglycerin (Nitro-Bid)
Isosorbide dinitrate (Isordil)
Erythrityl tetranitrate (Cardilate)
Pentaerythritol tetranitrate (Pentritol)

Calcium Blockers
Nifedipine (Procardia)
Verapamil (Calan)

Miscellaneous Coronary Vasodilators
Dipyridamole (Persantine)

Vasopressors
Phenylephrine
Norepinephrine
Dopamine
Metaraminol (Aramine)
Mephentermine (Wyamine)
Methoxamine (Vasoxyl)

Anticoagulants
Heparin
Dicumarol
Warfarin (Coumadin)

Diuretics
Acetazolamide (Diamox)
Mannitol (Osmitrol)
Chlorothiazide (Diuril)
Hydrochlorothiazide (Esidrix)
Chlorothalidone (Hygroton)
Cyclothiazide (Anhydron)
Furosemide (Lasix)
Ethacrynic acid (Edecrin)
Triamterene (Dyrenium)
Triamterene with hydrochlorothiazide (Dyazide)

NEUROMUSCULAR BLOCKING AGENTS

Nondepolarizing Neuromuscular Blocking Agents
Tubocurarine (*d*-tubocurarine)
Metocurine (Metubine)
Gallamine (Flaxedil)
Pancuronium (Pavulon)
Vecuronium (Norcuron)
Atracurium (Tracrium)

Depolarizing Neuromuscular Blocking Agents
Succinylcholine (Quelicin, Anectine)

SEDATIVES, HYPNOTICS, AND TRANQUILIZERS

Barbiturates

Long-acting Barbiturates
Barbital
Phenobarbital (Luminal)

Intermediate-acting Barbiturates
Pentobarbital (Nembutal)
Butabarbital (Butisol)
Amobarbital (Amytal)

Short-acting Barbiturate
Secobarbital (Seconal)

Ultra-short-acting Barbiturates
Thiopental (Pentothal)
Hexobarbital (Sombulex)

Nonbarbiturate Hypnotics

Paraldehyde
Chloral hydrate (Noctec)
Glutethimide (Doriden)
Ethchlorvynol (Placidyl)

Antianxiety Agents

Chlordiazepoxide hydrochloride (Librium)
Diazepam (Valium)
Flurazepam (Dalmane)
Oxazepam (Serax)
Meprobamate (Miltown, Equanil)
Lorazepam (Ativan)
Clorazepate (Tranxene, Azene)
Prazepam (Centrax)
Triazolam (Halcion)
Halazepam (Paxipam)
Alprazolam (Xanax)
Midazolam (Versed)

ANTIPSYCHOTIC AGENTS

Neuroleptics

Phenothiazines
Fluphenazine (Prolixin)
Trifluoperazine (Stelazine)
Prochlorperazine (Compazine)*
Thioridazine (Mellaril)
Chlorpromazine (Thorazine)*
Promazine (Sparine)*
Promethazine (Phenergan)*

Butyrophenones
Haloperidol (Haldol)

*Also used as antiemetic.

Miscellaneous Neuroleptics
Loxapine (Loxitane)
Molindone (Moban)
Reserpine

Antidepressants

Tricyclic Antidepressants
Amitriptyline (Elavil)
Imipramine (Tofranil)
Doxepin (Sinequan)
Trimipramine (Surmontil)
Nortriptyline (Aventyl)
Desipramine (Norpramin)
Protriptyline (Vivactil)
Amoxapine (Asendin)

Tetracyclic Antidepressants
Maprotiline (Ludiomil)

Monoamine Oxidase Inhibitors
Isocarboxazid (Marplan)
Phenelzine (Nardil)
Tranylcypromine (Parnate)

ANALGESICS

Narcotic Analgesics
Morphine
Codeine
Hydromorphone (Dilaudid)
Oxymorphone (Numorphan)
Levorphanol (Levo-Dromoran)
Pentazocine (Talwin)
Meperidine (Demerol)
Methadone (Dolophine)
Fentanyl (Sublimaze)
Propoxyphene (Darvon)
Butorphanol (Stadol)
Nalbuphine (Nubain)

Narcotic Antagonists
Nalorphine (Nalline)
Naloxone (Narcan)
Levallorphan (Lorfan)

Salicylates
Aspirin (acetylsalicylic acid)
Methyl salicylate

Aniline Derivatives
Phenacetin
Acetaminophen (Tempra, Tylenol)

Pyrazole Derivatives
Antipyrine
Amidopyrine
Phenylbutazone (Butazolidin)

Miscellaneous Analgesics
Indomethacin (Indocin)
Ibuprofen (Motrin)

RESPIRATORY STIMULANTS

Analeptics
Doxapram (Dopram)
Ethamivan (Emivan)
Nikethamide (Coramine)

Xanthines
Theophylline
Caffeine

Carbonic Anhydrase Inhibitors
Acetazolamide (Diamox)

Salicylates

Progesterone

HISTAMINE ANTAGONISTS

H$_1$ Antagonists

Ethanolamine Derivatives
Diphenhydramine (Benadryl)

Dimenhydrinate (Dramamine)
Carbinoxamine (Clistin)
Clemastine (Tavist)

Ethylenediamine Derivatives
Pyrilamine
Tripelennamine (Pyribenzamine)

Alkylamines
Chlorpheniramine (Chlor-Trimeton)
Brompheniramine (Dimetane)
Dexchlorpheniramine (Polaramine)
Triprolidine (Actidil)

Phenothiazines
Promethazine (Phenergan)
Trimeprazine (Temaril)

Piperazine Derivatives
Cyclizine (Marezine)
Meclizine (Antivert)
Hydroxyzine (Atarax, Vistaril)

Miscellaneous H$_1$ Antagonists
Terfenadine (Seldane)

H$_2$ Antagonists

Cimetidine (Tagamet)
Ranitidine (Zantac)

Appendix B

Applied Mathematics for Respiratory Care

Jon O. Nilsestuen, Ph.D., R.R.T.

SYMBOLS

TABLE B–1.

Gas Phase Symbols

PRIMARY GAS SYMBOLS		COMMON QUALIFYING SYMBOLS	
P	Pressure	I	Inspired
$\bar{P}$	Mean pressure	E	Expired
V	Volume	T	Tidal
$\dot{V}$	Volume per unit time	A	Alveolar
F	Fractional concentration	D	Dead space
f	Frequency	L	Lung
		B	Barometric
		STPD	Standard temperature and pressure dry (0°C, 760 mm Hg, dry)
		BTPS	Body temperature, ambient pressure saturated with water vapor
		ATPD	Ambient temperature and pressure dry
		ATPS	Ambient temperature and pressure saturated

TABLE B–2.

Blood Phase Symbols

PRIMARY BLOOD SYMBOLS		QUALIFYING SYMBOLS (LOWERCASE)	
Q	Blood volume	a	Arterial
$\dot{Q}$	Blood flow	c	Capillary
C	Concentration or content of gas in blood	v	Venous
S	Saturation of hemoglobin with oxygen	$\bar{v}$	Mixed venous

COMBINED SYMBOLS AND ABBREVIATIONS

Volume Measurements

V_T Tidal volume
V_A Alveolar volume
V_D Dead-space volume
V_L Actual volume of the lung

Measurements of Ventilation

$\dot{V}_I$ Inspired volume per minute (BTBS)

$\dot{V}_E$ Expired volume per minute (BTPS)

$\dot{V}_A$ Alveolar ventilation per minute (BTPS)

$\dot{V}_D$ Physiologic dead-space ventilation per minute (BTPS)

$\dot{V}_{O_2}$ Oxygen consumption per minute (STPD)

$\dot{V}_{CO_2}$ Carbon dioxide production per minute (STPD)

Gas Tension and Blood Gas Measurements

P_B Barometric pressure

$F_{I_{O_2}}$ Fractional concentration of inspired oxygen

$F_{E_{O_2}}, F_{E_{CO_2}}$ Fractional concentration of expired oxygen or carbon dioxide

$P_{A_{O_2}}, P_{A_{CO_2}}$ Partial pressure of oxygen or carbon dioxide in the alveolar gas

Pa_{O_2}, Pa_{CO_2} Arterial oxygen or carbon dioxide tensions

$P\bar{v}_{O_2}, P\bar{v}_{CO_2}$ Mixed venous oxygen or carbon dioxide tensions

Sa_{O_2} Arterial oxygen saturation

Cc'_{O_2} Oxygen content of pulmonary end-capillary blood

$P(A-a)_{O_2}$ Alveolar-arterial oxygen pressure difference

$C(a-\bar{v})_{O_2}$ Arterial-venous oxygen content difference

Measurements of Mechanics of Breathing

C   A general symbol for compliance measured as the volume change divided by the pressure change

Cdyn   Dynamic compliance measured at the point of zero gas flow at the mouth during active breathing

Cst   Static compliance measured during conditions of prolonged interruption of air flow

R   A general symbol for resistance measured as the pressure per unit flow

Cardiopulmonary Equations

Minute ventilation $\dot{V}_E = (V_A + V_D)\, f$

Alveolar gas equation $P_{A_{O_2}} = F_{I_{O_2}}(P_B - P_{H_2O}) - \dfrac{Pa_{CO_2}}{0.8}$

Bohr's equation $\dfrac{V_D}{V_T} = \dfrac{Pa_{CO_2} - P\bar{E}_{CO_2}}{Pa_{CO_2}}$

Respiratory quotient $R = \dfrac{\dot{V}_{CO_2}}{\dot{V}_{O_2}}$

Fick's equation $\dot{V}_{O_2} = \dot{Q}_T (Ca_{O_2} - C\bar{v}_{O_2})$

DRUG DOSAGE CALCULATIONS

In general, drug dosage calculations fall into one of three categories: (1) converting from one standard of measure to another, (2) calculating the amount of active ingredient or dosage in a prepared solution, and (3) diluting concentrated drugs to appropriate clinical concentrations. Each of the categories will be treated separately.

Units of Measurement

There are three systems of weights and measures: (1) the metric system, (2) the apothecary system, and (3) the avoirdupois (avdp) system. The following tables are presented to assist the reader in converting from one system of measurement to another.

Metric Length

1 meter (m)	= 10 decimeters (dm)
	= 100 centimeters (cm)
	= 1,000 millimeters (mm)
10 m	= 1 dekameter (dam)
100 m	= 1 hectometer (hm)
1,000 m	= 1 kilometer (km)

Metric Volume

1 liter (L)	= 10 deciliters (dl)
	= 100 centiliters (cl)
	= 1,000 milliliters (ml)
	= 1,000,000 microliters (μl)

Metric Weight

1 gram (gm)	= 10 decigrams (dg)
	= 100 centigrams (cg)
	= 1,000 milligrams (mg)
	= 1,000,000 micrograms (μg)
1,000 gm	= 1 kilogram (kg)

Apothecary Volume

1 minim* (amount of water that would weigh 1 grain)

60 minims = 1 fluid dram

*The minim is often used to mean approximately 1 drop.

8 fluid drams or 480 minims = 1 fluid ounce (oz)
16 fluid oz = 1 pint (pt)
2 pt = 1 quart (qt)
4 qt = 1 gallon (gal)

Apothecary Weight

1 grain (originally meant 1 grain of wheat)
60 grains = 1 dram
8 drams or 480 grains = 1 oz
12 oz or 5,760 grains = 1 pound (lb)

Avoirdupois System

1 grain (basic unit of weight)
437.5 grains = 1 oz
16 oz = 1 lb
7,000 grains = 1 lb

Conversions Between Systems

Since the metric system is the most standard or more common system, it will be used here as the basis for converting between systems. The following lists contain approximate equivalents.

Weight

1 gm = 15 grains
4 gm = 1 dram
30 gm = 1 oz
1 kg = 2.2 lb (avdp)

Volume

1 ml = 15 minims or 15 drops
4 ml = 1 fluid dram
30 ml = 1 fluid oz
473 ml = 1 pint
946 ml = 1 qt

Household Equivalents

4–5 ml = 1 teaspoon = 60 minims or drops
15 ml = 1 tablespoon = 3 teaspoons
30 ml = 1 fluid oz = 2 tablespoons
237 ml = 1 cup
473 ml = 1 pint
946 ml = 1 qt

SOLUTION PREPARATIONS

Definitions

Solute: The pure drug form that is dissolved in the solvent or solution.

Solvent: The liquid medium in which the drug (solute) is dissolved; most drugs are dissolved in water.

Solution: The mixture of solid solute and aqueous solvent.

Concentration or strength: The quantity of solute per unit of solution (solute plus solvent).

Types of Solution Preparations

1. *Weight to weight* (W/W): Expresses the number of grams of a drug or active ingredient in 100 gm of a mixture; used primarily in instances where a high degree of accuracy is required.

   W/W = Grams per 100 gm of mixture

2. *weight to volume* (W/V): Expresses the number of grams of a drug or active ingredient in 100 ml of a mixture or solution; commonly used in medicine and pharmacy.

   W/V = Grams per 100 ml of mixture

3. *Volume to volume* (V/V): Expresses the number of milliliters of drug or active ingredient in 100 ml of a mixture; sometimes used when mixing two liquids with different densities, such as alcohol and water, where alcohol weighs considerably less than water.

   V/V = Milliliters per 100 ml of mixture

4. *Solute-to-solvent ratio:* Respiratory therapy drugs are often expressed as a ratio of parts solute to parts solvent, generally gm/ml; however, other ratios are sometimes used as units of active ingredient per milliliter, such as penicillin or heparin.

Examples

1. W/V: Metaproterenol sulfate (Alupent) 5% solution:

$$5\% = \frac{5 \text{ gm}}{100 \text{ ml}} = \frac{5,000 \text{ mg}}{100 \text{ ml}} = 50 \text{ mg/ml.}$$

2. W/V: Isoetharine (Bronkosol) 1% solution:

$$1\% = \frac{1 \text{ gm}}{100 \text{ ml}} = \frac{1,000 \text{ mg}}{100 \text{ ml}} = 10 \text{ mg/ml.}$$

3. W/V: Sodium bicarbonate 2% solution:

$$2\% = \frac{2 \text{ gm}}{100 \text{ ml}} = \frac{2{,}000 \text{ mg}}{100 \text{ ml}} = 20 \text{ mg/ml.}$$

4. W/V: Racepinephrine (Micronefrin, Vaponefrin) 2.25%:

$$2.25\% = \frac{2.25 \text{ gm}}{100 \text{ ml}} = \frac{2{,}250 \text{ mg}}{100 \text{ ml}} = 22.5 \text{ mg/ml.}$$

5. W/V: Physiologic saline 0.9% NaCl solution:

$$0.9\% = \frac{0.9 \text{ gm}}{100 \text{ ml}} = \frac{900 \text{ mg}}{100 \text{ ml}} = 9 \text{ mg/ml.}$$

Ratio 1: Isoproterenol 1:200 solution:

$$\text{Ratio 1} = \frac{1 \text{ gm}}{200 \text{ ml}} = \frac{1{,}000 \text{ mg}}{200 \text{ ml}} = 5 \text{ mg/ml.}$$

Ratio 2: Aminophylline 0.25 gm in 20 ml or 0.2 gm/tablet:

$$\text{Ratio 2} = \frac{0.25 \text{ gm}}{20 \text{ ml}} = \frac{250 \text{ mg}}{20 \text{ ml}} = 12.5 \text{ mg/ml.}$$

Ratio 3: Theophylline elixir (Elixophyllin) 80 mg/15 ml:

$$\text{Ratio 3} = \frac{80 \text{ mg}}{15 \text{ ml}} = 5.3 \text{ mg/ml.}$$

DRUG DILUTION CALCULATIONS

Practitioners are sometimes asked to prepare various pharmacologic agents by diluting the original preparation to form a less concentrated mixture. This dilution can be done by adding solvent to pure solute or by adding solvent to a more concentrated mixture using the following formula:

(Diluted concentration) × (Diluted volume) = (Amount of solute)

Where:

F_{dil} = concentration of diluted solution
F_{con} = concentration of undiluted solution
V_{dil} = volume of diluted solution
V_{con} = volume of undiluted solution
W_{solute} = weight of the pure solute

$$F_{con} \times V_{con} = W_{solute}$$
$$F_{dil} \times V_{dil} = W_{solute}$$

Therefore:

$$F_{dil} \times V_{dil} = F_{con} \times V_{con}$$

Both of these equations are chemical formulas that simply state that the amount of pure solute that exists on either side of the equation is equal to the concentration times the amount of solution. In other words, adding solvent to a solution or to a pure active ingredient changes only the concentration of the solution without changing the amount of active ingredient.

Example 1.—How much active ingredient is there in 0.5 ml of a 1.0% (1 gm/100 ml) solution of isoetharine?
Where:
Concentration (F_{con}) = 1.0% or 1 gm/100 ml
Total amount of solution (V_{con}) = 0.5 ml.
Weight of active ingredient (W_{solute}) = ?

$$\begin{aligned} W_{solute} &= F_{con} \times V_{con} \\ &= \frac{1 \text{ gm}}{100 \text{ ml}} \times 0.5 \text{ ml} \\ &= \frac{1{,}000 \text{ mg}}{100 \text{ ml}} \times 0.5 \text{ ml} \\ &= 10 \text{ mg/ml} \times 0.5 \text{ ml} \\ &= 5 \text{ mg} \end{aligned}$$

Example 2.—How much of a 20% solution contains 3 mg of active ingredient?
Where:
Concentration (F_{con}) = 20% or 20 gm/100 ml or 0.20
Total amount of solution (V_{con}) = ?
Weight of active ingredient (W_{solute}) = 3 gm or 0.003 gm

$$\begin{aligned} F_{con} \times V_{con} &= W_{solute} \\ V_{con} &= \frac{W_{solute}}{F_{con}} \\ &= \frac{0.003 \text{ gm}}{20 \text{ gm/100 ml}} \\ &= \frac{0.003 \text{ gm} \times 100 \text{ ml}}{20 \text{ gm}} = 0.15 \text{ ml} \end{aligned}$$

Example 3.—How much active ingredient is there in 0.5 ml of a 1:200 solution of isoproterenol?

Where:

Concentration (F_{con}) = 1:200 or 0.5%
or 0.5 gm/100 ml
Total amount of solution (V_{con}) = 0.5 ml
Weight of active ingredient (W_{solute}) = ?

$$W_{solute} = F_{con} \times V_{con}$$
$$= \frac{0.5 \ gm}{100 \ ml} \times 0.5 \ ml$$
$$= \frac{500 \ mg}{100 \ ml} \times 0.5 \ ml$$
$$= 5 \ mg/ml \times 0.5 \ ml$$
$$= 2.5 \ mg$$

Example 4.—Calculate the number of milligrams of 1:1000 epinephrine HCl, that are contained in a 0.5 ml dose:

Where:

Concentration (F_{con}) = 1:1,000 or 1 gm/1,000 ml
Total amount of solution (V_{con}) = 0.5 ml
Weight of active ingredient (W_{solute}) = ?

$$W_{solute} = F_{con} \times V_{con}$$
$$= \frac{1 \ gm}{1,000 \ ml} \times 0.5 \ ml$$
$$= \frac{1000 \ mg}{1,000 \ ml} \times 0.5 \ ml$$
$$= 1 \ mg/ml \times 0.5 \ ml$$
$$= 0.5 \ mg$$

Example 5.—Determine how much isoproterenol (Isuprel) 1:200 solution is needed to give a dose of 2 mg:

Where:

Concentration (F_{con}) = 1:200 or 1 gm/200 ml
Total amount of solution (V_{con}) = ?
Weight of active ingredient (W_{solute}) = 2 mg

$$F_{con} \times V_{con} = W_{solute}$$
$$V_{con} = \frac{W_{solute}}{F_{con}}$$
$$= \frac{2 \ mg}{1 \ gm/200 \ ml}$$
$$= \frac{2 \ mg \times 200 \ ml}{1,000 \ mg} = 0.4 \ ml$$

Dilute Active Ingredient

Example 1.—How many milliliters of water must be added to 10 ml of a 20% solution of acetylcysteine to dilute it to a 10% solution?

Where:

Diluted concentration (F_{dil}) = 10% or 0.10

Volume of diluted solution (V_{dil}) = 10 ml + x
Active ingredient concentration (F_{con}) = 20% or 0.20
Amount of active solution (V_{con}) = 10 ml
Volume of H_2O (solvent to be added) = x

$$F_{dil} \times V_{dil} = F_{con} \times V_{con}$$
$$V_{dil} = \frac{F_{con} \times V_{con}}{F_{dil}}$$
$$x + 10 \ ml = \frac{0.20 \times 10 \ ml}{0.10}$$
$$x = 20 - 10 \ ml$$
$$= 10 \ ml \ (\text{volume of } H_2O$$
$$\text{to be added})$$

Example 2.—What would be the concentration of a new solution if 30 ml of water were added to 50 ml of a 60% solution?

Where:

Diluted concentration (F_{dil}) = ?
Volume of diluted solution (V_{dil}) = 50 + 30 ml or 80 ml
Active ingredient concentration (F_{con}) = 60% or 0.60
Amount of active solution (V_{con}) = 50 ml
Volume of H_2O (solvent added) = 30 ml

$$F_{dil} \times V_{dil} = F_{con} \times V_{con}$$
$$F_{dil} = \frac{F_{con} \times V_{con}}{V_{dil}}$$
$$= \frac{0.60 \times 50 \ ml}{80 \ ml}$$
$$= 0.37 \ or \ 37\%.$$

Example 3.—How much distilled water must be added to 40 ml of a 7.5% solution of sodium bicarbonate to obtain a new concentration of 5%?

Where:

Diluted concentration (F_{dil}) = 5% or 0.05
Volume of diluted solution (V_{dil}) = 40 ml + x
Active ingredient concentration (F_{con}) = 7.5%, or 0.075
Amount of active solution (V_{con}) = 40 ml
Volume of H_2O (solvent to be added) = x

$$F_{dil} \times V_{dil} = F_{con} \times V_{con}$$
$$V_{dil} = \frac{F_{con} \times V_{con}}{F_{dil}}$$
$$x + 40 \ ml = \frac{0.075 \times 40 \ ml}{0.05}$$
$$x = 60 - 40 \ ml$$
$$= 20 \ ml \ (\text{the volume of } H_2O$$
$$\text{to be added}).$$

SOLVING OXYGEN DELIVERY PROBLEMS

An interesting consequence of the chemical mixing or dilution formulas utilized in the previous section is their application to the solution of oxygen and air mixing problems. It is intuitively correct if one considers oxygen to be the pure active ingredient (remember, it is considered to be a drug) and air a less concentrated mixture of oxygen. With the use of the formula for diluted active ingredient, again, it is possible after appropriately representing the unknown variable to solve all of the different types of air-oxygen problems.

(Con × volume) + (Con × volume)
  (Source gas)   (Added gas)
           = Con desired × Total volume.
$$F_a(\dot{V}_a) + F_b(\dot{V}_b) = F_c(\dot{V}_a + \dot{V}_b).$$

Where:
F_a = Fractional concentration of source gas
F_b = Fractional concentration of added gas
F_c = Fractional concentration of delivered gas
$\dot{V}_a$ = volume of source gas
$\dot{V}_b$ = volume of added gas
$\dot{V}_c$ = volume of delivered gas

If source gas is 100% oxygen and the added gas is air, the equation can be rewritten:

$$\dot{V}O_2 + 0.21(\dot{V}_{air}) = FI_{O_2}(\dot{V}_{total}).$$

This equation states that the amount of active ingredient (oxygen) in the source gas plus the amount of active ingredient in air is equal to the total amount of active ingredient (oxygen) in the delivered mixture. A simple mnemonic is useful in helping to remember this formula:

Source + Added = Delivered.

Examples

Type 1.—A Venturi device is connected to an oxygen flow meter running at 10 L/min. If the device is to deliver a 50% mixture, how much room air must be entrained?
Where:
Source gas (oxygen) concentration = 100% O_2
Oxygen flow rate ($\dot{V}O_2$) = 10 L/min
Added gas concentration (F_{air}) = 0.21
  (21%, room air)
Total delivered gas = $\dot{V}_{air}$ + 10 L/min
Desired concentration of oxygen (FI_{O_2}) = 0.50
  (50%)
Room air entrainment ($\dot{V}_{air}$) = ?

$$FI_{O_2}(\dot{V}_{total}) = \dot{V}O_2 + 0.21(\dot{V}_{air})$$

$$0.5(\dot{V}_{air} + 10 \text{ L/min}) = 10 \text{ L/min} + 0.21(\dot{V}_{air})$$

$$0.5(\dot{V}_{air}) + 5 \text{ L/min} = 10 \text{ L/min} + 0.21(\dot{V}_{air})$$

$$0.29(\dot{V}_{air}) = 5 \text{ L/min}$$

$$\dot{V}_{air} = \frac{5 \text{ L/min}}{0.29} = 17 \text{ L/min}.$$

Type 2.—A similar kind of question involves determining the amount of oxygen that must be added to a nebulizer running off compressed air at 10 L/min to deliver a 24% mixture to the patient.
Where:
Desired concentration of O_2(FI_{O_2}) = 0.24(24% O_2)
Source gas (oxygen) concentration = 0.21 (21% oxygen)
Added gas concentration (O_2) = 1.00 (100% O_2)
Total delivered gas ($\dot{V}_{total}$) = $\dot{V}O_2$ + 10 L/min
Air flow rate ($\dot{V}_{air}$) = 10 L/min
Oxygen flow rate ($\dot{V}O_2$) = ?

$$FI_{O_2}(\dot{V}_{total}) = \dot{V}O_2 + 0.21(\dot{V}_{air})$$

$$0.24(\dot{V}O_2 + 10 \text{ L/min}) = \dot{V}O_2 + 0.21(10 \text{ L/min})$$

$$0.24(\dot{V}O_2) + 2.4 \text{ L/min} = \dot{V}O_2 + 2.1 \text{ L/min}$$

$$0.76(\dot{V}O_2) = 0.3 \text{ L/min}$$

$$\dot{V}O_2 = \frac{0.3 \text{ L/min}}{0.76} = 0.4 \text{ L/min}.$$

Type 3.—Both of the situations, types 1 and 2, may be used to calculate the air/oxygen entrainment ratios that are frequently asked for on examinations without memorizing the ratios. In the example in type 2, once the amounts of air and oxygen have been determined, the entrainment ratio is simply a matter of setting up the proper fraction.
Where:
Liters of air = 10
Liters of oxygen = 0.4

$$\frac{10 \text{ L/min}}{0.4 \text{ L/min}} = \frac{100}{4} = \frac{25}{1}.$$

On the other hand, if one is looking to determine a specific ratio for a given concentration, all that is required is to select some amount of oxygen or air and determine how much of the remaining gas must be added to give the desired concentration. For example, if we wanted to know the air/oxygen ratio for 60%, we would start by selecting a given amount of air or oxygen, say, 10 L/min of oxygen, and determine how much air to add to produce a 60% mixture.

Where:

Desired concentration = 60%
Amount of source gas (oxygen) = 10 L/min
Amount of room air = $\dot{V}_{air}$
Total amount of gas delivered = $10 + \dot{V}_{air}$

$$F_{I_{O_2}}(\dot{V}_{total}) = \dot{V}_{O_2} + 0.21(\dot{V}_{air})$$

$$0.6(10\ \text{L/min} + \dot{V}_{air}) = 10\ \text{L/min} + 0.21(\dot{V}_{air})$$

$$6\ \text{L/min} + 0.6(\dot{V}_{air}) = 10\ \text{L/min} + 0.21(\dot{V}_{air})$$

$$0.4(\dot{V}_{air}) = 4\ \text{L/min}$$

$$\dot{V}_{air} = \frac{4\ \text{L/min}}{0.4} = 10\ \text{L/min of room air.}$$

Therefore, the entrainment ratio = air/oxygen = 10/10 or 1/1.

Type 4.—The practitioner has been asked to set up a continuous positive-airway pressure (CPAP) device to deliver a 60% oxygen mixture at a minimum of 50 L/min. How much compressed air and how much oxygen should be mixed to give the desired concentration?

Where:

Desired concentration of delivered gas = 0.6 (60% O_2)
Amount of total gas to be delivered = 50 L/min
Source gas concentration = 1.00 (100% O_2)
Diluted gas concentration = 0.21 (21% O_2)
Amount of diluted gas (room air) = $\dot{V}_{air}$
Amount of source gas (oxygen) = $50 - \dot{V}_{air}$

$$F_{I_{O_2}}(\dot{V}_{total}) = \dot{V}_{O_2} + 0.21(\dot{V}_{air})$$

$$0.6(50\ \text{L/min}) = (50\ \text{L/min} - \dot{V}_{air}) + 0.21(\dot{V}_{air})$$

$$30\ \text{L/min} = 50\ \text{L/min} - 0.79(\dot{V}_{air})$$

$$0.79(\dot{V}_{air}) = 20\ \text{L/min}$$

$$\dot{V}_{air} = \frac{20\ \text{L/min}}{0.79} = 25\ \text{L/min of air}$$

$$\dot{V}_{O_2} = 50 - \dot{V}_{air}$$
$$= 50 - 25 = 25\ \text{L/min of oxygen.}$$

PATIENT ASSESSMENT PARAMETERS

Mean Blood Pressure

The mean blood pressure is the average pressure over the complete cardiac cycle. Mathematically it is expressed as the pressure-time integral over the systolic and diastolic pressure phases (Fig B–1) and can be determined electronically with a polygraph recorded. Under normal conditions, however, mean blood pressure can be approximated with reasonable accuracy by adding one third of the pulse pressure to the diastolic pressure. Pulse pressure is the difference between systolic and diastolic pressures:

$$\text{Mean blood pressure} = \text{Diastolic} + \frac{\text{Pulse pressure}}{3}.$$

Example.—Blood pressures recorded from a sphygmomanometer are systolic 122 mm Hg and diastolic 80 mm Hg:

$$\text{MBP} = 80 + \frac{(122 - 80)}{3} = 80 + 14 = 94\ \text{mm Hg.}$$

Heart Rate From Electrocardiogram

There are several methods for determining heart rate from an ECG. They are similar in most respects, however, and are based on an understanding of the design of the standard ECG paper and the speed at which the paper moves on the ECG machine.

Electrocardiogram paper is divided into two different subdivisions: small squares, each 1 mm in dimension, and larger squares outlined in bold print, each 5 mm in size (Fig B–2,A). Electrocardiogram machines have been standardized for the most part to move paper past the stylus at a rate of 25 mm/sec. At this standard rate, the paper will move the distance between five of the large bold squares (5 × 5

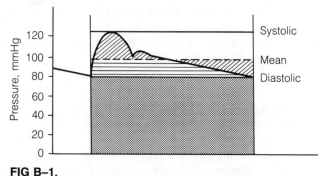

FIG B–1.
Estimation of mean blood pressure: Pulse pressure equals diastolic plus one third of the pulse pressure.

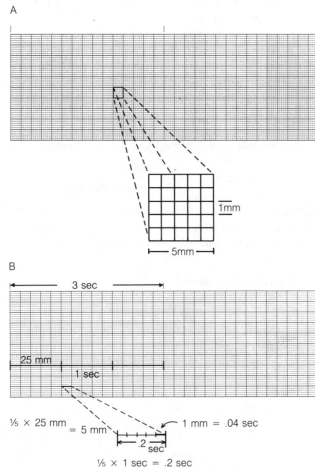

FIG B–2.
A and **B,** sample ECG graph paper.

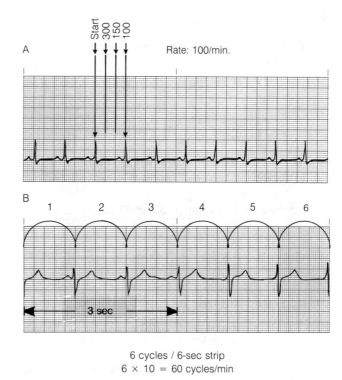

6 cycles / 6-sec strip
6 × 10 = 60 cycles/min

FIG B–3.
Calculating heart rate from an ECG. **A,** counting large squares; **B,** counting 6-second strips.

mm per square equals 25 mm) in 1 second or will move from one bold line to the next, the division of one bold square in one fifth of 1 second (0.2 seconds). In addition, since each bold square is further divided into five small squares, the paper will move past one small square in the equivalent of one fifth of 0.20 second, or 0.04 seconds (Fig B–2,B).

A common way of determining rate is to use the paper of the ECG machine that moves at rate of 25 mm/sec, or five bold spaces/sec. It follows that the paper will move five times 60, or 300 bold spaces in 1 minute. If a sample rhythm strip indicated that a complete cardiac cycle occurred during each bold space, the rate would be 300 cycles/min (Fig B–3,A). If the cardiac cycle occurred every second bold space, divide 300 by 2 and arrive at a rate of 150 cycles/min. Continuing this logic, one can determine the heart rate in cycles per minute by counting the number of bold spaces between cardiac cycles and dividing this number into 300. This is the basis for

the rate chart in Table B–3. The rate chart is worth memorizing because it provides a quick and rapid way of determining the heart rate under most clinical circumstances.

A second somewhat easier method of determining rate, particularly for irregular rhythms, is afforded by noting the small ticker marks, or notches, on the upper margin of the paper strip. Each of these marks is 3 seconds apart. If you count the number of cycles over two of these intervals, or 6 seconds, and then multiply this number by 10, you will have the number of cycles in 60 seconds, or 1 minute (Fig B–3,B).

TABLE B–3.

Heart Rate Determination Using ECG Paper

NO. OF LARGE SPACES BETWEEN CARDIAC CYCLES	HEART RATE, CYCLES/MIN
1	300
2	150
3	100
4	75
5	60
6	50

Temperature Conversion

Equations to Convert Between Fahrenheit and Celsius

$$F = \left[\frac{9}{5} \times C\right] + 32$$

$$C = \frac{5}{9} \times [F - 32]$$

Example.—Convert 0°C and 37°C to Fahrenheit:

$$F = \left[\frac{9}{5} \times 0\right] + 32 = 32° \text{ F}$$

$$= \left[\frac{9}{5} \times 37\right] + 32 = 98.6° \text{ F}$$

Example.—Convert 90° F and 212° F to Celsius:

$$C = \frac{5}{9} \times (90 - 32) = 32° \text{ C}$$

$$= \frac{5}{9} \times (212 - 32) = 100° \text{ C}$$

VENTILATION

Tidal Volume

The tidal volume is the amount of gas exhaled during one breath. For patients who are spontaneously breathing, the exhaled volume should be averaged over several breaths.

For patients receiving mechanical ventilation, the tidal volume should be measured at the patient's airway (endotracheal tube). If the gas is measured at the exhalation port, the volume compressed in the tubing or circuitry must be subtracted from this value, as the following illustrates.

Correction of Tidal Volume for Tubing Compliance

Measure tubing compliance:

1. With the patient disconnected from the ventilator, select a small tidal volume of about 100 to 200 ml.
2. Set the peak pressure limit to the maximum setting so that the ventilator will not pop off.
3. Adjust the flow setting to its minimum.
4. Plug the ventilator circuitry at the patient

connection site with a cork or occlude with a sterile alcohol swab.
5. Measure the peak airway pressure during several cycles to get an accurate reading of the peak pressure. You may want to add an inspiratory time delay to assure that there are no leaks in the circuitry and that your peak airway pressure is stable.
6. Calculate the tubing compliance by dividing the tidal volume by the pressure change:

$$\text{Compliance} = \frac{\text{Volume change } (\Delta V)}{\text{Pressure change } (\Delta P)}$$

This is the tubing compliance factor, which can now be used to calculate how much volume is compressed in the tubing during a single breath.

Correct tidal volume:

1. Remove the stopper from the patient circuitry, set the ventilator to the appropriate patient settings, and reconnect the patient.
2. Measure the peak airway pressure during several breaths with the patient connected.
3. Multiply the peak airway pressure by the tubing compliance factor to determine how much gas is compressed in the tubing during the patient breath. Subtract it from the tidal volume to determine how much volume the patient is actually receiving.

Example.—The calculated tubing compliance factor might be:

$$(200 \text{ ml}/50 \text{ cm } H_2O) = 4 \text{ ml/cm } H_2O$$

If the patient tidal volume was set on 1,000 ml and the peak airway pressure was measured to be 40 cm H_2O, the volume lost due to compression within the tubing was:

$$4 \text{ ml/cm } H_2O \times 40 \text{ cm } H_2O = 160 \text{ ml}$$

The actual volume that the patient received was:

$$1,000 \text{ ml} - 160 \text{ ml} = 840 \text{ ml}$$

Large tidal volumes are not greatly affected by compression within the tubing; however, small volumes are.

Example 1.—
1,500 ml delivered at 30 cm H_2O

$$V_{lost} = 4 \text{ ml/cm } H_2O \times 30 \text{ cm } H_2O = 120 \text{ ml}$$
$$V_T = 1,500 - 120 = 1,380 \text{ ml } (8\% \text{ loss})$$

Example 2.—
150 ml delivered at 30 cm H_2O

V_{lost} = 4 ml/cm H_2O × 30 cm H_2O = 120 ml
V_T = 150 − 120 = 30 ml (80% loss)

MINUTE VENTILATION

Minute ventilation is the volume of gas exhaled during 1 minute or the product of the tidal ventilation and the breathing frequency.

Minute ventilation ($\dot{V}_E$) equals tidal volume (V_T) times frequency (f):

$$\dot{V}_E = V_T \times f \qquad [1]$$

Tidal volume (V_T) is the combination of the alveolar volume (V_A) and the dead-space volume (V_D):

$$V_T = V_A + V_D \qquad [2]$$

Equation [1] can be rewritten by substituting ($V_A + V_D$) for V_T to derive either minute alveolar ventilation or minute dead-space ventilation:

$$\dot{V}_E = (V_A + V_D) \times f$$
$$= (V_A \times f) + (V_D \times f)$$
$$= \dot{V}_A + \dot{V}_D$$

Thus,

$$\dot{V}_A = \dot{V}_E - \dot{V}_D \qquad [3]$$

Or

$$\dot{V}_D = \dot{V}_E - \dot{V}_A \qquad [4]$$

ALVEOLAR VENTILATION

Practical Measurement of Alveolar Ventilation

The volume of gas that undergoes gas exchange in the lung can be estimated from equation [3] by measuring the total ventilation and then subtracting the dead-space ventilation. Dead-space ventilation can be roughly approximated by estimating 1 ml of anatomic dead space/lb of body ideal weight or more accurately using Fowler's method or the Bohr equation.

Example.—If the tidal volume is 700 ml, breathing frequency is 12/min, and weight is 150 lb:

Where:
Minute ventilation is 12/min × 700 ml = 8,400 ml/min
Dead-space volume is 1 ml/lb × 150 lb = 150 ml
Dead-space ventilation is 150 ml × 12/min = 1,800 ml/min
Alveolar ventilation is 8,400 − 1,800 = 6,600 ml/min

$$\dot{V}_E = \dot{V}_D + \dot{V}_A$$
$$8,400 \text{ ml} = 1.800 + 6,600$$

Precise Measurement of Alveolar Ventilation

A more physiologic way of measuring alveolar ventilation is through the collection of exhaled gases. Since only the alveolar gas is exposed to the pulmonary capillary blood, CO_2 can enter the exhaled gas only by crossing from the blood to the alveolar gas through the alveolar capillary membrane. Thus, all of the exhaled CO_2 must come from alveolar gas and not from the dead-space gas. Therefore, the total amount of CO_2 exhaled must be equal to the alveolar ventilation times the alveolar concentration of CO_2:

$$\dot{V}_{E_{CO_2}} = \dot{V}_A \times F_{A_{CO_2}} \qquad [5]$$

The CO_2 output ($\dot{V}_{E_{CO_2}}$) or the amount of CO_2 exhaled can be measured by collecting the expired gas over 1 minute, measuring the volume ($\dot{V}_E$) and analyzing the mixed expired CO_2 concentration ($F\bar{E}_{CO_2}$) with a gas analyzer:

$$\dot{V}_{E_{CO_2}} = \dot{V}_E \times F\bar{E}_{CO_2}$$

The fractional concentration of CO_2 in the alveolar gas can be analyzed using a rapid gas analyzer and sampling the gas from the final portion of a single expiration. Rearranging equation [5]:

$$\dot{V}_A = \frac{\dot{V}_{E_{CO_2}}}{F_{A_{CO_2}}} = \frac{\dot{V}_E \times F\bar{E}_{CO_2}}{F_{A_{CO_2}}} \qquad [6]$$

Example.—
Patient's collected minute ventilation is 7,000 ml
Mean expired CO_2 concentration is 4.5%
End tidal CO_2 concentration from CO_2 analyzer is 6%

$$\dot{V}_A = \frac{7,000 \text{ ml} \times 0.045}{0.06}$$
$$= 5,250 \text{ ml/min}$$

ADJUSTING VENTILATION TO ACHIEVE A DESIRED P_{CO_2}

A practical application of the measurement of alveolar ventilation as just shown is that it allows us to predict (with the addition of a blood gas) how much the arterial blood gases will change following any subsequent change in ventilation. Note that the partial pressure of CO_2 in the alveolar gas is proportional to the concentration of gas in the alveoli. The expression includes a constant that depends on the barometric pressure and water vapor pressure

$$P_{A_{CO_2}} = F_{A_{CO_2}} \times K$$

Substituting this expression in equation [6]:

$$\dot{V}_A = \frac{\dot{V}_{E_{CO_2}}}{F_{A_{CO_2}}}$$

$$= \frac{\dot{V}_{E_{CO_2}}}{P_{A_{CO_2}}} \times K$$

For normal subjects, the partial pressure of CO_2 in the alveolar gas and arterial blood are nearly the same, so that the arterial CO_2 can be used instead of the alveolar CO_2, thus:

$$\dot{V}_A = \frac{\dot{V}_{E_{CO_2}}}{P_{a_{CO_2}}} \times K \qquad [7]$$

After cross-multiplying:

$$\dot{V}_A \times P_{a_{CO_2}} = \dot{V}_{E_{CO_2}} \times K \qquad [8]$$

Since the production of CO_2 denoted by $\dot{V}_{E_{CO_2}}$ is determined by metabolism and is therefore relatively stable, the right side of equation [8] can be treated as a constant, and the left side can be used to predict changes in arterial CO_2 following change in ventilation:

$$\dot{V}_A \times P_{a_{CO_2}} = \dot{V}_{E_{CO_2}} \times K$$
$$\text{(Initial values)} \quad \text{(Constant)}$$

$$= \dot{V}_A \times P_{a_{CO_2}}$$
$$\text{(Desired values)}$$

Equation [8] can be applied under several different ways depending on whether the clinical circumstances warrant increasing or decreasing the $P_{a_{CO_2}}$ or even the addition of dead space. By substituting $(V_T - V_D)$ for alveolar ventilation, equation [8] can be written in its most useful form as:

$$(V_T - V_D) \times f \times P_{a_{CO_2}} = (V_T - V_D) \times f \times P_{a_{CO_2}}$$
$$\text{Known values} \qquad \text{Desired values} \qquad [9]$$

Before proceeding with sample problems, one should note that the decision to change alveolar ventilation can be accomplished by changing either frequency or tidal volume. As a clinical guideline, it is generally accepted that tidal volumes should be kept in the range of 10 to 15 ml/kg and frequencies in the range of 10 to 15 breaths/min. In addition, if the clinical situation warrants an increase in ventilation, the tidal volume should be increased up to the limit of 15 ml before the frequency is increased. The rationale for this sequence is that patients on mechanical ventilation tend to develop atelectasis. Maintenance of larger tidal volumes is therefore appropriate in the prevention of atelectasis and treatment of shunting and problems associated with maintaining oxygenation.

Example 1.—A 60-kg adult is receiving mechanical ventilation. The following parameters are recorded:

$$V_T = 900 \text{ ml}$$
$$P_{a_{CO_2}} = 50 \text{ mm Hg}$$
$$f = 9/\text{min}$$
$$\text{Weight} = 132 \text{ lb}$$
$$\text{Estimated anatomical dead space} = 132 \text{ ml}$$

The therapist wishes to stabilize the patient at a desired $P_{a_{CO_2}}$ of 40 mm Hg. Initial calculations reveal that the tidal volume is already set at the maximum of 15 ml/kg. The decision is made to increase the breathing frequency to reduce the arterial CO_2:

$$(V_T - V_D) \times f \times P_{a_{CO_2}} = (V_T - V_D) \times f \times P_{a_{CO_2}}$$
$$(900 - 132) \times 9 \times 50 = (900 - 132) \times (f) \times 40$$
$$\text{Known values} \qquad \text{Desired values}$$
$$f = \frac{(768)(9)(50)}{(768)(40)}$$
$$= 11/\text{min}$$

Therefore, an increase in the frequency from 9 to 11 breaths/min should reduce the $P_{a_{CO_2}}$ from 50 to 40 mm Hg.

Example 2.—The following parameters are recorded from a patient in acute ventilatory failure:

$$\text{Weight} = 70 \text{ kg (154 lb)}$$
$$V_T = 850 \text{ ml}$$
$$f = 12/\text{min}$$
$$P_{a_{CO_2}} = 70 \text{ mm Hg}$$
$$\text{Estimated anatomical dead space} = 154 \text{ ml}$$
$$\text{Desired } P_{a_{CO_2}} = 43 \text{ mm Hg}$$

The first step is to increase the tidal volume to 15 ml/kg or, in this case, from 850 to 1,050 ml. The second step is to increase the frequency to accommodate the additional need for ventilation:

$$(V_T - V_D) \times f \times Pa_{CO_2} = (V_T - V_D) \times f \times Pa_{CO_2}$$
$$(850 - 154) \times (12) \times (70) = (1,050 - 154) \times (f) \times 43$$

Known values Desired values

$$f = \frac{(696)\,(12)\,(70)}{(896)\,(43)}$$
$$= 15/min$$

Example 3.—A hypometabolic patient is returned from the operating room with the following parameters:

Weight = 60 kg (132 lb)
V_T = 600 ml
f = 10/min
Pa_{CO_2} = 32 mm Hg
Estimated anatomical dead space = 132 ml
Desired Pa_{CO_2} = 40 mm Hg

The initial observations indicate that the tidal volume is already in the lower range of normal. Any further reduction in the tidal volume in an attempt to decrease the CO_2 would likely cause problems with the oxygenation status. In addition, any further reduction in the breathing frequency would probably not be tolerated by the patient. The only remaining parameter that can be changed is the amount of dead space:

$$(V_T - V_D) \times f \times Pa_{CO_2}$$
$$= (V_T - V_D) \times f \times Pa_{CO_2}$$

Known values
$$(600 - 132) \times (10) \times (32)$$
$$= [(600 - 132) - \text{Added dead space}] \times (10) \times 40$$

Desired values
$$(468)\,(10)\,(32)$$
$$= (468 - \text{Added dead space})\,(400)$$
$$(468)\,(10)\,(32)$$
$$= (468)\,(400) - (\text{Added dead space})\,(400)$$

Added dead space
$$= \frac{(468)\,(400) - (468)\,(10)\,(32)}{400}$$
$$= 94 \text{ ml (or approximately two 5-in. sections of large-bore tubing)}$$

Dead-Space Ventilation

Dead-space ventilation is the portion of the minute ventilation that is not involved in the exchange of gases. It includes several kinds of dead space: (1) anatomical dead space, (2) alveolar dead space, (3) ventilation in excess of perfusion, and (4) physiologic dead space.

1. *Anatomical dead space:* Upper airway and the conducting airways; in practice, the anatomical dead space is usually approximated as 1 ml/lb of body weight.
2. *Alveolar dead space:* Alveoli that are ventilated but not perfused.
3. *Ventilation in excess of perfusion:* Alveoli that are ventilated out of proportion to their perfusion and therefore have a component of wasted ventilation; alveolar dead space and ventilation in excess of perfusion cannot be measured with conventional methods.
4. *Physiological dead space:* The combination of anatomical dead space, alveolar dead space, and ventilation in excess of perfusion; it represents the total amount of ventilation that is wasted or is not effective in gas exchange and can be calculated using the Bohr equation for the measurement of the dead space/tidal volume ratio.

Development of the Bohr Equation or V_D/V_T Ratio

The same assumption that was used in the development of the equation for the measurement of alveolar ventilation is used again for measurement of dead space, namely, that all of the expired CO_2 comes from alveolar gas and none from the dead-space gas. The total expired CO_2 can be measured by collecting the exhaled volume in a bag and multiplying the volume times the CO_2 concentration or fraction of expired CO_2 ($F\bar{E}_{CO_2}$) (equation [8]):

$$V_T \times F\bar{E}_{CO_2} = V_A \times FA_{CO_2}.$$

The tidal volume is the combination of the dead-space volume and the alveolar volume or:

$$V_T = V_D + V_A$$

Therefore, by substituting ($V_T - V_D$) for V_A in equation [8]:

$$V_T \times F\bar{E}_{CO_2} = (V_T - V_D) \times FA_{CO_2}$$
$$= (V_T \times FA_{CO_2}) - (V_D \times FA_{CO_2})$$

Rearranging:

$$(V_T \times F\bar{E}_{CO_2}) - (V_T \times FA_{CO_2}) = -(V_D \times FA_{CO_2})$$
$$V_T (F\bar{E}_{CO_2} - FA_{CO_2}) = -(V_D \times FA_{CO_2})$$

Multiplying both sides of the equation by unity (-1) gives you equation [9]:

$$V_T (FA_{CO_2} - F\bar{E}_{CO_2}) = (V_D \times FA_{CO_2})$$
$$\frac{V_D}{V_T} = \frac{FA_{CO_2} - F\bar{E}_{CO_2}}{FA_{CO_2}} \qquad [9]$$

Equation [9] can be further simplified by recognizing two other basic principles: (1) the fractional concentration of a gas (FA_{CO_2}) is proportional to the partial pressure of the gas (P_{CO_2}), and (2) under most circumstances the partial pressure of carbon dioxide in the alveolar gas is very closely approximated by the arterial carbon dioxide tension (Pa_{CO_2}). Incorporating these two principles in equation [9], we have:

$$\frac{V_D}{V_T} = \frac{Pa_{CO_2} - P\bar{E}_{CO_2}}{Pa_{CO_2}}$$

Note.—Only two easily obtainable parameters are necessary here to calculate the dead space/tidal volume ratio, an arterial blood gas and a sample of mixed expired gas. The mixed expired gas is usually collected over several minutes in an anesthesia bag connected to the exhalation port of the ventilator circuit.

As a key to understanding the use of the dead-space equation, remember that the amount of CO_2 produced by the body is dependent on the body's metabolism and is therefore relatively stable. This metabolic CO_2 is released into the lungs, where it becomes alveolar gas. The alveolar gas and the dead-space gas become mixed as they are collected in the reservoir bag. The degree of dilution of the CO_2 in the expired sample depends on how much of the tidal volume was alveolar ventilation and how much was dead-space ventilation. The larger the dead-space ventilation, the more the alveolar gas is diluted in the expired sample.

Example.—A patient has a tidal volume of 1,000 ml on a volume ventilator. Arterial blood gases are drawn with a Pa_{CO_2} of 40 mm Hg, and mixed expired gas sample is analyzed indicating a $P\bar{E}_{CO_2}$ of 30 mm Hg. Calculate the amount of dead-space ventilation:

$$\frac{V_D}{V_T} = \frac{Pa_{CO_2} - P\bar{E}_{CO_2}}{Pa_{CO_2}}$$

$$= \frac{40 - 30}{40} = 25\%$$

Therefore, 25% of the tidal volume, 250 ml, is dead-space ventilation.

GAS TRANSPORT

Oxygen Content

Oxygen exists in the blood in two forms: dissolved in the plasma and attached to hemoglobin.

Oxygen content refers to the sum of both forms of oxygen carried in a particular blood sample and is usually reported in volumes percent or the amount of oxygen in milliliters that is contained in 100 ml of blood.

Oxygen Solubility

The quantity of oxygen dissolved in the blood can be calculated from the Bunsen solubility coefficient. For every 100 ml of blood at BTPS, 0.003 ml of oxygen will be dissolved per 1 mm Hg of oxygen tension. Therefore, the amount of oxygen in volumes percent that is dissolved in a blood sample will be equal to the partial pressure of oxygen in the sample times the solubility coefficient or:

Volumes percent = P_{O_2} (mm Hg) $\times$ 0.003 ml/mm Hg.

Example 1.—How much oxygen will be carried as dissolved oxygen in a blood sample if the partial pressure of oxygen is 760 ml/mm Hg?

$$\text{vol}\% = 760 \text{ mm Hg} \times 0.003 \text{ ml/mm Hg}$$
$$= 2.3 \text{ ml}$$

Example 2.—How much oxygen will be carried in 100 ml of blood if the partial pressure of oxygen (Pa_{O_2}) is 95 mm Hg?

$$\text{vol}\% = 95 \text{ mm Hg} \times 0.003 \text{ ml/mm Hg}$$
$$= 0.28 \text{ ml}$$

Oxygen Bound to Hemoglobin

The amount of oxygen carried by hemoglobin can be derived from the knowledge of the chemical interaction between the two molecules and the application of Avogadro's law. Namely, 1 gm molecular weight of hemoglobin when fully saturated with oxygen combines with 4 gm molecular weights of oxygen, and 1 mole of any gas at standard temperature and pressure (0° C, 760 mm Hg) occupies 22.4 L:

1. $Hb + 4(O_2) = Hb(O_2)4$
2. Gram molecular weights of Hb = 64,457 gm
3. Volume of 4 moles of oxygen = 4 × 22.4 L = 89.6 L, or 89,600 ml
4. ml O_2/gm Hb = 89,600 ml/64,457 gm Hb = 1.39 ml/gm Hb

The value of 1.39 ml/gm of hemoglobin differs from the more traditional text book value of 1.34 ml/

gm of hemoglobin. However, several recent studies using hemolyzed blood rather than intact red blood cells have documented the newer value.

Oxygen Capacity

The previous discussion refers to the amount of oxygen that 1 gm of hemoglobin can carry when fully saturated, a condition known as the oxygen capacity. Not all hemoglobin, however, is fully saturated with oxygen or carries all four oxygen molecules. In fact, the degree of saturation is dependent on a number of factors, including the type of hemoglobin, the temperature, pH, and P_{CO_2} of the blood, the amount of 2,3-diphosphoglycerate (a metabolic by-product of glycolysis), and the partial pressure of oxygen in the blood. The actual saturation of the hemoglobin can be measured with a co-oximeter and the content or amount of oxygen bound to hemoglobin calculated as follows:

1. Oxygen bound to hemoglobin:

   Hb (gm%) × 1.39 ml O_2 × Hb sat = vol%.

2. Oxygen saturation:

   $$\text{Hb saturation} = \frac{O_2 \text{ combined to hemoglobin} \times 100}{O_2 \text{ capacity}}.$$

Example 1.—Calculate the oxygen content of an arterial blood sample with Hb content 15 gm%, Pa_{O_2} 100 mm Hg, Hb sat 100%:

1. Oxygen combined with hemoglobin:

   15 gm% × 1.39 ml/gm × 1.00 = 20.85 vol%.

2. Oxygen dissolved in the plasma:

   100 mm Hg × 0.003 ml/mm Hg = 0.30 vol%.

3. Total content:

   $$Ca_{O_2} = 20.85 + 0.30$$
   $$= 21.15 \text{ vol\%}.$$

Example 2.—Calculate the oxygen content of a venous blood sample with Hb content 15 gm%, $P\bar{v}_{O_2}$ 40 mm Hg, Hb sat 75%:

1. Oxygen combined with hemoglobin:

   15 gm% × 1.39 ml/gm × 0.75 = 15.64 vol%.

2. Oxygen dissolved in the plasma:

   40 mm Hg × 0.003 ml/mm Hg = 0.12 vol%.

3. Total content:

   $$C\bar{v}_{O_2} = 15.64 + 0.12$$
   $$= 15.76 \text{ vol\%}.$$

Oxygen Transport

Oxygen transport is the amount of oxygen delivered to the tissues by the arterial blood per unit time and is expressed in milliliters per minute. It is calculated simply as the product of the cardiac output and the arterial oxygen content. However, since the arterial oxygen content is expressed in volumes percent or the number of milliliters of oxygen per 100 ml of blood, we must convert the cardiac output into the number of 100-ml units of blood delivered per unit time:

Oxygen transport = Cardiac output ($\dot{Q}_T$) × Ca_{O_2}.

Example.—Calculate the oxygen transport from the following laboratory data: $\dot{Q}_T$, 6 L/min; Hb, 15 gm%; Pa_{O_2}, 100 mm Hg; and Hb sat, 98%.

1. Oxygen content:
   a. Oxygen combined with hemoglobin:

      15 gm% × 1.39 ml/gm × 0.98
      $$= 20.43 \text{ vol\%}.$$

   b. Oxygen dissolved in the plasma:

      100 mm Hg × 0.003 ml/mm Hg
      $$= 0.30 \text{ vol\%}.$$

   c. Total content:

      $$Ca_{O_2} = 20.43 + 0.30$$
      $$= 20.73 \text{ vol\%}.$$

2. Cardiac output:

   $$\dot{Q}_T = 6 \text{ L/min} \times \frac{(10) (100 \text{ ml units})}{L}$$
   $$= 60 (100 \text{ ml})/\text{min}.$$

3. Oxygen transport:

   O_2 transport = 60 (100 ml units)/min
   $$\times 20.73 \text{ vol\%}$$
   $$= 1,243.8 \text{ ml/min}.$$

Oxygen Consumption

Oxygen consumption can be calculated from the Fick equation:

$$\dot{V}_{O_2} = \dot{Q}_T (Ca_{O_2} - C\bar{v}_{O_2}),$$

which states that the amount of oxygen taken up by the blood from the lung or consumed by the tissues of the body is the product of the cardiac output ($\dot{Q}_T$) and the arterial-venous oxygen content differences ($CaO_2 - C\bar{v}O_2$). The equation just cited can be used in the clinic to calculate either the oxygen consumption or the cardiac output.

Example.—Determine the oxygen consumption from $\dot{Q}_T$, 4.5 L/min; CaO_2, 20.73 vol%; and $C\bar{v}O_2$, 15.73 vol%:

$$\begin{aligned} O_2 \text{ consumption} &= 4.5 \text{ L/min} \times 10(100 \text{ ml units/L}) \\ &\quad \times (20.73 - 15.73) \\ &= 45 \text{ (100 ml units)/min} \times 5 \text{ vol\%} \\ &= 225 \text{ ml/min.} \end{aligned}$$

Cardiac Output

From the Fick equation:

$$\dot{Q}_T = \frac{\dot{V}O_2}{CaO_2 - C\bar{v}O_2}$$

In this equation, the oxygen uptake can be measured by calculating the oxygen content difference between inspired and expired gases. It is accomplished by measuring the concentration of oxygen in the inspired and expired gases over a period of time and multiplying the concentration times the respective inspired or expired volumes. Inspired volumes can be measured with a Wright respirometer connected at the patient Y or with a pneumotachometer. Expired volumes are generally collected over time in an anesthesia bag and the mixed expired oxygen concentration measured with a rapid gas analyzer. Both measured volumes are corrected to STPD. The more recent use of metabolic carts has made this procedure relatively simple.

Example.—Determine the cardiac output from volume of inspired oxygen, 2.5 L/min; volume of expired oxygen, 2.25 L/min; and arterial venous oxygen content difference, 5 vol%:

$$\begin{aligned} \dot{Q}_T &= \frac{(2.5 \text{ L/min} - 2.25 \text{ L/min})}{5 \text{ vol\%}} \\ &= \frac{250 \text{ ml/min}}{5 \text{ ml/100 ml}} \\ &= 50 \text{ (100 ml)/min} \\ &= 5,000 \text{ ml/min, or 5 L/min.} \end{aligned}$$

VENTILATION PERFUSION RELATIONSHIPS

Respiratory Exchange Ratio

The respiratory exchange ratio (R) is the ratio of carbon dioxide production (CO_2 evolved from the lung) to oxygen consumption (oxygen taken up from the lung by the blood):

$$R = \frac{\dot{V}_{CO_2}}{\dot{V}_{O_2}}$$

In recent times the measurement of the respiratory exchange ratio has been made easy through the use of metabolic carts that measure CO_2 production and O_2 consumption. The R value for a given lung segment or unit is dependent on the ventilation perfusion ratio for that unit, as is the R value for the whole lung, which is dependent on the ventilation/perfusion ratio for the whole lung. In the steady state, R is referred to as the respiratory quotient, which reflects the same gas exchange ratio for the whole body. The respiratory quotient is determined by the type of fuel being metabolized by the body (carbohydrate R = 1.0; lipid R = 0.7; or protein R = 0.8). Usually we metabolize a combination of carbohydrate and lipid (or fat), giving us an R value of approximately 0.8.

Alveolar Gas Equation

The partial pressure of oxygen in the alveolus (PAO_2) can be calculated with reasonable accuracy using the following equation if the fractional concentration of inspired gas (FI_{O_2}) and the arterial CO_2 tension (Pa_{CO_2}) are known:

$$PAO_2 = FI_{O_2} (PB - PH_2O) - \frac{Pa_{CO_2}}{R}$$

Examples

Calculate the partial pressure of oxygen in the alveolus for a patient breathing the following oxygen concentrations:

Example 1.—For room air, PB is 760 mm Hg, and Pa_{CO_2} is 40 mm Hg:

$$\begin{aligned} PAO_2 &= 0.21 (760 - 47) - \frac{40}{0.8} \\ &= 0.21 (713) - 50 \\ &= 100 \text{ mm Hg} \end{aligned}$$

Example 2.—For 100% O_2, PB is 760 mm Hg, and Pa_{CO_2} is 40 mm Hg:

$$PAO_2 = 1.0 (760 - 47) - \frac{40}{0.8}$$
$$= 1.0 (713) - 50$$
$$= 663 \text{ mm Hg}$$

Example 3.—For 40% oxygen, PB is 757 mm Hg, and Pa_{CO_2} is 48 mm Hg:

$$PAO_2 = 0.4 (757 - 47) - \frac{48}{0.8}$$
$$= 0.4 (710) - 60$$
$$= 224 \text{ mm Hg}$$

Adjusting F_{IO_2} Using the PaO_2/PAO_2 Ratio

One of the common questions frequently asked in the clinical setting is what amount or concentration of oxygen should be given to a patient to achieve a desired arterial oxygen tension. In the past, the answer to this question has often depended predominantly on clinical judgment or experience rather than calculated values.

The $P(A-a)O_2$ has long been used to estimate the amount of pulmonary dysfunction due to $\dot{V}/\dot{Q}$ abnormality, shunt, or diffusion limitation; however, it is only of moderate assistance in deciding how much to increase the inspired oxygen concentration when treating the patient. Recently, the arterial/alveolar oxygen tension ratio has been used to more accurately predict the F_{IO_2} needed to achieve a desired oxygen tension using the following formula:

$$\frac{PaO_2 \text{ (known)}}{PAO_2 \text{ (calculated)}} = \frac{PaO_2 \text{ (desired)}}{PAO_2 \text{ (unknown)}}.$$

There are three steps involved in using this equation to predict the desired F_{IO_2}:

1. Use of the alveolar air equation to calculate the PAO_2 using the known inspired oxygen concentration.
2. Use of the arterial/alveolar ratio or proportion given to solve for the unknown PAO_2.
3. A second application of the alveolar air equation using the new PAO_2 to calculate the desired F_{IO_2}.

Example.—How much should the F_{IO_2} be increased to increase the PaO_2 to 75 mm Hg if F_{IO_2} is 0.30, PaO_2 is 45 mm Hg, Pa_{CO_2} is 40 mm Hg, and PB is 760 mm Hg?

1. $PAO_2 = 0.30 (760 - 47) - 40/0.8$
   $= 164 \text{ mm Hg.}$

2. $\dfrac{45 \text{ (known } PaO_2)}{164 \text{ (calculated } PAO_2)} = \dfrac{75 \text{ (desired } PaO_2)}{\text{unknown } PAO_2}.$

   $$\text{Unknown } PAO_2 = \frac{(75) (164)}{(45)}$$
   $$= 273 \text{ mm Hg.}$$

3. $273 \text{ new } PAO_2 = \text{Desired } F_{IO_2} (760 - 47)$
   $- 40/0.8.$
   $273 = \text{Desired } F_{IO_2} (713) - 50.$
   $\dfrac{273 + 50}{713} = \text{Desired } F_{IO_2}.$
   $0.45 = \text{Desired } F_{IO_2}.$

Shunt Equation

Several formulas are used for calculation of physiologic shunt. Although each of them may be applied under slightly different conditions, the essential concept depends on a thorough understanding of the basic shunt equation. Figure B–4 illustrates the basic concepts used in the derivation. The following observations are intuitively made from the diagram:

1. The total amount of oxygen leaving the lungs or entering the arterial system is equal to the total blood flow (Q_T) times the arterial oxygen content (CaO_2):

$$\dot{Q}_T \times CaO_2$$

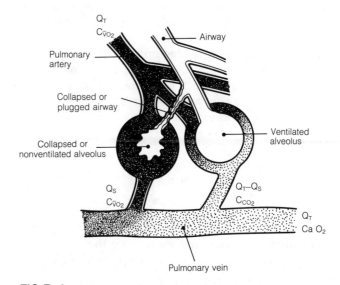

FIG B–4.
The effect of alterations of ventilation of ventilation-perfusion relationships on gas exchange.

2. The amount of oxygen carried by the shunted blood is equal to the shunted blood flow (Q_S) times the oxygen content of shunted blood ($C\overline{v}O_2$), which is the same as the oxygen content of mixed venous blood:

$$\dot{Q}_S \times C\overline{v}O_2$$

3. The amount of oxygen carried in the end-capillary blood is equal to the capillary blood flow ($Q_T - Q_S$) times the capillary oxygen content ($Cc'O_2$):

$$(\dot{Q}_T - \dot{Q}_S) \times Cc'O_2$$

Finally, the total amount of oxygen delivered to the arterial system in no. 1 must be equal to the sum of the amounts of oxygen in the shunted blood in no. 2 plus the amount of oxygen in the end-capillary blood in no. 3, or:

$$A = B + C$$

$$(\dot{Q}_T)(CaO_2) = (\dot{Q}_S)(C\overline{v}O_2) + (\dot{Q}_T - \dot{Q}_S)Cc'O_2$$

$$(\dot{Q}_T)(CaO_2) = (\dot{Q}_S)(C\overline{v}O_2) + (\dot{Q}_T)(Cc'O_2) - (\dot{Q}_S)(Cc'O_2)$$

$$(\dot{Q}_T)(CaO_2) - (\dot{Q}_T)(Cc'O_2) = (\dot{Q}_S)(C\overline{v}O_2) - (\dot{Q}_S)(Cc'O_2)$$

$$\dot{Q}_T(CaO_2 - Cc'O_2) = \dot{Q}_S(C\overline{v}O_2 - Cc'O_2)$$

$$\frac{\dot{Q}_S}{\dot{Q}_T} = \frac{Cc'O_2 - CaO_2}{Cc'O_2 - C\overline{v}O_2}$$

This classic shunt equation is somewhat difficult to use for two reasons: (1) the capillary O_2 content cannot be measured directly, although it is overcome by computing the $P_{C'O_2}$ form of the alveolar gas equation and using that value to calculate capillary O_2 content; and (2) the mixed venous oxygen content is not readily available unless a pulmonary artery catheter is in place. When mixed venous gases are available, however, it is the most correct form of the equation to use, and knowing the classic equation will help one to remember and understand the other alternative forms.

Clinical Shunt Equation

Because of the problems previously mentioned, another form of the shunt equation was introduced to help the clinician approximate shunt with the clinical data available. The classic equation was manipulated by adding and subtracting the arterial oxygen content from the denominator, as shown:

$$Cc'O_2 - C\overline{v}O_2 = (Cc'O_2 - C\overline{v}O_2) + (CaO_2 - CaO_2)$$
$$= (CaO_2 - C\overline{v}O_2) + (Cc'O_2 - CaO_2)$$

Therefore,

$$\frac{\dot{Q}_S}{\dot{Q}_T} = \frac{(Cc O_2 - CaO_2)}{(CaO_2 - C\overline{v}O_2) + (Cc O_2 - CaO_2)}.$$

In patients with stable cardiovascular function and a consistent metabolic rate, the term in the denominator for the arterial-venous oxygen difference may be approximated as 3.5 vol%. The equation then becomes:

$$\frac{\dot{Q}_S}{\dot{Q}_T} = \frac{(Cc'O_2 - CaO_2)}{3.5 + Cc'O_2 - CaO_2}$$

Alveolar to Arterial (A − a) Oxygen Tension Gradient: Second Form of the Clinical Shunt Equation

During clinical circumstances in which the PaO_2 is greater than 150 mm Hg, the hemoglobin molecule is considered to be 100% saturated. Under these conditions, the difference in oxygen content between alveolar capillary blood and arterial blood ($CcO_2 - CaO_2$) reduces to the amount of dissolved oxygen carried by the blood. The clinical shunt equation then becomes:

$$\frac{\dot{Q}_S}{\dot{Q}_T} = \frac{(PAO_2 - PaO_2)(0.003)}{(CaO_2 - C\overline{v}O_2) + (PAO_2 - PaO_2)(0.003)}.$$

This form of the shunt equation has limited use because most patients in the acute care setting have a PO_2 below 150 mm Hg. The standard form of the shunt equation is applicable in either case, and it is important to recognize that the shortened form is just a mathematical manipulation of the standard equation under the specific clinical criteria of a PaO_2 greater than 150 mm Hg.

One of the applications of this equation is that it has been used in a very general sense to approximate physiologic shunt by simply measuring the alveolar-arterial pressure gradient ($PAO_2 - PaO_2$) seen in both the numerator and the denominator. This gradient is commonly called the *A − a gradient*. As a very broad rule of thumb, when a patient is given 100% oxygen, for every 50 mm Hg of partial pressure difference in the A − a gradient, there is approximately a 2% shunt. The magnitude of the A − a gradient changes when the inspired oxygen concentration is changed. Therefore, the A − a gradient should be used only when: (1) there is cardiovascular stability, (2) the FIO_2 is constant, and (3) the PaO_2 is greater than 150 mm Hg.

Example 1.—The following laboratory data were obtained from a patient receiving mechanical ventilation:

Hb = 15 gm%
Pa_{O_2} = 65 mm Hg
$P\bar{v}_{O_2}$ = 30 mm Hg
Pa_{CO_2} = 50 mm Hg
Sa_{O_2} = 90%
$S\bar{v}_{O_2}$ = 60%
P_B = 760 mm Hg
$F_{I_{O_2}}$ = 0.70
R = 0.80

With this information, the PA_{O_2}, Cc'_{O_2}, and $C\bar{v}_{O_2}$ can be calculated:

1. PA_{O_2} = 0.70 (760 − 47) − 50/0.8
   = 0.70 (713) − 62.5
   = 499 − 63
   = 436
2. Cc'_{O_2} = (Hb × 1.39) 100% + (PA_{O_2} × 0.003)
   = (15 × 1.39) 1.0 + (436 × 0.003)
   = 20.85 + 1.31
   = 22.16
3. Ca_{O_2} = (Hb × 1.39 × sat) + (Pa_{O_2} × 0.003)
   = (15 × 1.39) 0.9 + (65 × 0.003)
   = 18.77 + 0.20
   = 18.97
4. $C\bar{v}_{O_2}$ = (Hb × 1.39 × sat) + ($P\bar{v}_{O_2}$) × 0.003
   = (15 × 1.39) 0.6 + (30 × 0.003)
   = 12.52 + 0.09
   = 12.61

From these results, the amount of physiologic shunt can now be calculated:

$$\frac{\dot{Q}_S}{\dot{Q}_T} = \frac{Cc'_{O_2} - Ca_{O_2}}{Cc'_{O_2} - C\bar{v}_{O_2}}$$
$$= \frac{22.16 - 18.97}{22.16 - 12.61}$$
$$= \frac{3.19}{9.55}$$
$$= 0.33, \text{ or } 33\%$$

Example 2.—A patient with a stable cardiovascular system is maintained on mechanical ventilation. Access to central venous gases is not possible because it was not necessary to place a pulmonary catheter. The following laboratory data, however, are available:

Pa_{O_2} = 160 mm Hg
Sat = 100%
Pa_{CO_2} = 45 mm Hg
P_B = 760 mm Hg
$F_{I_{O_2}}$ = 1.00
Hb = 14 gm%

The criteria for stable cardiovascular system, $P_{I_{O_2}}$ of 100% and P_{O_2} greater than 150 mm Hg, are met. First estimate the amount of shunt using the A − a gradient, and then compare the results with that obtained by using the second form of the clinical shunt equation.

A − a Gradient

1. PA_{O_2} = $F_{I_{O_2}}$ (P_B − PH_2O) − Pa_{CO_2}/R
   = 1.0 (760 − 47) − 45/0.8
   = 713 − 56
   = 657 mm Hg
2. A − a gradient = PA_{O_2} − Pa_{O_2}
   = 657 − 160
   = 497

A 2% shunt for every 50 mm Hg partial difference can be estimated; therefore, this example represents approximately a 20% shunt.

Clinical Form of the Shunt Equation

1. PA_{O_2} = 657 mm Hg (from the alveolar O_2 tension equation above)
2. Pa_{O_2} = 160 mm Hg (from clinical data)
3. Cc'_{O_2} − Ca_{O_2} = 3.5 vol% (from clinical estimate)

With this information, the amount of physiologic shunt can be estimated:

$$\frac{\dot{Q}_S}{\dot{Q}_T} = \frac{(PA_{O_2} - Pa_{O_2})(0.003)}{(Ca_{O_2} - C\bar{v}_{O_2}) + (PA_{O_2} - Pa_{O_2})(0.003)}$$
$$= \frac{(657 - 160)(0.003)}{3.5 + (657 - 160)(0.003)}$$
$$= \frac{1.49}{3.5 + 1.49}$$
$$= \frac{1.49}{4.99}$$
$$= 0.30, \text{ or } 30\%$$

PULMONARY MECHANICS

Compliance

Lung expansion requires that the elastic forces that tend to collapse the lung be overcome. The stronger the elastic forces resisting expansion, the greater the pressure required to expand or add volume to the lung. Compliance is the reciprocal of elastance ($C = 1/E$) or a measure of the ease of distensibility of the lung. If the addition of volume to the lung requires only a small amount of pressure, the lung is referred to as a compliant lung. On the other hand, if large pressures are needed to inflate the lung, the lung is referred to as a noncompliant lung. Compliance can be expressed as the relationship between volume and pressure or the volume change (ΔV) divided by the pressure change (ΔP):

$$\text{Compliance} = \frac{\text{Volume change }(\Delta V)}{\text{Pressure change }(\Delta P)}$$

Mechanical ventilation of the lung involves expansion of the lung as well as the chest wall. Therefore, several kinds of compliance can be defined:

1. *Lung compliance:* The compliance of the lung (C_L) by itself. The static pressure needed to expand the lung is measured as the pressure difference across the lung, referred to as the transpulmonary pressure (P_L), or the difference between alveolar pressure (P_A) and pleural pressure (Ppl):

$$P_L = P_A - Ppl$$
$$C_L = \frac{\text{Volume change}}{P_A - Ppl}$$

2. *Chest wall compliance:* The compliance of the chest wall (Ccw) alone. The pressure necessary to expand the chest wall (Pcw) is measured as the trans–chest wall pressure, or the pressure difference between the pleural space (Ppl) and the body surface (Pbs):

$$Pcw = Ppl - Pbs$$
$$Ccw = \frac{\text{Volume change}}{Ppl - Pbs}$$

3. *Respiratory compliance:* Compliance of the lungs and chest wall combined. The pressure needed to expand the respiratory system (rs) is the transthoracic pressure (Prs), or the pressure difference between the inside of the system (the alveolar pressure, P_A) and the

pressure outside of the system (the body surface pressure, Pbs):

$$Prs = P_A - Pbs$$
$$Crs = \frac{\text{Volume change}}{P_A - Pbs}$$

From a practical standpoint, usually only the respiratory system compliance is measured because both lung compliance and chest wall compliance require the measurement of pleural pressure. Pleural pressure may be measured with the use of a balloon placed in the esophagus, although it is rarely done in the clinical setting. It is possible, however, to measure pleural pressure in patients who have chest tubes in place.

Measurement of Respiratory System Compliance or Total Compliance

System compliance may be measured by recording the tidal volume and the airway pressure during mechanical ventilation (Fig B–5). The diagram in Figure B–5 represents a typical airway pressure tracing obtained during a tidal breath. The inspiratory plateau can be easily created by dialing in the inspiratory hold on current ventilators or by momentarily obstructing the expiratory valve (Fig B–6).

During inspiration, the peak pressure observed in the tracing is the pressure created in overcoming both resistive and compliance factors from the respiratory system and the ventilator circuit. During the plateau phase, however, airflow rapidly diminishes until the pressure that remains is predominantly produced by the elastic recoil properties of the system. The plateau pressure is therefore a reasonable estimate of the static pressure resulting from the system's elasticity. System compliance can then be calculated by dividing the tidal volume by the dif-

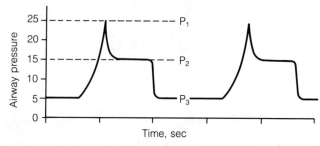

FIG B–5.
Diagram of a typical airway pressure tracing obtained during a tidal breath. An inspiratory plateau (P_2) can be created by dialing in an inspiration pause on a ventilator or by obstructing the exhalation valve momentarily.

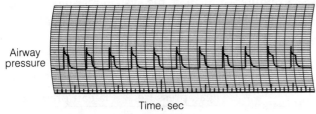

Time, sec

Actual laboratory pressure tracing

FIG B–6.
Actual laboratory pressure tracing of a tidal breath with an end-inspiratory pause.

ference between plateau pressure and baseline pressure:

System compliance

$$= \frac{\text{Tidal volume}}{\text{Plateau pressure} - \text{Baseline pressure}}$$

As a point of clarity, the term *effective dynamic compliance* (EDC) was often used in the clinic to refer to the compliance measured by dividing the volume change by the pressure difference between peak pressure and baseline pressure or end-expiratory pressure. Changes in peak pressure and, therefore, effective dynamic compliance are useful as an indication that some change has occurred in the system and are often monitored by ventilator peak pressure alarms. However, the measurement of effective dynamic compliance fails to distinguish between resistive and compliance changes and is thus misleading in any attempt to interpret such changes. Since the addition of the inspiratory plateau is a simple uncomplicated procedure, I would like to stress the importance of distinguishing between resistive or flow-dependent changes vs. changes in static system compliance and would encourage dropping the term EDC to avoid unnecessary confusion.

Example.—Calculate the system compliance using the following clinical data and the pressure values from Figure B–5:

Delivered tidal volume = 500 ml
Plateau pressure = 15 cm H_2O
PEEP or baseline pressure = 5 cm H_2O

$$\text{Compliance (Crs)} = \frac{\text{Tidal volume}}{\text{Plateau pressure}}$$

$$= \frac{500 \text{ ml}}{15 - 5 \text{ cm } H_2O}$$

$$= \frac{500 \text{ ml}}{10 \text{ cm } H_2O} = \frac{50 \text{ ml}}{1 \text{cm } H_2O}$$

$$= 0.05 \text{ L/cm } H_2O$$

Volume-Pressure Curve

The volume-pressure curve is included as a further explanation of the term compliance (Fig B–7). Although such curves are usually constructed only in the laboratory (because of the need to measure total lung volume), the curve is included here to illustrate how compliance changes with lung volume. By definition, compliance is the volume change divided by the pressure change, or the *slope* of the curve measured over a specific volume range. The slope of the curve, or the compliance, is seen to decrease at both low lung volumes and at very high lung volumes. Clinically it correlates with lung disorders that produce changes in functional residual capacity (FRC) either by diminishing the FRC, and therefore moving the volume pressure relationship to the left on the curve, or by overinflating the lung and therefore moving the system to the right on the volume pressure curve. Changes in compliance are often used as an indication of the therapeutic effectiveness of PEEP in the treatment of pulmonary insufficiency; the best PEEP, or the optimum PEEP, is determined by the level of end-expiratory pressure that achieves the highest system compliance.

Resistance

In contrast to compliance, which is a measure of the static elastic properties of the pulmonary system, resistance refers to the dynamic properties or the flow-dependent properties of the lung thorax sys-

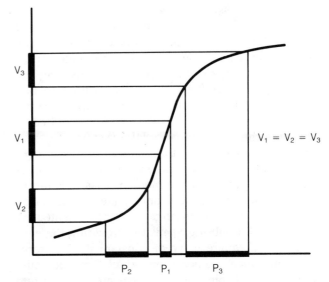

FIG B–7.
Volume-pressure curve illustrates how compliance changes with lung volume.

tem. Resistance to airflow within the system is calculated from the simultaneous measurement of airflow and the pressure difference required to produce the airflow. Pressure must be generated during breathing to overcome several kinds of resistance, including:

1. *Airway resistance:* Resistance specific to the movement of air through the conducting passages all the way from the mouth to the alveoli; for patients on mechanical ventilation, it includes the resistance of the ventilator circuitry and the endotracheal tube.
2. *Tissue viscous resistance:* The frictional resistance caused by the movement of the tissues of the lung and the chest wall.
3. *Inertia, or resistance to change in velocity or direction:* Inertial forces must be applied to accelerate the gas and the tissues that compose the system; physiologically, inertia has been found to be a negligible quantity during normal breathing.

Measurement of the Total System Resistance

Resistance is calculated from the general equation:

$$\text{Resistance} = \frac{\text{Pressure difference}}{\text{Flow}}.$$

Although it is possible to measure several different kinds of resistance, including airway resistance, pulmonary resistance (combination of airway and lung viscous resistance), and chest wall tissue resistance, the discussion here will refer to the resistance of the entire system, including the lung, the chest wall, and portions of the ventilator circuitry, depending on where the pressure manometer is located. Resistance can be calculated by dividing the pressure difference between peak pressure and plateau pressure by the airflow (see Fig B–5). Since the plateau pressure represents the pressure required to overcome the elastic forces of the system, it is reasonable to assume that the remaining pressure ($P_1 - P_2$) is the pressure required to overcome the resistance of the system at the moment airflow is terminated. Although airflow is not frequently measured on standard ventilators, it can be approximated by the flow setting on the ventilator providing the ventilator has a square wave or constant flow pattern. Resistance measurements on ventilators with sine wave or diminishing flow patterns are less accurate but can still be used as an indication of resistance changes, although they are somewhat less sensitive.

Example.—Calculate the system resistance using the following data:

Peak pressure   = 25 cm H_2O
Plateau pressure = 15 cm H_2O
Flow rate   = 40 L/min

$$\begin{aligned}
\text{Resistance} &= \frac{\text{Peak pressure} - \text{Plateau pressure}}{\text{Flow}} \\
&= \frac{25 - 15 \text{ cm } H_2O}{40 \text{ L/min}} \\
&= \frac{10 \text{ cm } H_2O}{40 \text{ L/min}} \\
&= 0.25 \text{ cm } H_2O/\text{L/min}.
\end{aligned}$$

BLOOD FLOW AND CARDIOVASCULAR MEASUREMENTS

General Considerations

Resistance equations appear several times in both pulmonary and cardiovascular physiology, such as airflow resistance (Poiseuille's law), pulmonary vascular resistance, and systemic vascular resistance. It is helpful to recognize that the same general formula applies to each of these calculations. The flow resistance offered by any system is calculated from the pressure differences across the system (the inlet minus the outlet pressure) divided by the flow through the system (Fig B–8):

$$\text{Resistance} = \frac{\text{Inlet pressure} - \text{Outlet pressure}}{\text{Flow}}$$

Pulmonary Vascular Resistance

Pulmonary vascular resistance (R) is calculated by dividing the pressure difference across the lung (mean pulmonary artery pressure [PAP] minus

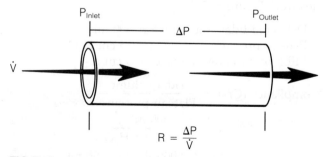

FIG B–8.
The resistance offered by any system is calculated from the pressure differences across the system.

mean left atrial pressure) by the cardiac output according to the following equation:

$$R = \frac{\text{Mean PAP} - \text{PCWP*}}{\text{Pulmonary blood flow}}$$
$$= \frac{14 - 5 \text{ mm Hg}}{6 \text{ L/min}}$$
$$= 1.5 \text{ mm Hg/L/min}$$

Systemic Vascular Resistance

The calculation of systemic vascular resistance (SVR) is very similar to that of pulmonary vascular resistance except for the magnitude of the driving pressure. For the systemic system, the driving pressure is approximately 10-fold greater than the pulmonary driving pressure.

$$\text{SVR}$$
$$= \frac{\text{Mean arterial} - \text{mean rt atrial pressure (or CVP)}}{\text{Cardiac output}}$$
$$= \frac{95 - 0 \text{ mm Hg}}{6 \text{ L/min}}$$
$$= 16 \text{ mm Hg/L/min}$$

Note.—Resistance measurements are sometimes reported in several different kinds of units. The units by which blood pressure and cardiac output are commonly reported in the clinic are millimeters of mercury and liters per minute. Some physiologists may prefer, however, to report blood flow in ml/sec, which then gives resistance units of mm Hg/ml/sec (a term called the *resistance unit*). Finally, in classic physical terms, pressure is measured in dynes per square centimeter (force per unit area) and flow is measured in cubic centimeters per second. Resistance then becomes:

$$\text{Resistance} = \frac{\text{Pressure}}{\text{Flow}}$$
$$= \frac{\text{dynes/cm}^2}{\text{cm}^3\text{/sec}}$$
$$= \frac{\text{dynes sec}}{\text{cm}^5}$$

Using the following conversions, one can convert mm Hg/L/min to dynes sec/cm⁵ where:

$$1 \text{ mm Hg} = 1,330 \text{ dynes/cm}^2$$
$$1 \text{ min} = 60 \text{ sec}$$
$$1 \text{ L} = 1,000 \text{ cm}^3$$

*The actual pressure in the outflow tract of the lung is the mean atrial pressure. Under most clinical conditions, it is approximated by the pulmonary capillary wedge pressure (PCWP).

$$R \text{ (dynes sec/cm}^5)$$
$$= \frac{\text{Pressure}}{\text{Flow}}$$
$$= \frac{\text{mm Hg} \times (1,330 \text{ dynes/cm}^2)/\text{mm Hg}}{\text{L} \times (1,000 \text{ cm}^3/\text{L}) \text{ min} \times (60 \text{ sec/min})}$$
$$= \frac{\text{mm Hg}}{\text{L/min}} \times 80$$
$$= \text{dynes sec/cm}^5$$

Ventricular Stroke Work

The work that the heart performs in moving the blood from the veins to the arteries can be expressed as the sum of the potential energy of pressure and the kinetic energy of blood flow. The latter usually represents only a small portion of the total cardiac work (about 5% during resting conditions) and will not be considered here. The majority of the work performed by the heart is done in the creation of pressure in the arterial system. This work, or potential energy of pressure, can be estimated by multiplying the stroke volume times the mean ventricular ejection pressure (e.g., mean pressure during the systolic phase of the cardiac cycle) (Fig B–9).

Left Ventricular Stroke Work (Fig B–10)

Work = Stroke volume
    × left ventricular mean ejection pressure

Right Ventricular Stroke Work

Work = Stroke volume
    × right ventricular mean ejection pressure

Mean aortic pressure or mean pulmonary artery pressure may be used as an approximation.

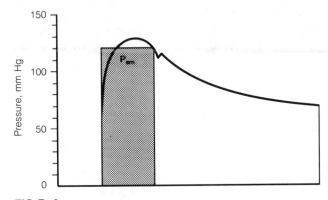

FIG B–9.
Diagram of an aortic pressure pulse illustrating the mean systolic pressure (P_{SM}).

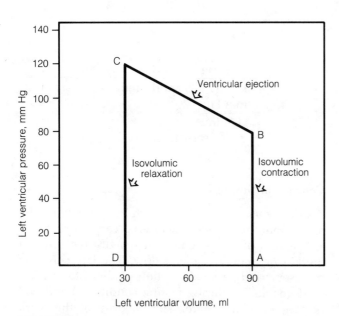

FIG B–10.
Diagram of the relationship between left ventricular pressure and volume for one cardiac cycle. The area *ABCDA* represents the total pressure-volume work.

Endocardial Viability Ratio

In nonspecific terms, the endocardial viability ratio (EVR) is an indicator of the ratio between myocardial blood flow and myocardial oxygen consumption or more simply the myocardial oxygen supply-demand relationship. The EVR is defined as the ratio of the diastolic pressure time index (DPTI) to the systolic pressure time index (SPTI):

$$EVR = DPTI/SPTI.$$

The DPTI is calculated by measuring the area under the aortic diastolic pressure curve and subtracting the area under the left ventricular diastolic pressure curve (see Fig B–10). It is generally done through use of a planimeter, a device that measures the area of a plane figure by tracing around the perimeter. The area measured, or the DPTI, is an

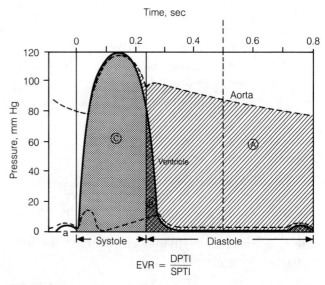

$$EVR = \frac{DPTI}{SPTI}$$

FIG B–11.
Endocardial viability rates can be determined by comparing area under systolic and diastolic pressure curves. *A*, area under aortic diastolic pressure curve; *B*, area under left ventricular diastolic pressure curve; *C*, systolic pressure time index.

expression of the pressure gradient across the myocardium and is an index of the coronary blood flow. The SPTI is similarly measured by planimetering the area under the systolic pressure curve. The area represents the amount of pressure work performed during systole and is an indicator of the myocardial oxygen consumption (Fig B–11).

Tension Time Index

The tension time index is a parameter of cardiac function that correlates with the myocardial oxygen demand. The parameter is calculated as the mean systolic pressure times the duration of systole times the heart rate. Although more specific indices of myocardial oxygen consumption, such as peak wall tension, are available, they are generally more difficult to obtain clinically.

Appendix C

Infection Control

Raymond S. Edge, Ed.D., R.R.T.

Respiratory care patients are at increased risk for nosocomial infections for a number of reasons. Many of our patients are among the most seriously ill of the hospitalized groups. Often these patients have therapeutic regimens or underlying conditions that compromise their defense systems, and many therapeutic or diagnostic techniques expose them to procedures that are invasive or that bypass host defense systems.

The linkage of respiratory care equipment and nosocomial infections is unfortunately well documented and clear, with one study showing that respiratory therapy equipment accounted for 11% of the infections associated with medical devices.[8] The nature of the respiratory care patient population and respiratory equipment that often harbors warm basins of liquid seemingly designed to promote microbial growth produce the framework for significant nosocomial problems. Reducing the risk of infection caused by environmental contamination depends on the individual practitioner adhering to tested protocols for appropriate practice at the bedside, coupled with quality control in cleaning and sterilization. In that 5% to 10% of the patients in America's hospitals, or approximately 2 million/year develop these infections, it is a problem of unbelievable impact on our health care system.[3, 5]

HANDWASHING

Handwashing is generally considered the single most important procedure for preventing nosocomial infections. Regardless of whatever benefits are ac-

crued by therapy or cleaning and sterilizing, it is all lost if the simple process of handwashing is overlooked.

Skin flora are categorized as either resident or transient. Resident flora survive and multiply on the skin and can be repeatedly cultured. These organisms are normally of low virulence and are associated with infections only when invasive procedures are used. Transient flora found on the hands are often high-virulence pathogens acquired from colonized or infected patients. These pathogens have been frequently implicated in nosocomial outbreaks.[6]

The long history of the association of respiratory care equipment to nosocomial infection has led to an awareness of practitioners to the need to wash their hands between patients. A 1981 study revealed that whereas less than 43% of the sampled physicians and nurses washed their hands after patient contact, compliance for respiratory care personnel was greater than 75%.[1] This increased awareness on the part of respiratory care personnel is gratifying, but, unfortunately, it leaves great room for improvement.

The recommended handwashing procedures depend on the purpose of the washing. In most situations, a vigorous brief washing with soap under a stream of running water is adequate to remove transient flora. Generally, simple handwashing with soap is performed when one is coming on duty, before and after contact with patients, and whenever the hands are soiled. In that the repeated washing with soap and disinfectants leaves the hands chafed and dry, it is recommended that hand creams be employed during off-duty hours. It would allow protection for the hands and yet avoid the possibility of recontamination from bacterial growth sometimes found in hand creams.

Antimicrobial handwashing procedures are indicated before all invasive procedures, during the care of patients in strict, respiratory, or enteric isolation, before entering special care units such as newborn nurseries and intensive care units, and in emergency situations where sinks are unavailable. The most commonly used agents are 70% isopropyl alcohol, iodophors, and chlorhexidine. Scrub regimens such as the povidone-iodine (Betadine) surgical scrub are appropriate for these areas (Table C–1). Since liquid soap containers have been shown to serve as reservoirs for microorganisms, they should be cleaned, dried, and refilled at least monthly.[4] Disposable liquid containers might be preferable to reduce the risk of contamination. When cake soap is used, they should be smaller bars and kept on racks that allow for complete drainage of water.

DEFINITIONS

The following definitions are useful for the remaining discussions of infection control:

1. *Antisepsis:* The process in which the destruction of pathogenic organisms in the vegetative state is accomplished on living tissue.
2. *Disinfection:* The process of destroying at least the pathogenic organisms and the destruction of their products.
   a. *Low-level disinfection:* Procedures that kill many viruses and vegetative bacteria but that cannot be relied on to kill resistant organisms such as the tuberculin bacillus and spores.
   b. *High-level disinfection:* Procedures capable of producing sterility if they are continued long enough; it can be said to have been accomplished when all but resistant spores are destroyed.
3. *Resident flora:* Bacteria that reside in the pore openings, cracks, and folds of the skin; they cannot be eliminated by simple handwashing and can be repeatedly cultured.
4. *Transient flora:* Bacteria that reside on the skin surface; they can usually be removed by simple handwashing techniques.
5. *Sanitize:* To reduce the population of microorganisms on inanimate objects to a safe level as judged by public health authorities.
6. *Sterility:* An absolute term referring to the destruction or removal of all microorganisms present; there is no degree of sterility.
7. *Surveillance:* Identification of baseline information in regard to frequency and type of infections to identify alterations from the baseline.

PHYSICAL AGENTS IN INFECTION CONTROL

For mechanical removal of microbes, the three key methods are scrubbing, filtration, and sedimentation. In respiratory care practice, mechanical scrubbing and filtration processes are commonly employed, whereas sedimentation has little current application. The most common nonmechanical physical agent used in the process of sterilization and disinfection is the application of heat. Depending on the desired result, heat may be applied dry or may be enhanced by the addition of moisture.

Scrubbing

Scrubbing is the basic process for disinfection and sterilization. In practice it is both mechanical and chemical. The physical act itself removes many microbes and is often augmented by soap, water, and antimicrobial agents.

Unless the microbes are of extreme virulence, contaminated equipment is first disassembled and scrubbed so that dirt, debris, and extraneous materials are removed. This first mechanical step is paramount if the later disinfection-sterilization processes are to be effective. Whether the contamination is of the hands, floors, or ventilator circuits, everything must, at a minimum, be clean.

TABLE C–1.
Povidone-Iodine (Betadine) Surgical Scrub Regimen*

1. Clean under nails. Keep fingernails short and clean.
2. Wet hands and forearms.
3. Apply two portions, about 5 ml of povidone-iodine, to hands.
4. Without adding water, wash hands and forearms thoroughly for 5 minutes. Use a brush if desired.
5. Use a sterile orange stick, clean under nails, add a little water for copious suds, and rinse thoroughly with running water.
6. Apply 5 ml from the dispenser to hands, repeat steps just given, and rinse with running water.

*Practitioners sensitive to iodine can substitute another disinfectant, such as hexachlorophene (pHisoHex).

Filtration

Filtration of bacteria is accomplished by passing a liquid or gas through a material whose pores are small enough to retain the microbes. In that liquid and gases are difficult to disinfect or sterilize, most commonly either is accomplished through the process of filtration. Materials most often used for bacterial filters are unglazed porcelain, diatomaceous earth, compressed asbestos, sintered glass, and cellulose membranes. Membrane filters of cellulose esters and other polymeric materials can be designed with pore sizes small enough to remove even certain virus types.

Filters interposed between the ventilator and breathing circuit effectively eliminate contaminants from the driving gas and prevent retrograde contamination. To remain efficient, they should be changed after 500 hours of use or according to the manufacturer's recommendation. One practical test is to cycle the ventilator to inspiration at 20 cm H_2O pressure and change the filter whenever the back pressure caused by resistance through the device is 4 cm H_2O pressure or greater.

Sedimentation

Sedimentation has little respiratory care application but is an important process in the purification of lakes, streams, and city water supplies. Suspended materials and bacteria settle to the bottom as a natural process.

Incineration

Incineration is the preferred method for materials contaminated with pathogens of extreme virulence or materials for which no further use is considered. To assure public safety, temperatures must be adequate to attain complete combustion to avoid air contamination.

Dry Heat

Dry heat is often used for powders, oils, and glassware that cannot withstand moist heat methods. The heat destroys the microorganisms through the effects of oxidation, dessication, and alteration in osmotic pressures. In that dry heat is conducted less well than moist and spores are resistant to dessication, high temperatures and extended time periods must be used. The standard range is 160°C to 180°C applied for 1 to 2 hours.

Boiling

Boiling is an age-old method for sanitization and low-level disinfection. In that resistant spores can withstand the 212°F (100°C) temperature of boiling water, sterilization in the true sense does not occur. At sea level, the minimal standard of exposure should be 30 minutes, with the time period adjusted upward 5 minutes per 1,000 feet of elevation above sea level. The efficiency of the process in killing spores can be increased by the addition of sodium bicarbonate (sal soda) sufficient to make a 2% solution or the addition of sodium hydroxide (caustic soda) so as to make a 0.1% solution. With the addition of these chemicals, bacterial spores are destroyed in 10 to 30 minutes.

Pasteurization

Pasteurization is an inexpensive and environmentally safe method of disinfection that has gained popularity in respiratory therapy departments. The process employs a mild heat to destroy vegetative pathogens. Essentially two separate standards are used: the *batch method*, where heat is applied at 62°C for 30 minutes; and the *flash,* or *HTST* (high temperature short time) *method*, which employs temperatures of 72°C for 15 seconds. The flash method has application in the assurance and safety of fresh milk but is not commonly used in respiratory care departments. With the current concern for environmental safety, pasteurization offers a low-cost, nontoxic alternative to glutaraldehyde or ethylene oxide in areas where disinfection alone is sufficient. Not all goods can be pasteurized; the heat and moisture cause some plastic devices to become deformed, and rubber products such as anesthesia masks and ventilator reservoir bags may deteriorate at an unacceptable rate due to the process.

As with liquid chemical disinfectants, devices that have undergone pasteurization are often recontaminated in the drying and repackaging phases. The use of a filtered air-drying chamber after the pasteurization process is recommended to avoid possible recontamination that might occur while the devices are drying in room air.

Autoclaving

Autoclaving is the application of steam and pressure to accomplish sterilization. Steam under 2 atmospheres of pressure has a temperature of 121°C. With this temperature and pressure, virtually all spores are killed within 15 minutes. If the pressure is increased to 3 atmospheres, the temperature is raised to 134°C, and sterilization is accomplished within 3 minutes. The moisture enhances the conduction of heat and the rate of killing. With autoclaving the microorganisms are destroyed by disruption of the cell membrane, the coagulation of the cell protoplasm, or both.

Autoclaving is the most commonly used, effective form of sterilization and is preferred unless the material is injured by temperature or pressure. At autoclave temperature (121°C), nearly all plastics except polycarbonate, polypropylene, nylon, and Teflon have a tendency to melt. This limitation is particularly problematic to respiratory care, because much of the equipment is rubber or plastic, which cannot withstand the process.

The efficiency of the sterilization is monitored by several methods. Thermocouples are inserted into the autoclave load to monitor temperatures, and heat-sensitive tape is often used to assure that 121°C is achieved in the chamber. These methods give only indirect assurance of the conditions of sterilization and are not as reliable as biologic indicators such as spores of *Bacillus stearothermophilus*. The storage or shelf life of the sterilized items is dependent on the wrap used and containment area (Table C–2).

The use of commercial biologic indicators is recommended at least once per week.[4] If the chamber contains implantable objects, the process should be monitored with each load and use of equipment delayed until culture results are obtained.

CHEMICAL AGENTS FOR STERILIZATION AND DISINFECTION

Disinfectants act to kill microorganisms by several methods: (1) oxidating microbial cells, (2) hydro-lyzing, (3) combining with microbial proteins to form salts, (4) coagulating the proteins of microbial cells, (5) denaturing enzymes, or (6) modifying cell wall permeability.

Certain criteria specify the ideal disinfectant for general use. At the present moment, no single agent matches all the qualities desired, and the selection is usually a compromise in the search for the ideal. The following are criteria to be considered in the selection of agents:

1. Should be effective against all forms of microorganisms
2. Should be rapid in action
3. Should be minimally toxic to body tissues; should not discolor or damage equipment being disinfected
4. Should not decompose when exposed to heat or light or be retarded by exposure to organic matter
5. Should dissolve in water to form a stable solution
6. Should have a pleasant or neutral odor
7. Should be readily available at a reasonable cost

The most important factors in selection should be the agent's ability to kill a broad range of microorganisms, its mildness to the skin and instruments, and its availability at a reasonable cost. When the criteria are narrowed to the list just given, there are several nearly ideal agents (Table C–3).

Aldehydes

The aldehydes contain some of the most commonly used antimicrobials in respiratory care practice. These agents, such as formaldehyde and glutaraldehyde, achieve their antimicrobial action through the alkylation of enzymes.

Formaldehyde has been used as a fumigant for decades. Its bactericidal effect is disappointing unless it is used at at least 70% relative humidity. Aqueous solutions are known as formalin. It is often combined as 8% formaldehyde to 70% isopropyl alcohol to form a rapid antimicrobial that achieves sterilization usually within 3 hours. The usefulness of this disinfectant-sterilant is limited due to the irritation caused by the formaldehyde fumes and its toxicity to tissue.

Glutaraldehyde is a chemical relative of formaldehyde and is somewhat more active. The cidal action of glutaraldehyde is accomplished by disruption

TABLE C–2.

Safe Storage Time for Sterile Packs

WRAPPING	DURATION OF STERILITY	
	CLOSED CABINET	OPEN SHELF
Single-wrapped muslin (two layers)	1 wk	2 days
Single-wrapped two-way crepe paper (single layer)	8 wk	3 wk
Single-wrapped muslin (two layers) sealed in 3-mil polyethylene	—	9 mo
Heat-sealed, paper-transparent plastic pouches	—	1 yr

TABLE C–3.

Common Antimicrobial Agents

	ETHYL ALCOHOL	ISOPROPYL ALCOHOL	IODOPHORS (POVIDONE-IODINE)	PHENOLICS (HEXACHLOROPHENE)	ACID GLUTARALDEHYDE	ALKALINE GLUTARALDEHYDE	CLORHEXIDENE
Suggested effective concentration, %	70–90	70–90	0.45	0.3	2	2	4
Bactericidal							
Staphylococcus aureus	+	+	+	+	+	+	+
Pseudomonas aeruginosa	+	+	+	+	+	+	+
Virucidal							
Lipophilic	+	+	+	+	+	+	+
Hydrophilic	–	–	+	–	–	+	+
Sporicidal							
Bacillus subtilis	–	–	–	–	–	+	+
Clostridium sporogenes	–	–	–	–	–	+	+
Instrument safe							
Rubber/plastic	–	–	–	–	–	+	+
Plated metal	+	+	–	–	+	+	+
Lensed	–	–	–	–	–	+	+
Contact dermatitis hazard	Safe	Safe	Relatively safe	Relatively safe	Gloves required	Gloves required	Safe

of the lipoproteins in the cell membrane and the cytoplasm of vegetative bacterial forms. This reaction between the chemical glutaraldehyde and cell proteins is dependent on both time and contact. Items to be disinfected must be free of material that would inhibit contact, and adequate contact time is needed for the chemical reaction to be completed.

Alkaline glutaraldehyde, buffered by a 0.3% bicarbonate agent, is used as a 2% solution. Once activated with the buffering solution, it is fully potent for approximately 14 days. This solution is bactericidal, virucidal, and tuberculocidal within 10 minutes and produces sterilization when applied for 10 to 20 hours. Equipment disinfected and sterilized with glutaraldehyde should be thoroughly rinsed and dried before use, because any residue would be irritating to mucous membranes. Personnel working with the solution should wear rubber gloves to avoid contact dermatitis.

Acid glutaraldehyde is bactericidal and virucidal within 20 minutes and produces sterilization in 1 hour if the solution is heated to 60°C. Once activated, it remains potent for approximately 28 days. These chemicals are extremely toxic, and all personnel handling them should wear rubber gloves and equipment must be thoroughly rinsed and dried before placing in use. Objects disinfected with these

agents must be rinsed in sterile water or water containing at least 10 mg/L of free residual chlorine (1:2500 dilution of household bleach that is 5.25% hypochlorite solution) to remove possible toxic or irritating residue. After rinsing, the equipment should be stored in protective wrappers to prevent recontamination.

Alcohols

Ethyl and isopropyl alcohols are perhaps the most commonly used disinfectants, with the latter being slightly superior and less expensive. Alcohols, as a chemical family, have many desirable characteristics needed in disinfectants. They are generally bactericidal and accomplish their bactericidal activity by damaging the cell wall membrane. They also have the ability to denature proteins, particularly enzymes called *dehydrogenases*. For alcohol to coagulate microbial proteins, water must be present. For this reason, traditionally 70% has been considered the critical dilution for alcohol, with a rapid loss of bactericidal activity with dilutions less than 50%. Both ethyl and isopropyl alcohols are rapidly effective against vegetative bacteria and tubercle bacilli but are not sporicidal.

Alcohols dissolve cement mountings on lensed

instruments and with long-term exposure harden and swell plastic tubing, including polyethylene. In practice, they have been found to be more useful as antiseptics than as disinfectants.

Phenols

Carbolic acid is the oldest of the germicides. Although the original chemical no longer is used, there are literally hundreds of compounds derived from it that constitute the class known as *phenolics*. Present-day disinfectants of this group can be roughly divided into two broad classes: (1) the alkyl and acryl phenols and (2) the halogenated phenols. The bactericidal effect of high-concentration phenol is due to its action as a protoplasmic poison, penetrating the cell wall and precipitating the cell protein. The derivatives of phenol usually act in low concentration by inactivation of the cell's essential enzyme systems. As a class, they are the most popular housekeeping disinfection agents. Phenolic preparations are good bactericides, including the tubercle bacillus, but are nonsporicidal. Not only are the phenolics good against vegetative bacteria, they have the desired property of residual effect and remain active over prolonged periods. Subsequent application of moisture to previously treated surfaces will redissolve the residual agent so that it can become active when in contact with organic material. It is for this reason that phenolics are the agents of choice for dealing with fecal contamination.

Examples of commonly used phenol compounds are hexachlorophene, 0-syl, and amphyl. Hexachlorophene is a very popular compound used for handwashing. Since 1972, its use has diminished, because it was found to be absorbed through the skin and to be neurotoxic.[8] In that there are equally efficacious substitutes, hexachlorophene has no distinct value for respiratory care services.

Halogens

Halogens comprise the iodine and iodophor agents. Tincture of iodine is simply iodine dissolved in alcohol. Although very popular as a skin preparation, it has the disadvantage of causing tissue necrosis in strong concentrations, leaving stains and, in certain individuals, causing allergic reactions. Free iodine is believed to form salts with bacterial protein, thus killing the cells. As a disinfectant, iodine is highly reactive and provides a broad spectrum of efficacy against vegetative bacteria, fungi, certain viruses, and spores.

Iodophors are compounds in which iodine is carried by a surface active solvent. Its active agent, iodine, is a potent broad-spectrum bactericide, including the tubercle bacillus. Common commercial examples are Wescodyne, Betadine, and Iosan. The elemental iodine in these preparations is lethal to microbes in that it produces alterations within the microbial protein. Although not as effective in their antimicrobial activity as tincture of iodine, the iodophors have the benefits of being nonstaining, nonallergic, and relatively nonirritating. The iodophors are effective in cold or lukewarm water. Hot water (100°C) will liberate free iodine from the solution and decrease its antimicrobial action.

Ethylene Oxide

Ethylene oxide (ETO) is a gas with a broad range of antimicrobial action. It is thought to destroy the microorganisms by aklylating cellular constituents. The gas is an odorless, poisonous, explosive agent used in combination with Freon or carbon dioxide to decrease the danger of fire or explosion. In that it kills both spores and bacteria, it has become a very popular method for sterilizing much of the heat- and moisture-sensitive respiratory care equipment. The gas is extremely penetrating and does not require high temperatures for activation. Sterilization of equipment is usually accomplished under conditions of 30% to 50% relative humidity and at temperatures of 50°C to 60°C. Under these conditions, it will effectively sterilize equipment within a 4-hour period. If the temperature is above 60°C, polymerization of the ETO takes place, and its efficacy as a sterilant is removed. For ETO sterilization to be effective, the equipment must be properly prepared and packaged. Materials to be sterilized must first be surgically clean and water free. All caps, plugs, valves, and stylettes should be removed to allow the gas free circulation. If syringes are to be sterilized, they must first be disassembled and packaged with the plungers outside their barrels.

Suitable wrapping materials include double-thickness muslin and paper wraps used with steam autoclaves. Some sealed pouches made of plastic films such as polyethylene are also permeable to ETO. Materials such as aluminum foil, nylon film, Saran, Mylar, cellophane, polyester, and polyvinylidene film should be avoided, because they often are impermeable to the sterilizing gases.

To avoid contact irritation from ETO, it is necessary that the residual gas be removed after sterilization is complete. Unless these trace gases are removed prior to the chamber opening, they represent a toxicologic hazard to the operator. Without the use of an aeration chamber, materials such as neoprene rubber and polyvinyl chloride (PVC) require extended aeration times up to 7 days. Heated aeration cabinets shorten the time required from more than 1 week at ambient temperature to 12 hours at 53°C.

The sterilization process is aided by moisture, but excess water combines with the gas to form ethylene glycol, a sticky residue that irritates tissue. Another toxic by-product is ethylene chlorohydrin formed in PVC following ETO sterilization. Formerly, it was thought to be associated with PVC previously gamma-irradiated, but the association has not proved to be true, and there is no reason to proscribe sterilization of previously gamma-irradiated PVC materials.

Successful sterilization with ETO is dependent on appropriate monitoring. The only way to ensure that the specified conditions of concentration, temperature, humidity, and time have been met is to use a biologic indicator, usually *B. subtilis*. Biologic indicators should be used routinely on at least a weekly basis and with each load that contains implantable materials.

In that ETO exposure has been associated with mutagenicity and carcinogenicity, great care should be used to assure compliance with exposure standards. The current U.S. standard for a worker's exposure to ETO is 1 ppm for an 8-hour time period. Following a recent court order, the Occupational Safety and Health Administration (OSHA) stated that it will propose to strictly limit worker exposure to the gas. The proposed regulation would establish a maximum limit for short-time exposure of between 5 to 10 ppm for a 15-minute period.[2]

ADVANTAGES AND DISADVANTAGES OF PHYSICAL AND CHEMICAL AGENTS IN INFECTION CONTROL

Infection control is of primary concern to all respiratory care practitioners and within the department several methods may be simultaneously used (Table C–4). Each available method of sterilization and disinfection, unfortunately, has its own set of attendant problems:

1. Irradiation is not economically feasible for most hospital use.
2. Autoclaving deteriorates rubber and destroys most plastics and delicate instruments such as respirometers.
3. Ethylene oxide is expensive, toxic, and time consuming due to the elongated aeration times.
4. Liquid chemicals are often toxic and expensive, and items disinfected can be recontaminated in drying and packaging phase.
5. Pasteurization is not appropriate for moisture-sensitive items, and items disinfected can be recontaminated in the drying and repackaging phase.

DECONTAMINATION PROCESS

After equipment has been used in a patient service area, it should be bagged and transported to the department decontamination area. No contaminated equipment should be carried open through the halls, and even large devices such as ultrasonic nebulizers and intermittent positive pressure breathing (IPPB) units should be covered before being transferred. Dirty and clean equipment should not be transferred on the same cart, or if it is necessary, there should be specifically designated areas of the cart for each so that mixing does not occur.

The basic layout of decontamination should be one that provides for a dirty entrance and clean exit with no cross-traffic flow between areas. The pathways for equipment flow through the cleaning process should allow no retrograde flow. The dirty and clean areas should be physically separated from each other and from other service areas such as the staff report area and lounge. Every piece of equipment used in the patient care area, unless grossly contaminated, is first disassembled and washed before the sterilization-disinfection process. The cleaning and disinfection area should have its own air exhaust capable of exchanging the air in the unit at least six times per hour. This exchange of air should not be recirculated to any other part of the hospital.

Usually an assembly and testing area is located between the cleaning and ready to use area. It is desirable but often not possible for these two areas to be staffed by different personnel. Where the same staff is used, care should be taken that they remove aprons, wipe shoes, wash hands, and take general precautions to assure that recontamination does not reoccur in the transfer between the dirty and clean areas. In the clean area, equipment is reassembled and processed for storage or use. Care should be

TABLE C–4.

Common Methods of Disinfection and Sterilization

METHOD	PROCESS	EQUIPMENT	ADVANTAGE	DISADVANTAGE
Autoclaving	High-temperature pressure, steam: 121°C for 15 min/2 atm or 134°C for 3 min/3 atm	Linens, surgical instruments	Is inexpensive, fast, efficient, nontoxic	Damages heat- and moisture-sensitive equipment
Pasteurization	Hot water, immersion: 62°C for 30 min or 72°C for 15 min	Rubber, plastic, metals	Is nontoxic, fast, easy, inexpensive	Recontamination can occur during processing; heat and moisture damage may occur
Acid glutaraldehyde	Low pH, liquid immersion, high-level disinfection/sterilization	Rubber, plastic, metals	Sterilizes in 1 hr; disinfects in 20 min at 60°C; lasts approximately 28 days	Forms toxic residue; recontamination can occur during processing; can cause contact dermatitis
Alkaline glutaraldehyde	High pH, liquid immersion, high-level disinfection/sterilization	Rubber, plastic, metals	Disinfects in 10 min; sterilizes in 10 hr; lasts approximately 2 wk at room temperature	Forms toxic residue; recontamination can occur during processing; can cause contact dermatitis
Gas sterilization	Relative humidity 30–50°, Temperature 50°C–56°C at 1 atm sterilizes in 4 hr	All items moisture or heat sensitive	Effectively sterilizes prewrapped materials	Is expensive and time consuming; aeration is needed to remove toxic residue
Boiling	Hot water, immersion: 100°C for 30 min	Home care items	Is inexpensive, simple	Is time consuming; does not produce sterility; damages moisture-sensitive equipment
Dry heat	170°C for 2 hr	Oils, powders	Is simple, inexpensive, nontoxic	Damages heat-sensitive equipment

taken that appropriate aeration times and other precautions are observed to assure that no toxic residuals remain on decontaminated equipment. All packaged equipment should be dated for shelf life before being sent for storage.

The monitoring of our disinfection-sterilization techniques is necessary to assure patient safety. A system of spot checking the equipment as part of the quality control process has often been recommended to detect breaks in the decontamination process and contamination of in-use equipment. This routine testing of effluent gases, swabbing, and rinsing equipment on a weekly basis does not seem cost effective and can often cause more problems than it resolves. Often several therapists are involved in the sampling process, and unless they are proficient in the culture-handling techniques, there is a greater risk of contaminating the sample than of finding an infectious organism on the selected equipment.

When there is a nosocomial infection outbreak, the hospital infection control team coordinates the department efforts. The investigation usually includes an analysis of patients' charts to detect similarities in modes of treatment, diagnostic procedures, and drug administration. Extensive samplings are taken within the patients' environment including objects and personnel. The infection control nurse usually interviews all employees who have had contact with the patient and reviews the procedures used. The solution to most nosocomial outbreaks is a team rather than a department effort.

For respiratory care personnel, infection control usually includes the maintenance and surveillance of health within the staff. It is vitally important that

TABLE C-5.
Decontamination Procedures

EQUIPMENT REUSABLE*	CHANGE TIME	SOAP AND WATER CLEAN	DISINFECTANT SPRAY	LIQUID DISINFECTANTS	PASTEURIZATION	ETO	STEAM AUTOCLAVE
Room humidifier	24 hr	Disassemble completely	–	+	+	Usually not cost effective	–
Venturi nebulizer	8–12 hr	Disassemble completely	–	–	–	+	–
Gas therapy humidifier	8–12 hr	Disassemble completely	–	–	–	+	–
USN generator	Between patients	Wipe down generator and fan unit, clean filters	Spray and wipe unit dry	Reusable filter	Reusable filter	–	–
USN medicine couplant	8–12 hr	+	–	+	+	–	–
IPPB units	Between patients	+	Spray and wipe dry	Reusable metal filters	Reusable metal filters	–	–
Portable spirometers	After PT use	–	Wipe down with 70% alcohol	–	–	+	–
Electrically powered ventilators	After PT use	Wash intake cooling fan filters; wipe and dry case	Case and wheels wiped and dry	–	–	–	Autoclave outer case as needed
Bag-mask units	After each use	–	–	–	–	+	–
Fiberoptic bronchoscopes	After each use	+	–	Submerge unit in chemical agent	–	–	–

*USN indicates ultrasonic nebulizer.

TABLE C–6.

Isolation Precautions

TYPE	HANDWASH	GOWNS	GLOVES	MASK	CLOSED DOORS	DOUBLE-BAGGED EQUIPMENT	DOUBLE-BAGGED TISSUE
Wound and skin	+	0	+	0	0	0	+
Enteric	+	0	+	0	0	0	+
Respiratory	+	0	0	+	+	+	+
Strict	+	+	+	+	+	+	+
Reverse	+	+	+	+	+	0	0

personnel report all acute infections so that those infected can be shifted toward non–patient care duties. Aseptic handwashing procedures, aseptic handling of supplies and equipment, and strict adherence to the principles of isolation are all techniques that should be monitored to assure staff compliance (Tables C–5 and C–6).

REFERENCES

1. Albert RK, Cardie F: Handwashing patterns in medical intensive care units. *N Engl J Med* 1981; 304:1465–1466.
2. *CMP Publications Health Week: The Newspaper for America's Health Industry.* Emoryville, Calif, CMP Publications, 1987, vol 1, pp 6–7.
3. Darin J: Respiratory therapy equipment in the development of nosocomial respiratory tract infections. *Curr Rev Respir Ther* 1985; 4:83.
4. Garner JS, Favero MS: CDC guidelines for the prevention and control of nosocomial infections. *Am J Infect Control* 1986; 14:110–129.
5. Halley WH: Nosocomial infections in United States hospitals. *Am J Med* 1981; 70:947.
6. Perkins JJ: *Principles and Methods of Sterilization.* Springfield, Ill, Charles C Thomas, Publishers, 1978, pp 346–348.
7. Schumann RM, Leech RW, Ellsworth CA: Neurotoxicity of hexaclorophene in the human. *Pediatrics* 1974; 54:689–695.
8. Stan W: Infections related to medical services. *Ann Intern Med* 1978; 89:764–769.

Appendix D

Referenced Self-Assessment Examination

Glen G. J. Low, M.Ed., R.R.T.

CHAPTER 1: PATIENT ASSESSMENT PROCEDURES

1. Which of the following components does the Weed system of standardized assessment involve?
   I. Patient assessment
   II. Patient's objective information
   III. Patient plan
   IV. Patient's subjective findings
   a. I
   b. III
   c. I and II
   d. I, III, and IV
   e. All of the above

2. Which of the following statements would reflect data relating to a patient's plan?
   a. "I am coughing less than yesterday."
   b. "The patient's temperature is 98°F, blood pressure is 125/72 mm Hg, and the pulse is 84 breaths/min."
   c. "The patient's asthma is worsening."
   d. "We will increase the inhaled bronchodilator to every 4 hours."
   e. None of the above

3. According to the U.S. Public Health Service, how many chronic complaints does each person have over age 55 years?
   a. 0.5
   b. 1.5
   c. 2.3
   d. 3.1
   e. 4.0

4. The major concern that patients arrive at the hospital with is referred to as:
   a. The major gripe
   b. The chief complaint
   c. The major illness
   d. The primary concern
   e. The primary discomfort

5. In most respiratory illnesses, what symptom accompanies the process?
   a. Shortness of breath
   b. Wheezing
   c. Cough
   d. Chest pain
   e. Hemoptysis

6. Calculate the pack-year history of a 28-year-old housewife who has smoked 2 packs/day for the past 12 years.
   a. 6 pack-years
   b. 12 pack-years
   c. 14 pack-years
   d. 24 pack-years
   e. 56 pack-years

7. What is the name for the sensation of difficult or uncomfortable breathing?
   a. Eupnea
   b. Tachypnea
   c. Hyperpnea
   d. Dyspnea
   e. Orthopnea

8. What type of chest pain is characterized by a "crushing tightness" often radiating to the neck, shoulders, and arms?
   a. Bronchitis
   b. Pleurisy
   c. Tsietze syndrome
   d. Angina pectoris
   e. Mediastinitis

9. Patients who have chronic pulmonary disease with swelling of the lower extremities may have:
   a. Cor pulmonale
   b. Malnutrition
   c. Fractured leg
   d. Shingles
   e. Tuberculosis

10. The term "compliance history" refers to:
    a. The change in tidal volume/change in pressure
    b. The change in pressure/change in tidal volume
    c. The long-term trend of lung compliance measurements
    d. How well a patient has been following his or her previously outlined treatment program
    e. None of the above

11. Who or what is the primary source of information about a patient?
    a. Head nurse
    b. Shift report
    c. Floor rounds
    d. Attending physician
    e. Hospital chart

12. What part of the chart describes the patient's date of birth, age, and marital status?
    a. Patient data
    b. Physician orders
    c. Intake-output record
    d. Laboratory reports
    e. History and physical examination

13. What part of the chart contains the shift-to-shift description of vital signs, temperature, pulse, and respiration?
    a. Patient data
    b. History and physical examination
    c. Clinical record
    d. Intake-output record
    e. Physician orders

14. What is the normal range of adult blood pressure?
    a. 60–90/30–50 mm Hg
    b. 80–100/50–70 mm Hg
    c. 110–130/70–80 mm Hg
    d. 120–140/90–100 mm Hg
    e. 130–150/100–110 mm Hg

15. Bradycardia is a heart rate less than:
    a. 60 beats/min
    b. 65 beats/min
    c. 70 beats/min
    d. 75 beats/min
    e. 80 beats/min

16. What is the normal inspiratory/expiratory (I/E) ratio in neonates?
    a. 2:1
    b. 1:1
    c. 1:1.5
    d. 1:2
    e. 1:3

17. Chest percussion is a useful diagnostic clinical tool in which of the following entities?
    I. Localization of small infiltrates
    II. Localization of small effusions
    III. Localization of small pneumothoraces
    IV. The level of diaphragmatic excursions
    a. I
    b. III
    c. IV
    d. I, III, and IV
    e. All of the above

18. In which clinical entities would hyperresonance over the thorax be heard?
    I. Pneumothorax
    II. Pleural thickening
    III. Pleural effusion
    IV. Atelectasis
    a. I
    b. III
    c. II and IV
    d. II, III, and IV
    e. All of the above

19. What breath pattern is the result of high-pitched, sibilant, piping or whistling sounds from partial obstruction of airways?
    a. Bronchial
    b. Vesicular
    c. Bronchovesicular
    d. Rales
    e. Wheeze

20. Who invented the stethoscope?
    a. René Laënnec
    b. Thomas Edison
    c. John Hammond
    d. Jack Emerson
    e. Leonardo DaVinci

CHAPTER 2: PULMONARY FUNCTION TESTING PROCEDURES

1. According to the 1979 statement of standardization of spirometry by the American Thoracic Society (ATS), spirometers must meet which of the following minimal standards for measuring vital capacity (VC)?
    I. Accumulate volume for at least 30 seconds
    II. Be capable of measuring volumes of at least 7 L
    III. Measure volume independent of flow between 0 and 12 L/sec
    IV. Have an accuracy of at least ±3% of reading or 50 ml, whichever is greater
    a. I
    b. II
    c. I and IV
    d. II, III, and IV
    e. All of the above

2. What is the minimal sampling rate for computer application of peak flow?
    a. 15 Hz
    b. 30 Hz
    c. 45 Hz
    d. 60 Hz
    e. 75 Hz

3. The practitioner calibrates a pulmonary function system with a large 3-L syringe. Which of the following are acceptable readings?
    I. 2.7 L
    II. 2.92 L
    III. 3.07 L
    IV. 3.15 L
    a. I and II
    b. II and III
    c. III and IV
    d. II, III, and IV
    e. All of the above

4. How should the adult patient be positioned when a pulmonary function test is performed?
    a. Sitting
    b. Standing
    c. Semi-Fowler's position
    d. Lying
    e. a or b

5. For forced vital capacity (FVC) reproducibility to be present according to ATS standards, what criteria must be met?
    a. The best two of three acceptable attempts should be within ±3% or 50 ml, whichever is greater.
    b. All three acceptable attempts should be within ±3% or 50 ml, whichever is greater.
    c. The best two of at least three acceptable attempts should be within ±5% or 100 ml, whichever is greater.
    d. All three acceptable attempts should be within ±5% or 100 ml, whichever is greater.
    e. None of the above

6. In what time period is the maximum voluntary ventilation (MVV) maneuver performed?
    a. 1 second
    b. 7 seconds
    c. 12 seconds
    d. 30 seconds
    e. 60 seconds

7. All actual spirometry values should be converted to:
    a. Ambient temperature and pressure saturated (ATPS)
    b. Body temperature, ambient pressure saturated with water vapor (BTPS)
    c. Kelvin
    d. Celsius
    e. Fahrenheit

8. The peak expiratory flow rate measurement on a patient should be repeated until the subject exerts what appears to be maximal effort and duplicates that value at least once to within:
   a. $\pm 3\%$
   b. $\pm 5\%$
   c. $\pm 7\%$
   d. $\pm 10\%$
   e. $\pm 15\%$

9. Which of the following lung capacities cannot be determined with direct spirometry methods?
   I. Total lung capacity (TLC)
   II. Inspiratory capacity (IC)
   III. VC
   IV. FRC
   a. I
   b. IV
   c. II and IV
   d. I and IV
   e. II, III, and IV

10. Which of the following methods can be used to determine FRC?
    I. Helium dilution
    II. Nitrogen washout
    III. Flow-volume loop
    IV. Body plethysmography
    a. I
    b. III
    c. II and IV
    d. I, II, and III
    e. I, II, and IV

11. What gas law describes how the body plethysmograph operates?
    a. Charles' law
    b. Henry's law
    c. Boyle's law
    d. Dalton's law
    e. Gay-Lussac's law

12. What gas analyzer measures concentration by actually counting the relative number of ionized molecules of each gas?
    a. Polarographic
    b. Thermal conductivity
    c. Gas chromatography
    d. Mass spectrometer
    e. Pulse oximeter

13. What gas collecting device is used to determine patient dead space?
    a. Wright respirometer
    b. Wright peak flowmeter
    c. Body plethysmography
    d. Bennett bellow spirometer
    e. Douglas bag

14. Oxygen uptake is defined as:
    a. $(\dot{V}_I \times F_{I_{O_2}}) - (\dot{V}_E \times F_{E_{O_2}})$
    b. $(\dot{V}_E \times F_{E_{O_2}}) - (\dot{V}_I \times F_{I_{O_2}})$
    c. $\dfrac{(\dot{V}_I \times F_{I_{O_2}})}{(\dot{V}_E \times F_{E_{O_2}})}$
    d. $\dfrac{(\dot{V}_E \times F_{E_{O_2}})}{(\dot{V}_I \times F_{I_{O_2}})}$
    e. $(\dot{V}_I \times F_{I_{O_2}}) \times (\dot{V}_E \times F_{E_{O_2}})$

15. Carbon dioxide output is defined as:
    a. $\dot{V}_E \times STPD \times F_{E_{CO_2}}$
    b. $\dfrac{\dot{V}_E}{STPD} \times F_{E_{CO_2}}$
    c. $\dfrac{\dot{V}_E}{F_{E_{CO_2}}} \times STPD$
    d. $\dfrac{F_{E_{CO_2}}}{\dot{V}_E} \times STPD$
    e. $\dfrac{STPD}{F_{E_{CO_2}}} \times \dot{V}_E$

16. The respiratory quotient is defined as:
    a. CO_2 production $\times$ O_2 consumption
    b. $\dfrac{CO_2 \text{ production}}{O_2 \text{ consumption}}$
    c. $\dfrac{O_2 \text{ consumption}}{CO_2 \text{ production}}$
    d. $\dfrac{\dot{V}_E}{O_2 \text{ consumption}}$
    e. $F_{E_{CO_2}} \times \dot{V}_E$

17. What type of oxygen electrode is in arterial blood gas analyzers?
    a. Polarographic
    b. Thermal conductivity
    c. Gas chromatography
    d. Mass spectrometer
    e. Fuel cell

18. When a blood sample is introduced into a blood gas analyzer, carbon dioxide diffuses across the membrane according to what gas law?
    a. Charles' law
    b. Henry's law
    c. Boyle's law
    d. Dalton's law
    e. Gay-Lussac's law

19. Quality assurance in blood gas analyzers through tonometered blood, commercially available materials, or both with known values of P_{O_2}, P_{CO_2}, and pH should lie within how many standard deviations of the limits?
    a. 0.5
    b. 1.5
    c. 2.0
    d. 2.5
    e. 3.0

20. Which of the following can be determined by spectrophotometry?
    I. pH
    II. P_{O_2}
    III. Carboxyhemoglobin
    IV. Methemoglobin
    a. II
    b. II and III
    c. III and IV
    d. II, III, and IV
    e. All of the above

CHAPTER 3: INTERPRETATION OF PATIENT ASSESSMENT DATA

1. A 60-year-old woman with a 45–pack-year smoking history is admitted to the emergency room with symptoms of chronic obstructive pulmonary disease (COPD). During coughing her complexion darkens; what might it indicate?
   a. Sun poisoning
   b. Oat cell carcinoma
   c. Hypercapnia
   d. Carbon monoxide poisoning
   e. Arterial desaturation

2. The findings of rhonchi during chest auscultation indicate?
   a. Atelectasis
   b. Pneumothorax
   c. Pulmonary edema
   d. Secretions in the larger airways
   e. Partial obstruction in the lower airways

3. Flattening of the diaphragms on chest x-ray are generally consistent with which clinical entity?
   a. Bronchiectasis
   b. Bronchiolitis
   c. Emphysema
   d. Sarcoidosis
   e. Scoliosis

4. What is the normal blood glucose level?
   a. 30–50 mg/dL
   b. 50–70 mg/dL
   c. 70–100 mg/dL
   d. 100–120 mg/dL
   e. 120–140 mg/dL

5. What is the normal blood creatinine level?
   a. 0.2–0.4 mg/dL
   b. 0.4–0.6 mg/dL
   c. 0.6–0.9 mg/dL
   d. 0.9–1.2 mg/dL
   e. 1.2–1.5 mg/dL

6. Which of the following media would produce the darkest x-ray?
   a. Right middle lobe pneumonia
   b. Left upper lobe pneumonia
   c. Diffuse pulmonary edema
   d. Air
   e. Heart

7. Which of the following statement(s) is/are true concerning portable chest x-rays?
   a. The variable distance between the tube and the cassette makes the magnification of the image change.
   b. There is poorer resolution.
   c. Portable x-rays are generally done anteroposteriorly.
   d. There is variability caused by the position of the patient.
   e. All of the above

8. What procedure uses x-ray imaging process whereby radiation produces an image on a fluorescent screen, allowing a "real time" image?
   a. Bronchoscopy
   b. Anteroposterior x-ray
   c. Fluoroscopy
   d. Ultrasound
   e. Nuclear magnetic resonance (NMR)

9. How long should a subject fast prior to a glucose level in the blood being taken?
   a. 2 hours
   b. 4 hours
   c. 8 hours
   d. 16 hours
   e. Not necessary

10. Which of the following functions do protein and albumin in the blood serve?
    I. H^+ ion buffer
    II. Transport media
    III. Osmotic homeostasis
    IV. Immunologic mechanisms
    a. I
    b. III
    c. I and IV
    d. II, III, and IV
    e. All of the above

11. What technique can be used to visually inspect the airways?
    a. Bronchoscopy
    b. Anteroposterior x-ray
    c. Fluoroscopy
    d. Ultrasound
    e. NMR

12. Which of the following can the results of pulmonary function testing be used for?
    I.   Identifying and classifying certain types of lung disease
    II. Evaluating the effectiveness of treatment
    III. Providing a yardstick for compensating the disabled
    IV. Documenting the progress of pulmonary disease
    a. I
    b. I and III
    c. II and IV
    d. I, III, and IV
    e. All of the above

13. All of the following are restrictive lung diseases except:
    a. Scoliosis
    b. Pneumonia
    c. Asthma
    d. Pulmonary fibrosis
    e. Neuromuscular disorder

14. A residual volume/total lung capacity (RV/TLC) ratio greater than _____ indicates a significant degree of obstructive lung disease?
    a. 15%
    b. 20%
    c. 25%
    d. 35%
    e. 45%

15. What does phase II of the single breath nitrogen elimination test indicate?

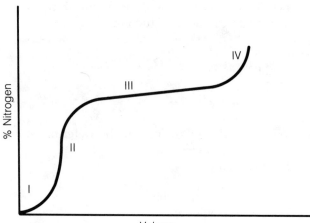

    a. FRC
    b. Tidal volume
    c. Anatomic dead space
    d. Mixing of inspired gases
    e. Closing volume

16. Which pulmonary function test should be used to evaluate the reversibility of small airway diseases?
    a. Helium dilution test
    b. Single breath nitrogen elimination
    c. Prebronchodilator-postbronchodilator study
    d. Body plethysmography
    e. CO diffusion test

17. What data can be obtained from a total static respiratory system compliance measurement?
    a. Lung compliance
    b. Thorax compliance
    c. Airway resistance
    d. a and b
    e. All of the above

18. Which of the following is/are considered risk(s) of anesthesia and surgery?
    I. Cigarette smoking
    II. Old age
    III. Obesity
    IV. Chronic lung disease
    a. I and II
    b. II and III
    c. I and IV
    d. II, III, and IV
    e. All of the above

19. Which of the following negative inspiratory force measurements would be acceptable for spontaneous ventilation?
    a. -5 cm H_2O
    b. -8 cm H_2O
    c. -12 cm H_2O
    d. -18 cm H_2O
    e. -32 cm H_2O

20. Calculate the expected Pa_{O_2} using the simplified alveolar gas equation with the following data: $F_{I_{O_2}}$ 0.4, P_{H_2O} 47 mm Hg, P_B 750 mm Hg, and Pa_{CO_2} 52 mm Hg.
    a. 218.8 mm Hg
    b. 234.2 mm Hg
    c. 282.8 mm Hg
    d. 312.4 mm Hg
    e. 345.6 mm Hg

CHAPTER 4: THE RESPIRATORY CARE PLAN

1. In which section of the medical record can an update on the patient's overall present condition be found?
   a. Patient data
   b. Medication orders
   c. Progress notes
   d. Respiratory care notes
   e. Laboratory data

2. The Joint Commission on Accreditation of Hospitals (JCAH) standards recommend the physician's order for respiratory care should specify:
   I. Type of treatment
   II. Frequency of treatment
   III. Duration of treatment
   IV. Type and dose of medication
   V. Type of diluent and oxygen concentration
   a. I and IV
   b. I, II, and IV
   c. I, III, and IV
   d. I, III, IV, and V
   e. All of the above

3. All of the following are types of information found in the respiratory care notes except:
   a. Names of the practitioners who have provided respiratory care
   b. Type of respiratory care being administered
   c. Frequency of the treatment
   d. Results of sputum culture and sensitivity
   e. Date, indications, times, and duration of respiratory therapy administered

4. The technique of assessing the patient's chest with a stethoscope is?
   a. Inspection
   b. Palpation
   c. Percussion
   d. Auscultation
   e. Ultrasound

5. Select the statement that most accurately describes respiratory care therapeutic objectives.
   a. They are found in the physician's order sheet.
   b. They are written after the practitioner administers therapy in the respiratory care notes.
   c. They are concise, measurable objectives identified for each therapeutic goal.
   d. They are a list of pulmonary problems.
   e. They are ventilator settings used for pressure support.

6. The need for timelines in evaluating therapeutic objectives include(s):
   I. Clarifies the physiologic parameters that need to be monitored
   II. Establishes a regular schedule for evaluating the level of pulmonary dysfunction
   III. Allows for timely modifications of the respiratory care being provided
   IV. Facilitates decisions on when treatments and modalities of care should be discontinued
   a. I
   b. III
   c. II and III
   d. II, III, and IV
   e. All of the above

7. A respiratory care quality assurance program would include all of the following except:
   a. Determine when patients are medically able to be discharged from the hospital
   b. Monitor the care being given
   c. Place priorities of respiratory care administration on the patient on the service
   d. Monitor how well practitioners meet criteria in completing flow sheets and respiratory care notes
   e. Evaluate the effectiveness of the established therapeutic objectives

8. A practitioner has administered intermittent positive pressure breathing (IPPB) at 20 cm H_2O of pressure with room air for 10 minutes to a 35-year-old postoperative abdominal surgery patient. All of the following would be important to document in the respiratory care notes except:
   a. Adverse reactions
   b. Medication administered
   c. Time and date treatment was administered
   d. Respiratory therapist's signature
   e. Scheduled time of next treatment

9. A practitioner has a physician order to administer 0.5 ml of 1% solution of isoetharine (Bronkosol) with 3 ml of normal saline to a mild asthmatic. The therapist notes a 40-beat increase in the patient's heart rate. The treatment is stopped at that time at the discretion of the practitioner. For a change in the medication to result, the practitioner should:
   a. Administer one half the dosage just as long as the medication is the same
   b. Change the medication to a less-potent drug
   c. Write in the order sheet for one half the dosage
   d. Contact the charge nurse and have him or her write the new order
   e. Contact the physician and have him or her write the new order

10. The respiratory care plan should be developed by:
    a. Identifying and quantifying levels of dysfunction
    b. Describing expected therapeutic outcomes
    c. Selecting the appropriate respiratory care to be administered
    d. Specifying a means and schedule for ongoing evaluation of the expected therapeutic outcomes
    e. All of the above

CHAPTER 5: OXYGEN AND MIXED GAS THERAPY

1. The amount of oxygen that dissolves in the plasma is directly dependent on what factor(s)?
   I. Solubility coefficient
   II. Pa_{CO_2}
   III. Hemoglobin level
   IV. Partial pressure of oxygen
   a. I
   b. III
   c. I and IV
   d. I and II
   e. I, III, and IV

2. For every 760 mm Hg of pressure, how many milliliters of oxygen are dissolved in 100 ml of blood?
   a. 1.3 vol%
   b. 1.8 vol%
   c. 2.3 vol%
   d. 2.6 vol%
   e. 3.1 vol%

3. For every 1 mm Hg of oxygen, how many milliliters of oxygen are dissolved per 100 ml of blood?
   a. 0.001 ml
   b. 0.003 ml
   c. 0.045 ml
   d. 0.2 ml
   e. 1.2 ml

4. How many milliliters of oxygen are capable of combining with 1 gm of hemoglobin?
   a. 0.003 ml
   b. 0.45 ml
   c. 0.82 ml
   d. 1.10 ml
   e. 1.34 ml

5. Calculate the total amount of oxygen transported in 100 ml of blood given the following data: Pa_{O_2} 132 mm Hg, Pa_{CO_2} 40 mm Hg, $P_{A_{O_2}}$ 148 mm Hg, hemoglobin 16 gm%, and saturation 98%.
   a. 0.396 ml
   b. 0.520 ml
   c. 21.01 ml
   d. 21.41 ml
   e. 21.45 ml

6. What condition(s) will cause the oxyhemoglobin curve to shift to the left?
   I.   Alkalotic pH
   II. Hypercarbia
   III. Increased temperature
   IV. Decreased temperature
   a. II and IV
   b. I and IV
   c. I and II
   d. I, II, and IV
   e. I and III

7. A patient is admitted to the emergency room with a chief complaint of shortness of breath. Laboratory results reveal the following: pH, 7.30; Pa_{O_2}, 100 mm Hg; Pa_{CO_2}, 30 mm Hg; arterial saturation, 97%; and O_2 content, 8 vol%. On the basis of these data, the practitioner can assume that which of the following condition(s) exist(s)?
   I.   Hypoxemia
   II. Anemia
   III. Carbon monoxide poisoning
   IV. Polycythemia
   a. II
   b. III
   c. I and II
   d. I, III, and IV
   e. I, II, and III

8. At a normal Pa_{O_2} (100 mm Hg), the arterial blood is approximately _____ percent saturated with oxygen?
   a. 82%
   b. 87%
   c. 94%
   d. 97%
   e. 100%

9. A P_{50} value of 24 mm Hg would indicate:
   I.   A left shift of the oxyhemoglobin curve
   II. A right shift of the oxyhemoglobin curve
   III. More O_2 released to the tissues
   IV. Less O_2 released to the tissues
   a. I and III
   b. I and IV
   c. II and III
   d. II and IV
   e. None of the above

10. The normal arterial oxygen content is approximately?
    a. 7.2 vol%
    b. 9.4 vol%
    c. 12.1 vol%
    d. 14.8 vol%
    e. 19.8 vol%

11. The normal mixed venous oxygen content is approximately?
    a. 6.8 vol%
    b. 7.2 vol%
    c. 12.2 vol%
    d. 14.8 vol%
    e. 16.3 vol%

12. Oxygen consumption is a function of which variables?
    a. Hemoglobin level $\times$ heart rate
    b. Heart rate $\times$ stroke volume
    c. Arteriovenous O_2 difference $\times$ cardiac output
    d. Hemoglobin levels $\times$ PaO_2
    e. Stroke volume/heart rate

13. Under normal conditions the O_2 consumption is:
    a. 180 ml/min
    b. 200 ml/min
    c. 250 ml/min
    d. 270 ml/min
    e. 300 ml/min

14. You are a practitioner working in the emergency room. A 72-year-old woman is admitted. She has been involved in an apartment fire after apparently falling asleep while smoking. Physical examination reveals tachypnea, tachycardia, pulmonary edema, no responsiveness to pain, cherry-red mucous membranes, and third-degree burns over 40% of her body. On the basis of the physical examination and following laboratory data, classify the hypoxia(s) present: FiO_2, 1.00; pH, 7.10; Hb, 16 gm%; $PaCO_2$, 28 mm Hg; PaO_2, 200 mm Hg; and SaO_2, 40%.
    I.   Anoxic hypoxia
    II. Anemic hypoxia
    III. Circulatory hypoxia
    IV. Histotoxic hypoxia
    a. I
    b. II
    c. IV
    d. I and II
    e. I and III

15. Cyanide poisoning is an example of:
    a. Anoxic hypoxia
    b. Anemic hypoxia
    c. Circulatory hypoxia
    d. Histotoxic hypoxia
    e. c and d

16. The brain functions are dependent on an adequate oxygenation level. Loss of consciousness will occur if the PaO_2 falls below what level?
    a. 30 mm Hg
    b. 35 mm Hg
    c. 40 mm Hg
    d. 45 mm Hg
    e. 50 mm Hg

17. Compensatory polycythemia results in:
    I.   Increased red blood cell (RBC) production
    II. Decreased O_2 carrying capacity
    III. Increased O_2 carrying capacity
    IV. Pulmonary hypertension
    a. I
    b. III
    c. IV
    d. I and II
    e. I, III, and IV

18. Acute respiratory failure as defined by arterial blood gases is described by which of the following?

	pH	Pa_{CO_2} (mm Hg)	PaO_2 (mm Hg)
a.	>7.50	>50	<50
b.	>7.50	<35	<50
c.	<7.35	<35	>50
d.	<7.35	>50	<50
e.	7.40	>50	<50

19. The goal(s) of oxygen therapy is/are?
    I.   Increase the PaO_2 by increasing the FiO_2
    II. Increase the PaO_2 by improving the distribution of gas in the lungs
    III. Decrease ventilatory work necessary to maintain the PaO_2 at a given level
    a. I
    b. II
    c. III
    d. I and III
    e. I, II, and III

20. The term "status asthmaticus" describes:
    a. Asthma during childhood
    b. A resolved asthmatic condition
    c. Asthma when bronchospasm no longer responds to bronchodilators
    d. An allergic asthmatic condition
    e. An emotional asthmatic trigger

CHAPTER 6: HUMIDITY AND AEROSOL THERAPY

1. Dew point can be defined as:
   a. The temperature at which the gas mixture becomes saturated, given the actual amount of water held as a gas in the mixture
   b. The actual mass or weight of water existing as a gas in milligrams per liter
   c. The actual absolute humidity as a percentage of the maximum absolute humidity as a given temperature
   d. Water in the vapor phase
   e. The process when a solid goes to a gas without passing through the liquid stage

2. How many milligrams of water are in 1 L of gas at room temperature (21°C) at 40% relative humidity?
   a. 7.3 mg/L
   b. 8.6 mg/L
   c. 12.4 mg/L
   d. 18.4 mg/L
   e. 22.25 mg/L

3. How many milligrams of water are in 1 L of gas at body temperature (37°C) at 100% relative humidity?
   a. 12.4 mg/L
   b. 18.35 mg/L
   c. 28.45 mg/L
   d. 38.2 mg/L
   e. 43.9 mg/L

4. Mouth breathing results in conditioning of inspired air to a relative humidity of _____ percent by the time it reaches the oropharynx?
   a. 40%
   b. 50%
   c. 60%
   d. 70%
   e. 80%

5. What is the average actual amount of water in milliliters per day contributed by the lung to saturate inspired gas?
   a. 200 ml
   b. 250 ml
   c. 300 ml
   d. 350 ml
   e. 400 ml

6. The amount of water the respiratory tract actually contributes to reach saturation at body temperature is called the:
   a. Humidity deficit
   b. Absolute humidity
   c. Relative humidity
   d. Dew point
   e. Sublimation

7. The addition of a supplemental humidity system should be used in all of the following situations except:
   a. Nasal cannula at 5 L/min
   b. Venturi mask
   c. Simple oxygen mask at 7 L/min
   d. Partial rebreathing mask at 7 L/min
   e. Non-rebreathing mask at 12 L/min

8. A clinical recommendation for the minimum amount of humidity a gas delivery system should have is:
   a. 8 mg/L
   b. 10 mg/L
   c. 12 mg/L
   d. 14 mg/L
   e. 16 mg/L

9. The National Conference on Oxygen Therapy of the American College of Chest Physicians (1984) recommends excluding supplemental humidity with cannulas and catheters if the flow rate is less than:
   a. 4 L/min
   b. 5 L/min
   c. 6 L/min
   d. 7 L/min
   e. 8 L/min

10. The inspired gas should be fully saturated and at a temperature range of _____ with intubated patients?
    a. 22°C–25°C
    b. 25°C–28°C
    c. 28°C–32°C
    d. 32°C–37°C
    e. 37°C–40°C

11. In which of the following patient situations is it most critical to supply properly heated and humidified gas?
    a. Premature neonate using an oxygen hood
    b. A 6-year-old in a croup tent
    c. An 18-year-old asthmatic with a nasal cannula at 4 L/min
    d. A 26-year-old trauma victim being ventilated with a manual resuscitator
    e. An intubated 48-year-old postoperative open heart surgery patient receiving mechanical ventilation

12. Which of the following methods can best decrease the amount of rainout in aerosol delivery tubing?
    a. Using the widest tubing available
    b. Setting the heater at the highest setting
    c. Filling the humidifier beyond the full mark
    d. Using heating wires inside delivery tubing
    e. Using water traps in the delivery tubing

13. For the pulmonary application of aerosols, the particles should be within what size?
    a. 0.2–0.8 μ
    b. 1–10 μ
    c. 20–30 μ
    d. 30–40 μ
    e. 45–50 μ

14. The "hygroscopic characteristics" of an aerosol refers to:
    a. The increase in the size of a particle due to condensation of humidity
    b. The decrease in the size of a particle due to condensation of humidity
    c. The increase in the size of a particle due to evaporation of humidity
    d. The decrease in the size of a particle due to evaporation of humidity
    e. A measure of the particles' terminal settling velocity under gravity, where the particle is assigned the diameter of a unit density sphere that has that identical settling velocity

15. The term "coalescence of aerosol particles" refers to:
    a. Leading to more but smaller aerosol particles
    b. Leading to more but larger aerosol particles
    c. Leading to fewer but smaller aerosol particles
    d. Leading to fewer but larger aerosol particles
    e. The number of particles per liter of gas

16. All of the following are considered hazards of aerosol therapy except:
    a. Bronchospasm
    b. Bacterial contamination
    c. Fluid overload
    d. Drug reaction
    e. Dehydration

17. Indications for bland unheated aerosol include which of the following clinical entities?
    I. Pediatric croup
    II. Postextubation
    III. Cystic fibrosis
    IV. Pneumonia
    a. I
    b. II
    c. I and II
    d. I, III, and IV
    e. All of the above

18. Approximately how many milliliters of water from an ultrasonic nebulizer can be deposited over the lung in a 24-hour period in an adult?
    a. 50 ml
    b. 75 ml
    c. 100 ml
    d. 150 ml
    e. 200 ml

19. Which of the following pharmacologic agents produce primary local vasoconstriction?
    I. Acetylcysteine (Mucomyst)
    II. Racemic epinephrine
    III. Phenylephrine
    IV. Corticosteroids
    a. I and IV
    b. I and II
    c. II and IV
    d. II and III
    e. II, III, and IV

20. Which of the following are indications for the use of aerosol therapy?
    I. Deposition of bronchoactive aerosols
    II. Enhancement of secretion clearance
    III. Sputum induction
    IV. Humidification of inspired gas
    a. I
    b. II
    c. II and III
    d. I, II, and IV
    e. All of the above

CHAPTER 7: CHEST PHYSICAL THERAPY AND AIRWAY CARE

1. Which of the following clinical entities warrants the use of prophylactic chest physical therapy
   I. 15-year-old patient with a fractured leg
   II. 52-year-old postoperative open heart surgery patient with a 60–pack-year smoking history
   III. 32-year-old postoperative gallbladder patient with no significant pulmonary history
   IV. 18-year-old postpartum woman
   a. II
   b. III
   c. I and II
   d. II and IV
   e. II, III, and IV

2. The results of postural drainage include which of the following?
   I. Facilitate the mucous flow
   II. Relieve bronchospasm
   III. Facilitate diaphragmatic movement
   IV. Impede venous return
   a. I and II
   b. II and III
   c. I
   d. I, II, and III
   e. All of the above

3. Breathing exercises result in:
   I. Increase in respiratory rate
   II. Decrease in respiratory rate
   III. Increased tidal volume
   IV. Increased lateral costal expansion
   a. I and III
   b. I and IV
   c. II and IV
   d. II and III
   e. II, III, and IV

4. A poor effort for a cough could be the result of:
   I. Decreased inspiratory volume
   II. Position
   III. Pain
   IV. Increased airway resistance
   a. I
   b. II
   c. II and III
   d. I, II, and IV
   e. All of the above

5. All of the following areas should be avoided when percussing a patient's chest except:
   a. Incisions
   b. Surface landmarks of the bronchial segment being drained
   c. Bony prominences
   d. Burns
   e. Open wounds

6. Vibrations applied to the chest wall should be done on:
   a. Inspiration
   b. Expiration
   c. Mid-expiration
   d. Mid-inspiration
   e. a and b

7. The chest physical therapy technique of shaking should be used on:
   I. Patients who have thick, difficult secretions
   II. Patients with osteoporosis
   III. Patients receiving long-term steroids
   IV. Patients who have a compliant chest wall
   a. I and II
   b. II and III
   c. I and IV
   d. I, III, and IV
   e. All of the above

8. The chest and related anatomy and physiology of an infant differs from an adult's in all of the following except:
   a. The child's chest has a greater airway resistance
   b. The child's chest is more circular
   c. The child's ribs angle more horizontally
   d. The child's larynx is lower
   e. The child has fewer collateral ventilatory channels

9. What is the primary hazard placing infants weighing less than 800 gm in the Trendelenberg position?
   a. Increased risk of intraventricular hemorrhage
   b. Increased risk of aspiration
   c. Increased risk of mucous plugging
   d. Increased risk of atelectasis
   e. Increased risk of apnea

10. Diaphragmatic breathing should be initially taught in which of the following positions?
    a. Trendelenberg's position
    b. Sitting
    c. Walking
    d. Standing
    e. Semi-Fowler's position with knees bent

11. Pursed lip breathing done inappropriately can lead to which of the following?
    a. Increased airway collapse
    b. Increased cardiovascular pressure
    c. Gas trapping
    d. Increased jugular vein distention
    e. All of the above

12. Which of the following are potential hazards of endotracheal suctioning?
    a. Infection
    b. Vagal stimulation
    c. Bradycardia
    d. Hypoxia
    e. All of the above

13. Order the steps of nasotracheal suctioning.
    I. Lubricate catheter with water-soluble gel.
    II. Inform the patient of the procedure.
    III. Check equipment and monitors.
    IV. Pull back catheter slightly, and then apply suction while withdrawing catheter.
    V. Repeat procedure if necessary.
    VI. Allow the patient to rest for several seconds, and then reoxygenate.
    VII. Limit aspiration time to 10 to 15 seconds total.
    VIII. Preoxygenate patient.
    IX. Place the patient's neck in mild extension.
    X. Pass catheter upward and backward with short increments until an obstruction is met.
    a. III, II, VIII, IX, I, X, IV, VII, VI, V
    b. II, VII, III, IX, I, X, IV, VII, VI, V
    c. II, III, IX, VIII, I, X, IV, VII, VI, V
    d. III, II, IX, VIII, I, X, IV, VII, VI, V
    e. X, IV, VII, VI, V, III, II, IX, VIII, I

14. Which of the following is true of nasotracheal airways?
    I. They can be difficult to suction due to the increased curvature of the tube.
    II. They are better tolerated for comfort.
    III. They are the airway of choice in an emergency.
    IV. A larger size can be used compared with an oral tube.

a. I
b. III
c. II and III
d. II and IV
e. I and II

15. Which of the following represents complications of tracheal intubation?
    a. Nasal bleeding
    b. Vocal cord hematomas
    c. Right main stem intubations
    d. Inability to adequately communicate
    e. All of the above

16. The volume of saline that should be instilled into a neonate prior to suctioning is:
    a. 0.1–0.2 ml
    b. 0.25–0.5 ml
    c. 0.5–1.0 ml
    d. 1.5–1.75 ml
    e. 1.75–2.0 ml

CHAPTER 8: INTERMITTENT POSITIVE-PRESSURE BREATHING

1. Which of the following should be included in an IPPB order?
    I. Preset pressure
    II. F_{IO_2}
    III. Pharmacologic agent
    IV. Duration and frequency
    a. I
    b. II and III
    c. I and III
    d. I, III, and IV
    e. All of the above

2. Which of the following are physiologic effects of IPPB?
    I. Increase in the mean airway pressure
    II. Decrease the work of breathing
    III. Manipulate the I/E ratio
    IV. Increase the tidal volume
    a. I
    b. IV
    c. I and III
    d. I, II, and III
    e. All of the above

3. Which of the following are potential side effects of increasing the transpulmonary pressure from IPPB?
   I. Increase left ventricle filling
   II. Decrease cardiac output
   III. Decrease pulmonary perfusion
   IV. Increase venous return
   a. II
   b. I and II
   c. II and III
   d. I and IV
   e. I, III, and IV

4. How long will the increase in tidal volume last after IPPB has been administered?
   a. As long as the treatment lasts
   b. 5 minutes
   c. 10 minutes
   d. 15 minutes
   e. 20 minutes

5. How much will IPPB increase the transpulmonary pressure over spontaneous breathing?
   a. 80%
   b. 95%
   c. 110%
   d. 125%
   e. 140%

6. What is the primary indication for IPPB?
   a. Improve cough
   b. Mobilize secretions
   c. Unable to inspire adequately
   d. Prevent atelectasis
   e. Improve the distribution and deposition of aerosol

7. An indication for IPPB would be a vital capacity less than:
   a. 15 ml/kg
   b. 20 ml/kg
   c. 25 ml/kg
   d. 30 ml/kg
   e. 35 ml/kg

8. Which of the following are recommended positions for the administration of IPPB?
   I. Sitting
   II. Standing
   III. Semi-Fowler's
   IV. Lying
   a. I
   b. II
   c. I and III
   d. II and III
   e. I, III, and IV

9. If adjustable, what should the sensitivity of an IPPB machine be set on?
   a. -2 to -4 cm H_2O
   b. -2 to 0 cm H_2O
   c. 0 cm H_2O
   d. $+1$ to $+2$ cm H_2O
   e. $+2$ to $+4$ cm H_2O

10. What should the exhaled tidal volume be when administering volume-oriented IPPB?
    a. 1–2 ml $\times$ ideal body weight (lb)
    b. 3–4 ml $\times$ ideal body weight (lb)
    c. 5–6 ml $\times$ ideal body weight (lb)
    d. 7–8 ml $\times$ ideal body weight (lb)
    e. 9–10 ml $\times$ ideal body weight (lb)

11. How long should a patient be encouraged to pause at the end of an inspiration when taking an IPPB treatment?
    a. 1–2 seconds
    b. 3–4 seconds
    c. 5–6 seconds
    d. 7–8 seconds
    e. No pause

12. All of the following are appropriate items to enter in a patient's chart after receiving an IPPB treatment except:
    a. Duration of therapy
    b. Peak pressure used
    c. Cost of the treatment
    d. Volume achieved
    e. Patient's response to therapy

13. Calculate the venous gradient given the following data: central venous pressure +15 cm H_2O, intrapleural pressure +10 cm H_2O, stroke volume 70 ml, and pulmonary artery pressure 25/10 mm Hg.
    a. 1.5 cm H_2O
    b. 5 cm H_2O
    c. 10 cm H_2O
    d. 25 cm H_2O
    e. 90 cm H_2O

14. A heart rate increase of greater than _____ beats/min over pretherapy levels should result in termination of IPPB therapy.
    a. 5
    b. 10
    c. 25
    d. 20
    e. 25

15. Which of the following are considered hazards associated with IPPB therapy?
    I.   Pneumothorax
    II. Hemoptysis
    III. Gastric insufflation
    IV. Respiratory alkalosis
    a. I
    b. II and III
    c. III and IV
    d. I, II, and IV
    e. All of the above

16. How often should IPPB breathing circuits be changed?
    a. Every day
    b. Every 2 days
    c. Every 3 days
    d. Every 4 days
    e. Every 5 days

17. What are the absolute contraindications to IPPB?
    I.   Tension pneumothorax
    II. Massive pulmonary hemorrhage
    III. Active tuberculosis
    IV. Intracranial injury
    a. I
    b. II
    c. I and II
    d. II and III
    e. I, II, and IV

CHAPTER 9: INCENTIVE SPIROMETRY AND OTHER AIDS TO LUNG INFLATION

1. The primary benefit of incentive spirometry is to:
   a. Prevent atelectasis
   b. Decrease airway resistance
   c. Increase compliance
   d. Increase anatomic dead space
   e. Increase cardiac output

2. Which of the following are identifiable risk groups prone to postoperative atelectasis?
   I.   Advanced age
   II. Smoking history
   III. Obesity
   IV. Sinus infection
   V.   COPD
   a. I and II
   b. II, III, and V
   c. II, III, IV, and V
   d. I, II, III, and V
   e. All of the above

3. What is/are the primary pathological factor(s) implicated in the etiology of atelectasis?
   a. Airway obstruction
   b. Altered sigh mechanism
   c. Increased pulmonary compliance
   d. a and b
   e. All of the above

4. What pulmonary function condition predisposes patients to bronchiolar collapse and atelectasis?
   a. When the FVC is greater than the FRC
   b. When the FRC is greater than the RV
   c. When the FRC is greater than the expiratory reserve volume (ERV)
   d. When the TLC is greater than the closing volume (CV)
   e. When the CV is greater than the ERV

5. Which of the following statements are true concerning a sigh?
   a. A sigh decreases the transpulmonary pressure.
   b. A sigh increases the transpulmonary pressure.
   c. An individual sighs approximately 10 times each hour.
   d. The sigh volume equals the anatomic dead space.
   e. b and c

6. Define LaPlace's law.
   a. P × V
   b. P/V
   c. P = ST/r
   d. ST = P/r
   e. P = ST/V

7. Referring to the illustration below which way will the gas flow if the stopcock is open?

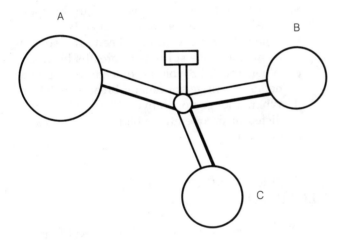

   a. A to B or C
   b. B to A or C
   c. C to A or B
   d. B to C only
   e. B and C to A

8. What is normal mean intrapulmonary pressure?
   a. +10 cm H_2O
   b. +5 cm H_2O
   c. 0 cm H_2O
   d. −5 cm H_2O
   e. −10 cm H_2O

9. Referring to the illustration below where is the intrapleural pressure the most negative?

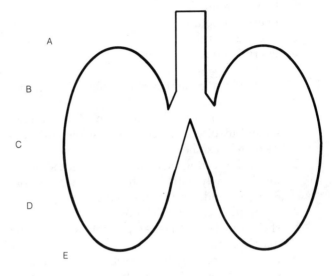

10. Which of the following would be clinical findings consistent with atelectasis?
    I.   Diminished lung volumes
    II. Decreased radiopacity
    III. Low-grade fever
    IV. Hyperresonant percussion note
    V.   Diminished breath sounds
    a. I and V
    b. II and III
    c. I, II, and IV
    d. I, III, and V
    e. I, II, IV, and V

11. What are the therapeutic goals for incentive spirometry?
    I.   Increase FRC
    II. Increase lung compliance
    III. Increase arterial oxygen tension
    IV. Increase work of breathing
    a. I
    b. II
    c. I and III
    d. I, II, and III
    e. All of the above

12. How long will a normal alveoli remain inflated?
    a. 5 minutes
    b. 10 minutes
    c. 20 minutes
    d. 40 minutes
    e. 60 minutes

13. How often should incentive spirometry be performed?
    a. Every 30 minutes
    b. Every 1 hour
    c. Every 1.5 hours
    d. Every 2 hours
    e. Every 2.5 hours

14. How should a patient perform sustained maximal inspiration (SMI) properly?
    a. From the resting RV position, the patient should inspire as quickly as possible and immediately exhale.
    b. From the resting position, the patient should inspire slowly with a postinspiratory pause of 3 to 5 seconds and then exhale.
    c. From the resting FRC position, the patient should inspire as fast as possible and immediately exhale.
    d. From the resting FRC position, the patient should inspire slowly with a postinspiratory pause of 3 to 5 seconds and then exhale.
    e. From TLC, the patient should exhale with a pause of 3 to 5 seconds and then inhale.

15. In which of the following situations would the patient be unable to perform incentive spirometry?
    I.   A 24-hour postoperative open heart patient
    II. A visually impaired patient
    III. A postoperative gallbladder patient
    IV. An 18-month bronchiolitis patient
    a. I
    b. III
    c. II and III
    d. II and IV
    e. I and III

16. Under preferable conditions, when is it most appropriate to initially teach a patient about SMI?
    a. Send a letter to the patient's house approximately 10 days prior to surgery explaining about the device.
    b. Mail the device to the patient's house with instructions 5 days prior to surgery.
    c. Provide preoperative teaching 24 hours prior to surgery.
    d. Provide preoperative teaching 1 hour after the preoperative medications for surgery have been given.
    e. Wait 24 hours after surgery.

17. How many breaths/hour should incentive spirometry be performed?
    a. 5
    b. 10
    c. 15
    d. 20
    e. 25

18. When should incentive spirometry breathing be terminated?
    a. When the patient can inspire 40% of the preoperative IC
    b. When the patient can inspire 60% of the preoperative IC
    c. When the patient can inspire 80% of the preoperative IC
    d. When the patient can inspire 70% of the preoperative FRC
    e. 24 hours postoperatively

19. When may IPPB be used instead of incentive spirometry?
    a. When the IPPB volume is equal to the spontaneous incentive spirometer breaths
    b. When the IPPB volume exceeds the spontaneous incentive spirometer breaths by 10%
    c. When the IPPB volume exceeds the spontaneous incentive spirometer breaths by 20%
    d. When the postoperative IC is 50% of predicted or preoperative volume
    e. b and d

CHAPTER 10: MECHANICAL VENTILATION

1. Which of the following are likely to lead to postoperative respiratory failure?
   I.   Cardiac surgery
   II. Upper abdominal surgery
   III. Hip reduction surgery
   IV. Thoracic surgery
   V.   Neurosurgery
   a. I and II
   b. II and III
   c. III, IV, and V
   d. I, II, IV, and V
   e. All of the above

2. Which of the following are a result of high carbon dioxide levels?
   I. High blood pressure
   II. Cerebral congestion
   III. Paresthesia
   IV. Tetanic muscle contraction
   V. Increased cerebrospinal fluid pressure
   a. I
   b. II
   c. III and IV
   d. I, II, and V
   e. I, II, IV, and V

3. What percentage is the pulmonary system oxygen consumption relative to the total?
   a. 2%–3%
   b. 5%–10%
   c. 12%–16%
   d. 17%–25%
   e. 28%–32%

4. Which of the following will result in a decreased mean intrathoracic pressure during mechanical ventilation?
   I. Intermittent mandatory ventilation (IMV)
   II. Decrease tidal volume
   III. Increase inspiratory time
   IV. Increase PEEP
   a. I
   b. III
   c. I and II
   d. II and IV
   e. II, III, and IV

5. What is the approximate pulmonary capillary blood volume?
   a. 90 ml
   b. 150 ml
   c. 200 ml
   d. 250 ml
   e. 500 ml

6. Which of the following represents metabolic compensation for respiratory alkalosis?
   a. Increased renal excretion of bicarbonate
   b. Retention of chloride
   c. Decreased ammonia production
   d. Decreased excretion of acid salts
   e. All of the above

7. What is the Coanda effect?
   a. Describes the phenomenon that states as the forward velocity of a gas increases the lateral pressure decreases
   b. Describes the phenomenon that causes a jet stream to attach to a nearby wall
   c. A synergistic drug response as a result of combining two similar drugs
   d. Describes the effect of increased gas velocity in relationship to airway resistance
   e. Describes the relationship between volume and compliance

8. Which of the following are true of the Emerson 3-PV Post-Operative ventilator?
   I. Single circuit
   II. Double circuit
   III. Sine wave flow pattern
   IV. Constant flow pattern
   V. Pneumatically driven
   a. I
   b. I and III
   c. II and III
   d. I, III, and V
   e. II, III, and V

9. Which of the following is an example of a linear drive constant flow rate ventilator?
   a. Bennett MA-1
   b. Puritan-Bennett 7200
   c. Bourns BP200
   d. Bourns LS104-150
   e. Siemens Servo Ventilator 900C

10. Which of the following statements best describes IMV?
   a. Mandatory breaths synchronized with the patient's own spontaneous breathing rate
   b. Mode of ventilation that allows the patient to breath spontaneously from the ventilator circuit in addition to receiving mandatory tidal breathing
   c. Mode of ventilation that must be triggered by the patient in order to receive a tidal volume
   d. Mode of ventilation that will allow only ventilation-initiated breaths
   e. Mode of ventilation that will deliver a mandatory tidal volume whenever the spontaneous ventilation is not adequate to reach a preset minute volume

11. Which of the following statements best describes pressure support?
    a. Mode of ventilation that allows a spontaneous breath to be assisted by a preset amount of constant pressure that is added to a baseline pressure throughout inspiration
    b. Mode of ventilation that allows the patient to breathe spontaneously from the ventilator circuit in addition to receiving mandatory tidal breathing
    c. Mode of ventilation that must be triggered by the patient to receive a tidal volume
    d. Mode of ventilation that will allow only ventilation-initiated breaths
    e. Mode of ventilation that will deliver a mandatory tidal volume whenever the spontaneous ventilation is not adequate to reach the preset minute volume

12. What is the average compliance factor for nondisposable ventilator circuits?
    a. 1 ml/cm H_2O
    b. 3 ml/cm H_2O
    c. 5 ml/cm H_2O
    d. 7 ml/cm H_2O
    e. 9 ml/cm H_2O

13. The use of PEEP during positive pressure ventilation results primarily in which of the following?
    a. Increased IC
    b. Increased TLC
    c. Decreased ERV
    d. Decreased tidal volume
    e. Increased FRC

14. Identify the fluidic element in the illustration below.

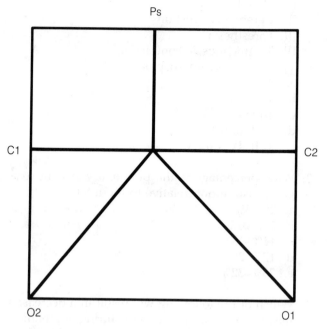

    a. Flip-flop
    b. OR/NOR gate
    c. AND/NAND gate
    d. Proportional amplifier
    e. Back pressure switch

15. Identify the fluidic element in the illustration below.

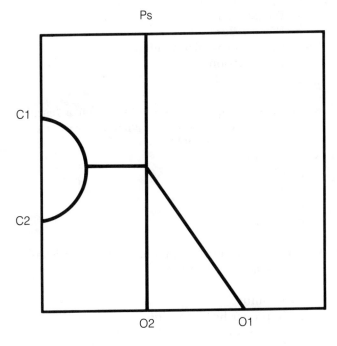

Ps

C1

C2

O2   O1

a. Schmitt trigger
b. OR/NOR gate
c. AND/NAND gate
d. Back pressure switch
e. Flip-flop

16. When mechanical ventilation is initiated on an adult patient, what respiratory rate is usually set?
    a. 6/min
    b. 10/min
    c. 14/min
    d. 18/min
    e. 22/min

17. Which of the following are true of the use of large tidal volumes for a patient on a mechanical ventilator?
    I. Reduces the alveolar-arterial O_2 gradient
    II. Results in small airway closure
    III. Aids in the internal stabilization of the chest wall
    IV. Results in right to left shunting of blood
    a. I
    b. II
    c. I and III
    d. II and III
    e. I, III, and IV

18. What is the minimum amount of PEEP indicated for use during mechanical ventilation?
    a. 3 cm H_2O
    b. 5 cm H_2O
    c. 7 cm H_2O
    d. 9 cm H_2O
    e. 12 cm H_2O

19. Which of the following factors will affect the size of the spontaneous tidal volume when a patient is receiving pressure support?
    I. The amount of pressure support provided
    II. The inspiratory time
    III. Whether the patient attempts to exhale prematurely, exceeding the upper pressure limit control
    IV. Prematurely cycling the ventilator into the expiratory phase
    a. I
    b. III
    c. II and IV
    d. I, II, and IV
    e. All of the above

20. Which of the following flow wave patterns results in a more physiologic flow and the least amount of pressure to deliver a tidal volume?
    a. Constant flow generators
    b. Accelerating flow generators
    c. Decelerating flow generators
    d. Sine wave flow generators
    e. Square wave flow generators

CHAPTER 11: CARDIOPULMONARY RESUSCITATION

1. Cardiac arrest is defined as:
   a. Drop in blood pressure to a point where the patient feels faint
   b. Drop in heart rate to less than 60 beats/min
   c. Cessation of cardiac output or a reduction of cardiac output to a point where it is ineffective in providing oxygenated blood
   d. Apnea with a heart rate of 60 beats/min
   e. Apnea with a drop in blood pressure to a point where a person feels faint

2. What F_{IO_2} does mouth to mouth resuscitation provide to the victim?
   a. 10%
   b. 12%
   c. 16%
   d. 18%
   e. 21%

3. In the adult patient, the ratio of compressions to ventilation for a two-person rescue team is:
   a. 2:1
   b. 5:1
   c. 10:1
   d. 12:1
   e. 15:1

4. In the adult patient, the ratio of compressions to ventilation for one rescuer is:
   a. 5:1
   b. 10:1
   c. 10:2
   d. 15:2
   e. 18:2

5. All of the following are true statements about the esophageal obturator except:
   a. The procedure requires a direct visualization of the vocal cords.
   b. The obturator consists of a mask attached to a cuffed tube.
   c. The obturator tube is cuffed to prevent gastric inflation and regurgitation.
   d. Vomiting and aspiration are potential complications when the tube is removed.
   e. Esophageal rupture is a potential complication.

6. The straight blade attachment of the laryngoscope:
   I.   Allows the tip of the blade to lift the epiglottis during intubation
   II. Allows the tip of the blade to fit in between the epiglottis and the base of the tongue
   III. Is used primarily for children
   IV. Is used primarily for adults
   a. I and III
   b. I and IV
   c. II and III
   d. II and IV
   e. I, III, and IV

7. Which of the following is/are associated with a high mortality rate following cardiopulmonary resuscitation (CPR)?
   a. Pneumonia
   b. Renal failure
   c. Cerebral vascular accident
   d. Hypotension
   e. All of the above

8. What is the approximate volume that a rescuer should deliver to an adult victim during a cardiopulmonary arrest?
   a. 350 ml
   b. 600 ml
   c. 800 ml
   d. 1,000 ml
   e. 1,200 ml

9. What is the most common course of resistance to ventilator during CPR?
   a. Dentures
   b. Vomitus
   c. Improper head position
   d. Laryngospasm
   e. Foreign body aspiration

10. What artery is used in the adult patient to assess circulatory adequacy?
    a. Radial
    b. Temporal
    c. Carotid
    d. Brachial
    e. Femoral

11. What is the percentage of cardiac output when compressions are performed adequately?
    a. 20%–25%
    b. 25%–30%
    c. 30%–35%
    d. 35%–40%
    e. 40%–45%

12. What depth should the rescuer compress on the adult victim's chest?
    a. ½–¾ in.
    b. ¾–1 in.
    c. 1–1½ in.
    d. 1½–2 in.
    e. 2–2½ in.

13. What is the minimum $F_{I_{O_2}}$ for a manual resuscitator according to the American National Standards Institute Z–79 subcommittee on resuscitators?
    a. 45%
    b. 60%
    c. 75%
    d. 85%
    e. 100%

14. What is the mandatory pressure limit on pediatric and neonatal resuscitators?
    a. 20 cm H_2O
    b. 30 cm H_2O
    c. 40 cm H_2O
    d. 50 cm H_2O
    e. None of the above

15. What is the recommended O_2 flow rate setting for a manual resuscitator?
    a. 5 L/min
    b. 10 L/min
    c. 15 L/min
    d. 20 L/min
    e. 25 L/min

16. Which of the following would lead to the highest $F_{I_{O_2}}$ delivery from a manual resuscitator attached to an O_2 flowmeter?
    I. Large tidal volumes
    II. Small tidal volumes
    III. Fast refill times
    IV. Slow refill times
    a. I and III
    b. I and IV
    c. II and III
    d. II and IV

17. What is the recommended dose for initial defibrillation of the adult according to the American Heart Association?
    a. 50 W-sec
    b. 100 W-sec
    c. 150 W-sec
    d. 200 W-sec
    e. 250 W-sec

18. Which of the following are factors influencing the success of defibrillation?
    a. Size of the paddles
    b. Paddle location
    c. Electrode gel
    d. Repeated defibrillations
    e. All of the above

19. For relief of a foreign body obstruction in an infant, which of the following techniques should be used?
    a. Heimlich maneuver
    b. Abdominal thrust
    c. Back blows
    d. Chest thrusts
    e. Finger sweep

20. All of the following are indications for the administration of intravenous epinephrine in the adult except:
    a. To treat premature ventricular contractions (PVCs)
    b. To treat ventricular asystole
    c. To convert fine ventricular fibrillation to coarse fibrillation
    d. To increase mean arterial pressure (MAP)
    e. To increase cardiac output

CHAPTER 12: EQUIPMENT FOR MIXED GAS AND OXYGEN THERAPY

1. Who was the individual responsible for the discovery of carbon dioxide?
    a. Joseph Black
    b. Leonardo DaVinci
    c. Joseph Priestly
    d. Carle Scheele
    e. Torbern Bergman

2. Who was the individual responsible for the discovery of oxygen?
    a. Jean Baptiste Van Helmont
    b. Leonardo DaVinci
    c. Joseph Priestly
    d. George Stahl
    e. Frances A. Lavoisier

3. What is the atomic weight of oxygen?
    a. 4
    b. 8
    c. 16
    d. 32
    e. 64

4. What is the density of oxygen?
    a. 1.43 gm/L
    b. 2.26 gm/L
    c. 3.82 gm/L
    d. 4.21 gm/L
    e. 5.62 gm/L

5. What is the relative speed with which CO_2 can diffuse between alveoli and pulmonary capillaries compared with oxygen?
   a. 7 times
   b. 14 times
   c. 21 times
   d. 28 times
   e. 32 times

6. What is the boiling point of oxygen?
   a. $+32°C$
   b. $+18°C$
   c. $-62°C$
   d. $-124°C$
   e. $-183°C$

7. Under normal circumstances what is the atmospheric concentration of carbon dioxide?
   a. 0.0015%
   b. 0.003%
   c. 0.01%
   d. 0.03%
   e. 0.045%

8. According to the Occupational Safety and Health Act (OSHA), what is the allowable exposure to carbon dioxide?
   I. 0.5% for 8 hours of continuous exposure
   II. 1.5% for 8 hours of continuous exposure
   III. 3% over a 10-minute period
   IV. 5% over a 10-minute period
   a. I
   b. II
   c. I and III
   d. II and III
   e. II and IV

9. What agency is responsible for the standards for construction of vessel safety of medical gas cylinders?
   a. Department of Transportation (DOT)
   b. Federal Aviation Association (FAA)
   c. American Society of Mechanical Engineers (ASME)
   d. National Fire Protection Agency (NFPA)
   e. Cryogenics Associates (CA)

10. The piping system for compressed gases is regulated by what agency?
    a. National Plumbing Association (NPA)
    b. National Welders Association (NWA)
    c. National Fire Protection Agency (NFPA)
    d. Compressed Gas Association (CGA)
    e. American Medical Association (AMA)

11. What type of material can be used in a hospital gas supply system?
    I. Seamless type K or L copper tubing
    II. Seamless type K or L brass tubing
    III. Seamless type L PVC tubing
    IV. Seamless type K steel tubing
    a. I
    b. I and IV
    c. I and II
    d. III and IV
    e. II, III, and IV

12. What is the maximum allowable amount of total water content in an air piping system under the federal specifications BB-A-1034?
    a. 0.3 mg/L
    b. 0.5 mg/L
    c. 0.8 mg/L
    d. 1.2 mg/L
    e. 1.5 mg/L

13. Name the agency that is responsible for proper storage of high-pressure medical gas cylinders?
    a. Department of Transportation
    b. Federal Aviation Association
    c. American Society of Mechanical Engineers
    d. National Fire Protection Agency
    e. Cryogenics Associates

14. Which of the following statements are true concerning the testing and checking of cylinders by governing agencies?
    I. All aluminum cylinders are inspected every 5 years.
    II. All aluminum cylinders are inspected every 10 years.
    III. High-quality alloy steel 3A and 3AA cylinders are inspected every 5 years.
    IV. High-quality alloy steel 3A and 3AA cylinders followed by a star are inspected every 10 years.
    a. I and IV
    b. II and III
    c. I and III
    d. I, III, and IV
    e. II, III, and IV

15. How many liters of gas are there in 1 cubic foot of gas?
    a. 16.2 L
    b. 18.4 L
    c. 22.4 L
    d. 26.2 L
    e. 28.3 L

16. How long will a one-half full E cylinder at 2 L/min last?
    a. 30 minutes
    b. 45 minutes
    c. 87 minutes
    d. 124 minutes
    e. 154 minutes

17. What temperature will the fusible metal plug in an oxygen cylinder melt at if exposed?
    a. 100°C
    b. 120°C
    c. 160°C
    d. 190°C
    e. 210°C

18. What agency is responsible for the indexing for the connections gas supply systems?
    a. Department of Transportation
    b. American Standards Association
    c. American Society of Mechanical Engineers
    d. National Fire Protection Agency
    e. Compressed Gas Association

19. What is the reduction in cylinder pressure given the following information: cylinder's high gas pressure (Pc) 2,200 psi, area subjected to high pressure (Ac) 2 mm^2, and area of a flexible diaphragm (Ar) 4 mm^2?
    a. 50 psi
    b. 110 psi
    c. 220 psi
    d. 810 psi
    e. 1,100 psi

20. Define Reynold's number.
    a. $\dfrac{\text{Density} \times \text{Velocity} \times \text{Radius}}{\text{Viscosity}}$
    b. $\dfrac{\text{Viscosity} \times \text{Velocity} \times \text{Radius}}{\text{Density}}$
    c. $\dfrac{\text{Viscosity} \times \text{Velocity} \times \text{Density}}{\text{Radius}}$
    d. $\dfrac{\text{Velocity} \times \text{Density}}{\text{Radius}}$
    e. $\dfrac{\text{Viscosity}}{\text{Velocity}}$

CHAPTER 13: AEROSOL GENERATORS AND HUMIDIFIERS

1. Which of the following devices will produce the largest particle size?
   a. Atomizer
   b. Jet nebulizer
   c. Ultrasonic nebulizer
   d. Small-volume nebulizer
   e. Hydrosphere nebulizer

2. Describe the type of nebulizer in the illustration below.

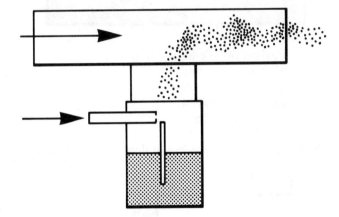

   a. Mainstream nebulizer
   b. Sidestream nebulizer
   c. Ultrasonic nebulizer
   d. Slipstream nebulizer
   e. Wick nebulizer

3. The F_{IO_2} from a handheld nebulizer is determined by:
   a. The F_{IO_2} of the source gas
   b. The patient's breathing pattern
   c. The patient's dead space
   d. a and b
   e. None of the above

4. What particle size range will be deposited in the small airways and alveoli?
   a. 0.25–1.0 μ
   b. 1.0–2.0 μ
   c. 2.0–3.5 μ
   d. 3.5–4.5 μ
   e. 4.5–5.5 μ

5. Describe the device in the illustration below.

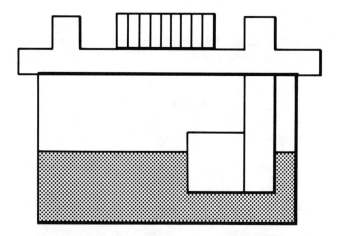

   a. Puritan Bubble-Jet humidifier
   b. Mainstream nebulizer
   c. Sidestream nebulizer
   d. Cascade humidifier
   e. Wick humidifier

6. Describe the device in the illustration below.

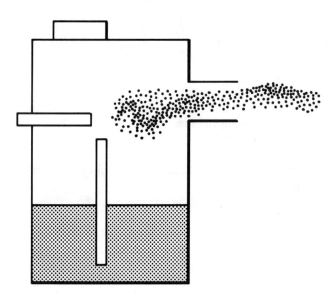

   a. Wick humidifier
   b. Babbington nebulizer
   c. Bubble humidifier
   d. Ultrasonic nebulizer
   e. Jet nebulizer

7. Describe the device in the illustration below.

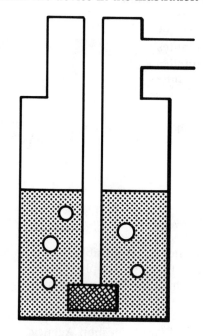

   a. Jet nebulizer
   b. Bubble humidifier
   c. Sidestream nebulizer
   d. Handheld nebulizer
   e. Atomizer

8. Describe the device in the illustration below.

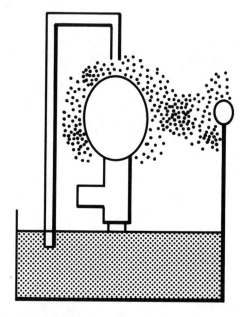

   a. Jet nebulizer
   b. Babbington nebulizer
   c. Sidestream nebulizer
   d. Ultrasonic nebulizer
   e. Atomizer

9. Which of the following will occur to a Venturi nebulizer setup if a large bolus of water settles in the tubing?
   I. F_{IO_2} increases
   II. F_{IO_2} decreases
   III. F_{IO_2} remains the same
   IV. Increase resistance in the setup
   V. Decrease resistance in the setup
   a. I and IV
   b. I and V
   c. II and IV
   d. II and V
   e. III and IV

10. What is the predicted total outflow from a nebulizer setup given the following data: oxygen flow 8 L/min and F_{IO_2} 0.40?
    a. 20 L/min
    b. 24 L/min
    c. 28 L/min
    d. 32 L/min
    e. 40 L/min

11. What is the range of outputs from heated nebulizers?
    a. 0.2–0.7 ml/min
    b. 0.7–1.3 ml/min
    c. 1.3–3.1 ml/min
    d. 3.1–5.2 ml/min
    e. 5.2–6.4 ml/min

12. What is the predicted total outflow from a nebulizer setup given the following data: oxygen flow 12 L/min and F_{IO_2} 0.80?
    a. 12 L/min
    b. 16 L/min
    c. 20 L/min
    d. 28 L/min
    e. 32 L/min

13. Which of the following factors will cause the fractional concentration of oxygen in a patient's hypopharynx (F_{HO_2}) to decrease if a patient is receiving oxygen via a face mask?
    I. Increased inspiratory flow
    II. Decreased inspiratory flow
    III. Increased tidal volume
    IV. Decreased nebulizer flow
    a. I and III
    b. II and IV
    c. III and IV
    d. II and III
    e. I, III, and IV

14. The gas flow exiting the reservoir tube on a T-piece aerosol should:
    a. Appear only during the initial one half of inspiration
    b. Appear only during inspiration
    c. Appear only during expiration
    d. b and c
    e. Not be visible during inspiration or expiration

15. On an ultrasonic nebulizer the aerosol output is dependent on which factor(s)?
    I. Amplitude of the frequency signal
    II. The frequency of the signal
    III. The velocity of the blower motor
    IV. The temperature of the couplant chamber
    a. I
    b. II
    c. I and II
    d. II, III, and IV
    e. All of the above

16. Which of the following aerosol generators is least likely to rain out in the tubing?
    a. Cascade humidifier
    b. Ultrasonic nebulizer
    c. Large mainstream nebulizer
    d. Bird inline micronebulizer
    e. Jet nebulizer

17. What are the approximate particle sizes produced from an ultrasonic nebulizer?
    a. 3 μ
    b. 7 μ
    c. 12 μ
    d. 16 μ
    e. 20 μ

18. What is the aerosol output of the Solo-Sphere nebulizer?
    a. 0.5 ml/min
    b. 1 ml/min
    c. 2 ml/min
    d. 3.5 ml/min
    e. 5 ml/min

19. What is acceptable water content reaching the patient according to the American National Standard for Humidifiers and Nebulizers for Medical Use (ANSI Z-79.9, 1979)?
    a. 15 mg/L, 80% relative humidity (RH) at 72°F
    b. 30 mg/L, 80% RH at 72°F
    c. 42 mg/L, 80% RH at 86°F
    d. 30 mg/L, 100% RH at 86°F
    e. 43 mg/L, 100% RH at 98°F

CHAPTER 14: INTERMITTENT POSITIVE-PRESSURE BREATHING DEVICES

1. What IPPB machine is known to have the "valve that breathes with the patient"?
   a. Bennett series
   b. Bird series
   c. Monaghan series
   d. Ohio series
   e. Cryogenic series

2. Below what flow rate will the Bennett valve counterweight close, resulting in exhalation?
   a. 0.5 L/min
   b. 1 L/min
   c. 1.5 L/min
   d. 2.5 L/min
   e. 4 L/min

3. How do you activate inspiration on a Bennett AP-4 series machine if the patient is not breathing?
   a. Push the manual breath button.
   b. Set a rate.
   c. Decrease the inspiratory time.
   d. Lift up the small handle on the Bennett valve.
   e. It cannot be achieved.

4. Which of the following IPPB machine(s) would be best suited for home care use?
   I. Bennett AP-4
   II. Bennett TA-1
   III. Bennett PR-2
   IV. Bird Mark 7
   a. I
   b. IV
   c. I and II
   d. II and III
   e. I, III, and IV

5. What is the maximum flow available through the Bennett valve on a PR-2?
   a. 45 L/min
   b. 55 L/min
   c. 65 L/min
   d. 80 L/min
   e. 100 L/min

6. What does the control pressure indicate on the Bennett PR-2?
   a. The pressure when a patient takes a controlled breath
   b. The pressure in the diluter regulator
   c. The pressure at the patient's mouth
   d. The pressure in the patient's circuit
   e. The pressure in the patient's airways

7. Which of the following statements are true on the Bennett PR-2 when the nebulizer control is turned on?
   I. FI_{O_2} decreases.
   II. FI_{O_2} stays the same.
   III. FI_{O_2} increases.
   IV. The tidal volume increases.
   V. The tidal volume decreases.
   a. I
   b. III
   c. III and IV
   d. I and V
   e. II and IV

8. The proper setting for the sensitivity on the Bennett PR-2 is:
   a. -0.5 cm H_2O
   b. -1 cm H_2O
   c. -1.5 cm H_2O
   d. -2 cm H_2O
   e. -2.5 cm H_2O

9. What is the purpose of the terminal flow control on the Bennett PR-2?
   a. It automatically terminates flow to the machine after 10 minutes.
   b. It automatically terminates flow to the machine after 20 minutes.
   c. It allows the practitioner to set a rate.
   d. It compensates for any leaks that may be in the circuit.
   e. It determines the amount of negative pressure the patient must generate to receive a breath.

10. What is the range of $F_{I_{O_2}}$ from the Bennett PR-2 when the air dilution control is on?
    a. 0.30–0.40
    b. 0.40–0.60
    c. 0.50–0.70
    d. 0.60–0.80
    e. 0.70–0.90

11. When the Bennett PR-2 is used for IPPB, the negative pressure control should be set at:
    a. -0.5 cm H_2O
    b. -1 cm H_2O
    c. -2.5 cm H_2O
    d. -3.5 cm H_2O
    e. Off

12. Before implementing an IPPB treatment on a patient with a Bennett PR-2, the practitioner cycles the machine on and pressurizes the circuit. The control pressure is set for 20 cm H_2O, and the practitioner notices that the system pressure is not being reached. The next step should be:
    a. To turn on the nebulizer
    b. To adjust the sensitivity
    c. To turn on the terminal flow
    d. To turn on the negative pressure
    e. To push in the air dilution

13. What control on the Bird Mark 7 controls the manual initiation of inspiration and halting of expiration?
    a. Manual inspiratory button
    b. Manual expiratory button
    c. a and b
    d. Flow rate control
    e. Manual timer rod

14. On the Bird Mark 7 what control allows a subambient pressure exerted by the patient to move the ceramic switch?
    a. Venturi gate
    b. Manual timer rod
    c. Expiratory termination cartridge
    d. Master diaphragm
    e. Sensitivity control

15. Which controls allow for adjustment of nebulization on the Bird Mark 7?
    a. Inspiratory nebulization control
    b. Expiratory nebulization control
    c. Continuous nebulization control
    d. a and b
    e. None of the above

16. What is the maximum attainable flow rate on the Bird Mark 7 with the air mix control on?
    a. 40 L/min
    b. 50 L/min
    c. 60 L/min
    d. 65 L/min
    e. 75 L/min

17. What is the maximum attainable flow rate on the Bird Mark 7 with the air mix control off?
    a. 20 L/min
    b. 30 L/min
    c. 40 L/min
    d. 50 L/min
    e. 60 L/min

18. The practitioner is giving an IPPB treatment to a patient using a Bird Mark 7. How will the performance of the machine be affected if the disposable circuit the patient is using does not have a bleed hole on the inspiratory service line to the nebulizer?
    a. The machine will immediately cycle into exhalation.
    b. The flow rate will double.
    c. The exhalation valve line will blow off.
    d. The machine will self-cycle.
    e. The patient pressure will increase by 10 cm H_2O.

19. What is the function of the inspiratory flow accelerator on the Bird Mark 10?
    a. It increases the $F_{I_{O_2}}$.
    b. It doubles the delivered tidal volume.
    c. If inspiration has not ended by a specified time, it causes a sudden increase in flow, resulting in a rise in pressure that will terminate inspiration.
    d. If inspiration has not ended by a specified time, it causes a sudden increase in flow, resulting in a decrease in pressure that will terminate inspiration.
    e. It allows a finer adjustment of sensitivity.

20. What is the adjustable range of sensitivity settings on the Monaghan 515?
    a. -0.5 to -1 cm H_2O
    b. -1 to -2 cm H_2O
    c. -2 to -3 cm H_2O
    d. -3 to -4 cm H_2O
    e. Not adjustable

CHAPTER 15: INCENTIVE SPIROMETERS AND SECRETION EVACUATION DEVICES

1. What is/are the main goal(s) of incentive spirometer devices?
   I. To actively remove secretions
   II. To decrease airway resistance
   III. To increase the patient's spontaneous tidal volume
   IV. To prevent atelectasis
   a. III
   b. I and III
   c. II and III
   d. III and IV
   e. All of the above

2. Another name of incentive spirometry is:
   a. SMI
   b. Deep breath augmentor
   c. Atelectasis removal device
   d. IPPB
   e. None of the above

3. What are correct instructions to a patient receiving incentive spirometry?
   a. Exhale normally to the end of residual volume, tightly seal his or her lips around the mouthpiece, slowly inspire to the end of normal tidal breathing, hold, then exhale.
   b. Exhale normally to the end of RV, tightly seal his or her lips around the mouthpiece, slowly inspire to the end of TLC, hold, then exhale.
   c. Exhale normally to the end-tidal expiratory volume, tightly seal his or her lips around the mouthpiece, slowly inspire to the end of TLC, hold, then exhale.
   d. Inhale normally to the end of TLC, tightly seal his or her lips around the mouthpiece, slowly exhale to the end-tidal volume level, hold, then repeat.
   e. Inhale normally to the end of normal tidal breathing, tightly seal his or her lips around the mouthpiece, slowly exhale to the end-tidal volume level, hold, then repeat.

4. How long should the practitioner instruct the patient to sustain an inspiratory hold when using the Triflo II incentive spirometer?
   a. 1 second
   b. 3 seconds
   c. 5 seconds
   d. 7 seconds
   e. 9 seconds

5. What is the acceptable range of flow rates the patient should try to inhale at when using an incentive spirometer to promote uniform distribution of gas?
   a. 100–300 ml/sec
   b. 300–600 ml/sec
   c. 600–900 ml/sec
   d. 900–1,200 ml/sec
   e. 1,200–1,500 ml/sec

6. Which of the following incentive spirometers are volume displacement devices?
   a. Triflo II
   b. Tru-Vol
   c. Volurex
   d. Spirocare
   e. b and c

7. Which of the following incentive spirometers' volumes are not influenced by inspiratory flow rates?
   a. Spirocare
   b. Triflo I
   c. Triflo II
   d. Volurex
   e. b and c

8. How long does the inspiratory hold remain lit on the Spirocare incentive breathing exercisers?
   a. 1.5 seconds
   b. 2.5 seconds
   c. 3.5 seconds
   d. 5.0 seconds
   e. 6.0 seconds

9. Which of the following are true statements about open-ended suction catheters?
   I. The entire negative pressure will be exerted on the tracheobronchial tree surface.
   II. One and one half times the set wall pressure is applied to the tracheobronchial tree surface.
   III. Faster removal of tracheobronchial secretions is accomplished.
   a. I
   b. II
   c. III
   d. I and III
   e. All of these

10. How many millimeters of mercury does 19 in. of mercury equal?
    a. 188.2 mm Hg
    b. 180.4 mm Hg
    c. 270.4 mm Hg
    d. 392.8 mm Hg
    e. 482.6 mm Hg

11. What type(s) of connections allow(s) for attachment of suction regulators to the wall outlets?
    I. Pin Index Safety System
    II. Quick Connect Outlet Connections
    III. Diameter Index Safety System
    IV. Negative Pressure Device Connection System
    a. I
    b. II and III
    c. III and IV
    d. I, III, and IV
    e. All of the above

CHAPTER 16: MECHANICAL VENTILATORS

1. What does Boyle's law state?
    a. A volume of gas varies inversely with the pressure provided the gas temperature is held constant.
    b. A volume of gas varies directly with the pressure provided the gas temperature is held constant.
    c. A volume of gas varies inversely with temperature provided the pressure is held constant.
    d. The pressure exerted by a volume of gas varies directly with temperature.

2. Compliance is defined as:
    a. Change in volume/change in pressure
    b. Change in volume times change in pressure
    c. Change in pressure/change in volume
    d. Change in volume/flow rate
    e. Change in pressure/flow rate

3. What physical law governs gas flow through a conduction system?
    a. Boyle's law
    b. Dalton's law
    c. Poiseuille's law
    d. Charles' law
    e. Beer's law

4. Who first described the iron lung as a body-enclosing respirator in which the patient sat upright?
    a. John Dalziel
    b. Philip Drinker
    c. Cecil Drinker
    d. John Emerson
    e. Greg Monaghan

5. Which of the following are true statements about the iron lung?
    I. Time cycled
    II. Electrically powered
    III. Pressure limit
    IV. Assist/control
    a. I
    b. I and II
    c. I and IV
    d. I, II, and III
    e. All of the above

6. What controls adjust the $F_{I_{O_2}}$ on an iron lung?
    a. Blender control
    b. Air-mix control
    c. Venturi control
    d. Inspiratory time
    e. None of the above

7. What physical law describes the gas movement in the iron lung?
    a. Dalton's law
    b. Charles' law
    c. Boyle's law
    d. Gay-Lussac's law
    e. Poiseuille's law

8. What controls will cause an increase of inspiratory time on the Bird Mark 7?
    I. Increase flow rate
    II. Decrease flow rate
    III. Increase pressure limit
    IV. Decrease pressure limit
    V. Increase the sensitivity
    a. I and III
    b. II and III
    c. I and IV
    d. I, III, and V
    e. II, IV, and V

9. What parameters will be affected if the peak inspiratory pressure is increased on the Bird Mark 7 ventilator?
   - I. Increased inspiratory pressure results in an increased controlled rate.
   - II. Increased inspiratory pressure results in a decreased controlled rate.
   - III. Decreased inspiratory pressure results in an increased controlled rate.
   - IV. Increased inspiratory pressure results in an increased F_{IO_2}.
   - V. Increased inspiratory pressure results in a decreased F_{IO_2}.
   - a. I and IV
   - b. II and IV
   - c. II and III
   - d. II, III, and IV
   - e. II, III, and V

10. Which control adjusts the control rate on the Emerson 3-PV ventilator?
    - I. Rate control
    - II. Inspiratory time
    - III. Expiratory time
    - IV. Percent of inspiratory time
    - a. I
    - b. II
    - c. III
    - d. II and III
    - e. II, III, and IV

11. What is the inspiratory flow wave pattern of the Emerson 3-PV ventilator?
    - a. Square wave
    - b. Accelerating square wave
    - c. Decelerating square wave
    - d. Sine wave
    - e. Sinusoidal wave

12. For the Emerson 3-PV ventilator circuit to be assured leak free:
    - a. The system should be pressurized for 2 seconds, and the pressure should not drop.
    - b. The system should be pressurized for 5 seconds, and the pressure should not drop.
    - c. The system should be pressurized for 10 seconds, and the pressure should not drop.
    - d. The system should be pressurized for 10 seconds, and the pressure should not drop more than 5 cm H_2O.
    - e. The system should be pressurized for 5 seconds, and the pressure should not drop more than 10 cm H_2O.

13. Classify the Bennett MA-1 ventilator.
    - I. Time cycled
    - II. Volume cycled
    - III. Pressure limited
    - IV. Assist/control modes
    - a. I and IV
    - b. I and II
    - c. I, III, and IV
    - d. II and IV
    - e. II, III, and IV

14. The oxygen system on the Bennett MA-1 ventilator monitors:
    - I. Set F_{IO_2}
    - II. Actual F_{IO_2}
    - III. Patient's exhaled F_{IO_2}
    - IV. Oxygen supply is pressurized
    - a. I
    - b. II
    - c. IV
    - d. I, II, and III
    - e. I, II, and IV

15. What monitoring alarm system on the Bennett MA-1 ventilator will be activated if the tidal volume, cycle rate, and peak flow setting result in a situation where the inspiratory phase is longer than the expiratory phase?
    - a. Sigh high-pressure alarm
    - b. Inverse I/E ratio
    - c. Low-oxygen pressure alarm
    - d. Disconnect alarm
    - e. None of the above

16. Which of the following operator selected alarms are on the BEAR-1 ventilator?
    - I. Low pressure
    - II. Low PEEP
    - III. Minimal exhaled volume
    - IV. Apnea
    - V. Ventilator inoperative
    - a. I and III
    - b. II, III, and IV
    - c. I, III, and V
    - d. II, III, IV, and V
    - e. All of the above

17. How do the characteristics of the delivered tidal volume change when the nebulizer control on the BEAR-I ventilator is turned on?
    I. The F_{IO_2} decreases unless set at 0.21.
    II. The F_{IO_2} increases.
    III. The F_{IO_2} stays the same.
    IV. The tidal volume increases.
    V. It does not change the performance of the ventilator.
    a. I
    b. V
    c. I and III
    d. II and IV
    e. III and IV

18. Which of the following modes is the Siemens-Elema Servo Ventilator 900C capable of operating?
    I. Volume control (assist/control)
    II. Synchronized intermittent mandatory ventilation (SIMV)
    III. Pressure support
    IV. Pressure control
    V. Manual
    a. I and II
    b. I, III, and V
    c. II, IV, and V
    d. III, IV, and V
    e. All of the above

19. Calculate a patient's flow rate on the Servo Ventilator 900C whose settings are minute volume 18.0 L/min, cycle rate 20 breaths/min, and inspiratory time percent 33%.
    a. 36 L/min
    b. 48 L/min
    c. 54 L/min
    d. 62 L/min
    e. 68 L/min

20. How is PEEP accomplished on the Bourns BP200 infant pressure ventilator?
    a. Spring-loaded disk
    b. A water column
    c. A pressurized mushroom valve
    d. A Venturi mechanism
    e. Weighted resistors

CHAPTER 17: ONGOING PATIENT ASSESSMENT

1. What is the rationale for continuous assessment and monitoring?
    I. Evaluate the patient's response to the care provided.
    II. Initiate and maintain therapy that has been prescribed.
    III. Provide a basis for documentation of care given.
    IV. Assure patient safety.
    a. I
    b. III
    c. I and III
    d. I, II, and IV
    e. All of the above

2. What is the most common site for evaluation of pulse?
    a. Carotid artery
    b. Radial artery
    c. Brachial artery
    d. Femoral artery
    e. Temporal artery

3. A bounding pulse may indicate which of the following?
    I. Hypoxemia
    II. Anemia
    III. Peripheral vasodilation
    IV. Hyperthyroidism
    a. I
    b. IV
    c. I and II
    d. I, II, and IV
    e. All of the above

4. Which of the following may be indicative of irregular heart rhythm?
    I. Anxiety
    II. Caffeine consumption
    III. Hypoxemia
    IV. Exercise
    a. I and IV
    b. II and III
    c. I and II
    d. I, II, and III
    e. All of the above

5. What is the most common cardiac rhythm associated with hypoxia?
   a. Sinus bradycardia
   b. Sinus tachycardia
   c. 1-degree heart block
   d. 3-degree heart block
   e. Ventricular tachycardia

6. Which of the following are possible contributing factors to systemic hypotension?
   I.   Peripheral vasodilation
   II. Low blood volume
   III. Increased peripheral vascular resistance
   IV. Increased ventricular contraction
   a. I
   b. II
   c. I and II
   d. I, III, and IV
   e. II, III, and IV

7. Which of the following are indications of compromised perfusion state?
   I.   Warm skin
   II. Dry skin
   III. Pale skin
   IV. Cold skin
   a. I
   b. III
   c. I and II
   d. II and III
   e. I, II, and III

8. What is the normal urine output in adults?
   a. 0.25–0.5 L/day
   b. 0.5–0.75 L/day
   c. 0.75–1.0 L/day
   d. 1.0–1.5 L/day
   e. 1.5–2.0 L/day

9. What primary factor(s) result(s) in urine filtration in the glomerulus of the kidneys?
   a. Blood pressure
   b. Blood volume
   c. Pa_{CO_2}
   d. pH
   e. a and b

10. How can positive-pressure ventilation affect renal function?
    I.   Increase in renal perfusion
    II. Decrease in renal perfusion
    III. Increase in antidiuretic hormone being released
    IV. Decrease in antidiuretic hormone being released
    V.   Increase retention of water
    a. I and III
    b. I and IV
    c. II and III
    d. II and IV
    e. II, III, and V

11. Which of the following thoracic deformities are characterized by sternal protrusion anteriorly?
    a. Kyphosis
    b. Scoliosis
    c. Kyphoscoliosis
    d. Pectus carinatum
    e. Pectus excavatum

12. The technique of chest wall palpation is used to evaluate all of the following except:
    a. Breath sounds
    b. Vocal fremitus
    c. Estimate symmetry of thoracic expansion
    d. Establish the position of the trachea
    e. Assess the skin and subcutaneous tissue

13. Which of the following would produce a decreased vocal fremitus?
    I.   Pneumothorax
    II. Pneumonia
    III. Emphysema
    IV. Pulmonary edema
    a. I
    b. I and III
    c. II and IV
    d. III and IV
    e. I, III, and IV

14. Which of the following are clinical entities resulting in a decreased thoracic expansion?
    a. Kyphosis
    b. Scoliosis
    c. Atelectasis
    d. Lobar pneumonia
    e. All of the above

15. Which of the following clinical entities would produce a dull or flat percussion note?
    I. Pleural Effusion
    II. Asthma
    III. Atelectasis
    IV. Pneumothorax
    a. I
    b. II
    c. I and III
    d. I, III, and IV
    e. All of the above

16. What breath sound is characterized by low-pitched continuous sounds often associated with the presence of excessive mucus in the airways?
    a. Vesicular
    b. Rhonchi
    c. Wheeze
    d. Bronchovesicular
    e. Decreased

17. What type of cough is associated with croup?
    a. Dry
    b. Barking
    c. Brassy
    d. Wheezy
    e. Hacking

18. What is the largest component of sputum?
    a. Water
    b. Lipoprotein
    c. Carbohydrate
    d. Lipids
    e. DNA

19. What breathing pattern is characterized by cyclic increases in tidal volume, followed by decreases in tidal volume?
    a. Eupnea
    b. Biot's respirations
    c. Tachypnea
    d. Cheyne-Stokes respirations
    e. Ataxic breathing

20. At what level of reversibility does a bronchodilator have a significant effect as determined by changes in the prebronchodilator and postbronchodilator studies of $FEF_{25\%-75\%}$ and $FEF_{.2-1.2L}$?
    a. 5%
    b. 10%
    c. 15%
    d. 20%
    e. 25%

CHAPTER 18: BLOOD GAS INTERPRETATION

1. Which of the following is considered the safest site of arterial puncture in an adult?
   a. Radial
   b. Brachial
   c. Femoral
   d. Dorsalis pedis
   e. Temporal

2. How long should it take for collateral circulation to be restored for Allen's test to be positive?
   a. 10–15 seconds
   b. 15–20 seconds
   c. 20–25 seconds
   d. 25–30 seconds
   e. 30–35 seconds

3. What gas law states that if O_2 makes up 21% of the atmosphere, it will exert an approximate partial pressure equal to 160 mm Hg if the atmospheric pressure is 760 mm Hg?
   a. Boyle's law
   b. Dalton's law
   c. Charles' law
   d. Henry's law
   e. Graham's law

4. What is the exchange of O_2 and CO_2 between the blood in the lungs and the gas exchange in the alveoli called?
   a. Dead space
   b. Shunt
   c. Internal respiration
   d. External respiration
   e. Respiratory quotient

5. Given the following information, calculate the alveolar O_2 tension: P_B, 755 mm Hg; F_{IO_2}, 0.40; P_{H_2O}, 47 mm Hg; R, 0.8; and Pa_{CO_2}, 48 mm Hg.
   a. 100 mm Hg
   b. 223 mm Hg
   c. 235 mm Hg
   d. 283 mm Hg
   e. 330 mm Hg

6. The P_{AO_2} increases above 100 mm Hg at a rate of approximately _____ mm Hg for every 0.01 increase in F_{IO_2} above 0.21?
   a. 2
   b. 7
   c. 15
   d. 20
   e. 25

7. What is the normal range of $P(A-a)O_2$, while breathing room air?
   a. 1–4 mm Hg
   b. 4–12 mm Hg
   c. 12–28 mm Hg
   d. 20–28 mm Hg
   e. 28–36 mm Hg

8. An increase in the $P(A-a)O_2$ would indicate which of the following?
   I.   Ventilation-perfusion mismatch
   II. Diffusion defect
   III. Shunt
   a. I
   b. II
   c. III
   d. II and III
   e. All of the above

9. At a P_{O_2} of 100 mm Hg for each volume percent of plasma, how much O_2 will be dissolved in the plasma?
   a. 0.003 ml
   b. 0.3 ml
   c. 1.34 ml
   d. 5.0 ml
   e. 20.0 ml

10. What would be considered a normal Pa_{O_2} for a 70-year-old patient?
    a. 55 mm Hg
    b. 60 mm Hg
    c. 65 mm Hg
    d. 70 mm Hg
    e. 80 mm Hg

11. What is the relationship between P_{O_2} and percent saturation of hemoglobin?
    a. Linear
    b. Accelerating linear
    c. Square
    d. Sigmoid
    e. Descending square wave

12. What is the normal P_{50} value at 37°C and a pH of 7.40?
    a. 1.34 mm Hg
    b. 15.2 mm Hg
    c. 26.6 mm Hg
    d. 52.8 mm Hg
    e. 81.2 mm Hg

13. Calculate the Ca_{O_2} given the following data: Pa_{O_2}, 110 mm Hg; hemoglobin saturation, 98%; pH, 7.42; Pa_{CO_2}, 36 mm Hg; and hemoglobin, 12 gm%.
    a. 16.1 vol%
    b. 16.4 vol%
    c. 17.2 vol%
    d. 17.6 vol%
    e. 18.1 vol%

14. Approximately how much O_2 is transported with hemoglobin compared to the amount in the plasma?
    a. 10 times
    b. 32 times
    c. 48 times
    d. 65 times
    e. 78 times

15. Calculate the systemic oxygen transport (SO_2T) given the following data: 90% sat; Pa_{O_2}, 80 mm Hg; hemoglobin, 12 gm%; pH, 7.35; Pa_{CO_2}, 45 mm Hg; stroke volume, 70 ml; and heart rate, 92/min.
    a. 912 ml/min
    b. 922 ml/min
    c. 947 ml/min
    d. 961 ml/min
    e. 987 ml/min

16. What mixed venous P_{O_2} indicates adequate tissue oxygenation?
    a. 7 mm Hg
    b. 12 mm Hg
    c. 26 mm Hg
    d. 32 mm Hg
    e. 40 mm Hg

17. In which of the following forms is CO_2 transported by the blood?
    I. Dissolved
    II. HCO_3^-
    III. Combined with protein in the form of carbamino compounds
    a. I
    b. II
    c. II and III
    d. I and III
    e. All of the above

18. What compound speeds up the reaction between CO_2 and H_2O inside the RBC?
    a. Carbonic acid
    b. Carbonic anhydrase
    c. Bicarbonate
    d. Enzymatic anhydrase
    e. Carbamino enzymatic

19. Approximately how much volatile acid is eliminated from the body each day by the lungs?
    a. 8,000–12,000 mEq
    b. 12,000–15,000 mEq
    c. 15,000–24,000 mEq
    d. 24,000–32,000 mEq
    e. 32,000–40,000 mEq

20. Interpret the following arterial blood gas data: pH, 7.41; Pa_{CO_2}, 30 mm Hg; Pa_{O_2}, 100 mm Hg; and HCO_3^-, 16 mEq/L.
    a. Acute respiratory acidosis
    b. Acute metabolic acidosis
    c. Partially compensated respiratory alkalosis
    d. Compensated respiratory alkalosis
    e. Metabolic and respiratory acidosis

CHAPTER 19: SYSTEMATIC MODIFICATION OF VENTILATORY SUPPORT

1. All of the following represent clinical entities resulting in increased Pa_{CO_2} except:
    a. Anxiety
    b. Retained secretions
    c. Pneumothorax
    d. Increased dead space
    e. Airway obstruction

2. Which of the following may occur when the patient fights the delivery of a positive pressure breath?
    I. Increased peak airway pressure
    II. Decreased intrathoracic pressure
    III. Decreased cardiac output
    IV. Development of pulmonary air leak
    a. I
    b. II
    c. III and IV
    d. I, III, and IV
    e. All of the above

3. What is the most common blood gas alteration in critically ill ventilator-dependent patients?
    a. Respiratory acidosis
    b. Respiratory alkalosis
    c. Metabolic alkalosis
    d. Metabolic acidosis
    e. Respiratory and metabolic acidosis

4. Critically ill ventilator-dependent patients lacking intake of solid food and undergoing diuretic and steroid therapy suffer from what type of electrolyte imbalance?
    I. Na^+ deficiencies
    II. K^+ excess
    III. K^+ deficiencies
    IV. Cl^- deficiencies
    V. HCO_3^- deficiencies
    a. I
    b. V
    c. II and IV
    d. III and IV
    e. I, II, and V

5. Which of the following would indicate that the patient maintained on IMV/SIMV mode can assume a greater role in the maintenance of spontaneous ventilation?
    a. Increased respiratory rate
    b. Decreased respiratory rate
    c. Increased tidal volume
    d. Decreased tidal volume
    e. Both a and d

6. Calculate the effective static compliance (CES) given the following data: exhaled tidal volume, 800 ml; plateau pressure, 42 cm H_2O; peak pressure, 50 cm H_2O; and PEEP, 10 cm H_2O.
   a. 18 ml/cm H_2O
   b. 22 ml/cm H_2O
   c. 25 ml/cm H_2O
   d. 28 ml/cm H_2O
   e. 30 ml/cm H_2O

7. Calculate the CES accounting for the loss of compressible volume given the following data: exhaled tidal volume, 700 ml; plateau pressure, 40 cm H_2O; peak pressure, 55 cm H_2O; PEEP, 8 cm H_2O, and compressible volume loss, 90 ml.
   a. 16 ml/cm H_2O
   b. 19 ml/cm H_2O
   c. 22 ml/cm H_2O
   d. 25 ml/cm H_2O
   e. 28 ml/cm H_2O

8. Calculate the dynamic compliance (Cdyn) given the following data: exhaled tidal volume 850 ml, peak pressure 60 cm H_2O, plateau pressure 52 cm H_2O, PEEP 10 cm H_2O, and compliance volume loss 126 ml.
   a. 14 ml/cm H_2O
   b. 17 ml/cm H_2O
   c. 23 ml/cm H_2O
   d. 26 ml/cm H_2O
   e. 29 ml/cm H_2O

9. A decrease in the CES may indicate which of the following?
   I.   Atelectasis
   II. Decompression of a pneumothorax
   III. Consolidation
   IV. Adult respiratory distress syndrome (ARDS)
   a. I
   b. II
   c. II and III
   d. I, III, and IV
   e. All of the above

10. Calculate the airway resistance (RA) given the following data: exhaled tidal volume (VT), 900 ml; peak pressure, 60 cm H_2O; plateau pressure, 50 cm H_2O; PEEP, 10 cm H_2O; compressible loss volume, 120 ml; and peak flow, 60 L/min.
    a. 0.08 cm H_2O/L/min
    b. 0.17 cm H_2O/L/min
    c. 0.32 cm H_2O/L/min
    d. 0.48 cm H_2O/L/min
    e. 0.54 cm H_2O/L/min

11. Calculate the inspiratory time (t_I) given the following data: tidal volume, 850 ml; peak pressure, 50 cm H_2O; plateau pressure, 40 cm H_2O; PEEP, 10 cm H_2O; and peak flow, 50 L/min.
    a. 0.5 second
    b. 1.0 second
    c. 1.4 seconds
    d. 1.8 seconds
    e. 2.2 seconds

12. What is the first organ system to respond to hypoxemia?
    a. Lungs
    b. Heart
    c. Kidneys
    d. Brain
    e. Liver

13. How much should the system pressure fluctuate if adequate flow is being provided to meet the patient's peak inspiratory demands?
    a. 0 cm H_2O
    b. ± 2 cm H_2O
    c. ± 4 cm H_2O
    d. ± 6 cm H_2O
    e. ± 8 cm H_2O

14. At what point of respiration should peak flow be measured in a continuous-flow IMV circuit to assure adequate flow?
    a. Beginning of inspiration
    b. Mid-inspiration
    c. Peak inspiration
    d. Beginning of exhalation
    e. Peak exhalation

15. If the patient's work of breathing increases beyond the capabilities of the demand valve on an IMV/SIMV mode of ventilation, which of the following should be done?
    I.   Increase the sensitivity of the demand valve.
    II. Increase the level of supported mechanical ventilation.
    III. Sedate the patient.
    IV. Change the ventilator to a continuous-flow IMV system.
    a. I
    b. II
    c. II and III
    d. II, III, and IV
    e. All of the above

16. Which of the following alarm systems represent the minimum that should be placed on a ventilator?
    I.   Ventilator disconnect
    II. High airway pressure
    III. Airway temperature
    IV. F_{IO_2}
    a. I
    b. II
    c. I and II
    d. II, III, and IV
    e. All of the above

17. System leaks can be identified by delivering a fixed volume of gas into the circuit with the high-pressure limit control set at maximum while preventing exhalation and occluding the patient Y. A pressure of _____ cm H_2O held for _____ seconds indicates a leak-free circuit.
    a. 40, 1
    b. 50, 1
    c. 70, 2–4
    d. 80, 1
    e. 80, 2–4

18. What is the allowable error for the rate setting and the tidal volume setting?
    a. ± 5%, ± 5%, respectively
    b. ± 10%, ± 5%, respectively
    c. ± 5%, ± 10%, respectively
    d. ± 10%, ± 10%, respectively
    e. ± 10%, ± 15%, respectively

19. At what setting should the peak airway pressure alarm be set when a patient is on a mechanical ventilator?
    a. 50 cm H_2O
    b. 70 cm H_2O
    c. 85 cm H_2O
    d. 10 cm H_2O above average airway pressure
    e. 20 cm H_2O above average airway pressure

20. At what setting should the loss of PEEP alarm be set when a patient is on a mechanical ventilator?
    a. −2 cm H_2O
    b. 0 cm H_2O
    c. 4 cm H_2O
    d. 1–2 cm H_2O below PEEP level
    e. 3–5 cm H_2O below PEEP level

CHAPTER 20: DETERIORATION DESPITE INTENSIVE RESPIRATORY CARE

1. Which of the following are clinically acceptable diagnostics for an acute myocardial infarction?
   I.   Serial ECGs
   II. Ultrasound
   III. Cardiac enzymes
   IV. Cardiac catheterization
   a. I
   b. II
   c. I and III
   d. II and IV
   e. I, III, and IV

2. Which of the following are likely to occur with congestive heart failure?
   I.   Increased pulmonary compliance
   II. Decreased pulmonary compliance
   III. Increased $P(A-a)O_2$
   IV. Decreased $P(A-a)O_2$
   V.   Progressive pulmonary infiltrates
   a. I and III
   b. I and IV
   c. II and III
   d. II and IV
   e. II, III, and V

3. Which of the following is the most common cause of iatrogenic congestive heart failure?
   a. Fluid overload
   b. Decreased ventricular contractility
   c. Mitral stenosis
   d. Pericardial effusion
   e. Systemic hypertension

4. Which of the following clinical signs and symptoms may occur with an intubated patient on a ventilator?
   I.   Decrease in dynamic compliance
   II. Increase in dynamic compliance
   III. Increase in cycling pressure
   IV. Hyperresonance percussion note over the affected area
   V.   Dull percussion note over the affected area
   a. I and III
   b. I, III, and IV
   c. I, III, and V
   d. II, III, and IV
   e. II, III, and V

5. Hypokalemia causes cardiac arrythmias and re-duced skeletal muscle contraction when serum potassium level falls below ____ mEq/L.
   a. 3.0
   b. 3.4
   c. 3.8
   d. 4.2
   e. 4.6

6. What is the compensation mechanism for an in-crease in HCO_3^-, PO_4^-, and Cl^-?
   a. Metabolic acidosis
   b. Metabolic alkalosis
   c. Alveolar hypoventilation
   d. Alveolar hyperventilation
   e. b and d

7. Which of the following are clinical signs and symptoms of overhydration while being sup-ported by mechanical ventilation?
   I. Decreasing pulmonary compliance
   II. Thickening of respiratory mucus
   III. Widening of alveolar-arterial oxygen gra-dient
   IV. Elevated wedge pressure
   V. Systemic hypertension
   a. I and III
   b. II and IV
   c. II, III, and IV
   d. I, III, and IV
   e. All of the above

8. What percentage of hospitalized patients in the United States suffer from malnutrition?
   a. 10%–20%
   b. 20%–30%
   c. 30%–40%
   d. 40%–50%
   e. 50%–60%

9. Which of the following represent clinical signs or symptoms of acute oxygen toxicity?
   I. Alveolar edema
   II. Atelectasis
   III. Hemorrhage
   IV. Fibroblastic proliferation
   V. Hyaline membrane formation
   a. I
   b. II
   c. II and IV
   d. I, II, and III
   e. I, II, III, and IV

10. Which of the following represent clinical signs or symptoms of pulmonary infection?
    I. Fever
    II. Change in sputum color
    III. Increase in esosinophil count
    IV. Increase in the osmotic pressure
    V. Infiltrate on chest x-ray
    a. I
    b. I and II
    c. II, III, and IV
    d. I, II, and V
    e. I, III, IV, and V

Chapter 1
1. e (p. 6)
2. d (p. 6)
3. c (p. 7)
4. b (p. 7)
5. c (p. 7)
6. d (p. 8)
7. d (p. 9)
8. d (p. 10)
9. a (p. 11)
10. d (p. 15)
11. e (p. 16)
12. a (p. 17)
13. c (p. 17)
14. c (p. 20)
15. a (p. 21)
16. b (p. 21)
17. c (p. 24)
18. a (p. 24)
19. e (p. 28)
20. a (p. 25)

Chapter 2
1. e (p. 35)
2. d (p. 38)
3. b (p. 41)
4. e (p. 42)
5. c (p. 45)
6. c (p. 46)
7. b (p. 47)
8. a (p. 54)
9. d (p. 54)
10. e (p. 54)
11. c (p. 68)
12. d (p. 71)
13. e (p. 75)
14. a (p. 76)
15. a (p. 76)
16. b (p. 77)
17. a (p. 79)
18. b (p. 79)
19. c (p. 82)
20. c (p. 82)

Chapter 3
1. e (p. 95)
2. d (p. 95)
3. c (p. 96)
4. c (p. 96)
5. c (p. 96)
6. d (p. 97)
7. e (p. 98)
8. c (p. 98)
9. c (p. 99)

10. e (p. 99)
11. a (p. 99)
12. e (p. 100)
13. c (p. 100)
14. e (p. 100)
15. c (p. 101)
16. c (p. 101)
17. d (p. 102)
18. e (p. 103)
19. e (p. 103)
20. a (p. 107)

Chapter 4
1. c (p. 110)
2. e (p. 110)
3. d (p. 111)
4. d (p. 120)
5. c (p. 121)
6. e (p. 121)
7. a (p. 122)
8. e (p. 122)
9. e (p. 122)
10. e (p. 126)

Chapter 5
1. c (p. 131)
2. c (p. 132)
3. b (p. 132)
4. e (p. 133)
5. d (p. 134)
6. b (p. 134)
7. c (p. 134)
8. d (p. 135)
9. b (p. 136)
10. e (p. 136)
11. d (p. 136)
12. c (p. 137)
13. c (p. 137)
14. d (p. 137)
15. d (p. 138)
16. a (p. 138)
17. e (p. 146)
18. d (p. 148)
19. e (p. 148)
20. c (p. 150)

Chapter 6
1. a (p. 165)
2. a (p. 166)
3. e (p. 166)
4. c (p. 166)
5. b (p. 166)
6. a (p. 166)
7. b (p. 167)

8. c (p. 167)
9. a (p. 167)
10. d (p. 168)
11. a (p. 168)
12. d (p. 169)
13. b (p. 169)
14. a (p. 171)
15. d (p. 171)
16. e (p. 177)
17. c (p. 174)
18. a (p. 176)
19. d (p. 174)
20. e (p. 174)

Chapter 7
1. a (p. 183)
2. c (p. 185)
3. e (p. 185)
4. e (p. 185)
5. b (p. 188)
6. b (p. 188)
7. c (p. 188)
8. d (p. 188)
9. a (p. 189)
10. e (p. 190)
11. e (p. 192)
12. e (p. 194)
13. a (p. 195)
14. e (p. 196)
15. e (p. 196)
16. c (p. 198)

Chapter 8
1. e (p. 201)
2. e (p. 201)
3. c (p. 201)
4. a (p. 202)
5. c (p. 202)
6. c (p. 203)
7. a (p. 203)
8. c (p. 203)
9. b (p. 203)
10. b (p. 204)
11. a (p. 204)
12. c (p. 204)
13. b (p. 205)
14. d (p. 205)
15. e (p. 205)
16. a (p. 206)
17. c (p. 206)

Chapter 9
1. a (p. 208)
2. d (p. 208)

3. d (p. 208)
4. e (p. 209)
5. e (p. 209)
6. c (p. 210)
7. e (p. 210)
8. d (p. 210)
9. a (p. 210)
10. d (p. 211)
11. d (p. 211)
12. e (p. 211)
13. b (p. 211)
14. d (p. 211)
15. d (p. 212)
16. c (p. 212)
17. b (p. 212)
18. c (p. 212)
19. c (p. 213)

Chapter 10
1. d (p. 216)
2. d (p. 217)
3. a (p. 218)
4. c (p. 218)
5. a (p. 218)
6. e (p. 219)
7. b (p. 235)
8. b (p. 224)
9. d (p. 225)
10. b (p. 226)
11. a (p. 226)
12. b (p. 230)
13. e (p. 231)
14. a (p. 236)
15. c (p. 237)
16. b (p. 240)
17. c (p. 241)
18. b (p. 241)
19. e (p. 240)
20. d (p. 243)

Chapter 11
1. c (p. 249)
2. c (p. 251)
3. b (p. 254)
4. d (p. 254)
5. a (p. 255)
6. a (p. 257)
7. e (p. 249)
8. c (p. 251)
9. c (p. 251)
10. c (p. 253)
11. b (p. 253)
12. d (p. 254)
13. d (p. 264)

14. c (p. 266)
15. c (p. 267)
16. d (p. 267)
17. d (p. 268)
18. e (p. 269)
19. c (p. 271)
20. a (p. 272)

Chapter 12
1. a (p. 287)
2. c (p. 285)
3. c (p. 288)
4. a (p. 289)
5. c (p. 290)
6. e (p. 290)
7. d (p. 291)
8. d (p. 291)
9. c (p. 293)
10. c (p. 296)
11. c (p. 296)
12. a (p. 298)
13. d (p. 299)
14. d (p. 299)
15. e (p. 301)
16. e (p. 301)
17. e (p. 302)
18. b (p. 302)
19. e (p. 305)
20. a (p. 309)

Chapter 13
1. a (p. 356)
2. b (p. 356)
3. d (p. 361)
4. a (p. 361)
5. d (p. 389)
6. e (p. 364)
7. b (p. 385)
8. b (p. 381)
9. a (p. 367)
10. d (p. 367)
11. c (p. 368)
12. b (p. 367)
13. e (p. 373)
14. d (p. 373)
15. a (p. 374)

16. b (p. 380)
17. a (p. 380)
18. c (p. 383)
19. d (p. 387)

Chapter 14
1. a (p. 406)
2. b (p. 406)
3. d (p. 407)
4. c (p. 407)
5. d (p. 408)
6. b (p. 409)
7. b (p. 409)
8. a (p. 409)
9. d (p. 409)
10. b (p. 409)
11. e (p. 409)
12. c (p. 409)
13. e (p. 410)
14. d (p. 410)
15. e (p. 411)
16. d (p. 411)
17. c (p. 411)
18. c (p. 411)
19. c (p. 412)
20. e (p. 416)

Chapter 15
1. d (p. 418)
2. a (p. 418)
3. c (p. 418)
4. b (p. 420)
5. c (p. 420)
6. e (p. 422)
7. d (p. 422)
8. b (p. 423)
9. a (p. 429)
10. e (p. 432)
11. b (p. 432)

Chapter 16
1. a (p. 438)
2. a (p. 439)
3. c (p. 439)
4. a (p. 440)
5. d (p. 440)
6. e (p. 440)

7. c (p. 440)
8. b (p. 441)
9. d (p. 442)
10. d (p. 443)
11. e (p. 443)
12. d (p. 444)
13. e (p. 445)
14. c (p. 447)
15. b (p. 447)
16. e (p. 451)
17. b (p. 454)
18. e (p. 454)
19. c (p. 456)
20. d (p. 466)

Chapter 17
1. e (p. 469)
2. b (p. 470)
3. d (p. 470)
4. d (p. 470)
5. b (p. 471)
6. c (p. 471)
7. b (p. 471)
8. d (p. 472)
9. e (p. 472)
10. e (p. 472)
11. d (p. 472)
12. a (p. 472)
13. b (p. 472)
14. e (p. 473)
15. c (p. 474)
16. b (p. 475)
17. b (p. 476)
18. a (p. 476)
19. d (p. 477)
20. c (p. 479)

Chapter 18
1. a (p. 497)
2. a (p. 498)
3. b (p. 498)
4. d (p. 499)
5. b (p. 499)
6. b (p. 499)
7. b (p. 499)
8. e (p. 499)

9. b (p. 500)
10. d (p. 500)
11. d (p. 501)
12. c (p. 502)
13. a (p. 502)
14. d (p. 502)
15. c (p. 504)
16. e (p. 505)
17. e (p. 505)
18. b (p. 505)
19. c (p. 506)
20. d (p. 507)

Chapter 19
1. a (p. 517)
2. d (p. 517)
3. c (p. 518)
4. c (p. 518)
5. c (p. 519)
6. c (p. 520)
7. b (p. 520)
8. a (p. 520)
9. d (p. 520)
10. b (p. 521)
11. b (p. 521)
12. b (p. 522)
13. b (p. 524)
14. c (p. 524)
15. d (p. 524)
16. c (p. 525)
17. e (p. 524)
18. b (p. 525)
19. d (p. 525)
20. e (p. 525)

Chapter 20
1. c (p. 537)
2. e (p. 536)
3. a (p. 536)
4. b (p. 537)
5. a (p. 538)
6. c (p. 538)
7. d (p. 538)
8. a (p. 539)
9. d (p. 540)
10. d (p. 542)

Appendix E

Pulmonary Function Normal Values

Richard K. Beauchamp, R.C.P.T., R.P.F.T.

Measures of pulmonary function are useful both to determine physiologic status at a given point in time and to monitor changes in status. Although, in the latter case, significant information may be provided by the magnitude of changes, or even by qualitative trends, meaningful application of pulmonary function data requires knowledge of whether the values in question are normal or abnormal. This determination implies, at least intuitively, a twofold process. First, the value that would be normal for the subject must be determined. Unfortunately in the case of pulmonary function testing (and unlike many other biologic analyses), most pulmonary function variables do not have a single normal value. Rather, the normal, or *predicted*, value for most of the variables is an interactive function of some combination of the subject's sex, height, age, weight, body surface area, or other anthropometrical data. Second, the significance of the subject's deviation from this predicted value must be determined. In this case, matters are complicated by the fact there is no completely satisfactory or universally accepted method for establishing the line between normal variants and abnormality for most variables.

Therefore, the present discussion will enumerate a few general points that the reader should bear in mind when attempting to determine whether a given value in a given subject is normal or abnormal. It will not be the purpose of this chapter to review all the available prediction equations for the various pulmonary function variables or to recommend any particular one of those equations for any variable. A number of equations for most variables are widely available.

The first point is that, with few exceptions, the predicted values for pulmonary function variables vary significantly with anthropometrical measurements and other factors. Accordingly, *one constant value should not be used as "the normal value"* unless it is known that the variable in question is one that does not vary with other factors. It is common practice, for example, to suggest that the normal value for oxygen intake is 250 ml/min, that normal lung compliance is 0.2 L/cm H_2O, or that the normal FEV_1/FVC ratio is anything greater than 0.70. These variables do vary with other factors, and using them or other constant values even as ballpark normals can be misleading.

The second point concerns the fact that, as already noted, multiple predicted regression equations are available for most pulmonary function variables. Not uncommonly, the values derived from different equations for the same variable in the same subject are quite different. Although there are a number of possible explanations for such differences, including the types of subjects tested and the methods used, the net effect is that a subject may be made to look normal or abnormal simply by the equation chosen to derive his or her predicted value. Accordingly, regression equations should be chosen carefully. One important step toward that end is to choose an equation derived from a population study that, as nearly as possible, matches the testing methods being used and the types of subjects being tested.

Finally, the question of how to determine what is an abnormal deviation from a predicted value needs to be answered. Historically, pulmonary function values were generally held to be abnormal below 80% of a predicted value, or in cases where increases are significant, above 120% of predicted.

More recently, this approach has come under attack as being arbitrary and without statistical basis. It is now widely suggested that more "meaningful" statistical approaches be taken to define the limits of normal in pulmonary function testing. More specifically, the suggestion often made is that limits of normal be defined in terms of standard deviations, meaning the limit of normal in cases where *only* a lower or an upper limit is important would be ±1.65 SD from the mean predicted values, whereas the limit of normal in cases where *both* a lower and upper limit are important would be ±1.96 (usually rounded to 2.0) SD from the mean value. However, despite the allure of characterizing data in terms of stringent statistical criteria, there are several points concerning this practice that should be considered.

The first point is that the data must exhibit a Gaussian or normal distribution (symmetrically bell-shaped curve) for application of standard deviations to be appropriate. Although it is probably true that the values for most pulmonary function variables are normally distributed in a given population, it may not be the case for all variables in all groups.[1]

The second point is that the conventional practice of defining normality as greater than 80% of predicted was not arbitrarily chosen. The practice arose from the fact that the coefficient of variation (or CV, which is the standard variation divided by the mean) for certain pulmonary function variables in early population studies was approximately 12%.[2] Thus, the value to be subtracted from the mean to determine the lower limit of normal was determined to be 12% × 1.65, or 20% of the mean. While not all subsequently described variables or populations exhibit the same 12% CV, it is important to realize that 80% was not simply pulled out of the air.

More important than any historical interest, however, this explanation also introduces the idea of using coefficients of variation rather than standard deviations. If a population study provides only one standard deviation value for the entire population, it is less meaningful the further from the mean it is applied. For example, let us suppose all females have a mean value and SD of 5.0 and 1.0, respectively, for a given pulmonary function variable that regresses with age and height. In a particular young

female subject whose individual predicted value is 4.65, defining the lower limit of normal as the mean minus 1.65 SD yields a value of 3.00, which is reasonable. On the other hand, in an elderly, short subject whose individual predicted value is 2.00, applying the same approach would set the lower limit of normal at 0.35, meaning a loss of 83% of function is required to make a call of abnormality, which is not reasonable. Although some population studies now provide standard deviations for different variables such as age and height, the ranges are usually relatively large, so that the problem is only partially negated. The more useful approach is the CV, which tailors the lower limit of normal to each subject. In the above example, the CV is 20% (1.0/5.0), meaning the lower limit of normal values (using the CV × 1.65) for the two subjects would be 3.12 and 1.34, respectively; the latter is obviously a more reasonable value.

The third point is that using standard deviations tends to be more *specific* in identifying abnormality, whereas using the conventional 80% of predicted tends to be more *sensitive*. Being more specific means the standard deviation approach is less likely to classify a normal subject as abnormal *(false-positives)*, whereas being more sensitive means the 80% of predicted approach is less likely to classify an abnormal subject as normal *(false-negatives)*. Accordingly, one factor to consider in choosing an approach to determine the significance of a subject's variance from a predicted value is the purpose for which the subject is being tested. Testing for the presence of early disease would probably benefit by use of the 80% of predicted approach, whereas testing in a situation where an abnormal finding might deny the subject employment or insurance would call for the use of the standard deviation approach.[1]

REFERENCES

1. Clausen JL: Prediction of normal values, in Clausen JL (ed): *Pulmonary Function Testing Guidelines and Controversies.* New York, Academic Press, 1982, pp 49–59.
2. Pennock BE, Cottrell JJ, Rodgers RM: Pulmonary function testing: What is "normal"? *Arch Intern Med* 1983; 143:2123–2127.

Index